EDITION 9

EXPLORING MEDICAL LANGUAGE

A STUDENT-DIRECTED APPROACH

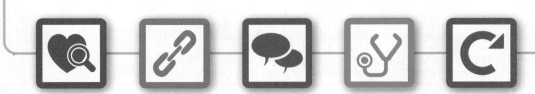

MYRNA LAFLEUR BROOKS, RN, BEd
Founding President
National Association of Health Unit Coordinators
Faculty Emeritus
Maricopa County Community College District
Phoenix, Arizona
Study Leader
Institute for Lifelong Education at Dartmouth (ILEAD)
Hanover, New Hampshire

DANIELLE LAFLEUR BROOKS, MEd, MATLA
Faculty, Allied Health and Medical Assisting
Community College of Vermont
Montpelier, Vermont

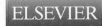

3251 Riverport Lane
St. Louis, Missouri 63043

ISBN: 978-0-323-11340-3

Content Strategist: Linda Woodard
Senior Content Development Specialist: Luke Held
Publishing Services Manager: Julie Eddy
Senior Project Manager: Andrea Campbell
Medical Illustrator: Jeanne Robertson
Design Direction: Jessica Williams

Printed in Canada

Last digit is the print number: 9 8 7 6 5 4 3 2 1

Working together
to grow libraries in
developing countries

www.elsevier.com • www.bookaid.org

What advice would you give to students just starting to learn medical terminology?

I remember, as a young medical student, having a reaction to some of these big words . . . feeling that some of the medical language was just too fancy, highbrow, or unnecessary at times. However, as I progressed I came to realize I was learning a language—a very precise language that I needed to understand so that I could properly communicate my intentions. For example, "diaphoresis" . . . why not just say "sweating?" Well, diaphoresis means sweating without exertion—from vagal stimulation maybe. Very different from sweating from normal exercise. If you fall outside of this you [may] become discredited and cannot communicate [effectively] with others in the field. So, if you can accept that this is a highly precise language . . . learn it . . . break it down . . . you'll find it an immense tool.

From an interview with Peter Goth, MD, FACEP, conducted by Michaella Warren, student, as part of a medical terminology class assignment.

CONTENTS

A complete list of the tables found throughout the text is located on the very last page of the book.

It can be difficult to determine, at a glance, all that is included in a chapter, so let's take a closer look at a typical body system chapter, Chapter 5, Respiratory System and Introduction to Diagnostic Procedures and Tests, pp. 138-206.

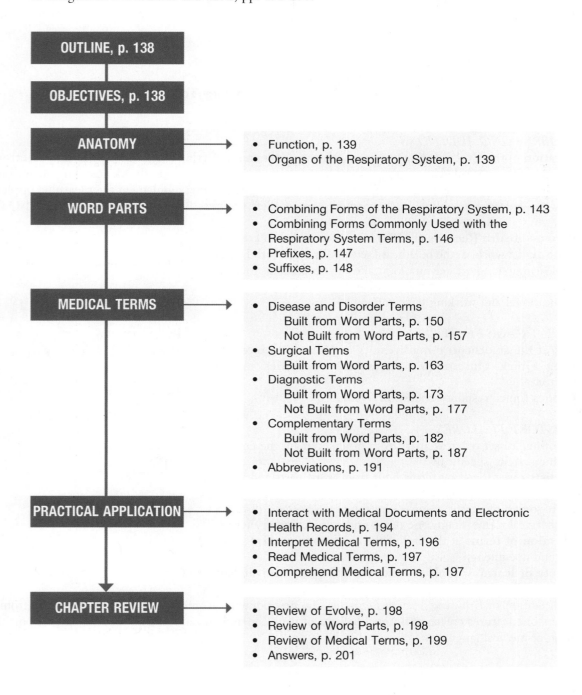

OUTLINE, p. 138

OBJECTIVES, p. 138

ANATOMY
- Function, p. 139
- Organs of the Respiratory System, p. 139

WORD PARTS
- Combining Forms of the Respiratory System, p. 143
- Combining Forms Commonly Used with the Respiratory System Terms, p. 146
- Prefixes, p. 147
- Suffixes, p. 148

MEDICAL TERMS
- Disease and Disorder Terms
    - Built from Word Parts, p. 150
    - Not Built from Word Parts, p. 157
- Surgical Terms
    - Built from Word Parts, p. 163
- Diagnostic Terms
    - Built from Word Parts, p. 173
    - Not Built from Word Parts, p. 177
- Complementary Terms
    - Built from Word Parts, p. 182
    - Not Built from Word Parts, p. 187
- Abbreviations, p. 191

PRACTICAL APPLICATION
- Interact with Medical Documents and Electronic Health Records, p. 194
- Interpret Medical Terms, p. 196
- Read Medical Terms, p. 197
- Comprehend Medical Terms, p. 197

CHAPTER REVIEW
- Review of Evolve, p. 198
- Review of Word Parts, p. 198
- Review of Medical Terms, p. 199
- Answers, p. 201

PREFACE

Medical terminology, like any living language, changes over time. The content of the ninth edition has been updated to reflect current use, ensuring the textbook remains an effective tool for those entering medical professions as well as those in related fields including software development, computer applications and support, insurance, law, equipment supply, pharmaceutical sales, and medical writing.

NEW CONTENT
- An expanded section on **diagnostic procedures and tests** in Chapter 5.
- Two new appendices introducing **Health Information Technology Terms** and **Dental Terms**.
- New and updated diagrams, tables, and sidebar boxes.

GROUNDBREAKING ADDITIONS
- **Integration** of the Evolve online program with chapter content, offering a **hybrid of print and electronic materials**. Callouts are threaded throughout the text for easy transition from **textbook learning** to **online learning**. Students may complete the Spelling and Pronunciation Exercises online; supplement their learning by playing Games or viewing Animations online; and review and assess their progress by completing Activities and Quick Quizzes online.
- **Electronic Health Records (EHRs)** have been added to keep up with the digital world in the healthcare setting. Practice with EHRs while learning medical terminology allows the student to gain familiarity with format and function, easing the transition between the educational and working environments.

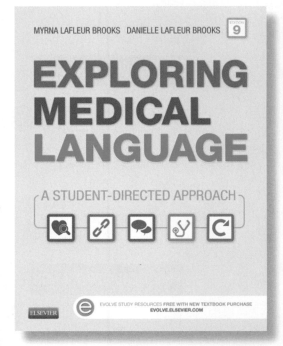

NEW ELECTRONIC FEATURES
- Ability of the student to **e-mail results** of Multiple Choice and Spelling **Quick Quizzes** and **Assessment Activities** to the instructor.
- **QR codes** (quick response codes) for Weblinks.

CORNERSTONE FEATURES
These continue to set our text apart from others, remain the core of our learning system, specifically:
- **Term lists** categorized by terms built from word parts and those not built from word parts
- **Subcategories of terms** grouped by topic: disease and disorder terms, surgical terms, diagnostic terms and complementary terms
- **Application of terms** at the end of the chapters in medical statements and documents
- A **variety of learning tools** to maximize effectiveness of student learning styles

In the 9th edition of *Exploring Medical Language*, the new content, groundbreaking additions of electronic materials, and cornerstone features create an optimal balance of hands on and virtual learning tools to best support the student's acquisition of medical language.

DEAR STUDENT

If you are reading this, you are probably already enrolled in a medical terminology course and preparing for your journey of learning medical language using this textbook. As you flip through the pages of *Exploring Medical Language* you may be thinking, "There is so much to learn. How will I do it?" or "Why are there so many exercises?" Let us assure you that you will be able to acquire the language in a quick and easy manner by doing all the exercises in the text. The exercises approach the terms from all angles: writing, spelling, pronunciation, and application. Chapter content flows from one chapter to the next in a repetitive manner, making the best use of one's time. You can acquire the language of medicine by using the textbook alone; however, it is totally integrated with the Evolve online supplemental learning review and assessment program to use as you wish.

On Evolve you can:
- hear terms pronounced
- practice spelling
- play games
- interact with electronic health records
- assess your preparedness for taking exams
- watch animations
- use electronic flash cards

We wish you the best as you embark on this journey. You will join a select group of students who have used *Exploring Medical Language* as a textbook for over 28 years.

We would like to hear of your experience with *Exploring Medical Language*. What exercises were most useful, suggestions for improvement, and so forth.

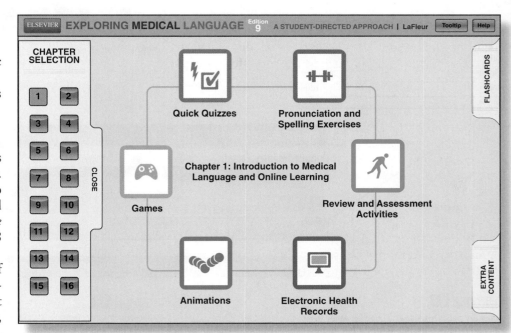

Reach us by e-mail at the following addresses:

danielle.lafleurbrooks@ccv.edu (Danielle)
myrnabrooks@comcast.net (Myrna)

Sincerely,
Myrna and Danielle

FEATURES

1 Employs a **learning system** utilizing Greek and Latin **word parts** to analyze, define, and build medical terms.

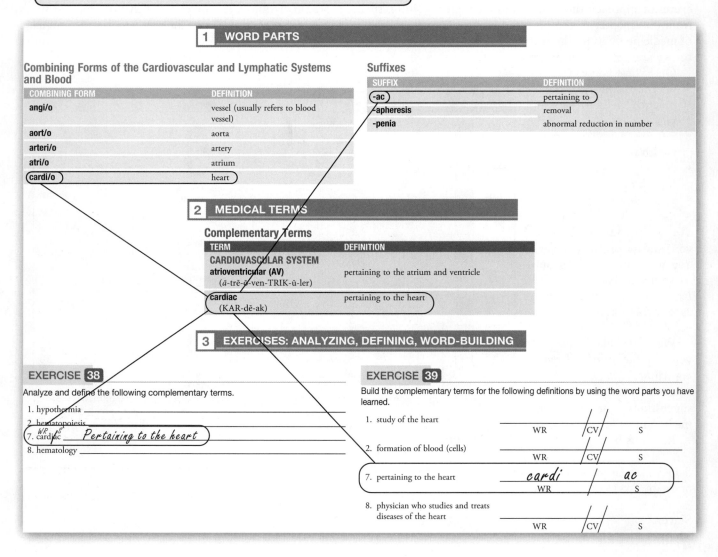

1 WORD PARTS

Combining Forms of the Cardiovascular and Lymphatic Systems and Blood

COMBINING FORM	DEFINITION
angi/o	vessel (usually refers to blood vessel)
aort/o	aorta
arteri/o	artery
atri/o	atrium
cardi/o	heart

Suffixes

SUFFIX	DEFINITION
-ac	pertaining to
-apheresis	removal
-penia	abnormal reduction in number

2 MEDICAL TERMS

Complementary Terms

TERM	DEFINITION
CARDIOVASCULAR SYSTEM	
atrioventricular (AV) (ā-trē-ō-ven-TRIK-ū-ler)	pertaining to the atrium and ventricle
cardiac (KAR-dē-ak)	pertaining to the heart

3 EXERCISES: ANALYZING, DEFINING, WORD-BUILDING

EXERCISE 38

Analyze and define the following complementary terms.

1. hypothermia _____
2. hematopoiesis _____
7. cardiac *Pertaining to the heart*
   WR S
8. hematology _____

EXERCISE 39

Build the complementary terms for the following definitions by using the word parts you have learned.

1. study of the heart
   _____ / ___ / _____
   WR   CV   S

2. formation of blood (cells)
   _____ / ___ / _____
   WR   CV   S

7. pertaining to the heart
   cardi / *ac*
   WR   S

8. physician who studies and treats diseases of the heart
   _____ / ___ / _____
   WR   CV   S

2 Divides terms into **categories** based on **learning methods**.

Medical Terms

Built from Word Parts	Not Built from Word Parts
1) Analyzing/Defining	1) Matching
2) Word Building	2) Recall
3) Pronunciation	3) Pronunciation
4) Spelling	4) Spelling

3 Introduces medical terms by **topic** (disease and disorder, surgical, diagnostic, and complementary), and then illustrates the use of terms in **practical application** exercises.

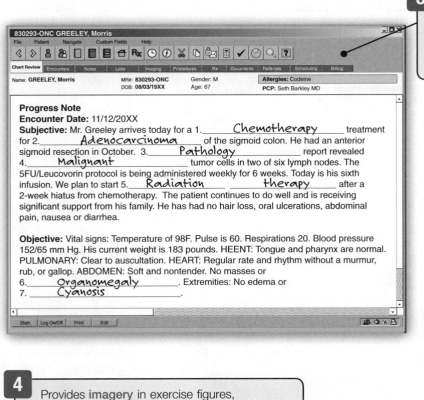

830293-ONC GREELEY, Morris

File   Patient   Navigate   Custom Fields   Help

Chart Review | Encounters | Notes | Labs | Imaging | Procedures | Rx | Documents | Referrals | Scheduling | Billing

Name: **GREELEY, Morris**   MR#: **830293-ONC**   Gender: M   **Allergies:** Codeine
                                 DOB: **08/03/19XX**   Age: 67   **PCP:** Seth Barkley MD

Progress Note
Encounter Date: 11/12/20XX
Subjective: Mr. Greeley arrives today for a 1.___Chemotherapy___ treatment for 2.___Adenocarcinoma___ of the sigmoid colon. He had an anterior sigmoid resection in October. 3.___Pathology___ report revealed 4.___Malignant___ tumor cells in two of six lymph nodes. The 5FU/Leucovorin protocol is being administered weekly for 6 weeks. Today is his sixth infusion. We plan to start 5.___Radiation___ ___therapy___ after a 2-week hiatus from chemotherapy. The patient continues to do well and is receiving significant support from his family. He has had no hair loss, oral ulcerations, abdominal pain, nausea or diarrhea.

Objective: Vital signs: Temperature of 98F. Pulse is 60. Respirations 20. Blood pressure 152/65 mm Hg. His current weight is 183 pounds. HEENT: Tongue and pharynx are normal. PULMONARY: Clear to auscultation. HEART: Regular rate and rhythm without a murmur, rub, or gallop. ABDOMEN: Soft and nontender. No masses or
6.___Organomegaly___. Extremities: No edema or
7.___Cyanosis___.

Start | Log On/Off | Print | Edit

4 Provides **imagery** in exercise figures, illustrations, and animations to depict the meaning of terms.
    Students label illustrations by using word parts.

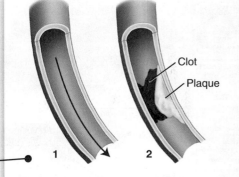

Clot
Plaque

1

2

1) Healthy artery with smooth blood flow.
2) Blocked artery due to:

Thromb	/	osis
(blood) clot		abnormal condition

and

ather	/ o /	sclerosis
fatty plaque	/CV/	hardening

Listen ◀)

Reset   Submit

5 Provides **audio** for **pronunciation and spelling** of terms. On the Evolve website, the student can hear, pronounce, and spell the terms until mastery is achieved.

INCIDENTALOMA

refers to a mass lesion involving an organ that is discovered unexpectedly by the use of ultrasound, computed tomography scan, or magnetic resonance imaging and has nothing to do with the patient symptoms or primary diagnos

🏛 SARCOMA

has been used since the time of ancient Greece to describe any fleshy tumor. Since the introduction of cellular pathology, the meaning has become **malignant connective tissue tumor**.

Often, an additional word root is used to denote the type of tissue involved, such as **oste** in **osteosarcoma**, which refers to a malignant tumor of the bone.

6 Anchors medical language in a **historical perspective** and **current usage** with side bars.

7 Identifies **online learning** opportunities, linking the textbook with the Evolve website.

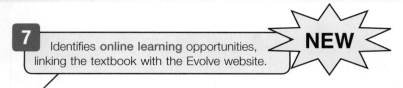
NEW

Look for the ⊖ as you work through chapters

- **Flash cards** for both word parts and abbreviations
- Spelling and Pronunciation **Exercises**
- Five fun, pedagogically sound **Games**
- Review and Assessment **Activities**
- NEW—**Electronic Health Records**
- **A & P Booster**
- **Quick Quizzes**
- **Animations**

⊖

For more practice with medical terms, go to evolve.elsevier.com. Select:
Chapter 5, **Activities**, Terms Not Built from Word Parts
                                    Hear It and Type It: Clinical Vignettes
Chapter 5, **Games**,   Term Explorer
                                    Termbusters
                                    Medical Millionaire

Refer to p. 10 for your Evolve Access Information.

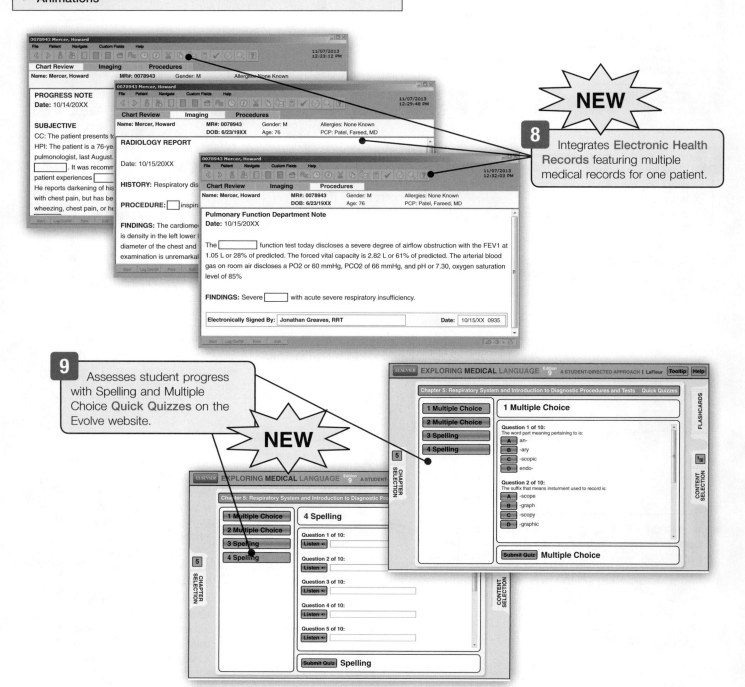

8 Integrates **Electronic Health Records** featuring multiple medical records for one patient.

NEW

9 Assesses student progress with Spelling and Multiple Choice **Quick Quizzes** on the Evolve website.

NEW

10 Introduces medical terms grouped by medical specialties in **Appendices**.

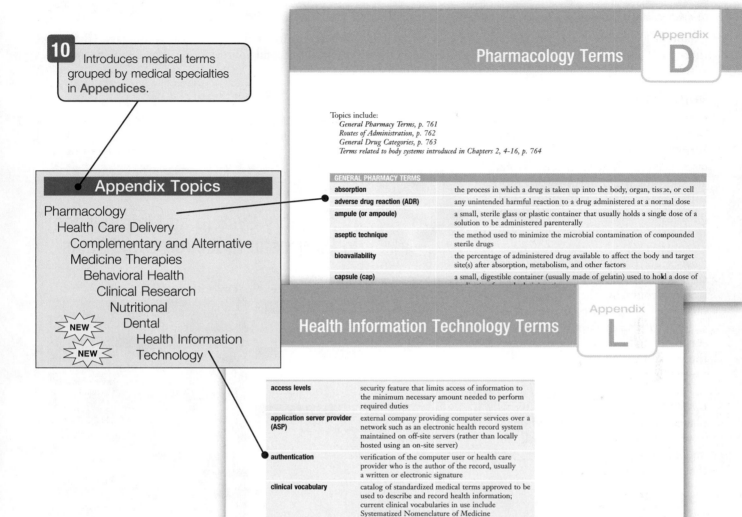

Appendix Topics

Pharmacology
Health Care Delivery
Complementary and Alternative
Medicine Therapies
Behavioral Health
Clinical Research
Nutritional
NEW Dental
Health Information
NEW Technology

Pharmacology Terms
Appendix **D**

Topics include:
General Pharmacy Terms, p. 761
Routes of Administration, p. 762
General Drug Categories, p. 763
Terms related to body systems introduced in Chapters 2, 4–16, p. 764

GENERAL PHARMACY TERMS

absorption	the process in which a drug is taken up into the body, organ, tissue, or cell
adverse drug reaction (ADR)	any unintended harmful reaction to a drug administered at a normal dose
ampule (or ampoule)	a small, sterile glass or plastic container that usually holds a single dose of a solution to be administered parenterally
aseptic technique	the method used to minimize the microbial contamination of compounded sterile drugs
bioavailability	the percentage of administered drug available to affect the body and target site(s) after absorption, metabolism, and other factors
capsule (cap)	a small, digestible container (usually made of gelatin) used to hold a dose of

Health Information Technology Terms
Appendix **L**

access levels	security feature that limits access of information to the minimum necessary amount needed to perform required duties
application server provider (ASP)	external company providing computer services over a network such as an electronic health record system maintained on off-site servers (rather than locally hosted using an on-site server)
authentication	verification of the computer user or health care provider who is the author of the record, usually a written or electronic signature
clinical vocabulary	catalog of standardized medical terms approved to be used to describe and record health information; current clinical vocabularies in use include Systematized Nomenclature of Medicine (SNOMED), Unified Medical Language System (UMLS), and Digital Imaging and Communications in Medicine (DICOM)
coding system, classification system	categorization of codes for medical terms grouped by related conditions, diseases, procedures, pharmaceuticals, and so forth. Currently used codes

WEB LINK

For more information about diseases and disorders of the digestive system and the latest treatments available, please visit the National Digestive Diseases Information Clearing House at *digestive.niddk.nih.gov.*

NEW

11 Provides fast access to more information using a smartphone with **QR codes** (quick response codes).

ORGANIZATION OF THE TEXTBOOK

Chapters 1 through 3 are introductory chapters, providing a foundation for building medical vocabulary. Chapters 4 through 16 are body systems chapters, presenting related word parts, terms, and abbreviations. The textbook concludes with a series of appendices designed to extend student learning as desired.

Introductory Chapters

Chapter 1 . . . may be the most important chapter in the text, because you will apply the knowledge you acquire here in the rest of the chapters to learn terms in an easy, quick fashion. You are introduced to the two **categories of terms**—those built from word parts and those which are not; each category is accompanied by different types of exercises. Also introduced in this chapter are **the four word parts**—word root, suffix, prefix, and combining vowel, which are the basis of terms built from word parts category.

Chapter 2 . . . introduces **body structure** and immediately provides practice in recognizing the two categories of terms along with corresponding exercises for each. You will likely be surprised at how fast you will learn the meaning and spelling of many medical terms.

Chapter 3 . . . covers directional terms, planes, positions, regions, and quadrants, providing a framework for understanding the body systems and their related terms.

Body System Chapters

Chapters 4 through 16 . . . introduce specific body systems with related word parts, terms, and abbreviations and follow a consistent format.

Appendices

Appendices A-D . . . appear in the textbook and provide a comprehensive lists of word parts, a list of error-prone abbreviations, and pharmacology terms.

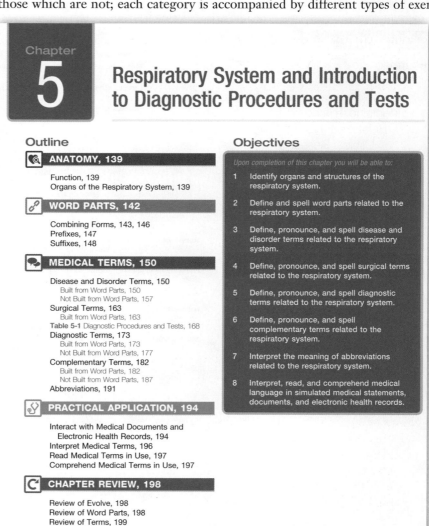

Chapter 5

Respiratory System and Introduction to Diagnostic Procedures and Tests

Outline

ANATOMY, 139

Function, 139
Organs of the Respiratory System, 139

WORD PARTS, 142

Combining Forms, 143, 146
Prefixes, 147
Suffixes, 148

MEDICAL TERMS, 150

Disease and Disorder Terms, 150
    Built from Word Parts, 150
    Not Built from Word Parts, 157
Surgical Terms, 163
    Built from Word Parts, 163
    Table 5-1 Diagnostic Procedures and Tests, 168
Diagnostic Terms, 173
    Built from Word Parts, 173
    Not Built from Word Parts, 177
Complementary Terms, 182
    Built from Word Parts, 182
    Not Built from Word Parts, 187
Abbreviations, 191

PRACTICAL APPLICATION, 194

Interact with Medical Documents and
    Electronic Health Records, 194
Interpret Medical Terms, 196
Read Medical Terms in Use, 197
Comprehend Medical Terms in Use, 197

CHAPTER REVIEW, 198

Review of Evolve, 198
Review of Word Parts, 198
Review of Terms, 199
Answers, 201

Objectives

Upon completion of this chapter you will be able to:

1 Identify organs and structures of the respiratory system.

2 Define and spell word parts related to the respiratory system.

3 Define, pronounce, and spell disease and disorder terms related to the respiratory system.

4 Define, pronounce, and spell surgical terms related to the respiratory system.

5 Define, pronounce, and spell diagnostic terms related to the respiratory system.

6 Define, pronounce, and spell complementary terms related to the respiratory system.

7 Interpret the meaning of abbreviations related to the respiratory system.

8 Interpret, read, and comprehend medical language in simulated medical statements, documents, and electronic health records.

HOW WILL I LEARN MEDICAL TERMS USING *EXPLORING MEDICAL LANGUAGE*?

You will learn medical terms by completing the many and varied exercises, activities, and games, using all learning styles. Upon completion, you will be able to speak and write the language of medicine, preparing you to understand and be understood in a medical setting.

Let's travel through Chapter 5, Respiratory System, and explore how you will acquire this new language.

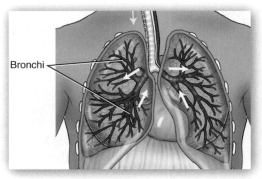

Anatomy

If you have not previously studied anatomy, this section is for you. You will learn the content by:

- Reading content, example p. 139
- Studying diagrams, example p. 140
- Completing exercises and checking answers, example, pp. 142, 201
- Using the **online** A & P Booster, example box p. 141

Word Parts

Many medical terms are made up of Greek and Latin word parts. By learning their meaning and spelling, you will be able to define the many terms built from word parts included in this text and many more.

You will learn the meaning and spelling of word parts by:

- Reading each word part and its definition, example p. 143
- Labeling anatomic diagrams with word parts, example p. 144
- Completing exercises and checking answers, example pp. 145, 201
- Using paper or **online** flashcards
- Completing online activities indicated in the callout boxes throughout the section

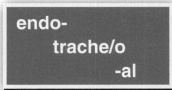

Medical Terms Built from Word Parts

Medical terms built from word parts are constructed from word parts learned in the word part section mentioned above. You will apply this newfound knowledge in learning the meaning and spelling of these terms.

You will learn to speak and write medical terms built from word parts by:

- Reading each of the terms and its definition, example p. 143
- Referring to diagrams demonstrating disease processes, surgery, or diagnostic studies, example p. 150
- Referring to tables and boxes on use of terms, historical and clinical contexts, and tips to navigate the material, example p. 150
- Filling in word parts to label the Exercise Figures, example p. 153
- Pronouncing each of the terms and hearing them **online**, example box p. 153
- Completing analyzing and defining exercises and checking answers, example pp. 154, 201
- Completing word-building exercises and checking answers, example p. 155
- Completing spelling exercises by in-person or **online** dictation, example p. 157
- Completing online activities indicated in the callout boxes throughout the section

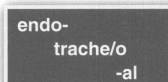

Medical Terms Not Built from Word Parts

Terms appearing in the "Not Built from Word Parts" lists may indeed contain recognizable word parts; however, they cannot be easily defined through the meanings of the word parts. Memorization is the method used to learning these terms.

You will learn to speak and write these terms not built from word parts by:

- Reading each of the terms and its definition, example, p. 157
- Referring to tables and boxes on use of terms, historical and clinical contexts, and tips to navigate the material, examples p. 157
- Referring to diagrams demonstrating disease processes, surgery, or diagnostic studies, example p. 159
- Pronouncing each of the terms and hearing them **online**, example, p. 160
- Completing fill-in-the-blank and matching exercises, and checking answers, example pp. 160–162, 203
- Completing the spelling exercises by in-person or **online** dictation, example p. 162
- Completing online activities indicated in the callout boxes throughout the section

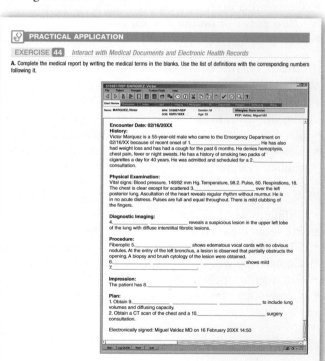

Abbreviations

Abbreviations are frequently used in healthcare settings.

You will learn abbreviations by:

- Reading each abbreviation and its definition, example pp. 191–192
- Completing the exercises and checking answers, example pp. 192–193, 206
- Completing online activities indicated in the callout boxes throughout the section

Practical Application

Practical application offers an opportunity for you to apply your newfound knowledge in clinical situations and with medical documents.

You will apply what you have learned by:

- Interacting with medical documents and electronic health records, example p. 194
- Interpreting medical terms, example p. 196
- Reading medical terms in use, in the text and **online**, p. 197
- Comprehending medical terms, p. 197
- Completing online activities indicated in the callout boxes throughout the section

Chapter Review

Online and Textbook chapter review summarizes the textbook and online chapter content, p. 198

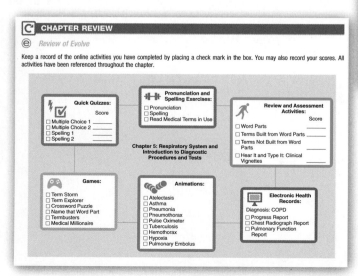

DEAR INSTRUCTOR

If you are new to teaching medical terminology, we offer a wide variety of teaching resources you can use to prepare for classes, including lesson plans, handouts, PowerPoint presentations, and test bank questions. **TEACH, an online supplement, is the primary instructional resource for EML**, providing one place to view all of these teaching materials. It is chapter objective-based and can be used as is, or may be altered to suit your teaching needs. See Online Resources below.

If you are a veteran instructor and have your classroom materials developed, you might choose to add the **Tournament of Terminology** game, which can be played by the whole class to prepare for exams, or weave **illustrations from the image collection** into your PowerPoint presentations. All resources are easily accessible on the Evolve website for *Exploring Medical Language* (EML). New to this edition is the **option for students to e-mail to the instructor the results of the assessment portion of the activities** and the results of the **Quick Quizzes**, which includes both multiple choice and spelling.

We are dedicated to supporting your teaching efforts and look forward to hearing from you. We welcome your comments and questions. Danielle currently teaches both online and classroom courses and is eager to share, especially ideas and materials for online learning. We can be reached at the following addresses.

danielle.lafleurbrooks@ccv.edu (Danielle)
myrnabrooks@comcast.net (Myrna)

Sincerely,
Myrna and Danielle

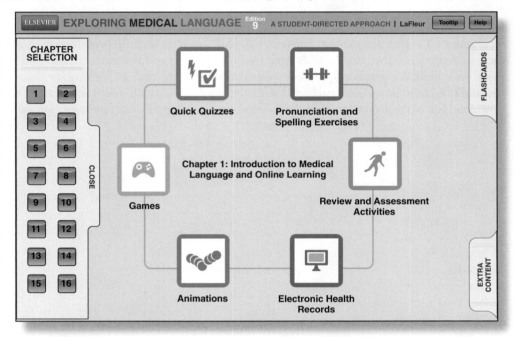

ONLINE TEACHING RESOURCES

- **Chapter Pretests** for measuring pre- and post-chapter knowledge
- **Materials and Resources Lists** for classroom preparation
- **Assessment and Critical Thinking Questions** to use as an introduction to lectures
- **Lesson Plans** that correlate chapter objectives with textbook content and teaching resources
- **Classroom Handouts, Discussion Questions, and Suggested Classroom Activities** organized by chapter objective
- **PowerPoint presentations** for each chapter for use as lecture aids
- **Performance Evaluation** plan for monitoring and evaluating student progress

Teaching Tools:
- **ExamView Test Bank** with objective-based questions for each chapter (also available as RTF files)
- **Image Collection** from the textbook to download for use in the classroom
- **Tournament of Terminology**, a Jeopardy-like game for exam preparation by reviewing chapter content
- **Electronic Flashcards** for classroom use, accessible through the Student site
- **Spanish/English glossary**, accessible through the Student site
- **Electronic Health Records**, accessible through the Student site

Course Management Tools:
- **Online discussion boards**
- **Online calendar**
- **Outline of course syllabus, outlines, and lecture notes**
- **Sample course outline and syllabus**
- **Web links**

ALSO AVAILABLE

Mosby's Medical Terminology Online

Mosby's Medical Terminology Online to accompany *Exploring Medical Language* is a great resource to supplement your textbook. This web-delivered course supplement provides a range of visual, auditory, and interactive elements to reinforce your learning and synthesize concepts presented in the text. Objective-based quizzes at the end of each section and an end-of-module exam provide you with self-testing tools. In addition, related Internet resources may be accessed by links provided throughout the program. This online course supplement may be accessed if you have purchased the pincode packaged with your book. If you did not purchase the pincode, ask your instructor for information or visit http://evolve.elsevier.com/LaFleur/Exploring/ to purchase it.

Instructors interested in *Mosby's Medical Terminology Online*, please contact your sales rep, call Faculty Support at 1-800-222-9570, or visit http://evolve.elsevier.com/LaFleur/Exploring/ for more information.

Audio CDs and iTerms

The audio CDs that accompany *Exploring Medical Language* include pronunciations and definitions. Because the CDs include definitions, they are an additional tool for learning and reviewing terms. The CDs are especially helpful when using your book is impractical, such as when you are driving in a car, walking, or doing daily chores. You may purchase the audio CDs separately or packaged with the book for a small additional cost. This audio product is available for download for MP3 players and is called *iTerms for Exploring Medical Language, 9th edition.*

William W. Bohnert, MD, FACS
Urologist
Arizona Urologic Specialists
Scottsdale, Arizona
Electronic Health Records—Chapters 6-7 (Evolve website)

Richard K. Brooks, MD, FACP, FACG
Internal Medicine and Gastroenterology
Mayo Clinic (retired)
Scottsdale, Arizona
Margin boxes

Catherine J. Cerulli, MEd
Director
Interwoven Healing Arts
Montpelier, Vermont
Appendix G—Complementary and Alternative Medicine Therapies (Evolve website)

Christine Costa, GCM, HUC
Geriatric Care Manager
Tempe, Arizona
Appendix A—Combining Forms, Prefixes, and Suffixes Alphabetized According to Word Part
Appendix B—Combining Forms, Prefixes, and Suffixes Alphabetized According to Definition
Appendix C—Abbreviations
Appendix E—Additional Combining Forms, Prefixes, and Suffixes (Evolve website)
Quick Quizzes (Evolve website)

Cynthia Heiss, PhD, RD
Professor
Department of Healthcare Professions
Metropolitan State University of Denver
Denver, Colorado
Appendix J—Nutritional Terms (Evolve website)

Marjorie "Meg" A. Holloway, MS, RN, APRN
Instructor, Medical Strand Leader
Center for Advanced Professional Studies
Blue Valley School District
Overland Park, Kansas
Chapter 6—Urinary System
Chapter 7—Male Reproductive System
Chapter 8—Female Reproductive System
Chapter 9—Obstetrics and Neonatology
Chapter 10—Cardiovascular, Immune, Lymphatic Systems and Blood
Chapter 14—Musculoskeletal System
Chapter 15—Nervous System and Behavioral Health

Erinn Kao, PharmD, BCNP
GE Medical
St. Louis, Missouri
Appendix D—Pharmacology Terms

Dale Levinsky, MD
Associate Medical Director
Genova Clinical Research, Inc.
Tucson, Arizona
Electronic Health Records—Chapters 9, 10, 12, 13, 15, 16 (Evolve website)

Caroline M. Murphy, DDS
General Practice Dentist
Montpelier, Vermont
Appendix K—Dental Terms (Evolve website)

Cheryl A. Sullivan, BSN, MA, RN (Retired)
Nurse Manager, Behavioral Health Department
Shawnee Mission Medical Center
Shawnee, Kansas
Appendix H—Behavioral Health Terms (Evolve website)

Sharon Tompkins Luczu, RN, MA, MBA
Program Director
Health Services Management
Gateway Community College
Phoenix, Arizona
Appendix F—Health Care Delivery Terms (Evolve website)

Cris E. Wells, EdD, MBA, CCRP, RT(R)(M)
Assistant Professor/Director of Interprofessional Programs and the Clinical Research Management Master of Science Program
Arizona State University, College of Nursing and Health Innovation
Phoenix, Arizona
Appendix I—Clinical Research Terms (Evolve website)

Christine Costa, GCM, HUC
Geriatric Care Manager
Tempe, Arizona

Heather Drake, RN
Nursing Lab Manager and Allied Health
    Instructor
Southern West Virginia Community and
    Technical College
Mt. Gay, West Virginia

**Mary M. Fabick, MSN, MEd, RN-BC,
    CEN**
Associate Professor of Nursing
Milligan College
Milligan, Tennessee

Brian J. Gennero, DC
Adjunct Faculty
Baker College
Clinton Township, Michigan

**Sharon Guthrie, PhD, ARNP, CPNP,
    NCSN**
Assistant Professor
Mount Mercy University
Cedar Rapids, Iowa

**Janie E. Jackson, RT(R)(M)(CT), BS,
    CMRT, LVN**
Assistant Professor
Tarrant County College District—Trinity
    River East Campus
Health Care Professions Division
Radiography Program
Fort Worth, Texas

Stephanie L. Jansen
Educator
Business, Marketing, and Information
    Technology Department
Muskego Norway School District
Muskego, Wisconsin

**Barbara Jareo, RN, BSN, ADN, CEN,
    CCM**
Adjunct Instructor
Davenport University
Flint, Michigan

Nancy Klein, MS, OTR/L
Adjunct Professor
St. Louis Community College
St. Louis, Missouri

**Amanda Elizabeth Lasseter, PT, DPT,
    COMT**
Physical Therapist, Certified Orthopedic
    and Manual Therapist
Select Physical Therapy
Tempe, Arizona

Dale M. Levinsky, MD
Board Certified by American Board of
    Family Medicine
Member of American Academy of Family
    Physicians
Tucson, Arizona

**Jennifer Mai, PT, DPT, PhD, MHS,
    NCS**
Associate Professor of Physical Therapy
Clarke University
Dubuque, Iowa

Rosalee (Lee) C. Means
Teacher
Mukwonago School District
Mukwonago High School
Mukwonago, Wisconsin

Sandra Metcalf, ME
Professor
Grayson County College
Denison, Texas

Jacalyn O'Hara
Computer and Business Technology/
    Medical Administrative Specialist
Elkhart Area Career Center
Elkhart, Indiana

Karen O'Neill, BA
Essex Junction, Vermont

Joseph D. Patrico Jr., BA, MS, DC
Chiropractic Physician and Nutritionist
Adjunct Professor
Baker College
Clinton Township, Michigan

ACKNOWLEDGMENTS

We depend on so many to assist us in keeping the textbook and electronic content current and accurate, in incorporating the latest learning styles and technologies, and in having the printed pages and electronic screens appeal to the learner. We are indebted to the following:

Luke Held, senior content development specialist, who guided us through the revision process, all the while demonstrating exceptional patience, follow-through, and dedication.

Jessica Williams, book designer, who worked with us to create an attractive and engaging book.

Andrea Campbell, senior project manager, who seemed to effortlessly bring our vision of the print pages to fruition.

Linda Woodard, content strategist, whose deep understanding of all things related to medical terminology publication guided us to a crisp, current and concise 9th edition.

Contributors listed on pages xvii–xviii and **Reviewers and Advisors** listed on pages xix–xx who shared with us their expertise, knowledge, and precious time.

Meg Holloway, who joined us as a contributor and skillfully applied her knowledge and clinical resources to revising Chapters 6-10, 14, and 15, the test bank, and to writing the EHR for Chapter 8.

Chris Costa, who assisted with the revision of the Evolve program content and Appendices A-D, as well as spending many hours adroitly searching through the manuscript with a tireless concern for the accuracy of the printed word.

Carolyn Kruse, for using her linguistic knowledge and pleasing voice for updating pronunciation, both in print and audio.

Richard K. Brooks, MD, my husband, who reviewed and assisted with revisions for all content in the text and who was willing to be there for us every step of the way.

Winifred K. Starr (1921-1993), who was my first coauthor and whose creative contributions remain in the text today.

Faculty, who have adopted the text to use in their classrooms, and have used their valuable time to give us feedback.

Students, who over the years have worn thin the pages of previous editions to acquire their own language of medicine.

Each page of the 9th Edition is better because of your collective contributions. Thank you.

Chapter

1

Introduction to Medical Language and Online Learning

Outline

Objectives

Upon completion of this chapter you will be able to:

1 Create an account and register on the Evolve website.

2 Describe four origins of medical language.

3 Define two categories of medical terms.

4 Identify and define the four word parts and the combining form.

5 Analyze and define medical terms.

6 Build medical terms for given definitions.

Online Learning

Mastery of medical language can be achieved by textbook learning alone. For those who want more or different learning strategies, an integrated online supportive learning program has been made available on the Evolve companion website, indicated throughout the text by this icon ⊜. **You will find pronunciation and spelling exercises, games, animations, electronic health records, plus quick quizzes and review and assessment activities that may be used to evaluate your progress and/or prepare for examinations (Figure 1-1).**

Create an Account and Register

To use the Evolve companion website, follow the steps below to create an account and register.

> Future enhancements to Evolve may require a change in these steps. For problem solving, go to **evolvesupport.elsevier.com** or call **1-800-222-9570**.

EXERCISE 1

Place a check mark next to the step once you have completed it.

- ☐ 1. Go to **evolve.elsevier.com/LaFleur/exploring**.

- ☐ 2. Click **Register for This Now** **REGISTER FOR THIS NOW**.

- ☐ 3. If you purchased a new textbook, go to the inside front cover to retrieve your access code to access your Evolve resources. Then click **I have an access code**, **enter the code** in the box, and click **Apply** to verify the code.

     If you purchased a used textbook and the code on the inside front cover has been used, click on **I want access to purchase a pin code**.

- ☐ 4. Click **Redeem/Checkout** **REDEEM/CHECKOUT >**.

- ☐ 5. Create an account by **filling out the fields** requested and then selecting **Continue**. A confirmation email will be sent to you to verify the information you entered plus an assigned username.

     Record your information for future use:
     Username: _____
     Password: _____

- ☐ 6. View and accept the Registered User Agreement, then click **Submit**.

- ☐ 7. Click **Get Started** just below the confirmation, or **My Evolve** tab in the top left corner of the screen.

     Congratulations! You are now registered with the Evolve website for *Exploring Medical Language*. To login to the website, refer to p. 10 for your **Evolve Access Information**.

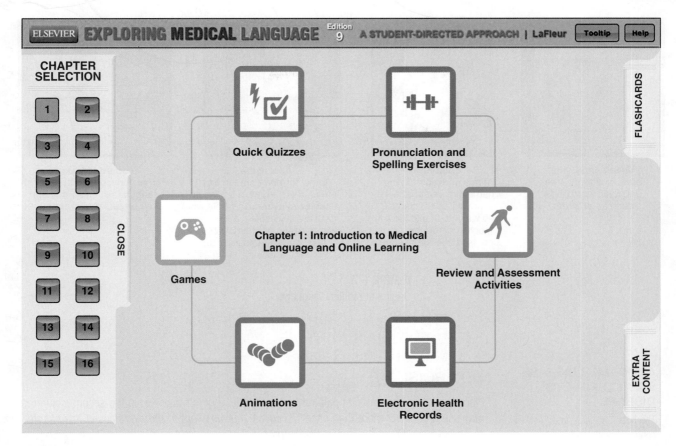

FIGURE 1-1
Main menu for Evolve *Exploring Medical Language* website online activities. Click on the icon or tab to gain access to the activities. **Career Videos, A&P Booster, Dictionary with Audio, English/Spanish Glossary, Appendices, and Textbook Answers are located under the Extra Content tab.**

Origins of Medical Language

Medicine has a language of its own, and its vocabulary includes terms built from **Greek and Latin word parts, eponyms, acronyms, and modern language** (Figure 1-2). Like any language, medical language is dynamic and develops over time. As clinical settings, current practice, technology, and medical knowledge evolve with scientific advancement, medical language changes. Some terms drop out of usage, the meanings of others are altered, and new terms come into use.

The majority of medical terms in use today are composed of **Greek and Latin word parts,** some of which were used by Hippocrates and Aristotle more than 2400 years ago. Many can be translated literally to find their meaning. In **Exploring Medical Language**, these terms are taught through a step-by-step word-building process that includes learning the meanings of word parts and how they fit together to form medical terms. Acquiring this skill will enable you to learn scores of medical terms quickly, and it will give you the tools you need to understand new terms you encounter in school or on the job.

Medical terms that are **eponyms, acronyms,** or **based on modern language** need to be learned by memorization. Medical terms composed of Greek and Latin word parts that cannot be literally translated through the meanings of their word parts will also be learned by memorization. Illustrations, notes on current use, historical information, and learning tips will be presented with these terms to help you become familiar with their meanings as easily as possible. Although it takes effort, memorization is a fundamental step that allows you to create a foundation of knowledge. You will find that Exploring Medical Language creates multiple opportunities for you to practice, and practice itself will help you internalize the meanings and use of medical terms.

USING MEDICAL TERMS

Using medical terms to communicate allows for concise and accurate communication. For example, using the medical term **osteoarthritis,** which means **inflammation of the bone and joint,** offers clear and concise written or verbal communication using one word instead of six.

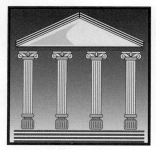

Greek and Latin
Terms built from Greek
and Latin word parts
such as *arthritis*

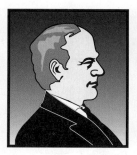

Eponyms
Terms derived from the
name of a person, often
a physician or scientist
who was the first to identify
a technique or condition,
such as *Alzheimer disease*

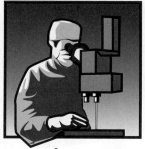

Acronyms
Terms formed from the first
letters of the words in a phrase
that can be spoken as a whole word
and usually contain a vowel,
such as *laser* (light amplification
by stimulated emission of
radiation)

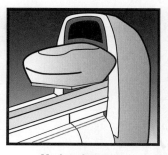

Modern language
Terms derived from the English
language such as *nuclear
medicine scanner*

FIGURE 1-2
Origins of medical language.

ALZHEIMER DISEASE VS. ALZHEIMER'S DISEASE

The need for clarity and consistency in medical language has resulted in the **modern trend to eliminate the possessive form of eponyms and use instead the non-possessive form**. The non-possessive form is observed by the American Association for Medical Transcription, the American Medical Association's Manual of Style, in most medical dictionaries, and is the style used throughout this textbook. With either use, the noun that follows is not capitalized.

EXERCISE 2

Place the letter from the first column to identify the origin of the term in the second column. You may use an answer more than once. *To check your answers to the exercises in this chapter, go to Answers, p. 17, at the end of the chapter.*

a. components of Greek and Latin word parts
b. eponym
c. acronym
d. modern language

  B 1. Parkinson disease
  A 2. hepatitis
  C 3. MRSA (methicillin-resistant *Staphylococcus aureus*)
  d 4. posttraumatic stress disorder
  a 5. arthritis
  d 6. nuclear medicine scanner
  C 7. AIDS (acquired immunodeficiency syndrome)
  B 8. Alzheimer disease

Categories of Medical Terms and Learning Methods

All medical terms in the text are divided into two categories arranged according to the learning method of each (Table 1-1):

1. terms built from word parts
2. terms not built from word parts

Terms built from word parts can be translated literally to find their meaning. **Analyzing, defining,** and **building** terms using word parts are used as learning methods. Terms not built from word parts cannot be translated literally. **Memorization** of terms, using many exercises, is used as the learning method.

TABLE 1-1 Categories of Medical Terms and Learning Methods

CATEGORY	ORIGIN	EXAMPLE	LEARNING METHODS
Terms Built from Word Parts (can be translated literally to find their meaning)	1. Word parts of Greek and Latin origin put together to form words that can be translated literally to find their meanings	1. arthr/itis	1. Analyzing terms 2. Defining terms 3. Building terms
Terms Not Built from Word Parts (cannot be easily translated literally to find their meaning)	1. Eponyms, terms derived from the name of a person 2. Acronyms, terms formed from the first letters of a phrase that can be spoken as a whole word and usually contains a vowel 3. Modern language, terms derived from the English language 4. Terms of Greek and Latin word parts that cannot be easily translated to find their meanings	1. Alzheimer disease 2. MRSA (methicillin-resistant *Staphylococcus aureus*) 3. complete blood count and differential 4. orthopedics	1. Memorizing terms

EXERCISE 3

Complete the following. *To check your answers, go to p. 17 .*

Medical terms _built from word parts_ _____ can be translated literally to find their meaning, whereas medical terms _not built from word parts_ _____ _____ cannot be easily translated literally to find their meaning.

Medical Terms Built from Word Parts

Terms built from word parts are composed of Greek and Latin **word roots, prefixes,** and **suffixes** and can be translated literally to find their meanings. A **combining vowel** is often added to ease pronunciation. Techniques to learn these terms are **analyzing, defining,** and **building** medical terms.

Four Word Parts

Most medical terms built from word parts consist of some or all of the following components:

1. Word root
2. Prefix
3. Suffix
4. Combining vowel

Word Root

The word root is the word part that is the core of the word. The word root contains the fundamental meaning of the word.

EXAMPLES

In the word	play/er, *play* is the word root.
In the medical term	arthr/itis, *arthr* (which means *joint*) is the word root.
In the medical term	hepat/itis, *hepat* (which means *liver*) is the word root.

The word root is the core of the word; therefore, each medical term contains one or more word roots.

EXERCISE 4

Complete the following: *To check your answers, go to p. 17.*

A word root is *core of the word*.

Suffix

The suffix is a word part attached to the end of the word root to modify its meaning.

SUFFIXES

frequently indicate:

- **procedures,** such as *-scopy*, meaning visual examination, or *-tomy*, meaning incision
- **conditions,** such as *-itis*, meaning inflammation
- **diseases,** such as *-oma*, meaning tumor.

EXAMPLES

In the word	play/er, *-er* is the suffix.
In the medical term	hepat/ic, *-ic* (which means *pertaining to*) is the suffix. *Hepat* is the word root for *liver*; therefore, *hepatic* means *pertaining to the liver.*
In the medical term	hepat/itis, *-itis* (which means *inflammation*) is the suffix. The medical term *hepatitis* means *inflammation of the liver.*

 The suffix is used to modify the meaning of a word. Most medical terms have a suffix.

EXERCISE 5

Complete the following: *To check your answers, go to p. 17.*

The suffix is *word part at end of word*.

Prefix

PREFIXES

often indicate:

- **number** such as *bi-*, meaning two
- **position,** such as *sub-*, meaning under
- **direction,** such as *intra-*, meaning within
- **time,** such as *brady-*, meaning slow
- **negation,** such as *a-*, meaning without

The prefix is a word part attached to the beginning of a word root to modify its meaning.

EXAMPLES

In the word	re/play, *re-* is the prefix.
In the medical term	sub/hepat/ic, *sub-* (which means *under*) is the prefix. *Hepat* is the word root for *liver*; and *-ic* is the suffix for *pertaining to*. The medical term *subhepatic* means *pertaining to under the liver.*
In the medical term	intra/ven/ous, *intra-* (which means *within*) is the prefix, *ven* (which means *vein*) is the word root, and *-ous* (which means *pertaining to*) is the suffix. The medical term *intravenous* means *pertaining to within the vein.*

A prefix can be used to modify the meaning of a word. Many medical terms do not have a prefix.

EXERCISE 6

Complete the following: *To check your answers, go to p. 17.*

The prefix is *word part attached to beggining*

Combining Vowel

The combining vowel is a word part, usually an o, used to ease pronunciation (Table 1-2).

The combining vowel is:

- Placed to connect two word roots
- Placed to connect a word root and a suffix
- **Not** placed to connect a prefix and a word root

VOWELS

are speech sounds represented by the letters *a, e, i, o, u,* and sometimes *y.*

EXAMPLES

In the medical term	oste/o/arthr/itis, *o* is the combining vowel used between two word roots *oste* (which means bone) and *arthr* (which means joint).
In the medical term	arthr/o/pathy, *o* is the combining vowel used between the word root *arthr* and the suffix-*pathy* (which means *disease*).
In the medical term	sub/hepat/ic, the combining vowel is not used between the prefix *sub-* and the word root *hepat*.

> ⚙ The combining vowel is used to ease pronunciation; therefore *not all medical terms have combining vowels.* Medical terms introduced throughout the text that have combining vowels other than *o* are highlighted at their introduction.

Four Guidelines for Using Combining Vowels

Learning the four guidelines for using combining vowels will assist you in correctly spelling medical terms built from word parts. Refer to Table 1-2, as you build terms in the following chapters until the guidelines are a part of your memory.

Guideline One

When connecting a word root and a suffix, a combining vowel is used if the suffix does not begin with a vowel.

EXAMPLE

In the medical term	arthr/o/pathy, the suffix -*pathy* does not begin with a vowel; therefore, a combining vowel is used.

Guideline Two

When connecting a word root and a suffix, a combining vowel is usually **not** used if the suffix begins with a vowel.

EXAMPLE

In the medical term	hepat/ic, the suffix -*ic* begins with the vowel *i*; therefore, a combining vowel is not used.

Guideline Three

When connecting two word roots, a combining vowel is usually used even if vowels are present at the junction.

EXAMPLE

In the medical term oste/o/arthr/itis,

o is the combining vowel used, even though the word root *oste* ends with the vowel *e*, and the word root *arthr* begins with the vowel *a*.

Guideline Four

When connecting a prefix and a word root, a combining vowel is **not** used.

EXAMPLE

In the medical term sub/hepat/ic,

the combining vowel is not used between the prefix *sub-* and the word root *hepat.*

EXERCISE 7

Complete the following: *To check your answers, go to p. 17.*

1. A combining vowel is _usually an "O" to ease pronunciation_

2. When connecting a word root and a suffix, a combining vowel is _used_ if the suffix does not begin with a vowel.

3. When connecting a word root and a suffix, a combining vowel is usually not used if the suffix begins with a _vowel_.

4. When connecting two _word roots_, a combining vowel is usually used, even if vowels are present at the junction.

5. When connecting a prefix and a word root, a combining vowel is _not_ used.

TABLE 1-2 Guidelines for Using Combining Vowels

COMBINING VOWEL GUIDELINES	EXAMPLE
1. When connecting a word root and a suffix, **a combining vowel Is Used if the suffix Does Not Begin with a vowel.**	arthr/**o**/pathy
2. When connecting a word root and a suffix, **a combining vowel Is Usually Not Used if the suffix Begins with a vowel.**	hepat/ic
3. When connecting two word roots, **a combining vowel Is Usually Used even if vowels are present at the junction.**	oste/**o**/arthr/itis
4. When connecting a prefix and a word root, **a combining vowel Is Not Used.**	sub/hepat/ic

Combining Form

A combining form is a word root with the combining vowel attached, separated by a slash (Table 1-3).

EXAMPLES

arthr/o

oste/o

ven/o

The combining form is not a word part per se; rather it is the word root and the combining vowel. *For learning purposes, word roots are presented together with their combining vowels as **combining forms** throughout the text.*

Word roots are presented as combining forms throughout the text.

EXERCISE 8

Complete the following: *To check your answers, go to p. 17.*

A combining form is *a word root w/ combining vowel attached, separated by a slash* .

EXERCISE 9

Match the phrases in the first column with the correct terms in the second column. *To check your answers, go to p. 17.*

B 1. attached at the beginning
A 2. usually an *o*
D 3. all medical terms built from word parts contain at least one
E 4. attached at the end of a word root
C 5. word root with combining vowel attached

a. combining vowel
b. prefix
c. combining form
d. word root
e. suffix

EXERCISE 10

Answer *T* for true and *F* for false. *To check your answers, go to p. 17.*

F 1. There are always prefixes at the beginning of medical terms.
F 2. A combining vowel is always used when connecting a word root and a suffix that begins with the letter *o*.
T 3. A prefix modifies the meaning of the word.
T 4. A combining vowel is used to ease pronunciation.
F 5. *I* is the most commonly used combining vowel.
T 6. The word root is the core of a medical term.
F 7. A combining vowel is used between a prefix and a word root.
F 8. A combining form is a word part.
T 9. A combining vowel is used when connecting a word root and a suffix if the suffix begins with the letter *g*.

TABLE 1-3 Word Parts and Combining Form

Word root	The core of the word	**hepat**/itis
Suffix	Attached at the end of a word root to modify its meaning	hepat/**itis**
Prefix	Attached at the beginning of a word root to modify its meaning	**sub**/hepatic
Combining vowel	Usually an "o" used to ease pronunciation	hepat/**o**/megaly
Combining form	Word root with a combining vowel attached, separated by a slash	**hepat/o**

Following is your first invitation to use the integrated online learning program. You have already created an account by completing Exercise 1 on p. 2.

For review and/or assessment, go to evolve.elsevier.com.
Select: Chapter 1, **Activities,** Word Parts and Combining Form.

Refer to p. 10 for your Evolve Access Information.

Evolve Access Information

Use the following steps for accessing the Evolve website to complete online activities, designated by , that appear throughout each textbook chapter.

> ☼ Future enhancements to Evolve may require a change to these steps. For problem solving, go to **evolvesupport.elsevier.com** or call **1-800-222-9570**.

1. Go to **evolve.elsevier.com**.
2. Click **Login** at the upper right hand corner
3. **Login** using your username and password created in Exercise 1, p. 2. For future reference, record this information in the spaces below.

   a. Username: _____

   b. Password: _____

   If you did not already register for the Evolve Resources for Exploring Medical Language, 9th edition, see Exercise 1, page 2.
4. Click **Evolve Resources for Exploring Medical Language 9th edition**. Chose the listing marked **"Resources"**.
5. Click **Student Resources** under Course Content.
6. Click **Student Resources** (in red) under Table of Contents.
7. Choose a chapter and begin. Have fun and learn at the same time!

Techniques for Learning Medical Terms Built from Word Parts

Analyzing, defining, and **building** medical terms are used in this text to learn medical terms built from word parts. You will use them many times to complete exercises in the following chapters. Refer to Table 1-4, p. 14, as often as needed until you become familiar with these techniques.

Analyzing Medical Terms

To analyze medical terms, divide them into word parts and label each word part and each combining form (Table 1-4 on p. 14). Follow the procedure below:

1. **Divide the term** into word parts with vertical slashes.

   EXAMPLE: oste / o / arthr / o / pathy
2. **Label each word part** by using the following abbreviations.

   WR Word Root
   P   Prefix
   S   Suffix
   CV Combining Vowel

               WR CV WR CV   S
   EXAMPLE: oste / o /arthr / o / pathy
3. **Label each combining form.**

               WR CV WR CV   S
   EXAMPLE: oste / o / arthr / o / pathy
                      CF   CF

EXERCISE 11

Analyze the following medical term. Use the word part list on p. 11 as a reference: *To check your answers, go to p. 17.*

o s t e o p a t h y

EXERCISE 12

Complete the following. *To check your answers, go to p. 17.*

Three steps to analyze medical terms are:

1. *Divide term into word parts w/ vertical slashes.*
2. *Label each word part.*
3. *Label each combing form*

> For review and/or assessment, go to evolve.elsevier.com.
> Select: Chapter 1, **Activities**, Analyze Medical Terms.
> ──
> Refer to p. 10 for your Evolve Access Information.

Defining Medical Terms

To define medical terms, apply the meaning of each word part contained in the term.

EXERCISE 13

Define the medical term: *To check your answers, go to p. 17.*

oste/o/arthr/o/pathy

Use the Word Part List below as a reference.

1. Begin by defining the suffix, *-pathy*. Write the definition on the line below.
2. Move to the beginning of the term, define the word roots *oste* and *arthr*. Write the definitions on the line below, continuing the definition of the term.

oste/o/arthr/o/pathy means _____ of the _____ and _____
                                                    -pathy   oste   arthr

> Most medical terms built from word parts can be defined by beginning with the meaning of the suffix; however, this does not always apply.

Word Part List

WORD ROOTS	DEFINITION	SUFFIXES	DEFINITION
arthr	joint	-itis	inflammation
hepat	liver	-ic	pertaining to
ven	vein	-ous	pertaining to
oste	bone	-pathy	disease
		-megaly	enlargement
PREFIXES		**COMBINING VOWEL**	
intra-	within	o	
sub-	under		

EXERCISE 14

Complete the following: *To check your answers, go to p. 17.*

To define medical terms built from word parts, _____

Divide into word parts w/ slashes, label word part, & label combining vowel

EXERCISE 15

Using the Word Part List on p. 11 to identify the word parts and their meanings, analyze and define the following terms. *To check your answers, go to p. 17.*

          WR   CV   WR   CV   S

EXAMPLE: oste / o / arthr / o / pathy   disease of the bone and joint

1. arthritis   *arthr/itis - inflammation of the joint*
2. hepatitis   *hepat/itis - inflammation of the liver*
3. subhepatic   *sub/hepat/ic - pertaining to under the liver*
4. intravenous   *intra/ven/ous - pertaining to within the vein*
5. arthropathy   *arthr/o/pathy - disease of the joint*
6. osteitis   *oste/itis - inflammation of the bone*
7. hepatomegaly   *hepat/o/megaly - enlargement of the liver*

> (e) For review and/or assessment, go to http://evolve.elsevier.com.
> Select: Chapter 1, **Activities**, Define Medical Terms.
>
> Refer to p. 10 for your Evolve Access Information.

Building Medical Terms

To build medical terms, place word parts together to form words.

EXERCISE 16

Build the medical term for the following. *To check your answers, go to p. 17.*

disease of a joint

Use the Word Part List on p. 11 as a reference. *To check your answers, go to p. 17.*

1. Find the word part for *disease*. Write the word part in the correct space below.
2. Find the word part for *joint*. Write the word part in the correct space below.
3. Insert the combining vowel *o* in the correct space below. (*A combining vowel is needed because the suffix does not begin with a vowel.*)

     arthr / *o* / *pathy*
     WR   /CV/   S

EXERCISE 17

Complete the following: *To check your answers, go to p.17.*

To build medical terms means *place word parts together to form words*.

> ☼ Keep in mind that the beginning of the definition usually indicates the suffix.

EXERCISE 18

Using the Word Part List on p. 11 as a reference, build medical terms for the following definitions. *To check your answers, go to p. 17.*

EXAMPLE: disease of a joint

arthr	/ o /	pathy
WR	/CV/	S

1. inflammation of a joint

arthr / itis
WR / S

2. pertaining to the liver

hepat / ic
WR / S

3. pertaining to <u>under</u> the liver

sub/ hepat / ic
P / WR / S

4. pertaining to <u>within</u> the vein

intra / ven / ous
~~sub~~
P / WR / S

5. inflammation of the bone

oste / itis
WR / S

6. inflammation of the liver

hepat / itis
WR / S

7. disease of the bone and joint

oste/o/arthr/o/
WR /CV/ WR /CV/ S

8. enlargement of the liver

hepat /o/ megaly
WR /CV/ S

EXERCISE FIGURE A

Fill in the blanks to complete labeling of the diagram. *To check your answers, go to p. 17.*

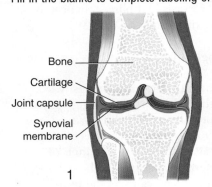

Bone
Cartilage
Joint capsule
Synovial membrane

1

1. Normal knee joint

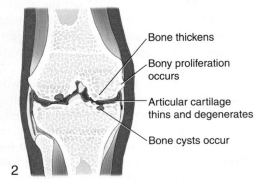

Bone thickens
Bony proliferation occurs
Articular cartilage thins and degenerates
Bone cysts occur

2

2. Knee joint showing

oste/o/arthr/itis
bone /cv/ joint / inflammation

> At this time, do not be concerned about which word root goes first when building a term that contains two word roots. The order is usually dictated by common practice; for surgical or diagnostic terms, word roots are sometimes arranged by the order of function or by the order in which an instrument may encounter a structure. As you practice and learn, you will become accustomed to the accepted order.

For review and/or assessment, go to evolve.elsevier.com.
Select: Chapter 1, **Activities,** Build Medical Terms.

Refer to p. 10 for your Evolve Access Information.

TABLE 1-4 Techniques to Learn Medical Terms Built from Word Parts

• Analyzing	1. Divide medical terms into word parts	oste / o / arthr / o / pathy
	2. Label each word part	WR CV WR CV S oste / o / arthr / o / pathy
	3. Label each combining form	WR CV WR CV S oste / o / arthr / o / pathy CF CF
• Defining	1. Apply the meaning of each word part contained in the term (*begin by defining the suffix, then move to the beginning of the term*) oste / o / arthr / o / pathy WR WR S	 **disease** of the **bone** and **joint**
• Building	1. Place word parts together to form terms (*the beginning of the definition usually indicates the suffix*) **disease** of the **bone** and **joint** 2. Add **combining vowels** as needed	 oste / / arthr / / pathy WR WR S oste / o / arthr / o / pathy WR CV WR CV S

Medical Terms Not Built from Word Parts

Medical terms not built from word parts are terms that cannot be easily translated to find their meanings. Many exercises using memorization are presented in each chapter to assist in learning these terms. Origins of terms not built from word parts are:

1. **eponyms,** terms derived from the name of a person, such as Alzheimer disease
2. **acronyms,** terms formed from the first letter of words in a phrase that can be spoken as a whole word and usually contains a vowel, such as MRSA (methicillin-resistant *Staphylococcus aureus*)
3. **modern language,** terms derived from the English language such as complete blood count and differential
4. **terms made up of Greek and Latin word parts that cannot be easily translated to find their meaning,** such as orthopedic. Orth/o/ped/ic is made up of three word parts: orth/o meaning straight, ped/o meaning child or foot, and -ic meaning pertaining to. Translated literally, **orthopedic** means **pertaining to a straight child or foot,** whereas its meaning as used today is a **branch of medicine dealing with the study and treatment of diseases and abnormalities of the musculoskeletal system.** As you can see, the term orthopedic cannot be translated literally to find its meaning.

EXERCISE 19

Place a check mark in the space provided to identify terms not built from word parts. This may be the first time you have seen some of these terms. Apply your newly acquired knowledge and see how you do. *To check your answers, go to p. 17.*

1. _____ arthritis
2. __✓__ upper respiratory infection
3. __✓__ Lyme disease
4. __✓__ AIDS
5. __✓__ macular degeneration

6. _____ hepatitis
7. __✓__ nuclear medicine scanner
8. __✓__ malignant
9. _____ osteopathy
10. __✓__ Alzheimer disease

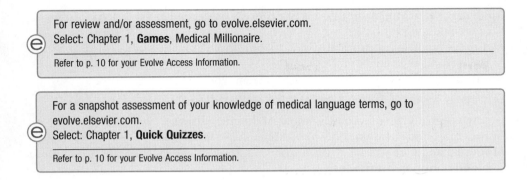

For review and/or assessment, go to evolve.elsevier.com.
Select: Chapter 1, **Games**, Medical Millionaire.

Refer to p. 10 for your Evolve Access Information.

For a snapshot assessment of your knowledge of medical language terms, go to evolve.elsevier.com.
Select: Chapter 1, **Quick Quizzes**.

Refer to p. 10 for your Evolve Access Information.

Chapter Review

Review of Evolve

Keep a record of activities you have completed by placing a check in the box. You may also record your scores. All activities have been referenced throughout the text.

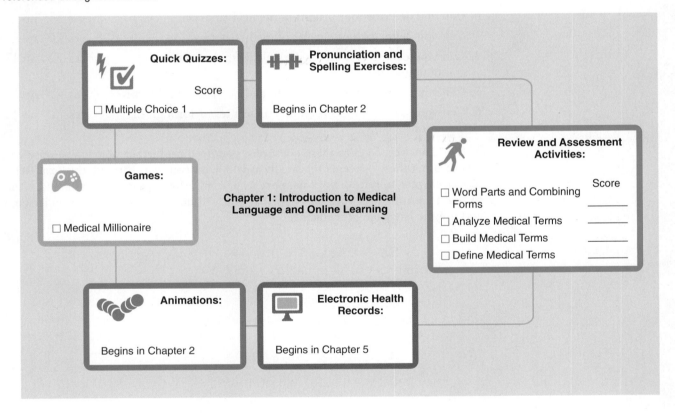

Review of Categories of Medical Terms

Terms built from word parts—can be translated literally to find their meaning
Terms not built from word parts—cannot be translated literally to find their meaning

Review of Medical Terms Built from Word Parts

Word root—core of a word; example, **hepat**
Suffix—attached at the end of a word root to modify its meaning; example, **-ic**
Prefix—attached at the beginning of a word to modify its meaning; example, **sub-**
Combining vowel—usually an o used between two word roots or a word root and suffix to ease pronunciation; example, hepat **o** pathy
Combining form—word root plus combining vowel separated by a vertical slash; example, **hepat/o**

Analyzing—dividing medical terms into word parts, then labeling each word part and combining form

Defining—applying the meaning of each word part contained in the medical term to derive its meaning

Building—placing word parts together to form words

Review of Medical Terms Not Built from Word Parts

Eponyms—name of a person; example, **Alzheimer disease**

Acronyms—from first letter of words, example, **MRSA**

Modern Language—terms derived from the English language, example, **complete blood count and differential**

Terms not easily translated from word parts—example, **orthopedic**

Review of Objectives

To complete this chapter successfully, you do not need to know what the word parts, such as *arthr*, mean. You will learn these in subsequent chapters. **It is important that you have met these objectives:**

1. Can you access the Evolve website?	yes ☐	no ☐
2. Can you describe four origins of medical language?	yes ☐	no ☐
3. Can you define two categories of medical terms?	yes ☐	no ☐
4. Can you identify and define the four word parts and combining form?	yes ☐	no ☐
5. Can you use word parts to analyze and define medical terms?	yes ☐	no ☐
6. Can you use word parts to build medical terms for a given definition?	yes ☐	no ☐

If you answered yes to these questions, you need no further practice because you will be using these concepts repeatedly as you work your way through this text. Refer to this chapter to refresh your memory as needed. Move on to Chapter 2 and begin to build your medical vocabulary so that you will be better prepared to understand and use the language of medicine.

ANSWERS

ANSWERS TO CHAPTER 1 EXERCISES
Exercise Figure
Exercise Figure
A. oste/o/arthr/itis

Exercise 1
Online Activity

Exercise 2
1. b
2. a
3. c
4. d
5. a
6. d
7. c
8. b

Exercise 3
built from word parts; not built from word parts

Exercise 4
a word part that is the core of the word

Exercise 5
a word part attached to the end of the word root to modify its meaning

Exercise 6
a word part attached at the beginning of a word root to modify its meaning

Exercise 7
1. a word part, usually an o, used to ease pronunciation
2. used
3. vowel
4. word roots
5. not

Exercise 8
a word root with the combining vowel attached, separated by a vertical slash

Exercise 9
1. b
2. a
3. d
4. e
5. c

Exercise 10
1. *F*, a medical term may begin with the word root and have no prefix.
2. *F*, if the suffix begins with a vowel, the combining vowel is usually not used.
3. *T*
4. *T*
5. *F*, *o* is the combining vowel most often used.
6. *T*
7. *F*, a combining vowel is used between two word roots or between a word root and a suffix to ease pronunciation.
8. *F*, a combining form is a word root with a combining vowel attached and is not one of the four word parts.
9. *T*

Exercise 11
Note: The combining form is identified by italic and bold print.

WR CV S
oste/o/pathy
  CF

Exercise 12
(1) divide the term into word parts; (2) label each word part; and (3) label each combining form

Exercise 13
disease of the bone and joint

Exercise 14
apply the meaning of each word part contained in the term

Exercise 15
Note: The combining form is identified by italic and bold print.

1. WR S
  arthr/itis
  inflammation of a joint

2. WR S
  hepat/itis
  inflammation of the liver

3. P WR S
  sub/hepat/ic
  pertaining to under the liver

4. P WR S
  intra/ven/ous
  pertaining to within the vein

5. WR CV S
  arthr/o/pathy
     CF
  disease of a joint

6. WR S
  oste/itis
  inflammation of the bone

7. WR CV S
  hepat/o/megaly
     CF
  enlargement of the liver

Exercise 16
arthr/o/pathy

Exercise 17
to place word parts together to form words

Exercise 18
1. arthr/itis
2. hepat/ic
3. sub/hepat/ic
4. intra/ven/ous
5. oste/itis
6. hepat/itis
7. oste/o/arthr/o/pathy
8. hepat/o/megaly

Exercise 19
Check marks for numbers 2, 3, 4, 5, 7, 8, 10

Answers for all chapters are on the Evolve website located under the tab **Extra Content.** They can be printed in one document for easy use to check answers.

Chapter

2

Body Structure, Color, and Oncology

Outline

 ANATOMY, 19

Objectives

Upon completion of this chapter you will be able to:

1. Identify anatomic structures of the human body.

2. Define and spell word parts related to body structure, color, and oncology.

3. Define, pronounce, and spell disease and disorder oncology terms.

4. Define, pronounce, and spell body structure terms.

5. Define, pronounce, and spell complementary terms related to body structure, color, and oncology.

6. Identify and use singular and plural endings.

7. Interpret the meaning of abbreviations related to body structure and oncology.

8. Interpret, read, and comprehend medical language in simulated medical statements and documents.

ANATOMY

Organization of the Body

The structure of the human body falls into the following four categories: cells, tissues, organs, and systems. Each structure is a highly organized unit of smaller structures (Exercise Figure A).

TERM	DEFINITION
cell	basic unit of all living things (Figure 2-1). The human body is composed of trillions of cells, which vary in size and shape according to function.
cell membrane	forms the boundary of the cell
cytoplasm	gel-like fluid inside the cell
nucleus	largest structure within the cell, usually spherical and centrally located. It contains chromosomes for cellular reproduction and is the control center of the cell.
chromosomes	located in the nucleus of the cell. There are 46 chromosomes in all normal human cells, with the exception of mature sex cells, which have 23.
genes	regions within the chromosome. Each chromosome has several thousand genes that determine hereditary characteristics.
DNA (deoxyribonucleic acid)	comprises each gene; is a genetic material that regulates the activities of the cell
tissue	group of similar cells that performs a specific function (Exercise Figure B)
muscle tissue	composed of cells that have a special ability to contract, usually producing movement
nervous tissue	found in the nerves, spinal cord, and brain. It is responsible for coordinating and controlling body activities.
connective tissue	connects, supports, penetrates, and encases various body structures. Adipose (fat), osseous (bone) tissues, and blood are types of connective tissue.
epithelial tissue	the major covering of the external surface of the body; forms membranes that line body cavities and organs and is the major tissue in glands
organ	two or more kinds of tissues that together perform special body functions. For example, the skin is an organ composed of epithelial, connective, muscle, and nerve tissue.
system	group of organs that work together to perform complex body functions. For example, the cardiovascular system consists of the heart, blood vessels, and blood. Its function is to transport nutrients and oxygen to the cells and remove carbon dioxide and other waste product (Table 2-1).

For clinical research terms, go to evolve.elsevier.com.
Select: **Extra Content,** Appendix I, Clinical Research Terms.

Refer to p. 10 for your Evolve Access Information.

MEDICAL GENOMICS

A **genome** is the complete set of genes for all the cells of a specific organism. **Genomics** is the study of the genome and its products and interactions.

Medical genomics is the study of the genome and how it can be used to determine the cause, treatment, and prevention of disease. Medical genomics will alter twenty-first century medicine.

Gene therapy is any therapeutic procedure in which genes are intentionally introduced into human body cells to achieve gene repair, gene suppression, or gene addition. Gene therapy is still in its infancy. The first human gene transfer was performed on a patient with malignant melanoma in 1989.

STEM CELLS

Hematopoietic stem cells are immature cells found in the bone marrow and peripheral blood. They have the potential to develop into mature cells of any type of body tissue or form mature blood cells. Hematopoietic stem cells for transplantation may be obtained from the patient (**autologous**), from an identical twin (**synergetic**), or from a sibling or other individual (**allogenic**).

Embryonic stem cells are derived from the earliest stage of development of the embryo and have the potential to develop into mature body cells.

Stem cell transplantation is used to treat **leukemia** (cancer involving the white blood cells), **aplastic anemia** (disease in which there is inadequate production of blood cells), **multiple myeloma** (cancer that forms tumors in the bone marrow), **lymphoma** (cancer involving lymphoid cells), and **immune deficiency disorders**.

🏛 CHROMOSOME
is derived from the Greek **chromos**, meaning **color**, and **soma**, meaning **body**. German anatomist Waldeyer first used the term in 1888.

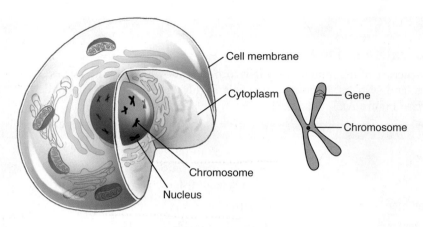

FIGURE 2-1
Body cell.

Table 2-1
Body Systems

BODY SYSTEMS	ORGANS AND FUNCTION
INTEGUMENTARY SYSTEM	Composed of skin, nails, and glands. Forms a protective covering for the body, regulates body temperature, and helps manufacture vitamin D.
RESPIRATORY SYSTEM	Composed of nose, pharynx (throat), larynx (voice box), trachea (windpipe), bronchial tubes, and lungs. Performs respiration which provides for the exchange of oxygen and carbon dioxide within the body.
URINARY SYSTEM	Composed of kidneys, ureters, bladder, and urethra. Removes waste material (urine) from the body, regulates fluid volume, and maintains electrolyte concentration.
REPRODUCTIVE SYSTEM	Female reproductive system is composed of ovaries, uterine tubes, uterus, vagina, and mammary glands. Male reproductive system is composed of testes, urethra, penis, prostate gland, and associated tubes. Responsible for heredity and reproduction.
CARDIOVASCULAR SYSTEM	Composed of the heart and blood vessels. Pumps and transports blood throughout the body.
LYMPHATIC SYSTEM	Composed of a network of vessels, ducts, nodes, and organs. Provides for defense against infection and drainage of extracellular fluid.
DIGESTIVE SYSTEM	Composed of the gastrointestinal tract which includes the mouth, esophagus, stomach, large and small intestine plus accessory organs, liver, gallbladder, and pancreas. Prepares food for use by the body cells and eliminates waste.
MUSCULOSKELETAL SYSTEM	Composed of muscle, bones, and joints. Provides movement and framework for the body, protects vital organs such as the brain, stores calcium, and produces red blood cells.
NERVOUS SYSTEM	Composed of the brain, spinal cord, and nerves. Regulates body activities by sending and receiving messages.
ENDOCRINE SYSTEM	Composed of glands that secrete hormones. Hormones regulate many body activities.

Body Cavities

The body is not a solid structure as it appears on the outside, but has five cavities (Figure 2-2), each containing an orderly arrangement of the internal organs.

TERM	DEFINITION
cranial cavity	space inside the skull (cranium) containing the brain
spinal cavity	space inside the spinal column containing the spinal cord
thoracic, or chest, cavity	space containing the heart, aorta, lungs, esophagus, trachea, bronchi, and mediastinal area
abdominal cavity	space containing the stomach, intestines, kidneys, adrenal glands, liver, gallbladder, pancreas, spleen, and ureters
pelvic cavity	space containing the urinary bladder, certain reproductive organs, parts of the small and large intestine, and the rectum
abdominopelvic cavity	both the pelvic and abdominal cavities

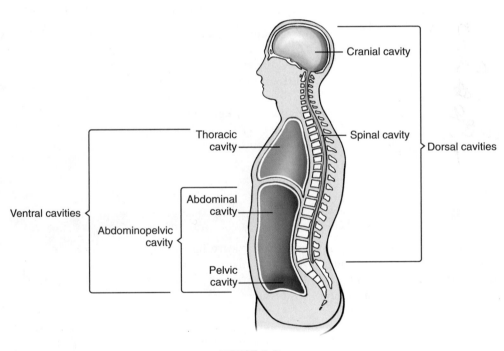

FIGURE 2-2
Body cavities.

For more anatomy and physiology, go to evolve.elsevier.com.
Select: **Extra Content**, A & P Booster, Chapter 2.

Refer to p. 10 for your Evolve Access Information.

EXERCISE 1

Match the anatomic terms in the first column with the correct definitions in the second column.
To check your answers to the exercises in this chapter, go to Answers, p. 59, at the back of the chapter.

h	1. chromosomes	a.	type of connective tissue
e	2. nucleus	b.	regions within the chromosome
d	3. cytoplasm	c.	covers external body surface, lines body cavities and organs
k	4. cell	d.	gel-like fluid inside the cell
g	5. muscle tissue	e.	contains chromosomes
f	6. nerve tissue	f.	coordinates body activities
c	7. epithelial tissue	g.	usually produces movement
a	8. bone	h.	contain genes
b	9. genes	i.	chest cavity
j	10. DNA	j.	genetic material that regulates the activities of the cell
		k.	basic unit of all living things

EXERCISE 2

Match the anatomic terms in the first column with the correct definitions in the second column.

h	1. spinal cavity	a.	group of organs functioning together
b	2. thoracic cavity	b.	chest cavity
c	3. organ	c.	composed of two or more tissues
e	4. cranial cavity	d.	found in the skin
g	5. pelvic cavity	e.	space inside the skull
a	6. system	f.	contains the stomach
f	7. abdominal cavity	g.	contains the urinary bladder
		h.	contains the spinal cord

🔗 WORD PARTS

Begin building your medical vocabulary by learning the word parts listed next. The list may appear long to you; however, the many exercises that follow are designed to help you understand and remember the word parts. Also, many of the word parts will be repeatedly used throughout this text.

> 🔅 Use the flashcards accompanying this text or electronic flashcards to assist you in memorizing the word parts for this chapter.

To use electronic flashcards, go to evolve.elsevier.com.
Select: Chapter 2, **Flashcards**.

Refer to p. 10 for your Evolve Access Information.

Combining Forms of Body Structure

COMBINING FORM	DEFINITION
aden/o	gland
cyt/o	cell
epitheli/o	epithelium
fibr/o	fiber
hist/o	tissue
kary/o	nucleus
lip/o	fat
my/o	muscle
neur/o	nerve
organ/o	organ
sarc/o	flesh, connective tissue
system/o	system
viscer/o	internal organs

> ☼ Reminder: the word root is the core of the word. The combining form is the word root with the combining vowel attached, separated by a vertical slash.

> 🏛 **EPITHELIUM**
> originally meant **surface over the nipple. Epi** means **upon,** and **thela** means **nipple** (or projecting surfaces of many kinds).

EXERCISE FIGURE A

Fill in the blanks with combining forms in this diagram of the organization of the body. *To check your answers, go to p. 59.*

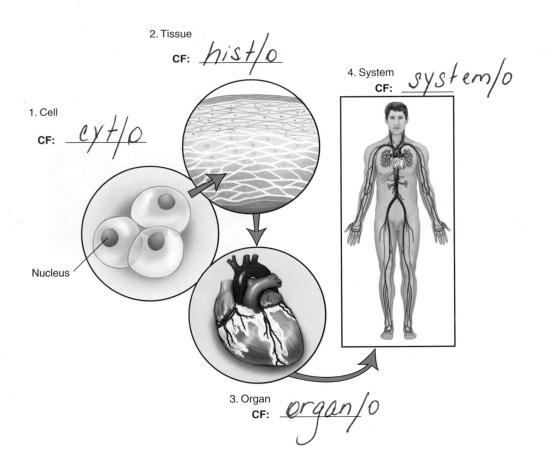

2. Tissue
CF: _hist/o_

4. System
CF: _system/o_

1. Cell
CF: _cyt/o_

Nucleus

3. Organ
CF: _organ/o_

EXERCISE 3

Write the definitions of the following combining forms.

1. sarc/o _flesh, connective tis_
2. lip/o _fat_
3. kary/o _nucleus_
4. viscer/o _internal organs_
5. cyt/o _cell_
6. hist/o _tissue_
7. my/o _muscle_
8. neur/o _nerve_
9. organ/o _organ_
10. system/o _system_
11. epitheli/o _epithelium_
12. fibr/o _fiber_
13. aden/o _gland_

EXERCISE FIGURE B

Fill in the blanks with combining forms in this diagram of types of tissues.

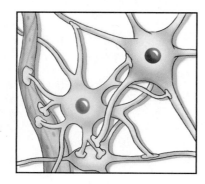

1. Nerve
CF: _neur/o_

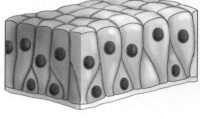

2. Epithelium
CF: _epitheli/o_

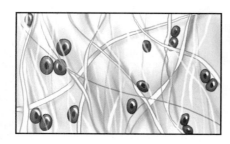

3. Connective
CF: _sarc/o_

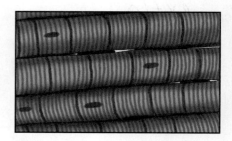

4. Muscle
CF: _my/o_

EXERCISE 4

Write the combining form for each of the following.

1. internal organs _viscer/o_
2. epithelium _epitheli/o_
3. organ _organ/o_
4. nucleus _kary/o_
5. cell _cyt/o_
6. tissue _hist/o_
7. nerve _neur/o_

8. muscle _my/o_
9. fat _lip/o_
10. system _system/o_
11. flesh, connective tissue _sarc/o_
12. fiber _fibr/o_
13. gland _aden/o_

Combining Forms Commonly Used with Body Structure Terms

COMBINING FORM	DEFINITION
cancer/o, carcin/o	cancer (a disease characterized by the unregulated, abnormal growth of new cells)
eti/o	cause (of disease)
gno/o	knowledge
iatr/o	physician, medicine (also means treatment)
lei/o	smooth
onc/o	tumor, mass
path/o	disease
rhabd/o	rod-shaped, striated
somat/o	body

🏛 CANCER

Carcin and cancer are derived from Latin and Greek words meaning crab. They originated before the nature of malignant growth was understood. One explanation was that the swollen veins around the diseased area looked like the claws of a crab.

EXERCISE 5

Write the definitions of the following combining forms.

1. onc/o _tumor, mass_
2. carcin/o _cancer_
3. eti/o _cause of disease_
4. path/o _disease_
5. somat/o _body_

6. cancer/o _cancer_
7. rhabd/o _red shaped, striated_
8. lei/o _smooth_
9. gno/o _knowledge_
10. iatr/o _physician/medicine_

EXERCISE 6

Write the combining form for each of the following.

1. disease _path/o_
2. tumor, mass _onc/o_
3. cause (of disease) _eti/o_
4. cancer a. _cancer/o_
          b. _carcin/o_

5. body _somat/o_
6. smooth _lei/o_
7. rod-shaped, striated _rhabd/o_
8. knowledge _gno/o_
9. physician, medicine _iatr/o_

Combining Forms that Describe Color

COMBINING FORM	DEFINITION
chlor/o	green
chrom/o	color
cyan/o	blue
erythr/o	red
leuk/o	white
melan/o	black
xanth/o	yellow

🏛 ERYTHRO

Aristotle noted "two colors of blood" and applied the term **erythros** to the dark red blood.

EXERCISE 7

Write the definitions of the following combining forms.

1. cyan/o _blue_
2. erythr/o _Red_
3. leuk/o _white_
4. xanth/o _yellow_
5. chrom/o _color_
6. melan/o _black_
7. chlor/o _green_

EXERCISE 8

Write the combining form for each of the following.

1. blue _cyan/o_
2. red _erythr/o_
3. white _leuk/o_
4. black _melan/o_
5. yellow _xanth/o_
6. color _chrom/o_
7. green _chlor/o_

Reminder: prefixes are placed at the beginning of word roots to modify their meanings.

Prefixes

PREFIX	DEFINITION
dia-	through, complete
dys-	painful, abnormal, difficult, labored
hyper-	above, excessive
hypo-	below, incomplete, deficient, under
meta-	after, beyond, change
neo-	new
pro-	before

EXERCISE 9

Write the definitions of the following prefixes.

1. neo- *New*
2. hyper- *Above, excessive*
3. meta- *after, beyond, change*
4. hypo- *below, incomplete, under deficient*
5. dys- *painful, abnormal, difficult, labored*
6. dia- *through, complete*
7. pro- *before*

EXERCISE 10

Write the prefix for each of the following.

1. new *Neo-*
2. above, excessive *hyper-*
3. below, incomplete, deficient, under *hypo-*
4. after, beyond, change *meta-*
5. painful, abnormal, difficult, labored *dys-*
6. through, complete *dia-*
7. before *pro-*

Suffixes

SUFFIX	DEFINITION
-al, -ic, -ous	pertaining to
-cyte (NOTE: the combining form for cell is cyt/o; the suffix for cell is -cyte, ending with an e.)	cell
-gen	substance or agent that produces or causes
✳ -genic	producing, originating, causing
-logist	one who studies and treats (specialist, physician)
-logy	study of
-megaly	enlargement
-oid	resembling
-oma	tumor, swelling
-osis	abnormal condition (means **increase** when used with blood cell word roots)
-pathy	disease
✳ -plasia	condition of formation, development, growth
-plasm	growth, substance, formation
-sarcoma	malignant tumor
-sis	state of
✳ -stasis	control, stop, standing

Reminder: suffixes are placed at the end of word roots to modify their meanings.

The suffix -**logist** may indicate a specialist such as in **psychologist who is not a physician** or a specialist such as in **oncologist who is a physician.** For learning purposes in the text, if the specialist is a physician, it will be indicated in the definition such as **oncologist … a physician who studies and treats (malignant) tumors.** Also, some physicians, such as pathologists, do not treat. The definition of -logist will vary.

> Some suffixes are made of a word root plus a suffix; they are presented as suffixes for ease of learning. For example, **-pathy** is made up of the word root **path** and the noun ending **-y.** When analyzing a medical term, divide the suffixes as learned. For example, **somatopathy** should be divided somat/o/pathy and **not** somat/o/path/y.

 Refer to **Appendix A** and **Appendix B** for alphabetized lists of word parts and their meanings.

EXERCISE 11

Match the suffixes in the first column with their correct definitions in the second column.

i	1. -logy	a.	producing, originating, causing
l	2. -osis	b.	cell
q	3. -pathy	c.	specialist, physician
f m	4. -plasm	d.	new
g	5. -al, -ic, -ous	e.	enlargement
	6. -stasis	f.	growth, substance, formation
h	7. -oid	g.	pertaining to
b	8. -cyte	h.	resembling
c	9. -logist	i.	study of
n	10. -oma	j.	control, stop, standing
a	11. -gen	k.	substance that produces
p	12. -sarcoma	l.	abnormal condition
m	13. -plasia	m.	condition of formation, development, growth
a	14. -genic	n.	tumor, swelling
o	15. -sis	o.	state of
e	16. -megaly	p.	malignant tumor
		q.	disease

EXERCISE 12

Write the definitions of the following suffixes.

1. -logist *one who studys or treats*
2. -pathy *disease*
3. -logy *Study of*
4. -ic *pertaining to*
5. -stasis *Control, stop, standing*
6. -cyte *cell*
7. -osis *abnormal conditions*
8. -ous *pertaining to*
9. -plasm *condition of, formation,*

10. -al _pertaining to_
11. -plasia _condition of formation, development_
12. -oid _Resembling_
13. -gen _Substance that produces or causes_
14. -genic _producing, orginating, causing_
15. -oma _tumor_
16. -sarcoma _(malignant_
17. -sis _State of_
18. –megaly _enlargment_

For review and/or assessment, go to evolve.elsevier.com. Select:
Chapter 2, **Activities**, Word Parts
Chapter 2, **Games**, Name that Word Part

Refer to p. 10 for your Evolve Access Information.

🗨 **MEDICAL TERMS**

Oncology

Oncology is the study of tumors. Tumors develop from excessive growth of cells from a body part. Tumors, or masses, are benign (noncancerous) or malignant (cancerous). The names of tumors are often made of the word root for the body part and the suffix **-oma,** as in the term *my/oma,* which means "tumor composed of muscle."

Oncology terms are introduced in this chapter because of their relation to cells and cell abnormalities. This is an introductory list only. **More oncology terms appear in subsequent chapters and are presented with the introduction of the related body systems.**

Disease and Disorder Oncology Terms

Built from Word Parts

The following terms are built from word parts you have already learned and can be translated literally to find their meanings. Further explanation of terms beyond the definition of their word parts, if needed, is included in parentheses. *At first the list of terms may seem long to you; however, many of the word parts are repeated in many of the terms. You will soon find that knowing parts of the terms makes learning the words easy. Analyzing, defining,* and **building exercises** are used to learn these terms.

TERM	DEFINITION
adenocarcinoma (*ad*-e-nō-*kar*-si-NŌ-ma)	cancerous tumor of glandular tissue
adenoma (ad-e-NŌ-ma)	tumor composed of glandular tissue (benign)
carcinoma (CA) (*kar*-si-NŌ-ma)	cancerous tumor (malignant) (Exercise Figure C)
chloroma (klo-RŌ-ma)	tumor of green color (malignant, arising from myeloid tissue)
epithelioma (*ep*-i-*thē*-lē-Ō-ma)	tumor composed of epithelium (may be benign or malignant)

🏛 Practice two things in your dealings with disease: either help or do not harm the patient.
—**Hippocrates** 460–375 BC

TNM STAGING SYSTEM OF CANCER

AJCC (American Joint Committee on Cancer) has devised a classification widely used to stage certain types of cancer properly.

T refers to size and the extent of the primary tumor (ranked 0-4).

N denotes the involvement of the lymph nodes (ranked 0-4).

M defines whether there is metastasis (0 = none; 1 = present).

For example, T$_2$ N$_1$ M$_0$

T$_2$ refers to the primary tumor of 2 cm.

N$_1$ means spread of tumor to ipsilateral (same side) lymph nodes.

M$_0$ means no distant metastasis.

This system helps communicate the extent of cancer and is frequently cited by oncologists, surgeons, and radiation oncologists.

Disease and Disorder Oncology Terms—cont'd

Built from Word Parts

INCIDENTALOMA

refers to a mass lesion involving an organ that is discovered unexpectedly by the use of ultrasound, computed tomography scan, or magnetic resonance imaging and has nothing to do with the patient's symptoms or primary diagnosis.

TERM	DEFINITION
fibroma (fi-BRŌ-ma)	tumor composed of fiber (fibrous tissue) (benign)
fibrosarcoma (fi-brō-sar-KŌ-ma)	malignant tumor composed of fiber (fibrous tissue)
leiomyoma (*lī*-ō-mī-Ō-ma)	tumor composed of smooth muscle (benign)
leiomyosarcoma (*lī*-ō-*mī*-ō-sar-KŌ-ma)	malignant tumor of smooth muscle
lipoma (li-PŌ-ma)	tumor composed of fat (benign tumor)
liposarcoma (*lip*-ō-sar-KŌ-ma)	malignant tumor of fat
melanocarcinoma (*mel*-a-nō-*kar*-si-NŌ-ma)	cancerous black tumor (malignant)
melanoma (mel-a-NŌ-ma)	black tumor (primarily of the skin) (Exercise Figure C)
myoma (mī-Ō-ma)	tumor composed of muscle (benign)
neoplasm (NĒ-ō-plazm)	new growth (of abnormal tissue, benign or malignant)
neuroma (nū-RŌ-ma)	tumor composed of nerve (benign)
rhabdomyoma (*rab*-dō-mī-Ō-ma)	tumor composed of striated muscle (benign)
rhabdomyosarcoma (*rab*-dō-*mī*-ō-sar-KŌ-ma)	malignant tumor of striated muscle (Exercise Figure C)
sarcoma (sar-KŌ-ma) *(NOTE: sarc/o also is presented in this chapter as a word root.)*	tumor of connective tissue (such as bone or cartilage) (highly malignant) (Exercise Figure C)

🏛 **SARCOMA**

has been used since the time of ancient Greece to describe any fleshy tumor. Since the introduction of cellular pathology, the meaning has become **malignant connective tissue tumor.**

Often, an additional word root is used to denote the type of tissue involved, such as **oste** in **osteosarcoma**, which refers to a malignant tumor of the bone.

ⓔ To watch animations go to evolve.elsevier.com. Select:
Chapter 2, **Animations,** Neoplasms

Refer to p. 10 for your Evolve Access Information.

EXERCISE 13

Practice saying aloud each of the disease and disorder oncology terms built from word parts on pp. 29–30. Use Table 2-2, p. 31, for explanation of the pronunciation guide.

ⓔ To hear the terms, go to evolve.elsevier.com. Select: Chapter 2, **Exercises,** Pronunciation.

Refer to p. 10 for your Evolve Access information.

☐ Place a check mark in the box when you have completed this exercise.

Table 2-2
Pronunciation Key

GUIDELINES	EXAMPLES
1. Words are distorted minimally to indicate proper phonetic sound.	doctor (dok-tor)
2. The macron (ˉ) indicates the long vowel sound.	donate (dō-nāte) ā as in say ē as in me ī as in spine ō as in no ū as in cute
3. Vowels with no markings should have a short sound.	medical (med-i-cal) a as in sad e as in get i as in sit o as in top u as in cut
4. Primary accents are indicated by capital letters; the secondary accent (which is stressed, but not as strongly as the primary accent) is indicated by italics. *There may be geographical variations in pronunciation.*	altogether (*all*-tū-GETH-er) pancreatitis (*pan*-krē-a-TĪ-tis)

EXERCISE 14

Analyze and define the following disease and disorder oncology terms. Refer to Chapter 1, pp. 10–11 to review analyzing and defining techniques. **This is an important exercise; do not skip any portion of it.**

```
         WR  CV   WR  CV    S
EXAMPLE: lei / o /  my / o / sarcoma   malignant tumor of smooth muscle
            ‿          ‿
            CF         CF
```

1. sarcoma _____ *sar* _____
2. melanoma _____
3. epithelioma _____
4. lipoma _____
5. neoplasm _____
6. myoma _____
7. neuroma _____
8. carcinoma _____
9. melanocarcinoma _____
10. rhabdomyosarcoma _____
11. leiomyoma _____
12. rhabdomyoma _____
13. fibroma _____
14. liposarcoma _____
15. fibrosarcoma _____
16. adenoma _____
17. adenocarcinoma _____
18. chloroma _____

EXERCISE FIGURE **C**

Fill in the blanks to complete labeling of these diagrams of types of cancers.

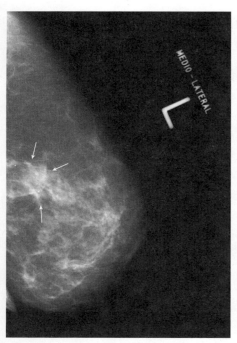

carcinjoma of the breast

1.   cancer / tumor

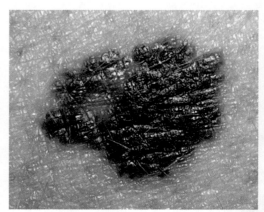

melanjoma

2.   black / tumor

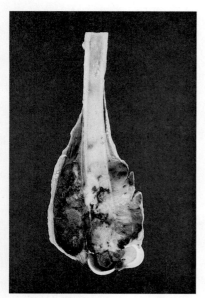

chist joma of the femur

3.   connective / tumor
     tissue

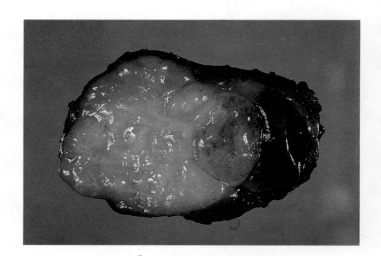

joj my joj

4.   striated /cv/ muscle /cv/ malignant tumor

EXERCISE 15

Build medical disease and disorder oncology terms for the following definitions by using the word parts you have learned. If you need help, refer to Chapter 1, pp. 10–11, to review medical term building techniques. **Once again, this is an integral part of the learning process; do not skip any part of this exercise.**

EXAMPLE: tumor composed of fat $\dfrac{\text{lip}}{\text{WR}} \Big/ \dfrac{\text{oma}}{\text{S}}$

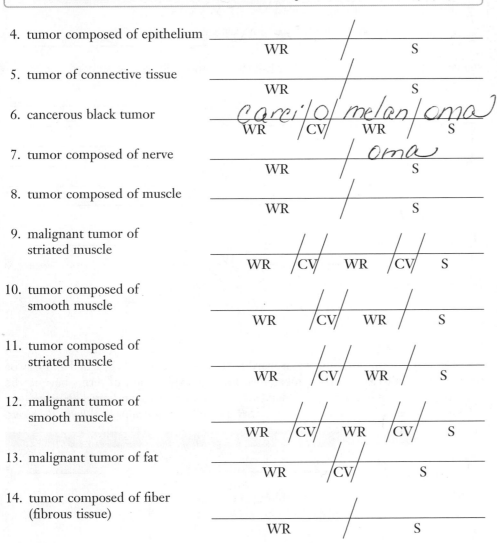

1. black tumor $\dfrac{\text{melan}}{\text{WR}} \Big/ \dfrac{\text{oma}}{\text{S}}$

2. cancerous tumor $\dfrac{\text{carcin}}{\text{WR}} \Big/ \dfrac{\text{oma}}{\text{S}}$

3. new growth $\dfrac{\text{neo}}{\text{P}} \Big/ \dfrac{\text{plasm}}{\text{S(WR)}}$

> When analyzing medical terms that have a suffix containing a word root, it may appear, as in the word **neoplasm,** that the term is composed of only a prefix and a suffix. Keep in mind that the word root is embedded in the suffix and is indicated in the *Building Medical Terms* exercises by S(WR).

4. tumor composed of epithelium $\dfrac{}{\text{WR}} \Big/ \dfrac{}{\text{S}}$

5. tumor of connective tissue $\dfrac{}{\text{WR}} \Big/ \dfrac{}{\text{S}}$

6. cancerous black tumor $\dfrac{\text{carci}}{\text{WR}} \Big/ \dfrac{\text{o}}{\text{CV}} \Big/ \dfrac{\text{melan}}{\text{WR}} \Big/ \dfrac{\text{oma}}{\text{S}}$

7. tumor composed of nerve $\dfrac{}{\text{WR}} \Big/ \dfrac{\text{oma}}{\text{S}}$

8. tumor composed of muscle $\dfrac{}{\text{WR}} \Big/ \dfrac{}{\text{S}}$

9. malignant tumor of striated muscle $\dfrac{}{\text{WR}} \Big/ \dfrac{}{\text{CV}} \Big/ \dfrac{}{\text{WR}} \Big/ \dfrac{}{\text{CV}} \Big/ \text{S}$

10. tumor composed of smooth muscle $\dfrac{}{\text{WR}} \Big/ \dfrac{}{\text{CV}} \Big/ \dfrac{}{\text{WR}} \Big/ \text{S}$

11. tumor composed of striated muscle $\dfrac{}{\text{WR}} \Big/ \dfrac{}{\text{CV}} \Big/ \dfrac{}{\text{WR}} \Big/ \text{S}$

12. malignant tumor of smooth muscle $\dfrac{}{\text{WR}} \Big/ \dfrac{}{\text{CV}} \Big/ \dfrac{}{\text{WR}} \Big/ \dfrac{}{\text{CV}} \Big/ \text{S}$

13. malignant tumor of fat $\dfrac{}{\text{WR}} \Big/ \dfrac{}{\text{CV}} \Big/ \text{S}$

14. tumor composed of fiber (fibrous tissue) $\dfrac{}{\text{WR}} \Big/ \dfrac{}{\text{S}}$

15. malignant tumor of fiber
    (fibrous tissue)

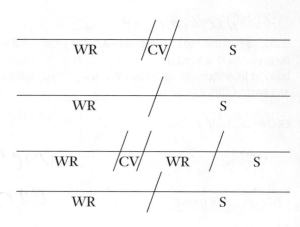

————————————————————
    WR   /CV/   S

16. tumor composed of
    glandular tissue

————————————————————
    WR   S

17. cancerous tumor of
    glandular tissue

————————————————————
    WR   /CV/   WR   /   S

18. tumor of green color

————————————————————
    WR   /   S

EXERCISE 16

Spell each of the disease and disorder oncology terms built from word parts on pp. 29–30 by having someone dictate them to you.

To hear and spell the terms, go to evolve.elsevier.com. Select: Chapter 2, **Exercises,** Spelling.

Refer to p. 10 for your Evolve Access Information.

☐ Place a check mark in the box if you have completed this exercise online.

You may type the terms on the screen or write them below in the spaces provided.

1. _____   11. _____
2. _____   12. _____
3. _____   13. _____
4. _____   14. _____
5. _____   15. _____
6. _____   16. _____
7. _____   17. _____
8. _____   18. _____
9. _____   19. _____
10. _____

Body Structure Terms

Built from Word Parts

The following terms are built from word parts you have already learned and can be translated literally to find their meanings. Further explanation of terms beyond the definition of their word parts, if needed, is included in parentheses. *By analyzing, defining, and building the terms in the exercises that follow, you will come to know the terms.*

TERM	DEFINITION
cytogenic (sī-tō-JEN-ik)	producing cells
cytoid (SĪ-toid)	resembling a cell
cytology (sī-TOL-o-jē)	study of cells

TERM	DEFINITION
cytoplasm (SĪ-tō-plazm)	cell substance
dysplasia (dis-PLĀ-zha)	abnormal development (Figure 2-6, p. 44)
epithelial (*ep*-i-THĒ-lē-al)	pertaining to epithelium
erythrocyte (RBC) (e-RITH-rō-sīt)	red (blood) cell (Exercise Figure D)
erythrocytosis (e-*rith*-rō-sī-TŌ-sis)	increase in the number of red (blood) cells
histology (his-TOL-o-jē)	study of tissue
hyperplasia (*hī*-per-PLĀ-zha)	excessive development (number of cells) (Exercise Figure E) (see Figure 2-6, p. 44)
hypoplasia (hī-pō-PLĀ-zha)	incomplete development (of an organ or tissues)
karyocyte (KĂR-ē-ō-sīt)	cell with a nucleus
karyoplasm (KĂR-ē-ō-*plazm*)	substance of a nucleus
leukocyte (WBC) (LŪ-kō-sīt)	white (blood) cell (Exercise Figure D)
leukocytosis (*lū*-kō-sī-TŌ-sis)	increase in the number of white (blood) cells
lipoid (LIP-oid)	resembling fat
myopathy (mī-OP-a-thē)	disease of the muscle
neuroid (NŪ-rōyd)	resembling a nerve
organomegaly (*or*-ga-nō-MEG-a-lē)	enlargement of an organ
somatic (sō-MAT-ik)	pertaining to the body
somatogenic (*sō*-ma-tō-JEN-ik)	originating in the body (organic as opposed to psychogenic)
somatopathy (*sō*-ma-TOP-a-thē)	disease of the body
somatoplasm (sō-MAT-ō-plazm)	body substance
systemic (sis-TEM-ik)	pertaining to a (body) system (or the body as a whole)
visceral (VIS-er-al)	pertaining to the internal organs

Ellipsis is the practice of omitting an essential part of a word by common consent. Note this practice in the terms **erythrocyte** (red **blood** cell) and **leukocyte** (white **blood** cell). The word root for blood is omitted.

EXERCISE FIGURE D

Fill in the blanks to label this diagram of blood cells.

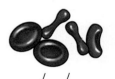

1. _____ / cv / cell(s)
        red

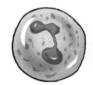

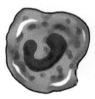

2. _____ / cv / cell(s)
        white

EXERCISE FIGURE E

Fill in the blanks to label the diagram.

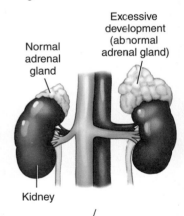

Normal adrenal gland

Excessive development (abnormal adrenal gland)

Kidney

_____ / development
excessive

EXERCISE 17

Practice saying aloud each of the body structure terms built from word parts on pp. 34–35.

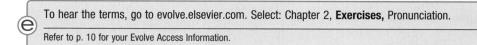

To hear the terms, go to evolve.elsevier.com. Select: Chapter 2, **Exercises,** Pronunciation.

Refer to p. 10 for your Evolve Access Information.

☐ Place a check mark in the box when you have completed this exercise.

EXERCISE 18

Analyze and define the following body structure terms.

```
                 WR  CV    S
EXAMPLE:     cyt / o / genic    producing cells
                  \___/
                   CF
```

1. cytology _____
2. histology _____
3. visceral _____
4. karyocyte _____
5. karyoplasm _____
6. systemic _____
7. cytoplasm _____
8. somatic _____
9. somatogenic _____
10. somatoplasm _____
11. somatopathy _____
12. neuroid _____
13. myopathy _____
14. erythrocyte _____
15. leukocyte _____
16. epithelial _____
17. lipoid _____
18. hyperplasia _____
19. erythrocytosis _____
20. leukocytosis _____
21. hypoplasia _____
22. cytoid _____
23. dysplasia _____
24. organomegaly _____

EXERCISE 19

Build medical terms for the following body structure definitions by using the word parts you have learned.

EXAMPLE: Example: producing cells $\dfrac{\text{cyt} / \text{o} / \text{genic}}{\text{WR} / \text{CV} / \text{S}}$

1. cell substance   _____ / _____ / _____
   WR   CV   S

2. substance of a nucleus   _____ / _____ / _____
   WR   CV   S

3. pertaining to the body   _____ / _____
   WR   S

4. disease of the muscle   _____ / _____ / _____
   WR   CV   S

5. body substance   _____ / _____ / _____
   WR   CV   S

6. pertaining to the internal organs   _____ / _____
   WR   S

7. originating in the body   _____ / _____ / _____
   WR   CV   S

8. disease of the body   _____ / _____ / _____
   WR   CV   S

9. red (blood) cell   _____ / _____ / _____
   WR   CV   S

10. resembling a nerve   _____ / _____
    WR   S

11. pertaining to a (body) system   _____ / _____
    WR   S

12. white (blood) cell   _____ / _____ / _____
    WR   CV   S

13. cell with a nucleus   _____ / _____ / _____
    WR   CV   S

14. resembling fat   _____ / _____
    WR   S

15. study of cells   _____ / _____ / _____
    WR   CV   S

16. excessive development (of cells)   _____ / _____
    P   S(WR)

17. resembling a cell   _____ / _____
    WR   S

18. pertaining to epithelium   _____ / _____
    WR   S

19. study of tissue

_____/_/_____
WR   /CV/   S

20. increase in the number
of red (blood) cells

_____/_/_____/_____
WR   /CV/   WR   /   S

21. incomplete development
(of an organ or tissue)

_____/_____
P   /   S(WR)

22. increase in the number of
white (blood) cells

_____/_/_____/_____
WR   /CV/   WR   /   S

23. abnormal development

_____/_____
P   /   S(WR)

24. enlargement of an organ

_____/_/_____
WR   /CV/   S

EXERCISE 20

Spell each of the body structure terms built from word parts on pp. 34–35 by having someone dictate them to you.

> To hear and spell the terms, go to evolve.elsevier.com. Select: Chapter 2, **Exercises,** Spelling.
>
> Refer to p. 10 for your Evolve Access Information.
>
> ☐ Place a check mark in the box if you have completed this exercise online.

1. _____   14. _____

2. _____   15. _____

3. _____   16. _____

4. _____   17. _____

5. _____   18. _____

6. _____   19. _____

7. _____   20. _____

8. _____   21. _____

9. _____   22. _____

10. _____   23. _____

11. _____   24. _____

12. _____   25. _____

13. _____

Complementary Terms

 Complementary terms complete the vocabulary presented in the chapter by describing **signs, symptoms, medical specialties, specialists,** and **related words.**

Built from Word Parts

The following terms are built from word parts you have already learned and can be translated literally to find their meanings. Further explanation of terms beyond the definition of their word parts, if needed, is included in parentheses.

TERM	DEFINITION
cancerous (KAN-ser-us)	pertaining to cancer
carcinogen (kar-SIN-o-jen)	substance that causes cancer
carcinogenic (*kar*-sin-ō-JEN-ik)	producing cancer
cyanosis (sī-a-NŌ-sis)	abnormal condition of blue (bluish discoloration, especially of the skin, caused by inadequate supply of oxygen in the blood) (Figure 2-3)
diagnosis (Dx) (*dī*-ag-NŌ-sis)	state of complete knowledge (identifying a disease)
etiology (ē-tē-OL-o-jē)	study of causes (of diseases)
iatrogenic (ī-*at*-rō-JEN-ik)	produced by a physician (the unexpected results from a treatment prescribed by a physician)
iatrology (ī-a-TROL-o-jē)	study of medicine
metastasis (pl. metastases) (mets) (me-TAS-ta-sis) (me-TAS-ta-sēz)	beyond control (transfer of cells from one organ to another, as in malignant tumors) (Figure 2-4)
oncogenic (*ong*-kō-JEN-ik)	causing tumors
oncologist (ong-KOL-o-jist)	physician who studies and treats (malignant) tumors
oncology (ong-KOL-o-jē)	study of tumors (a branch of medicine concerned with the study of malignant tumors)
organic (or-GAN-ik)	pertaining to an organ
pathogenic (path-ō-JEN-ik)	producing disease
pathologist (pa-THOL-o-jist)	physician who studies diseases (examines biopsies and performs autopsies to determine the cause of disease or death)
pathology (pa-THOL-o-jē)	study of disease (a branch of medicine dealing with the study of the causes of disease and death)

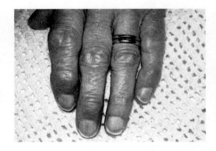

Complementary Terms—cont'd
Built from Word Parts

TERM	DEFINITION
prognosis (Px) (prog-NŌ-sis)	state of before knowledge (prediction of the outcome of disease)
xanthochromic (*zan*-thō-KRŌ-mik)	pertaining to yellow color
xanthosis (zan-THŌ-sis)	abnormal condition of yellow (discoloration)

🏛 **PROGNOSIS**
was used by Hippocrates to mean the same then as now: **to foretell the course of a disease.**

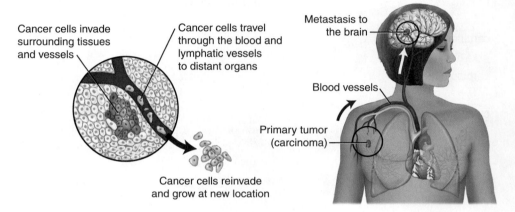

FIGURE 2-4
Metastasis.

EXERCISE 21

Practice saying aloud each of the complementary terms built from word parts on pp. 39–40.

> ⓔ To hear the terms, go to evolve.elsevier.com. Select: Chapter 2, **Exercises,** Pronunciation.
>
> Refer to p. 10 for your Evolve Access Information.

☐ Place a check mark in the box when you have completed this exercise.

EXERCISE 22

Analyze and define the following complementary terms.

         WR CV S
EXAMPLE: path / o / genic <u>producing disease</u>
           CF

1. pathology _____

2. pathologist _____

3. metastasis _____

4. oncogenic _____

5. oncology _____

6. cancerous _____

7. carcinogenic _____

8. cyanosis _____

9. etiology _____

10. xanthosis _____

11. xanthochromic _____

12. carcinogen _____

13. oncologist _____

14. prognosis _____

15. organic _____

16. diagnosis _____

17. iatrogenic _____

18. iatrology _____

EXERCISE 23

Build medical terms for the following definitions of complementary terms by using the word parts you have learned.

EXAMPLE: producing disease $\dfrac{\text{path} \;/\; \text{o} \;/\; \text{genic}}{\text{WR} \;/\text{CV}/\; \text{S}}$

1. pertaining to yellow color $\dfrac{}{\text{WR} \quad /\text{CV}/ \quad \text{WR} \quad / \quad \text{S}}$

2. beyond control $\dfrac{}{\text{P} \qquad / \qquad \text{S(WR)}}$

3. study of the cause (of disease) $\dfrac{}{\text{WR} \quad /\text{CV}/ \quad \text{S}}$

4. study of tumors $\dfrac{}{\text{WR} \quad /\text{CV}/ \quad \text{S}}$

5. study of diseases $\dfrac{}{\text{WR} \quad /\text{CV}/ \quad \text{S}}$

6. physician who studies diseases $\dfrac{}{\text{WR} \quad /\text{CV}/ \quad \text{S}}$

7. abnormal condition of yellow $\dfrac{}{\text{WR} \qquad / \qquad \text{S}}$

8. causing tumors $\dfrac{}{\text{WR} \quad /\text{CV}/ \quad \text{S}}$

9. pertaining to cancer $\dfrac{}{\text{WR} \qquad / \qquad \text{S}}$

10. abnormal condition of blue $\dfrac{}{\text{WR} \qquad / \qquad \text{S}}$

11. producing cancer $\dfrac{}{\text{WR} \quad /\text{CV}/ \quad \text{S}}$

12. substance that causes cancer $\dfrac{}{\text{WR} \quad /\text{CV}/ \quad \text{S}}$

13. physician who studies and
    treats tumors

    _____
    WR   /CV/   S

14. study of medicine

    _____
    WR   /CV/   S

15. pertaining to an organ

    _____
    WR   /   S

16. state of complete knowledge

    _____
    P   /   WR   /   S

17. produced by a physician

    _____
    WR   /CV/   S

18. state of before knowledge

    _____
    P   /   WR   /   S

EXERCISE 24

Spell each of the complementary terms built from word parts on pp. 39–40 by having someone dictate them to you.

> To hear and spell the terms, go to evolve.elsevier.com. Select: Chapter 2, **Exercises,** Spelling.
>
> Refer to p. 10 for your Evolve Access Information.
>
> ☐ Place a check mark in the box if you have completed this exercise online.

1. _____   11. _____
2. _____   12. _____
3. _____   13. _____
4. _____   14. _____
5. _____   15. _____
6. _____   16. _____
7. _____   17. _____
8. _____   18. _____
9. _____   19. _____
10. _____

> For review and/or assessment, go to evolve.elsevier.com. Select:
> Chapter 2, **Activities**, Analyze Medical Terms
>   Terms Built from Word Parts
> Chapter 2, **Games,**   Term Storm
>
> Refer to p. 10 for your Evolve Access Information.

Complementary Terms
Not Built from Word Parts

> 🔆 *Medical terms not built from word parts cannot be translated literally to find their meanings. The terms are learned by memorizing the whole word by using recall and spelling exercises.*

The terms in this list are not built from word parts. The terms are commonly used in the medical world and you will need to know them. In some of the words, you may recognize a word part; however, these terms cannot be literally translated to find the meaning. New knowledge may have changed the meanings of the terms since they were coined; some terms are eponyms, some are acronyms, and some have no apparent explanation for their names. Memorization is used in the following exercises to learn the terms.

TERM	DEFINITION
apoptosis (*ap*-op-TŌ-sis)	programmed cell death, a mechanism for cell deletion to regulate cell population, or destroy damaged or defective cells. Some cancers disrupt apoptosis; cells lose their ability to die and live forever.
benign (be-NĪN)	not malignant, nonrecurrent, favorable for recovery (Figure 2-7)
biological therapy (bī-ō-LOJ-i-kel) (THER-a-pē)	treatment of cancer with biological response modifiers (BRM) that work with the immune system. (Also called **biotherapy** or **immunotherapy**)
carcinoma in situ (kar-si-NŌ-ma) (in SĪ-too)	cancer in the early stage before invading surrounding tissue (Figure 2-6)
chemotherapy (chemo) (kē-mō-THER-a-pē)	treatment of cancer with drugs (Figure 2-8)
encapsulated (en-KAP-sū-lā-ted)	enclosed within a capsule, as with benign or malignant tumors that have not spread beyond the capsule of the organ in which it originated (Figure 2-5)
exacerbation (eg-zas-er-BĀ-shun)	increase in the severity of a disease or its symptoms
hospice (HOS-pis)	provides palliative or supportive care for terminally ill patients and their families
idiopathic (id-ē-ō-PATH-ik)	pertaining to disease of unknown origin
inflammation (in-fla-MĀ-shun)	localized protective response to injury or tissue destruction characterized by redness, swelling, heat, and pain
in vitro (in) (VĒ-trō)	within a glass, observable within a test tube
in vivo (in) (VĒ-vō)	within the living body

NECROSIS/ APOPTOSIS

Necrosis is an abnormal, detrimental cell death caused by external conditions such as trauma, infection, or toxins. **Apoptosis** is a normal, beneficial cell death occurring within the body to eliminate damaged or unneeded cells. In an average adult 50-70 billion cells die each day.

🏛 **BENIGN AND MALIGNANT**
Benign is derived from the Latin word root **bene**, meaning **well** or **good**, as used in **benefit** or **benefactor**. **Malignant** is derived from the Latin word root **mal** meaning **bad**, as used in **malicious**, **malaise**, **malady**, and **malign**.

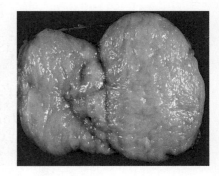

FIGURE 2-5
An encapsulated benign tumor.

> 🔆 Inflammatory **and** inflammation **are spelled with two** *m's. Inflame* **and** *inflamed* **have one** *m.*

🏛 **SITU**
is from the Latin term **situs**, which means **position** or **place**. Think of **in situ** as meaning "in place" or "not wandering around."

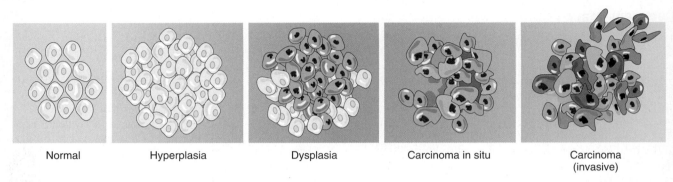

| Normal | Hyperplasia | Dysplasia | Carcinoma in situ | Carcinoma (invasive) |

FIGURE 2-6
Progression of cell growth.

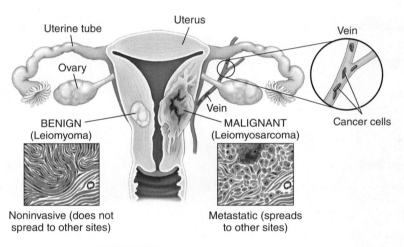

FIGURE 2-7
Examples of benign and malignant tumors.

Complementary Terms—cont'd

Not Built from Word Parts

TERM	DEFINITION
malignant (ma-LIG-nant)	tending to become progressively worse and to cause death, as in cancer (Figure 2-7)
morbidity (mor-BID-i-tē)	state of being diseased or unwell; incidence of illness in a population
mortality (mor-TAL-i-tē)	state of being mortal (death); incidence of the number of deaths in a population
palliative (PAL-ē-a-tiv)	providing relief but not cure
radiation therapy (XRT) (rā-dē-Ā-shun) (THER-a-pē)	treatment of cancer with a radioactive substance, x-ray, or radiation (also called **radiation oncology** and **radiotherapy**) (Figure 2-9)
remission (rē-MISH-un)	improvement or absence of signs of disease

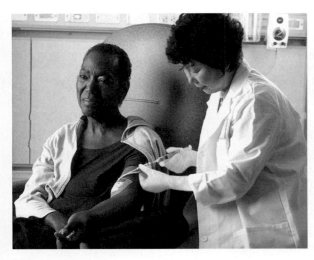

FIGURE 2-8
A patient receiving intravenous chemotherapy. Chemotherapy may also be administered orally in pill form.

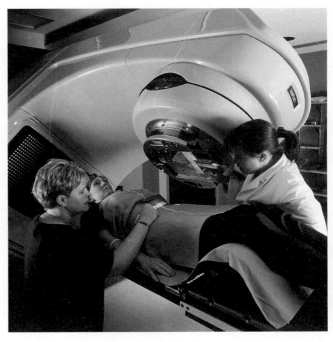

FIGURE 2-9
Radiation therapist preparing the patient for radiation therapy.

Table 2-3
Cancer Therapies

THERAPY	DESCRIPTION
Neoadjuvant therapy	a cancer treatment that precedes other treatment, such as administering chemotherapy or radiation therapy to a patient before surgery.
Adjuvant chemotherapy	the use of chemotherapy after or in combination with another form of cancer treatment such as administering chemotherapy after surgery or with radiation therapy.
Brachytherapy	the use of radiotherapy in which the source of radiation is placed within or close to the area being treated, such as implantation of radiation sources into the breast to treat cancer (as shown in the illustration).
Biological therapy	the treatment of cancer with the use of man-made biological response modifiers (BRM) that occur naturally in the body. They alter the immune system's interaction with cancer cells to restore, direct, or boost the body's ability to fight disease. For example, an agent called **rituximab (Rituxan),** a monoclonal antibody, is used to treat some lymphomas. Other biologic agents are **thalidomide,** which is used to treat multiple myeloma, and **interferon,** which is used in the treatment of lymphomas.

Table 2-4
Hospice Care/Palliative Care

THERAPY	DESCRIPTION
Hospice and Palliative Medicine	a medical subspecialty recognized by the American Board of Medical Specialties.
Hospice care	a facility or program that provides a caring environment to meet the physical and emotional needs of the terminally ill and their families. Medicare, Medicaid, and other payers offer services to patients who have a prognosis of six months or less if the disease follows its natural course, and the patient agrees to forego curative forms of treatment. A team-based palliative care approach is used in an out-of-hospital setting, usually in the patient's home.
Palliative care	provides symptom management to relieve suffering in all stages of disease and is not limited to care at the end of life. The care provided honors the patient's values and preferences throughout his or her illness. Palliative care is available to the patient at the same time as curative or life prolonging treatment. Hospice care involves palliative care; not all of palliative care is hospice care.

To watch animations, go to evolve.elsevier.com. Select:
Chapter 2, **Animations**, Breast Cancer Metastasis
                             Chemotherapy
                             Radiation Therapy

Refer to p. 10 for your Evolve Access Information.

EXERCISE 25

Practice saying aloud each of the complementary terms not built from word parts on pp. 43–44.

To hear the terms, go to evolve.elsevier.com. Select: Chapter 2, **Exercises,** Pronunciation.

Refer to p. 10 for your Evolve Access Information.

☐ Place a check mark in the box when you have completed this exercise.

EXERCISE 26

Write the definitions for the following terms.

1. benign _____

2. malignant _____

3. remission_____

4. idiopathic _____

5. inflammation _____

6. chemotherapy_____

7. radiation therapy _____

8. encapsulated _____

9. in vitro_____

10. in vivo _____

11. carcinoma in situ _____

12. exacerbation _____

13. palliative _____

14. mortality _____

15. morbidity _____

16. hospice _____

17. biological therapy _____

18. apoptosis _____

EXERCISE 27

Match the complementary terms in the first column with the correct definitions in the second column. *To check your answers, go to p. 59.*

_____ 1. remission

_____ 2. in vivo

_____ 3. in vitro

_____ 4. hospice

_____ 5. idiopathic

_____ 6. palliative

_____ 7. apoptosis

_____ 8. benign

_____ 9. malignant

a. within a glass
b. disease of unknown origin
c. providing relief but not cure
d. programmed cell death
e. nonrecurrent
f. absence of signs and symptoms
g. palliative and supportive care
h. becoming progressively worse
i. within the living body

EXERCISE 28

Match the complementary terms in the first column with the correct definitions in the second column. *To check your answers, go to p. 59.*

_____ 1. encapsulated

_____ 2. biological therapy

_____ 3. radiation therapy

_____ 4. chemotherapy

_____ 5. morbidity

_____ 6. mortality

_____ 7. exacerbation

_____ 8. inflammation

_____ 9. carcinoma in situ

a. treatment of cancer with a radioactive substance
b. state of being diseased
c. protective response to injury
d. treatment of cancer that works with the immune system
e. increase in severity of disease
f. enclosed within a capsule
g. carcinoma in the early stage
h. state of being mortal (death)
i. treatment of cancer with drugs

EXERCISE 29

Spell each of the complementary terms not built from word parts on pp. 43–44 by having someone dictate them to you.

> (e) To hear and spell the terms, go to evolve.elsevier.com. Select: Chapter 2, **Exercises**, Spelling.
>
> Refer to p. 10 for your Evolve Access Information.
>
> ☐ Place a check mark in the box if you have completed this exercise online.

1. _____
2. _____
3. _____
4. _____
5. _____
6. _____
7. _____
8. _____
9. _____
10. _____
11. _____
12. _____
13. _____
14. _____
15. _____
16. _____
17. _____
18. _____

> (e) For review and/or assessment, go to evolve.elsevier.com. Select:
> Chapter 2, **Activities**, Terms Not Built from Word Parts
>   Hear It and Type It: Clinical Vignettes
> Chapter 2, **Games**,   Term Explorer
>   Termbusters
>   Medical Millionaire
>
> Refer to p. 10 for your Evolve Access Information.

Refer to **Appendix D** for pharmacology terms related to oncology.

Plural Endings for Medical Terms

> 💡 Because of common usage, some plural forms of medical terms will add an "s" rather than use Greek or Latin plural endings. **Carcinomas** rather than **carcinomata** is frequently seen in medical literature.

In the English language plurals are formed by simply adding an "s" or "es" to the end of a word. For example, hand becomes plural by adding an "s" to form hands. Likewise, box becomes boxes by adding "es." In the language of medicine, many terms have Latin or Greek suffixes, and forming plurals for these terms is not quite as easy. Table 2-3, Common Plural Endings, lists the most common singular and plural endings used in medical terminology. When appropriate, both singular and plural endings are included in the word lists throughout the text, such as metastasis/metastases on p. 39.

Table 2-5
Common Plural Endings for Medical Terms

SINGULAR ENDINGS	SINGULAR FORM		PLURAL FORMATION	PLURAL FORM	
-a	verteb**ra**		-ae	verteb**rae**	
-ax	thor**ax**		-aces	thor**aces**	
-is	test**is**		-es	test**es**	
-ix	append**ix**		-ices	append**ices**	
-ma	carcino**ma**		-mata	carcino**mata**	
-on	gangli**on**		-a	gangli**a**	
-sis	metasta**sis**		-ses	metasta**ses**	
-um	ov**um**		-a	ov**a**	
-us	fung**us**		-i	fung**i**	
-nx	lary**nx**		-nges	lary**nges**	
-y	biops**y**		-ies	biops**ies**	

Complete the following exercises to become familiar with how plurals are formed. Do not be concerned about the meaning of these terms; concentrate only on the plural endings.

EXERCISE 30

Convert each of the following terms from singular to plural. Refer to Table 2-5, Common Plural Endings for Medical Terms, on p. 49 for guidance.

1. etiology _____
2. staphylococcus _____
3. cyanosis _____
4. bacterium _____
5. nucleus _____
6. pharynx _____
7. sarcoma _____
8. carcinoma _____
9. anastomosis _____
10. pubis _____
11. prognosis _____
12. spermatozoon _____
13. fimbria _____
14. thorax _____
15. appendix _____

EXERCISE 31

Circle the correct singular or plural form in each sentence.

1. During a colonoscopy the gastroenterologist noted that the patient had several (**diverticula, diverticulum**) in his transverse colon.
2. Bronchogenic carcinoma was diagnosed in the patient's left (**bronchus, bronchi**).
3. Bilateral (two sides) orchiditis is inflammation of the (**testes, testis**).
4. The light brown mole with notched borders turned out to be a (**melanomata, melanoma**).
5. Multiple (**embolus, emboli**) were observed on the lung scan.
6. Many (**diagnosis, diagnoses**) of benign tumors are picked up during whole-body scanning.
7. Diagnostic studies have shown (**metastasis, metastases**) of the patient's carcinoma of the breast to both her lungs and brain.

For review and/or assessment of plural endings, go to evolve.elsevier.com. Select: Chapter 2, **Activities**, Plural Endings

Refer to p. 10 for your Evolve Access Information.

Abbreviations

Abbreviations are frequently used verbally and in writing to communicate in the medical and healthcare setting. Abbreviations of the terms included in the chapter are listed below.

ABBREVIATION	DEFINITION
CA	carcinoma
chemo	chemotherapy
Dx	diagnosis
mets	metastases
Px	prognosis
RBC	red blood cell
XRT	radiation therapy
WBC	white blood cell

 Abbreviations that are easily misinterpreted and may lead to medication errors are reported to the Institute for Safe Medication Practice. A list of these abbreviations is in Appendix C along with The Joint Commission's "do not use" list of abbreviations.

 Refer to **Appendix C** for a complete list of abbreviations.

EXERCISE 32

Write the term for each of the abbreviations in the following paragraph.

A 55-year-old woman was admitted to the oncology unit with a **Dx** _____ of **CA** _____ of the breast, **mets** _____ to the lung and brain. Her **Px** _____ was guarded. Laboratory tests, including **RBC**

_____ _____ _____ and **WBC** _____

_____ _____ counts, were ordered. She will receive both

chemo _____ and **XRT**

_____ _____.

For practice with abbreviations, go to evolve.elsevier.com. Select:
Chapter 2, **Flashcards**
Chapter 2, **Games**, Crossword Puzzle

Refer to p. 10 for your Evolve Access Information.

PRACTICAL APPLICATION

EXERCISE 33 *Interact with Medical Documents*

A. Below is a physician's progress note. Complete the record by writing the medical terms in the blanks that correspond to the numbered definitions.

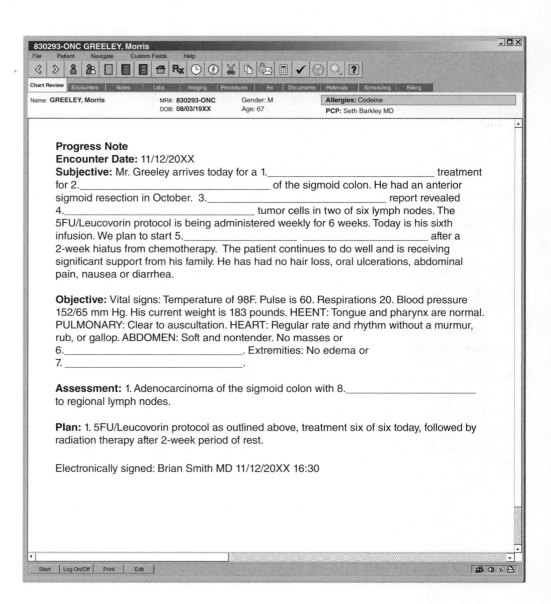

830293-ONC GREELEY, Morris

File | Patient | Navigate | Custom Fields | Help

Chart Review | Encounters | Notes | Labs | Imaging | Procedures | Rx | Documents | Referrals | Scheduling | Billing

Name: **GREELEY, Morris** MR#: **830293-ONC** Gender: M **Allergies:** Codeine
DOB: **08/03/19XX** Age: 67 **PCP:** Seth Barkley MD

Progress Note
Encounter Date: 11/12/20XX
Subjective: Mr. Greeley arrives today for a 1._____ treatment
for 2._____ of the sigmoid colon. He had an anterior
sigmoid resection in October. 3._____ report revealed
4._____ tumor cells in two of six lymph nodes. The
5FU/Leucovorin protocol is being administered weekly for 6 weeks. Today is his sixth
infusion. We plan to start 5._____ _____ after a
2-week hiatus from chemotherapy. The patient continues to do well and is receiving
significant support from his family. He has had no hair loss, oral ulcerations, abdominal
pain, nausea or diarrhea.

Objective: Vital signs: Temperature of 98F. Pulse is 60. Respirations 20. Blood pressure
152/65 mm Hg. His current weight is 183 pounds. HEENT: Tongue and pharynx are normal.
PULMONARY: Clear to auscultation. HEART: Regular rate and rhythm without a murmur,
rub, or gallop. ABDOMEN: Soft and nontender. No masses or
6._____. Extremities: No edema or
7. _____.

Assessment: 1. Adenocarcinoma of the sigmoid colon with 8._____
to regional lymph nodes.

Plan: 1. 5FU/Leucovorin protocol as outlined above, treatment six of six today, followed by
radiation therapy after 2-week period of rest.

Electronically signed: Brian Smith MD 11/12/20XX 16:30

Start | Log On/Off | Print | Edit

1. Treatment of cancer by using drugs
2. Cancerous tumor of glandular tissue
3. Study of disease
4. Tending to become progressively worse
5. Treatment of cancer by using radioactive substance, x-rays, or radiation
6. Abnormal condition of blue appearing
7. Beyond control

B. Read the office visit report and answer the following questions.

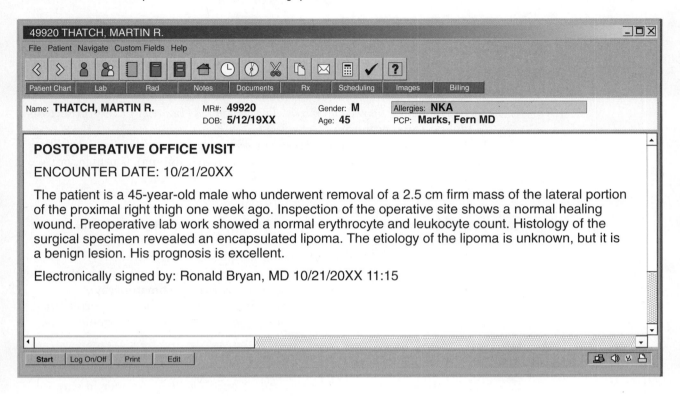

49920 THATCH, MARTIN R.	_ □ ☒

File Patient Navigate Custom Fields Help

| Patient Chart | Lab | Rad | Notes | Documents | Rx | Scheduling | Images | Billing |

Name: **THATCH, MARTIN R.**   MR#: **49920**   Gender: **M**   Allergies: **NKA**
DOB: **5/12/19XX**   Age: **45**   PCP: **Marks, Fern MD**

POSTOPERATIVE OFFICE VISIT

ENCOUNTER DATE: 10/21/20XX

The patient is a 45-year-old male who underwent removal of a 2.5 cm firm mass of the lateral portion of the proximal right thigh one week ago. Inspection of the operative site shows a normal healing wound. Preoperative lab work showed a normal erythrocyte and leukocyte count. Histology of the surgical specimen revealed an encapsulated lipoma. The etiology of the lipoma is unknown, but it is a benign lesion. His prognosis is excellent.

Electronically signed by: Ronald Bryan, MD 10/21/20XX 11:15

| Start | Log On/Off | Print | Edit |

1. The firm mass was confirmed as a lipoma from the surgical specimen in which area of study?
   a. cell
   b. tissue
   c. blood
   d. plasma
2. The lipoma was
   a. spreading.
   b. enclosed in a capsule.
   c. inflamed.
   d. blue in color.

3. Erythr and leuk refer to the _____ of cells.
   a. size
   b. shape
   c. amount
   d. color
4. Write the plural form of
   a. prognosis _____
   b. lipoma _____
   c. histology _____

EXERCISE 34 *Interpret Medical Terms*

To test your understanding of the terms introduced in this chapter, circle the words that correctly complete each sentence. The italicized words refer to the correct answer.

1. Mr. Roberts was diagnosed as having a cancerous *tumor of connective tissue*, or (**sarcoma, melanoma, lipoma**). The doctor said the tumor was *becoming progressively worse*; that is, it was (**benign, malignant, pathogenic**).
2. The blood test showed an *increased amount of red blood cells*, or (**erythrocytosis, leukocytosis, cyanosis**).
3. (**Organic, Visceral, Systemic**) means *pertaining to internal organs*.
4. A *tumor composed of fat*, or (**neuroma, carcinoma, lipoma**), is benign, or (**recurrent, nonrecurrent, cancerous**).
5. Many substances are thought to be *cancer producing*, or (**carcinogenic, carcinogen, cancerous**).
6. *Etiology* is the study of (**the causes of disease, tissue disease, the causes of tumors**).
7. A *tumor* may be called a (**cytoplasm, neoplasm, karyoplasm**).
8. The pain *originated in the body*, or was (**somatogenic, oncogenic, pathogenic**).
9. Any *disease of a muscle* is called (**myoma, myopathy, somatopathy**).
10. The term for *abnormal development* is (**hypoplasia, dysplasia, hyperplasia**).
11. The term that means *produced by a physician* is (**diagnosis, iatrogenic, prognosis**).
12. The incidence of malignant *black tumor* (**fibrosarcoma, fibroma, melanoma**) is increasing in the white population. One *study of disease* (**pathology, pathogenic, liposarcoma**) finding influencing *state of before knowledge* (**cancer in situ, in vitro, prognosis**) may be tumor thickness.
13. The term that means *within the living organism* is (**in vitro, in vivo, encapsulated**).
14. A (**liposarcoma, fibroma, myoma**) is a *malignant tumor.*
15. (**DNA, RBC, WBC**) regulates the *activities of a cell.*
16. The term for *programmed cell death*, a natural occurrence within the body, is (**dysplasia, apoptosis, xanthosis**).
17. (**Hospice, palliative, biological therapy**) provides *palliative and supportive care for terminally ill patients and their families.*
18. The overall survival and acceptable *state of being diseased* (**mortality, morbidity, prognosis**) justifies performing a therapeutic lymphadenectomy for nodal metastatic melanoma.

EXERCISE 35   *Read Medical Terms in Use*

Practice pronunciation of terms by reading aloud the following medical document.

Use the pronunciation key after each medical term to assist you in saying the words. The script contains medical terms not yet presented. Treat them as information only; you will learn more about them as you continue to study. Or, if desired, look for their meanings in your medical dictionary.

To read and hear the terms, go to evolve.elsevier.com.
Select: Chapter 2, **Exercises,** Read Medical Terms in Use.

Refer to p. 10 for your Evolve Access Information.

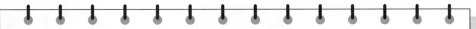

A 54-year-old woman presented to the office with a 3-week history of bloody diarrhea. She had been diagnosed with ulcerative colitis at age 25 years. She was referred for a colonoscopy. The examination revealed a suspicious lesion in the transverse colon. A biopsy was performed and a **cytology** (sī-TOL-o-jē) specimen was obtained. The **pathologist** (pa-THOL-o-jist) made a **diagnosis** (dī-ag-NŌ-sis) of **carcinoma** (kar-si-NŌ-ma) of the colon. Advanced **dysplasia** (dis-PLĀ-zha) and **inflammation** (in-fla-MĀ-shun) existed in the specimen. The patient underwent surgery and was found to have no evidence of **metastasis** (me-TAS-ta-sis). Her entire colon was removed because of a high risk for developing a **malignant** (ma-LIG-nant) lesion in the remaining colon. She made an uneventful recovery and was referred to an **oncologist** (ong-KOL-o-jist) for consideration of **chemotherapy** (kē-mō-THER-a-pē). Her **prognosis** (prog-NŌ-sis) is generally positive. **Radiation therapy** (rā-dē-Ā-shun) (THER-a-pē) or **biological therapy** (bī-ō-LOJ-i-kel) (THER-a-pē) were not indicated in this case.

 WEB LINK

For additional information on cancer visit the **National Cancer Institute** at *http://www.nci.nih.gov.*

EXERCISE 36   *Comprehend Medical Terms in Use*

Test your comprehension of terms in the previous medical document by answering *T* for true and *F* for false.

_____ 1. The cancer has spread from the colon to other surrounding organs.

_____ 2. The specimen is described as having abnormal development.

_____ 3. The patient's prognosis is carcinoma of the colon.

_____ 4. The patient's colon was removed to avoid development of a malignant lesion in the remaining colon.

_____ 5. The patient was referred to a pathologist for consideration of treatment for the cancer with drugs.

For a snapshot assessment of your knowledge of body structure, color, and oncology terms, go to evolve.elsevier.com.

Select: Chapter 2, **Quick Quizzes**

Refer to p. 10 for your Evolve Access Information.

CHAPTER REVIEW

Review of Evolve

Keep a record of the online activities you have completed by placing a check mark in the box. You may also record your scores. All activities have been referenced throughout the text.

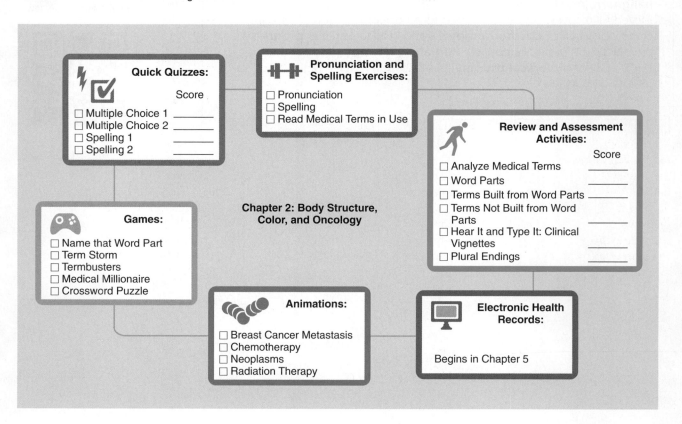

Quick Quizzes:

Score

☐ Multiple Choice 1 _____
☐ Multiple Choice 2 _____
☐ Spelling 1 _____
☐ Spelling 2 _____

Pronunciation and Spelling Exercises:

☐ Pronunciation
☐ Spelling
☐ Read Medical Terms in Use

Review and Assessment Activities:

Score

☐ Analyze Medical Terms _____
☐ Word Parts _____
☐ Terms Built from Word Parts _____
☐ Terms Not Built from Word Parts _____
☐ Hear It and Type It: Clinical Vignettes _____
☐ Plural Endings _____

Games:

☐ Name that Word Part
☐ Term Storm
☐ Termbusters
☐ Medical Millionaire
☐ Crossword Puzzle

Chapter 2: Body Structure, Color, and Oncology

Animations:

☐ Breast Cancer Metastasis
☐ Chemotherapy
☐ Neoplasms
☐ Radiation Therapy

Electronic Health Records:

Begins in Chapter 5

Review of Word Parts

Can you define and spell the following word parts?

COMBINING FORMS

aden/o	erythr/o	leuk/o	rhabd/o
cancer/o	eti/o	lip/o	sarc/o
carcin/o	fibr/o	melan/o	somat/o
chlor/o	gno/o	my/o	system/o
chrom/o	hist/o	neur/o	viscer/o
cyan/o	iatr/o	onc/o	xanth/o
cyt/o	kary/o	organ/o	
epitheli/o	lei/o	path/o	

PREFIXES / SUFFIXES

PREFIXES	SUFFIXES		
dia-	-al	-logist	-pathy
dys-	-cyte	-logy	-plasia
hyper-	-gen	-megaly	-plasm
hypo-	-genic	-oid	-sarcoma
meta-	-ic	-oma	-sis
neo-		-osis	-stasis
pro-		-ous	

Review of Terms

Can you define, spell, and pronounce the following terms *built from word parts*?

ONCOLOGY	BODY STRUCTURE	COMPLEMENTARY
adenocarcinoma	cytogenic	cancerous
adenoma	cytoid	carcinogen
carcinoma (CA)	cytology	carcinogenic
chloroma	cytoplasm	cyanosis
epithelioma	dysplasia	diagnosis (Dx)
fibroma	epithelial	etiology
fibrosarcoma	erythrocyte (RBC)	iatrogenic
leiomyoma	erythrocytosis	iatrology
leiomyosarcoma	histology	metastasis (mets)
lipoma	hyperplasia	oncogenic
liposarcoma	hypoplasia	oncologist
melanocarcinoma	karyocyte	oncology
melanoma	karyoplasm	organic
myoma	leukocyte (WBC)	pathogenic
neoplasm	leukocytosis	pathologist
neuroma	lipoid	pathology
rhabdomyoma	myopathy	prognosis (Px)
rhabdomyosarcoma	neuroid	xanthochromic
sarcoma	organomegaly	xanthosis
	somatic	
	somatogenic	
	somatopathy	
	somatoplasm	
	systemic	
	visceral	

Can you define, pronounce, and spell the following terms *not built from word parts?*

COMPLEMENTARY

apoptosis
biological therapy
benign
carcinoma in situ
chemotherapy (chemo)
encapsulated
exacerbation
hospice
idiopathic
inflammation
in vitro
in vivo
malignant
morbidity
mortality
palliative
radiation therapy (XRT)
remission

For a complete list of CAM terms, go to evolve.elsevier.com.
Select: **Extra Content,** Appendix G, Complementary and Alternative Medical Therapies

Refer to p. 10 for your Evolve Access Information.

COMPLEMENTARY AND ALTERNATIVE MEDICINE (CAM)

According to the National Center for Complementary and Alternative Medicine (NCCAM) Institute of the National Institutes of Health (NIH), **Complementary and Alternative Medicine (CAM)** is defined as "a group of diverse medical and health care systems, practices, and products that are not generally considered part of conventional medicine."

Complementary medicine is used in conjunction with conventional medicine.

Alternative medicine is used in place of conventional medicine.

Integrative medicine is the combination of mainstream medical therapies and evidence-based CAM therapies. Use of CAM has increased dramatically in recent years as healthcare consumers search for a variety of ways to treat illness and promote wellness.

Look for evidence-based CAM therapies throughout the text.

ANSWERS

ANSWERS TO CHAPTER 2 EXERCISES

Exercise Figures

Exercise Figure
A. 1. cell: cyt/o
2. tissue: hist/o
3. organ: organ/o
4. system: system/o

Exercise Figure
B. 1. neur/o
2. epitheli/o
3. sarc/o
4. my/o

Exercise Figure
C. 1. carcin/oma
2. melan/oma
3. sarc/oma
4. rhabd/o/my/o/sarcoma

Exercise Figure
D. 1. erythr/o/cyte
2. leuk/o/cyte

Exercise Figure
E. hyper/plasia

Exercise 1
1. h
2. e
3. d
4. k
5. g
6. f
7. c
8. a
9. b
10. j

Exercise 2
1. h
2. b
3. c
4. e
5. g
6. a
7. f

Exercise 3
1. flesh, connective tissue
2. fat
3. nucleus
4. internal organs
5. cell
6. tissue
7. muscle
8. nerve
9. organ
10. system
11. epithelium
12. fiber
13. gland

Exercise 4
1. viscer/o
2. epitheli/o
3. organ/o
4. kary/o
5. cyt/o
6. hist/o
7. neur/o
8. my/o
9. lip/o
10. system/o
11. sarc/o
12. fibr/o
13. aden/o

Exercise 5
1. tumor, mass
2. cancer
3. cause (of disease)
4. disease
5. body
6. cancer
7. rod-shaped, striated
8. smooth
9. knowledge
10. physician, medicine

Exercise 6
1. path/o
2. onc/o
3. eti/o
4. a. cancer/o
   b. carcin/o
5. somat/o
6. lei/o
7. rhabd/o
8. gno/o
9. iatr/o

Exercise 7
1. blue
2. red
3. white
4. yellow
5. color
6. black
7. green

Exercise 8
1. cyan/o
2. erythr/o
3. leuk/o
4. melan/o
5. xanth/o
6. chrom/o
7. chlor/o

Exercise 9
1. new
2. above, excessive
3. after, beyond, change
4. below, incomplete, deficient, under
5. painful, abnormal, difficult, labored
6. through, complete
7. before

Exercise 10
1. neo-
2. hyper-
3. hypo-
4. meta-
5. dys-
6. dia-
7. pro-

Exercise 11
1. i
2. l
3. q
4. f
5. g
6. j
7. h
8. b
9. c
10. n
11. k
12. p
13. m
14. a
15. o
16. e

Exercise 12
1. one who studies and treats (specialist, physician)
2. disease
3. study of
4. pertaining to
5. control, stop, standing
6. cell
7. abnormal condition
8. pertaining to
9. growth, substance, formation
10. pertaining to
11. condition of formation, development, growth
12. resembling
13. substance or agent that produces or causes
14. producing, originating, causing
15. tumor, swelling
16. malignant tumor
17. state of
18. enlargement

Exercise 13
Pronunciation Exercise

Exercise 14
Note: The combining form is identified by italic and bold print.
1. WR   S
   sarc/oma
   tumor composed of connective tissue
2. WR   S
   melan/oma
   black tumor
3. WR   S
   epitheli/oma
   tumor composed of epithelium
4. WR   S
   lip/oma
   tumor composed of fat
5. P   S(WR)
   neo/plasm
   new growth
6. WR   S
   my/oma
   tumor composed of muscle
7. WR   S
   neur/oma
   tumor composed of nerve
8. WR   S
   carcin/oma
   cancerous tumor

9. WR CV WR   S
    melan/o/carcin/oma
         CF
    cancerous black tumor

10. WR CV WR CV S
    rhabd/o/my/o/sarcoma
         CF   CF
    malignant tumor of striated muscle

11. WRCVWR S
    lei/o/my/oma
       CF
    tumor composed of smooth muscle

12. WR   CV WR S
    rhabd/o/my/oma
         CF
    tumor composed of striated muscle

13. WR   S
    fibr/oma
    tumor composed of fiber (fibrous
    tissue)

14. WR CV   S
    lip/o/sarcoma
       CF
    malignant tumor of fat

15. WR CV   S
    fibr/o/sarcoma
        CF
    malignant tumor of fiber (fibrous
    tissue)

16. WR   S
    aden/oma
    tumor composed of glandular tissue

17. WR CV WR   S
    aden/o/carcin/oma
         CF
    cancerous tumor composed of
    glandular tissue

18. WR   S
    chlor/oma
    tumor of green color

Exercise 15

1. melan/oma
2. carcin/oma
3. neo/plasm
4. epitheli/oma
5. sarc/oma
6. melan/o/carcin/oma
7. neur/oma
8. my/oma
9. rhabd/o/my/o/sarcoma
10. lei/o/my/oma
11. rhabd/o/my/oma
12. lei/o/my/o/sarcoma
13. lip/o/sarcoma
14. fibr/oma
15. fibr/o/sarcoma
16. aden/oma
17. aden/o/carcin/oma
18. chlor/oma

Exercise 16
Spelling Exercise; see text p. 34.

Exercise 17
Pronunciation Exercise

Exercise 18
*Note: The combining form is identified by
italic and bold print.*

1. WR CV S
    cyt/o/logy
        CF
    study of cells

2. WR CV S
    hist/o/logy
        CF
    study of tissue

3. WR   S
    viscer/al
    pertaining to internal organs

4. WR CV S
    kary/o/cyte
         CF
    cell with a nucleus

5. WR CV   S
    kary/o/plasm
         CF
    substance of a nucleus

6. WR   S
    system/ic
    pertaining to a (body) system

7. WR CV S
    cyt/o/plasm
        CF
    cell substance

8. WR   S
    somat/ic
    pertaining to the body

9. WR CV S
    somat/o/genic
          CF
    originating in the body

10. WR CV S
    somat/o/plasm
          CF
    body substance

11. WR CV S
    somat/o/pathy
          CF
    disease of the body

12. WR   S
    neur/oid
    resembling a nerve

13. WR CV S
    my/o/pathy
         CF
    disease of the muscle

14. WR CV S
    erythr/o/cyte
          CF
    red (blood) cell

15. WR CV S
    leuk/o/cyte
          CF
    white (blood) cell

16. WR   S
    epitheli/al
    pertaining to epithelium

17. WR S
    lip/oid
    resembling fat

18. P   S(WR)
    hyper/plasia
    excessive development (of cells)

19. WR   CV WR S
    erythr/o/cyt/osis
          CF
    increase in the number of red
    (blood) cells

20. WR CV WR S
    leuk/o/cyt/osis
          CF
    increase in the number of white
    (blood) cells

21. P   S(WR)
    hypo/plasia
    incomplete development (of an
    organ or tissue)

22. WR S
    cyt/oid
    resembling a cell

23. P   S(WR)
    dys/plasia
    abnormal development

24. WR CV   S
    organ/o/megaly
           CF
    enlargement of an organ

Exercise 19

1. cyt/o/plasm
2. kary/o/plasm
3. somat/ic
4. my/o/pathy
5. somat/o/plasm
6. viscer/al
7. somat/o/genic
8. somat/o/pathy
9. erythr/o/cyte
10. neur/oid
11. system/ic
12. leuk/o/cyte
13. kary/o/cyte
14. lip/oid
15. cyt/o/logy
16. hyper/plasia

17. cyt/oid
18. epitheli/al
19. hist/o/logy
20. erythr/o/cyt/osis
21. hypo/plasia
22. leuk/o/cyt/osis
23. dys/plasia
24. organ/o/megaly

Exercise 20
Spelling Exercise; see text p. 38.

Exercise 21
Pronunciation Exercise

Exercise 22
Note: The combining form is identified by italic and bold print.

1. WR CV S
   path/o/logy
      CF
   study of disease

2. WR CV S
   path/o/logist
      CF
   a physician who studies diseases

3. P   S(WR)
   meta/stasis
   beyond control (transfer of disease)

4. WR CV S
   onc/o/genic
      CF
   causing tumors

5. WR CV S
   onc/o/logy
      CF
   study of tumors

6. WR   S
   cancer/ous
   pertaining to cancer

7. WR   CV S
   carcin/o/genic
         CF
   producing cancer

8. WR   S
   cyan/osis
   abnormal condition of blue (bluish discoloration of the skin)

9. WR CV S
   eti/o/logy
      CF
   study of causes (of disease)

10. WR   S
    xanth/osis
    abnormal condition of yellow

11. WR CV WR S
    xanth/o/chrom/ic
         CF
    pertaining to yellow color

12. WR CV S
    carcin/o/gen
         CF
    substance that causes cancer

13. WR CV S
    onc/o/logist
         CF
    physician who studies and treats tumors

14. P WR S
    pro/gno/sis
    state of before knowledge

15. WR   S
    organ/ic
    pertaining to an organ

16. P WR S
    dia/gno/sis
    state of complete knowledge

17. WR CV S
    iatr/o/genic
         CF
    produced by a physician

18. WR CV S
    iatr/o/logy
         CF
    study of medicine

Exercise 23
1. xanth/o/chrom/ic
2. meta/stasis
3. eti/o/logy
4. onc/o/logy
5. path/o/logy
6. path/o/logist
7. xanth/osis
8. onc/o/genic
9. cancer/ous
10. cyan/osis
11. carcin/o/genic
12. carcin/o/gen
13. onc/o/logist
14. iatr/o/logy
15. organ/ic
16. dia/gno/sis
17. iatr/o/genic
18. pro/gno/sis

Exercise 24
Spelling Exercise; see text p. 42.

Exercise 25
Pronunciation Exercise

Exercise 26
1. not malignant, nonrecurrent, favorable for recovery
2. tending to become progressively worse and to cause death, as in cancer
3. improvement or absence of signs of disease
4. pertaining to disease of unknown origin
5. localized protective response to injury or tissue destruction; signs are redness, swelling, heat, and pain
6. treatment of cancer with drugs
7. treatment of cancer with radioactive substance, such as x-ray or radiation
8. enclosed within a capsule, as in benign or malignant tumors
9. within a glass, observable within a test tube
10. within the living body
11. cancer in the early stage before invading the surrounding tissue
12. increase in the severity of a disease or its symptoms
13. providing relief but not cure
14. state of being mortal (death); incidence of the number of deaths in a population
15. state of being diseased or unwell; incidence of illness in a population
16. provides palliative and supportive care for terminally ill patients and their families
17. treatment of cancer with biological response modifiers that work with the immune system
18. programmed cell death

Exercise 27
1. f
2. i
3. a
4. g
5. b
6. c
7. d
8. e
9. h

Exercise 28
1. f
2. d
3. a
4. i
5. b
6. h
7. e
8. c
9. g

Exercise 29
Spelling Exercise; see text p. 48.

Exercise 30
1. etiologies
2. staphylococci

3. cyanoses
4. bacteria
5. nuclei
6. pharynges
7. sarcomata
8. carcinomata
9. anastomoses
10. pubes
11. prognoses
12. spermatozoa
13. fimbriae
14. thoraces
15. appendices

Exercise 31
1. diverticula
2. bronchus
3. testes
4. melanoma
5. emboli
6. diagnoses
7. metastases

Exercise 32
diagnosis; carcinoma; metastasis; prognosis; red blood cell; white blood cell; chemotherapy; radiation therapy

Exercise 33
A. 1. chemotherapy
2. adenocarcinoma
3. pathology
4. malignant
5. radiation therapy
6. organomegaly
7. cyanosis
8. metastases
B. 1. b
2. b
3. d
4. a. prognoses
b. lipomata
c. histologies

Exercise 34
1. sarcoma, malignant
2. erythrocytosis
3. visceral
4. lipoma, nonrecurrent
5. carcinogenic
6. causes of disease
7. neoplasm
8. somatogenic
9. myopathy
10. dysplasia
11. iatrogenic

12. melanoma, pathology, prognosis
13. in vivo
14. liposarcoma
15. DNA
16. apoptosis
17. hospice
18. morbidity

Exercise 35
Reading Exercise

Exercise 36
1. *F*, "no evidence of metastasis" (transfer of disease from one organ to another) means the cancer has not spread to surrounding organs.
2. *T*
3. *F*, prognosis means "prediction of the outcome of disease"; diagnosis means "identifying a disease."
4. *T*
5. *F*, an oncologist treats patients with cancer; a pathologist studies body changes caused by disease usually from a specimen in a laboratory setting.

Directional Terms, Planes, Positions, Regions, and Quadrants

Outline

Objectives

Upon completion of this chapter you will be able to:

1 Define and spell word parts related to directional terms.

2 Define, pronounce, and spell terms used to describe directions with respect to the body.

3 Define, pronounce, and spell terms used to describe anatomic planes.

4 Define, pronounce, and spell terms used to describe body positions.

5 Define, pronounce, and spell terms used to describe abdominopelvic regions.

6 Identify and spell the four abdominopelvic quadrants.

7 Interpret the meaning of abbreviations presented in this chapter.

8 Interpret, read, and comprehend medical language in simulated medical statements and documents.

Types of body movement are presented in Chapter 14, Musculoskeletal System, on page 579. Terms related to body movement are: *abduction, adduction, inversion, eversion, extension, flexion, pronation, supination,* and *rotation.*

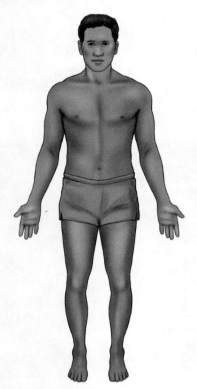

FIGURE 3-1
Anatomic position.

 ANATOMIC POSITION

In the description and use of body directions and planes, the body is assumed to be in the standard, neutral frontal position of reference called the anatomic position. In this position, the body is viewed as standing erect, arms at the side, palms of the hands facing forward, and feet placed side by side pointed anteriorly (Figure 3-1).

 WORD PARTS

Combining Forms of Directional Terms

Word parts you need to learn to complete this chapter are listed on the following pages. The exercises at the end of each list will help you learn their definitions and spelling.

> Use the flashcards accompanying this text or electronic flashcards to assist you in memorizing the word parts for this chapter.

> (e) To use electronic flashcards, go to evolve.elsevier.com. Select: Chapter 3, **Flashcards**.
> Refer to p. 10 for your Evolve Access Information.

COMBINING FORM	DEFINITION
anter/o	front
caud/o	tail (downward)
cephal/o	head (upward)
dist/o	away (from the point of attachment of a body part)
dors/o	back
infer/o	below
later/o	side
medi/o	middle
poster/o	back, behind
proxim/o	near (the point of attachment of a body part)
super/o	above
ventr/o	belly (front)

> Do not be concerned about which combining form to use for front or back. As you continue to study and use medical terms, you will become familar with common usage of each word part.

EXERCISE **1**

Write the definitions for the following combining forms. *To check your answers to the exercises in this chapter, go to Answers, p. 90, at the end of the chapter.*

1. ventr/o _____

2. cephal/o _____

3. later/o _____

4. medi/o _____

5. infer/o _____

6. proxim/o _____

7. super/o_____

8. dist/o _____

9. dors/o _____

10. caud/o _____

11. anter/o_____

12. poster/o _____

EXERCISE FIGURE **A**

Fill in the blanks with directional combining forms. *To check your answers, go to p. 90.*

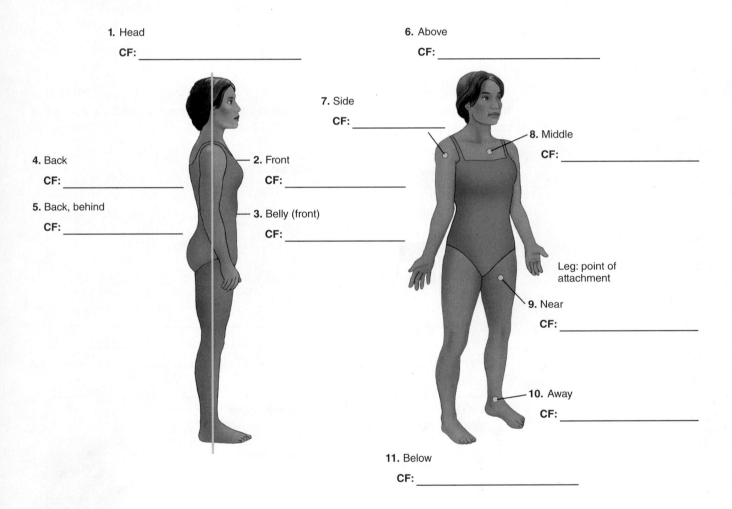

1. Head

    CF: _____

6. Above

    CF: _____

7. Side

    CF: _____

8. Middle

    CF: _____

4. Back

    CF: _____

2. Front

    CF: _____

5. Back, behind

    CF: _____

3. Belly (front)

    CF: _____

Leg: point of attachment

9. Near

    CF: _____

10. Away

    CF: _____

11. Below

    CF: _____

Prefixes

PREFIX	DEFINITION
bi-	two
uni-	one

Suffixes

SUFFIX	DEFINITION
-ad	toward
-ior	pertaining to

No test

 Refer to Appendix A and Appendix B for alphabetized lists of word parts and their meanings.

Many suffixes mean **pertaining to.** You have already learned three of them in Chapter 2: **-al, -ic,** and **-ous.** You will learn more in subsequent chapters. With practice, you will learn which suffix is most commonly used with a particular word root or combining form.

EXERCISE 2

Match the prefixes and suffixes in the first column with their correct definitions in the second column.

_____ 1. -ad
_____ 2. -ior
_____ 3. bi-
_____ 4. uni-

a. one
b. pertaining to
c. toward
d. two

EXERCISE 3

Write the definitions of the following prefixes and suffixes.

1. -ior _____
2. -ad _____
3. bi- _____
4. uni- _____

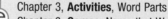

For review and/or assessment, go to evolve.elsevier.com. Select:
Chapter 3, **Activities**, Word Parts
Chapter 3, **Games**, Name that Word Part

Refer to p. 10 for your Evolve Access Information.

💬 MEDICAL TERMS

Directional Terms

The following terms are built from word parts you have already learned and can be translated literally to find their meanings. Further explanation of terms beyond the definition of their word parts, if needed, is included in parentheses.

TERM	DEFINITION
caudad (KAW-dad)	toward the tail (or the inferior portion of the trunk; downward)
cephalad (SEF-a-lad)	toward the head (upward) (Figure 3-2)
lateral (lat) (LAT-er-al)	pertaining to a side (Figure 3-2)
medial (med) (MĒ-dē-al)	pertaining to the middle (Figure 3-3)
unilateral (ū-ni-LAT-er-al)	pertaining to one side (only)
bilateral (bī-LAT-er-al)	pertaining to two sides
mediolateral (mē-dē-ō-LAT-er-al)	pertaining to the middle and to the side
distal (DIS-tal)	pertaining to away (from the point of attachment of a body part) (Figure 3-4)
proximal (PROK-si-mal)	pertaining to near (to the point of attachment of a body part) (Figure 3-4)
inferior (inf) (in-FĒR-ē-or)	pertaining to below (Figure 3-5)
superior (sup) (sū-PĒR-ē-or)	pertaining to above (Figure 3-5)
caudal (KAW-dal)	pertaining to the tail (synonymous with **inferior** in human anatomy when specifying location in the trunk of the body)
cephalic (se-FAL-ik)	pertaining to the head
anterior (ant) (an-TĒR-ē-or)	pertaining to the front (Figure 3-5)
posterior (pos-TĒR-ē-or)	pertaining to the back (Figure 3-5)
dorsal (DOR-sal)	pertaining to the back (Figure 3-5)
ventral (VEN-tral)	pertaining to the belly (front) (Figure 3-5)
anteroposterior (AP) (an-ter-ō-pos-TĒR-ē-or)	pertaining to the front and to the back (see Exercise Figure C)
posteroanterior (PA) (pos-ter-ō-an-TĒR-ē-or)	pertaining to the back and to the front (see Exercise Figure C)

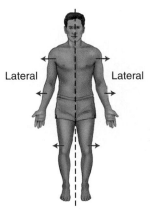

FIGURE 3-2
Lateral.

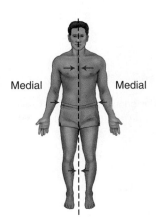

FIGURE 3-3
Medial.

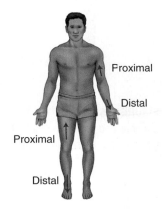

FIGURE 3-4
Distal and proximal.

To watch animations, go to evolve.elsevier.com.
Select: Chapter 3, **Animations**, Directions of the Body

Refer to p. 10 for your Evolve Access Information.

EXERCISE 4

Practice saying aloud each of the directional terms on p. 67.

 To hear the terms, go to evolve.elsevier.com. Select: Chapter 3, **Exercises**, Pronunciation.

Refer to p. 10 for your Evolve Access Information.

☐ Place a check mark in the box when you have completed this exercise.

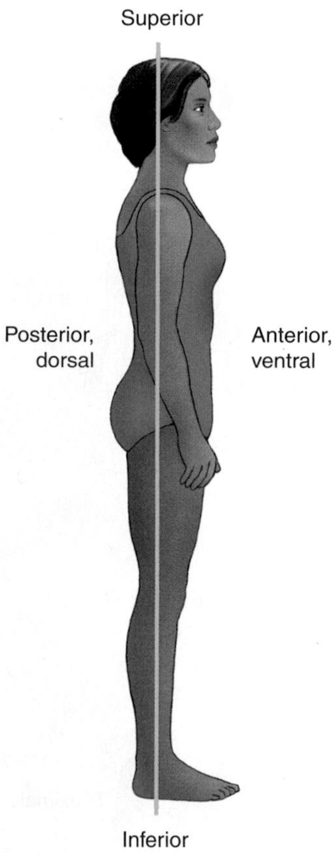

EXERCISE 5

Analyze and define the following directional terms.

1. cephalad_____

2. cephalic _____

3. caudad _____

4. caudal_____

5. anterior _____

6. posterior _____

7. dorsal_____

8. superior _____

9. inferior_____

10. proximal _____

11. distal _____

12. lateral_____

13. medial _____

14. ventral _____

15. posteroanterior_____

16. unilateral _____

17. mediolateral _____

18. anteroposterior_____

19. bilateral _____

Superior

Posterior,
dorsal

Anterior,
ventral

Inferior

FIGURE 3-5
Superior and inferior, posterior
and anterior, dorsal and ventral.

EXERCISE FIGURE **B**

Fill in the blanks to label the diagram.

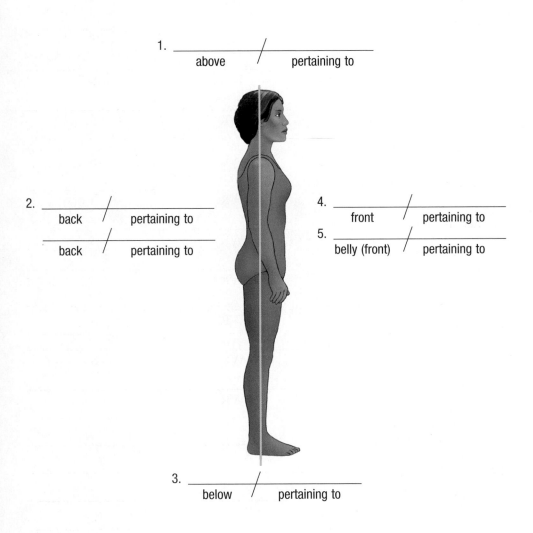

1. _____/_____
   above / pertaining to

2. _____/_____
   back / pertaining to

   _____/_____
   back / pertaining to

4. _____/_____
   front / pertaining to

5. _____/_____
   belly (front) / pertaining to

3. _____/_____
   below / pertaining to

EXERCISE 6

Build directional terms for the following definitions by using the word parts you have learned.

1. toward the head (upward)   _____ / _____
   WR   S

2. pertaining to the head   _____ / _____
   WR   S

3. pertaining to the tail   _____ / _____
   WR   S

4. pertaining to the front   _____ / _____
   WR   S

5. pertaining to the back   _____ / _____
   WR   S

   _____ / _____
   WR   S

6. pertaining to above   _____ / _____
   WR   S

7. pertaining to below   _____ / _____
   WR   S

8. pertaining to near   _____ / _____
   WR   S

9. pertaining to away   _____ / _____
   WR   S

10. pertaining to a side   _____ / _____
    WR   S

11. pertaining to the middle   _____ / _____
    WR   S

12. toward the tail (downward)   _____ / _____
    WR   S

13. pertaining to the belly   _____ / _____
    WR   S

14. pertaining to the back
    and to the front   _____ / ____ / _____ / _____
    WR   CV   WR   S

15. pertaining to the middle
    and to the side   _____ / ____ / _____ / _____
    WR   CV   WR   S

16. pertaining to one side (only)   _____ / _____ / _____
    P   WR   S

17. pertaining to the front
    and to the back   _____ / ____ / _____ / _____
    WR   CV   WR   S

18. pertaining to two sides   _____ / _____ / _____
    P   WR   S

EXERCISE FIGURE **C**

Fill in the blanks to label the diagram.

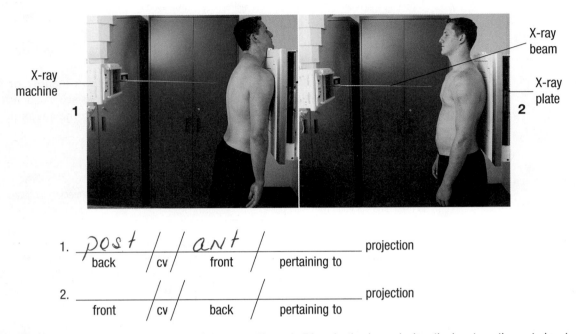

X-ray machine   **1**

X-ray beam

X-ray plate   **2**

1. $\underset{\text{back}}{pos\,t}$ / $\underset{\text{cv}}{}$ / $\underset{\text{front}}{a\,N\,t}$ / $\underset{\text{pertaining to}}{}$ projection

2. $\underset{\text{front}}{}$ / $\underset{\text{cv}}{}$ / $\underset{\text{back}}{}$ / $\underset{\text{pertaining to}}{}$ projection

Organs closest to the x-ray plate look the most accurate on a radiograph. PA projection is used when the heart or other anterior structures are the focus of the diagnostic study. AP projection is used when the spine is the primary focus.

EXERCISE **7**

Spell each of the directional terms on p. 67 by having someone dictate them to you.

> To hear and spell the terms, go to evolve.elsevier.com. Select: Chapter 3, **Exercises**, Spelling.
>
> Refer to p. 10 for your Evolve Access Information.
>
> ☐ Place a check mark in the box if you have completed this exercise online.

1. _____
2. _____
3. _____
4. _____
5. _____
6. _____
7. _____
8. _____
9. _____
10. _____

11. _____
12. _____
13. _____
14. _____
15. _____
16. _____
17. _____
18. _____
19. _____

For review and/or assessment, go to evolve.elsevier.com. Select:
Chapter 3, **Activities**, Analyze Medical Terms
Terms Built from Word Parts

Refer to p. 10 for your Evolve Access Information.

Anatomic Planes

Planes are imaginary flat fields used as points of reference to identify or view the location of organs and anatomical structures. Anatomic planes are frequently used in diagnostic imaging and surgery. The body is assumed to be in the anatomic position unless specified otherwise (Table 3-1).

> ☀ MIDLINE
> is an imaginary line that separates the body, or body parts, into halves. In medical language, midline is used as a common reference point.

> ☀ **Sagittal** describes vertical planes dividing the body into right and left sides. **Midsagittal** and **parasagittal** planes are both sagittal planes with the midsagittal plane dividing the body equally into halves and the parasagittal plane dividing the body into unequal sides.

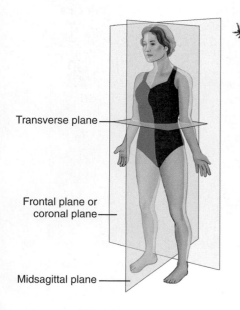

Transverse plane

Frontal plane or
coronal plane

Midsagittal plane

FIGURE 3-6
Anatomic planes.

TERM	DEFINITION
frontal or coronal (FRON-tal) (ko-RŌN-al)	vertical plane passing through the body from side to side, dividing the body into anterior and posterior portions (Figure 3-6)
midsagittal (mid-SAJ-i-tal)	vertical plane passing through the body from front to back at the midline, dividing the body equally into right and left halves (Figure 3-6)
parasagittal (*par*-a-SAJ-i-tal)	vertical plane passing through the body from front to back, dividing the body into unequal left and right sides
sagittal (SAJ-i-tal)	vertical plane passing through the body from front to back, dividing the body into right and left sides (any plane parallel to the midsagittal plane)
transverse (trans-VERS)	horizontal plane dividing the body into superior and inferior portions (Figure 3-6)

Table 3-1

Anatomic Planes and Diagnostic Images

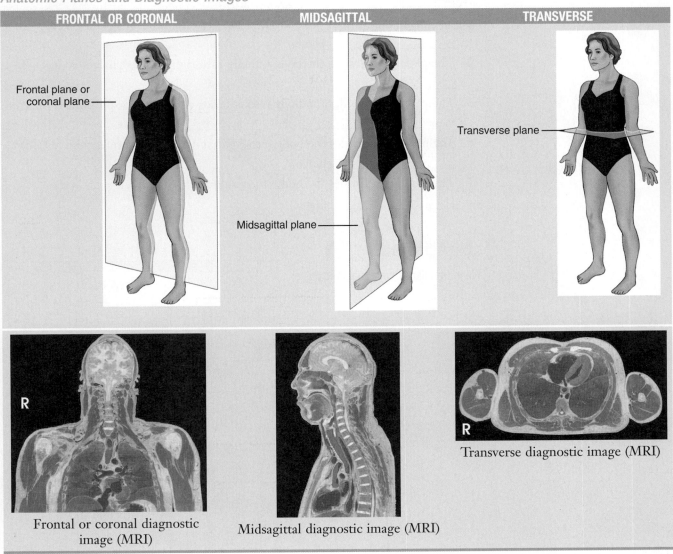

FRONTAL OR CORONAL	MIDSAGITTAL	TRANSVERSE

Frontal plane or coronal plane

Midsagittal plane

Transverse plane

R

Frontal or coronal diagnostic image (MRI)

Midsagittal diagnostic image (MRI)

R

Transverse diagnostic image (MRI)

EXERCISE 8

Practice saying aloud each of the anatomic planes on p. 72.

To hear the terms, go to evolve.elsevier.com. Select: Chapter 3, **Exercises**, Pronunciation.

Refer to p. 10 for your Evolve Access Information.

☐ Place a check mark in the box when you have completed this exercise.

EXERCISE 9

Fill in the blanks with the correct terms.

1. The plane that divides the body into superior and inferior portions is the
    _____ plane.
2. The plane that divides the body **equally** into right and left halves is the
    _____ plane.
3. The plane that divides the body into anterior and posterior portions is referred
    to as _____ or _____ plane.
4. Any plane that divides the body into right and left sides is referred to as a(n)
    _____ plane.
5. The plane that divides the body into **unequal** right and left sides is the
    _____ plane.

EXERCISE FIGURE D

Fill in the blanks with anatomic planes.

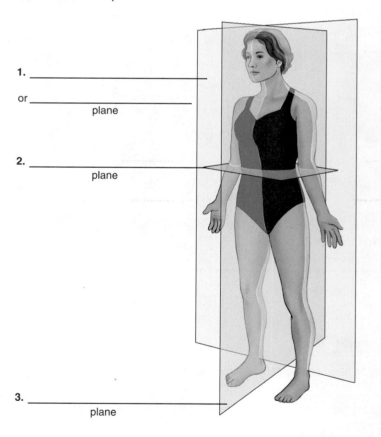

1. _____
   or _____
      plane

2. _____
      plane

3. _____
      plane

EXERCISE 10

Spell each of the anatomic plane terms on p. 72 by having someone dictate them to you.

> To hear and spell the terms, go to evolve.elsevier.com. Select: Chapter 3, **Exercises**, Spelling.
>
> Refer to p. 10 for your Evolve Access Information.
>
> ☐ Place a check mark in the box if you have completed this exercise online.

1. _____   4. _____

2. _____   5. _____

3. _____   6. _____

Body Positions

Position terms are used in health care settings to communicate how the patient's body is placed for physical examination, diagnostic procedures, surgery, treatment, and recovery.

TERM	DEFINITION
Fowler position (FOW-ler) (pe-ZISH-en)	semi-sitting position with slight elevation of the knees (Exercise Figure F)
lithotomy position (lith-OT-o-mē) (pe-ZISH-en)	lying on back with legs raised and feet in stirrups, hips and knees flexed, thighs abducted and externally rotated (Exercise Figure G)
orthopnea position (or-THOP-nē-a) (pe-ZISH-en)	sitting erect in a chair or sitting upright in bed supported by pillows behind the head and chest (also called **orthopneic position**)
prone position (prōn) (pe-ZISH-en)	lying on abdomen, facing downward (head may be turned to one side) (Exercise Figure E)
recumbent position (rē-KUM-bent) (pe-ZISH-en)	lying down in any position
Sims position (simz) (pe-ZISH-en)	lying on left side with right knee drawn up and with left arm drawn behind, parallel to the back (Exercise Figure G)
supine position (SOO-pine) (pe-ZISH-en)	lying on back, facing upward (Exercise Figure E)
Trendelenburg position (tren-DEL-en-berg) (pe-ZISH-en)	lying on back with body tilted so that the head is lower than the feet (Exercise Figure F)

FOWLER POSITION

indicates the patient is in a sitting position with the head of the bed raised between 30° and 90°. Variations in the angle are denoted by **high Fowler**, indicating an upright position at approximately 90°, **Fowler** indicating an angle between 45° and 60°, **semi-Fowler**, 30° to 45°, and **low Fowler**, where the head is slightly elevated.

EXERCISE 11

Practice saying aloud each of the body position terms above.

> To hear the terms, go to evolve.elsevier.com. Select: Chapter 3, **Exercises**, Pronunciation.
>
> Refer to p. 10 for your Evolve Access Information.

☐ Place a check mark in the box when you have completed this exercise.

EXERCISE 12

Match the body position terms in the first column with their correct definitions in the second column.

_____ 1. orthopnea position
_____ 2. Fowler position
_____ 3. lithotomy position
_____ 4. prone position
_____ 5. supine position
_____ 6. recumbent position
_____ 7. Sims position
_____ 8. Trendelenburg position

a. lying on back with legs raised and feet in stirrups, hips and knees flexed, thighs abducted and externally rotated
b. lying down in any position
c. lying on back, facing upward
d. lying on back with body tilted so that the head is lower than the feet
e. sitting erect in a chair or sitting upright in bed supported by pillows behind the head and chest
f. lying on left side with right knee drawn up and with left arm drawn behind, parallel to the back
g. semi-sitting position with slight elevation of the knees
h. lying on abdomen, facing downward (head may be turned to one side)

EXERCISE FIGURE E

Label the following diagrams by writing the term for the corresponding definition.

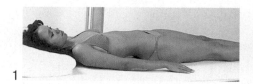

1 ____

1. _____ _____, lying on back, facing upward

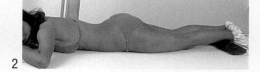

2 ____

2. _____ _____, lying on abdomen, facing downward

EXERCISE FIGURE F

Label the following diagrams by writing the term for the corresponding definition.

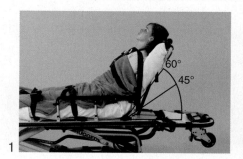

1 ____

1. _____ _____, semi-sitting position with slight elevation of the knees

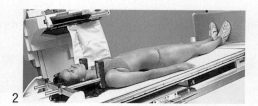

2 ____

2. _____ _____, lying on back with body tilted so that the head is lower than the feet

EXERCISE FIGURE G

Label the following diagrams by writing the term for the corresponding definition.

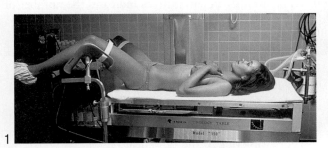

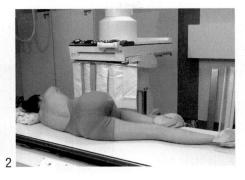

1. Modified _____,
lying on back with legs raised (notice legs are supported
under the knees rather than by stirrups)

2. Modified _____ _____, lying
on left side with right knee drawn up (notice the
arm is placed in front, rather than behind the
body)

EXERCISE 13

Spell each of the body position terms on p. 75 by having someone dictate them to you.

To hear and spell the terms, go to evolve.elsevier.com. Select: Chapter 3, **Exercises**, Spelling.

Refer to p. 10 for your Evolve Access Information.

☐ Place a check mark in the box if you have completed this exercise online.

1. _____   5. _____

2. _____   6. _____

3. _____   7. _____

4. _____   8. _____

Abdominopelvic Regions (9)

To assist in locating medical problems with greater accuracy and for identification purposes, the abdomen and pelvis are divided into nine regions (Figure 3-7). Abdominopelvic regions are often used in relation to physical examination and medical history to describe signs and symptoms. The number in parentheses indicates the number of regions.

TERM	DEFINITION
umbilical region (1) (um-BIL-i-kal) (RĒ-jun)	around the navel (umbilicus)
lumbar regions (2) (LUM-bar) (RĒ-junz)	to the right and left of the umbilical region, near the waist
epigastric region (1) (*ep*-i-GAS-trik) (RĒ-jun)	superior to the umbilical region
hypochondriac regions (2) (*hī*-pō-KON-drē-ak) (RĒ-junz)	to the right and left of the epigastric region
hypogastric region (1) (*hī*-pō-GAS-trik) (RĒ-jun)	inferior to the umbilical region
iliac regions (2) (IL-ē-ak) (RĒ-junz)	to the right and left of the hypogastric region, near the groin (also called **inguinal regions**)

🏛 **UMBILICUS**
is a term derived from the Latin **umbo,** which denoted the boss, or protuberant part, of a shield. Around the first century the term was used to designate either a raised or a depressed spot in the middle of anything.

🏛 **HYPOCHONDRIAC**
is derived from the Greek **hypo,** meaning **under,** and **chondros,** meaning **cartilage.** This ancient term was used by Hippocrates to refer to the region just below the cartilages of the ribs. In 1765, the term was first used to refer to people who experienced discomfort or painful sensations in this area but had no organic findings. Now, a person who falsely believes he or she has an illness is referred to as a **hypochondriac.**

🏛 **CYBERCHONDRIA**
emerged in 2000 as a term describing a pattern of using Internet research to self-diagnose symptoms, fueling health anxiety and worry.

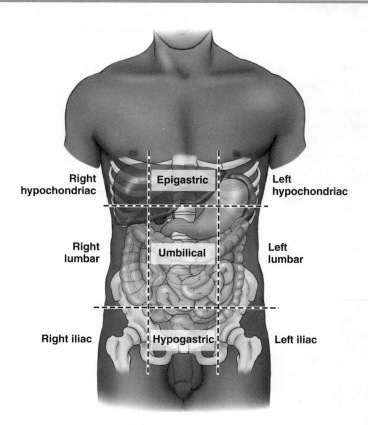

FIGURE 3-7
Abdominopelvic regions.

 To watch animations, go to evolve.elsevier.com. Select: Chapter 3, **Animations**, Epigastric Pain.

Refer to p. 10 for your Evolve Access Information.

EXERCISE 14

Practice saying aloud each of the abdominopelvic region terms on p. 78.

> To hear the terms, go to evolve.elsevier.com. Select: Chapter 3, **Exercises**, Pronunciation.
>
> Refer to p. 10 for your Evolve Access Information.

☐ Place a check mark in the box when you have completed this exercise.

EXERCISE FIGURE H

Fill in the blanks with abdominopelvic regions.

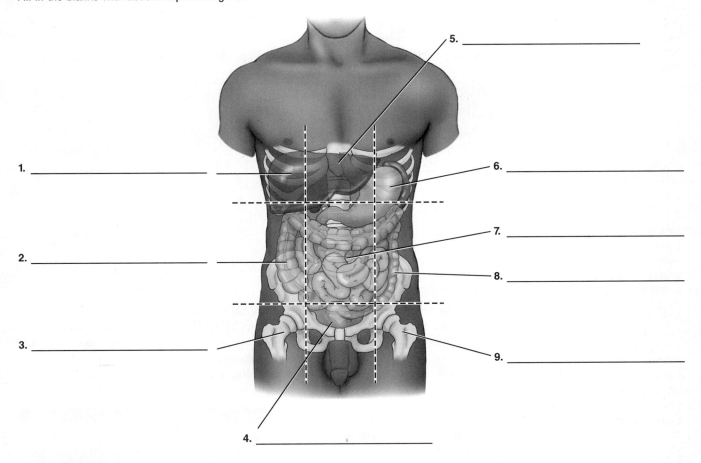

5. _____

1. _____

6. _____

7. _____

2. _____

8. _____

3. _____

9. _____

4. _____

EXERCISE 15

Fill in the blanks with the correct terms.

1. The regions to the right and left of the hypogastric region, near the groin, are the _____ regions.
2. The _____ region is superior to the umbilical region.
3. Inferior to the umbilical region is the _____ region.
4. The _____ are the regions to the right and left of the epigastric region.
5. Superior to the hypogastric region is the _____ region.
6. To the right and the left of the umbilical region, near the waist, are the _____ regions.

EXERCISE 16

Match the terms in the first column with the correct definitions in the second column.

_____ 1. epigastric

_____ 2. hypochondriac

_____ 3. hypogastric

_____ 4. iliac

_____ 5. lumbar

_____ 6. umbilical

a. inferior to the umbilical region

b. superior to the umbilical region

c. right and left of the umbilical region, near the waist

d. right and left of the epigastric region

e. right and left of the hypogastric region, near the groin

f. inferior to the hypogastric region

g. inferior to the epigastric region

EXERCISE 17

Spell each of the abdominopelvic region terms on p. 78 by having someone dictate them to you.

> To hear and spell the terms, go to evolve.elsevier.com. Select: Chapter 3, **Exercises**, Spelling.
>
> Refer to p. 10 for your Evolve Access Information.
>
> ☐ Place a check mark in the box if you have completed this exercise online.

1. _____   4. _____

2. _____   5. _____

3. _____   6. _____

Abdominopelvic Quadrants

The abdominopelvic area can also be divided into four quadrants by using imaginary vertical and horizontal lines that intersect at the umbilicus. These divisions are used by healthcare professionals to specify the location of pain, incisions, markings, lesions, and so forth. The quadrants provide a more general denotation than the abdominopelvic regions, and they are used in describing the location of findings from the physical examination and medical history (Figure 3-8).

TERM	DEFINITION
right upper quadrant (RUQ) (KWOD-rant)	refers to the area encompassing the right lobe of the liver, the gallbladder, medial portion of the pancreas, and portions of the small and large intestines
left upper quadrant (LUQ) (KWOD-rant)	refers to the area encompassing the left lobe of the liver, the stomach, the spleen, lateral portion of the pancreas, and portions of the small and large intestines
right lower quadrant (RLQ) (KWOD-rant)	refers to the area encompassing portions of the small and large intestines, the appendix, the right ureter, and the right ovary and uterine tube in women or the right spermatic duct in men
left lower quadrant (LLQ) (KWOD-rant)	refers to the area encompassing portions of the small and large intestines, the left ureter, and the left ovary and uterine tube in women or the left spermatic duct in men

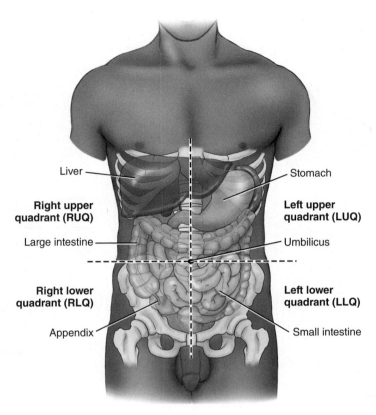

FIGURE 3-8
Abdominopelvic quadrants.

To watch **animations**, go to evolve.elsevier.com. Select:
Chapter 3, **Animations**, LLQ Pain
                            LUQ Pain
                            RLQ Pain
                            RUQ Pain
                            Quadrants of the Body

Refer to p. 10 for your Evolve Access Information.

EXERCISE 18

Write the abbreviation for the abdominopelvic quadrant associated with the following organs.

_____ 1. appendix
_____ 2. right lobe of the liver
_____ 3. left spermatic duct in men
_____ 4. the stomach and the spleen
_____ 5. right ovary and uterine tube in women
_____ 6. gallbladder
_____ 7. right ureter

EXERCISE FIGURE ▮▮

Fill in the blanks with abdominopelvic quadrants and the abbreviations for each.

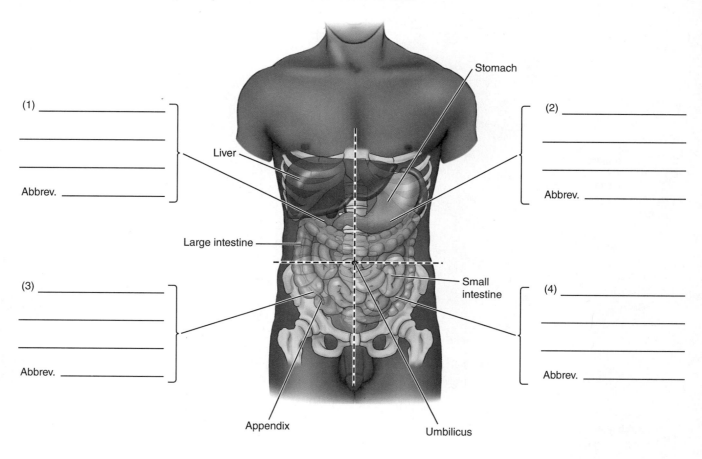

(1) _____

_____

_____

Abbrev. _____

Stomach

Liver

Large intestine

(3) _____

_____

_____

Abbrev. _____

Appendix

(2) _____

_____

_____

Abbrev. _____

Small
intestine

(4) _____

_____

_____

Abbrev. _____

Umbilicus

EXERCISE 19

Spell each of the abdominopelvic quadrant terms on p. 80 by having someone dictate them to
you.

> To hear and spell the terms, go to evolve.elsevier.com. Select: Chapter 3, **Exercises**, Spelling.
>
> Refer to p. 10 for your Evolve Access Information.
>
> ☐ Place a check mark in the box if you have completed this exercise online.

1. _____   3. _____

2. _____   4. _____

> For review and/or assessment, go to evolve.elsevier.com. Select:
> Chapter 3, **Activities**, Terms Not Built from Word Parts
>   Hear It and Type It: Clinical Vignettes
> Chapter 3, **Games**,   Medical Millionaire
>
> Refer to p. 10 for your Evolve Access Information.

Abbreviations

ABBREVIATION	MEANING
ant	anterior
AP	anteroposterior
inf	inferior
lat	lateral
LLQ	left lower quadrant
LUQ	left upper quadrant
med	medial
PA	posteroanterior
RLQ	right lower quadrant
RUQ	right upper quadrant
sup	superior

For practice with abbreviations, go to evolve.elsevier.com. Select:
Chapter 3, **Flashcards**
Chapter 3, **Games**, Crossword Puzzle

Refer to p. 10 for your Evolve Access Information.

Refer to Appendix C for a complete list of abbreviations.

EXERCISE 20

Write the meaning of each abbreviation in the space provided.

1. sup _____

2. ant _____

3. inf _____

4. PA _____

5. AP _____

6. med _____

7. lat _____

PRACTICAL APPLICATION

A. Complete the physician's progress note by writing the medical terms in the blanks. Use the list of definitions with corresponding numbers following the document.

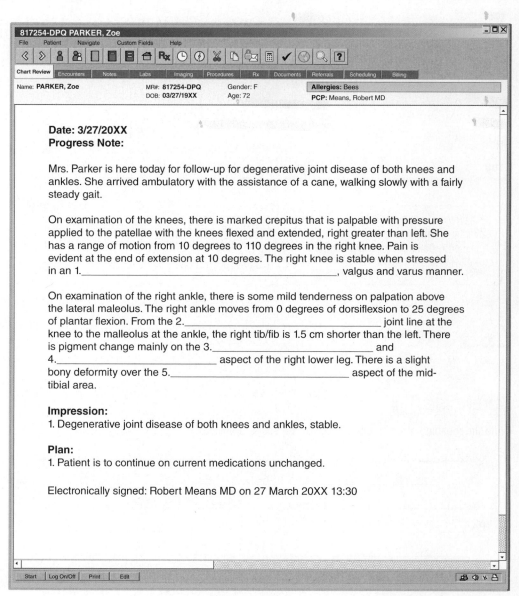

817254-DPQ PARKER, Zoe

File   Patient   Navigate   Custom Fields   Help

Chart Review | Encounters | Notes | Labs | Imaging | Procedures | Rx | Documents | Referrals | Scheduling | Billing

Name: **PARKER, Zoe**   MR#: **817254-DPQ**   Gender: F   **Allergies:** Bees
                 DOB: **03/27/19XX**   Age: 72   **PCP:** Means, Robert MD

Date: 3/27/20XX
Progress Note:

Mrs. Parker is here today for follow-up for degenerative joint disease of both knees and ankles. She arrived ambulatory with the assistance of a cane, walking slowly with a fairly steady gait.

On examination of the knees, there is marked crepitus that is palpable with pressure applied to the patellae with the knees flexed and extended, right greater than left. She has a range of motion from 10 degrees to 110 degrees in the right knee. Pain is evident at the end of extension at 10 degrees. The right knee is stable when stressed in an 1._____, valgus and varus manner.

On examination of the right ankle, there is some mild tenderness on palpation above the lateral maleolus. The right ankle moves from 0 degrees of dorsiflexsion to 25 degrees of plantar flexion. From the 2._____ joint line at the knee to the malleolus at the ankle, the right tib/fib is 1.5 cm shorter than the left. There is pigment change mainly on the 3._____ and 4._____ aspect of the right lower leg. There is a slight bony deformity over the 5._____ aspect of the mid-tibial area.

Impression:
1. Degenerative joint disease of both knees and ankles, stable.

Plan:
1. Patient is to continue on current medications unchanged.

Electronically signed: Robert Means MD on 27 March 20XX 13:30

Start | Log On/Off | Print | Edit

1. pertaining to the front and to the back
2. pertaining to the side
3. pertaining to the back
4. pertaining to the middle
5. pertaining to the front

B. Read the procedure for palpating arterial pulses and answer the questions following it.

PROCEDURE FOR PALPATING ARTERIAL PULSES

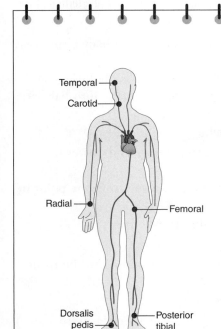

Palpate arteries with the distal pads of the first two fingers. The fingertips are used because they are the most sensitive parts of the hand. Unless contraindicated, simultaneous palpation is preferred.

Temporal: Palpate over the temporal bone on each side of the head, lateral to each eyebrow.

Carotid: Palpate the anterior edge of the sternocleidomastoid muscle, just medial and inferior to the angle of the jaw. To avoid reduction of blood flow, do not palpate right and left carotid pulses simultaneously.

Radial: Palpate lateral and anterior side of wrist, proximal to the first metacarpal phalangeal joint.

Femoral: This pulse is inferior to the inguinal ligament; the pulse is found midway between anterior superior iliac spine and pubic tubercle.

Dorsalis pedis: Lightly palpate the dorsal surface of the foot, with the foot slightly dorsiflexed.

Posterior tibial: This pulse is found posterior and slightly inferior to the medial malleolus of the ankle.

1. The **temporal pulse** is palpated
   a. just above the eyebrow.
   b. to the side of the eyebrow.
   c. below the eyebrow.
   d. to the middle of the eyebrow.

2. The **radial pulse** is palpated on the
   a. lateral and front of the wrist.
   b. lateral and back of the wrist.
   c. medial and back of the wrist.
   d. medial and front of the wrist.

3. The **femoral pulse** is located
   a. below the inguinal ligament.
   b. above the inguinal ligament.
   c. to the front of the inguinal ligament.
   d. to the back of the inguinal ligament.

4. When used with the foot, the directional term *dorsal* has a slightly different meaning. With the use of your medical dictionary or an online resource, describe the dorsal surface of the foot. Hint: try *dorsum* and *dorsal pedis* as search terms.

   The dorsal surface of the foot is _____ _____.

EXERCISE 22   *Interpret Medical Terms*

To test your understanding of the terms introduced in this chapter, complete the sentence by filling in the blank with the term that corresponds to the definition provided.

1. The _____ plane is a general term specifying the vertical plane running through the body from front to back. (**dividing the body into right and left sides**)

2. The terms _____ plane and _____ plane more specifically describe the sagittal plane by indicating whether the body is divided in half or in unequal portions. (**dividing the body equally into halves**) (**dividing the body into unequal sides**)

3. Images for computed tomography (CT) scanning can be produced from the sagittal plane, the frontal or _____ plane, and the _____ plane. (**dividing the body into anterior and posterior portions**) (**dividing the body into superior and inferior portions**)

4. A polyp was found in the colon _____ to the splenic flexure. (**pertaining to away from the point of attachment of a body part**)

5. The drainage catheter is placed over the right _____ pelvis. (**pertaining to the front**)

6. The incision was made at the _____ pole of the lesion. (**pertaining to above**)

7. A(n) _____ chest radiograph is taken from the _____ position. (**pertaining to the front and to the back**) (**dividing the body into anterior and posterior portions**)

8. The patient complained of _____ pain. (**superior to umbilical region**)

9. A _____ chest radiograph displays the anatomy in the _____ plane. (**pertaining to a side**) (**divides the body into right and left sides**)

10. The patient was scheduled for an ultrasound-guided _____ thoracentesis. (**pertaining to two [both] sides**)

11. The doctor's order indicated that the patient with dyspnea was to be placed in the _____ position to facilitate breathing. (**sitting erect or upright**)

12. The patient being treated for cardiovascular shock was placed in the _____ position. (**lying on back with the head lower than the feet**)

13. Gallbladder pain is likely to be in the _____ _____ _____. (**abbreviated as RUQ**)

14. _____ is often used to describe the back of the hand or upper surface of the foot. (**pertaining to the back**)

15. Just before birth, the fetus shifted to a _____ presentation. (**pertaining to the head**)

16. _____ epidural steroid injection may be performed to relieve chronic low back pain. (**pertaining to the tail**)

17. The pathology report for the patient with a palpable right breast lump included the following sections:
    a. Right axillary sentinel lymph node, biopsy;
    b. Right breast, _____ margin biopsy (**pertaining to above**);
    c. Right breast, _____ margin, biopsy (**pertaining to below**);
    d. Right breast, deep margin, biopsy;
    e. Right breast, _____ margin, biopsy (**pertaining to the middle**); and
    f. Right breast, _____ margin, biopsy (**pertaining to a side**).

EXERCISE 23   *Read Medical Terms in Use*

Practice pronunciation of terms by reading aloud the following medical document. Use the pronunciation key following the medical term to assist you in saying the word. The script contains medical terms not yet presented. Treat them as information only; you will learn more about them as you continue to study. Or, if desired, look for their meanings in your medical dictionary.

> To hear these terms, go to evolve.elsevier.com. Select:
> Chapter 3, **Exercises**, Read Medical Terms in Use.
>
> Refer to p. 10 for your Evolve Access Information.

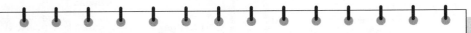

The patient presented to her physician with pain in the right **lumbar** (LUM-bar) **region** and right **unilateral** (ū-ni-LAT-er-al) leg pain. The pain was felt in the **posterior** (pos-TĒR-ē-or) portion of the leg and radiated to the **distal** (DIS-tal) **lateral** (LAT-er-al) portion of the extremity. There was some **proximal** (PROK-si-mal) muscle weakness reported of the affected leg. A lumbar spine radiograph was normal. If the pain does not respond to antiinflammatory medication, she will be referred to an orthopedist.

EXERCISE 24   *Comprehend Medical Terms in Use*

Test your comprehension of terms in the previous medical document by answering T for true and F for false.

_____ 1. The patient had pain on both sides of her leg and to the right of the hypogastric region.

_____ 2. The pain was felt at the back of the leg and radiated away from this point to the side of the extremity.

_____ 3. The muscle weakness was felt near the point of attachment.

> For a snapshot assessment of your knowledge, go to evolve.elsevier.com. Select:
> Chapter 3, **Quick Quizzes**.
>
> Refer to p. 10 for your Evolve Access Information.

CHAPTER REVIEW

e *Review of Evolve*

Keep a record of the online activities you have completed by placing a check mark in the box. You may also record your scores. All activities have been referenced throughout the text.

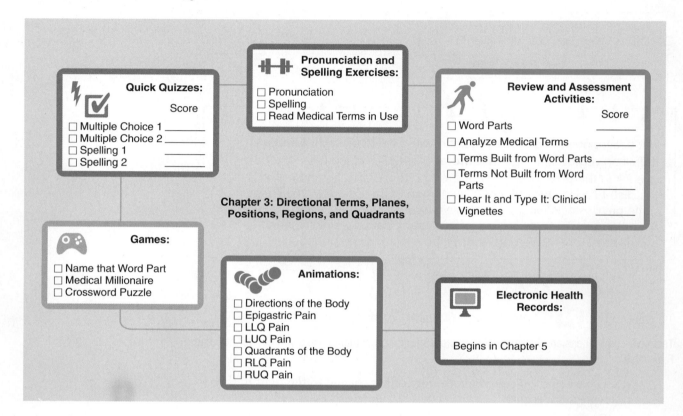

Review of Word Parts

Can you define and spell the following word parts?

COMBINING FORMS		PREFIXES	SUFFIXES
anter/o	medi/o	bi-	-ad
caud/o	poster/o	uni-	-ior
cephal/o	proxim/o		
dist/o	super/o		
dors/o	ventr/o		
infer/o			
later/o			

Review of Terms

Can you define, pronounce, and spell the following terms?

DIRECTIONAL TERMS	ANATOMIC PLANES	BODY POSITIONS	ABDOMINOPELVIC REGIONS	ABDOMINOPELVIC QUADRANTS
anterior (ant)	frontal or	Fowler position	epigastric region	left lower quadrant
anteroposterior (AP)	coronal	lithotomy position	hypochondriac regions	(LLQ)
bilateral	midsagittal	orthopnea position	hypogastric region	left upper quadrant
caudad	parasagittal	prone position	iliac regions	(LUQ)
caudal	sagittal	recumbent position	lumbar regions	right lower quadrant
cephalad	transverse	Sims position	umbilical region	(RLQ)
cephalic		supine position		right upper quadrant
distal		Trendelenburg position		(RUQ)
dorsal				
inferior (inf)				
lateral (lat)				
medial (med)				
mediolateral				
posterior				
posteroanterior (PA)				
proximal				
superior (sup)				
unilateral				
ventral				

> *Types of body movement* are presented in Chapter 14, Musculoskeletal System, on page 579. Terms related to body movement are: *abduction, adduction, inversion, eversion, extension, flexion, pronation, supination,* and *rotation.*

ANSWERS

ANSWERS TO CHAPTER 3 EXERCISES

Exercise Figures

Exercise Figure

A.
1. head: cephal/o
2. front: anter/o
3. belly: ventr/o
4. back: dors/o
5. back, behind: poster/o
6. above: super/o
7. side: later/o
8. middle: medi/o
9. near: proxim/o
10. away: dist/o
11. below: infer/o

Exercise Figure

B.
1. super/ior
2. poster/ior, dors/al
3. infer/ior
4. anter/ior
5. ventr/al

Exercise Figure

C.
1. poster/o/anter/ior
2. anter/o/poster/ior

Exercise Figure

D.
1. frontal or coronal plane
2. transverse plane
3. midsagittal plane

Exercise Figure

E.
1. supine position
2. prone position

Exercise Figure

F.
1. Fowler position
2. Trendelenburg position

Exercise Figure

G.
1. lithotomy position
2. Sims position

Exercise Figure

H.
1. right hypochondriac
2. right lumbar
3. right iliac
4. hypogastric
5. epigastric
6. left hypochondriac
7. umbilical
8. left lumbar
9. left iliac

Exercise Figure

I.
1. right upper quadrant (RUQ)
2. left upper quadrant (LUQ)
3. right lower quadrant (RLQ)
4. left lower quadrant (LLQ)

Exercise 1
1. belly (front)
2. head (upward)
3. side
4. middle
5. below
6. near (point of attachment of a body part)
7. above
8. away (from the point of attachment of a body part)
9. back
10. tail (downward)
11. front
12. back, behind

Exercise 2
1. c
2. b
3. d
4. a

Exercise 3
1. pertaining to
2. toward
3. two
4. one

Exercise 4
Pronunciation Exercise

Exercise 5
Note: The combining form is noted by italic and bold print.

1. WR   S
   cephal/ad
   toward the head

2. WR   S
   cephal/ic
   pertaining to the head

3. WR   S
   caud/ad
   toward the tail

4. WR   S
   caud/al
   pertaining to the tail

5. WR   S
   anter/ior
   pertaining to the front

6. WR   S
   poster/ior
   pertaining to the back

7. WR   S
   dors/al
   pertaining to the back

8. WR   S
   super/ior
   pertaining to above

9. WR   S
   infer/ior
   pertaining to below

10. WR   S
    proxim/al
    pertaining to near

11. WR   S
    dist/al
    pertaining to away

12. WR   S
    later/al
    pertaining to a side

13. WR   S
    medi/al
    pertaining to the middle

14. WR   S
    ventr/al
    pertaining to the belly (front)

15. WR CV WR   S
    poster/o/anter/ior
         CF
    pertaining to the back and to the front

16. P   WR   S
    uni/later/al
    pertaining to one side

17. WR CV WR   S
    medi/o/later/al
         CF
    pertaining to the middle and to the side

18. WR CV WR   S
    anter/o/poster/ior
         CF
    pertaining to the front and to the back

19. P   WR   S
    bi/later/al
    pertaining to two sides

Exercise 6
1. cephal/ad
2. cephal/ic
3. caud/al

4. anter/ior
5. poster/ior, dors/al
6. super/ior
7. infer/ior
8. proxim/al
9. dist/al
10. later/al
11. medi/al
12. caud/ad
13. ventr/al
14. poster/o/anter/ior
15. medi/o/later/al
16. uni/later/al
17. anter/o/poster/ior
18. bi/later/al

Exercise 7
Spelling Exercise; see text p. 71.

Exercise 8
Pronunciation Exercise

Exercise 9
1. transverse
2. midsagittal
3. frontal or coronal
4. sagittal
5. parasagittal

Exercise 10
Spelling Exercise; see text p. 75.

Exercise 11
Pronunciation Exercise

Exercise 12
1. e
2. g
3. a
4. h
5. c
6. b
7. f
8. d

Exercise 13
Spelling Exercise; see text p. 77.

Exercise 14
Pronunciation Exercise

Exercise 15
1. iliac
2. epigastric
3. hypogastric
4. hypochondriac
5. umbilical
6. lumbar

Exercise 16
1. b
2. d
3. a
4. e
5. c
6. g

Exercise 17
Spelling Exercise; see text p. 80.

Exercise 18
1. RLQ
2. RUQ
3. LLQ
4. LUQ
5. RLQ
6. RUQ
7. RLQ

Exercise 19
Spelling Exercise; see text p. 82.

Exercise 20
1. superior
2. anterior
3. inferior
4. posteroanterior
5. anteroposterior
6. medial
7. lateral

Exercise 21
A. 1. anteroposterior
2. lateral
3. posterior or dorsal
4. medial
5. anterior
B. 1. b
2. a
3. a
4. answers may vary: the upper surface of the foot; the surface opposite the sole

Exercise 22
1. sagittal
2. midsagittal, parasagittal
3. coronal, transverse
4. distal
5. anterior
6. superior
7. anteroposterior; frontal (or coronal)
8. epigastric
9. lateral; sagittal
10. bilateral
11. orthopnea
12. Trendelenburg
13. right upper quadrant
14. dorsal
15. cephalic
16. caudal
17. a. no answer, b. superior, c. inferior, d. no answer, e. medial, f. lateral

Exercise 23
Reading Exercise

Exercise 24
1. *F*, "unilateral" means one side; "bilateral" means two sides. The right lumbar region is to the right of the umbilical region.
2. *T*
3. *T*

Integumentary System

Outline

Objectives

Upon completion of this chapter you will be able to:

1 Identify organs and structures of the integumentary system.

2 Define and spell word parts related to the integumentary system.

3 Define, pronounce, and spell disease and disorder terms related to the integumentary system.

4 Define, pronounce, and spell surgical terms related to the integumentary system.

5 Define, pronounce, and spell complementary terms related to the integumentary system.

6 Interpret the meaning of abbreviations related to the integumentary system.

7 Interpret, read, and comprehend medical language in simulated medical statements and documents.

The remaining chapters are organized according to body systems; therefore, they present material in a consistent format. The better you understand the format, the quicker and easier you will learn the material. Take time now to review How I Will Learn Medical Terms using *Exploring Medical Language*, pp. xiii–xiv in the Front Matter to reacquaint yourself with the finer points of using this textbook to its ultimate potential.

ANATOMY

The integumentary system is composed of the skin, glands, hair, and nails.

🏛 **INTEGUMENTARY**
is derived from the Latin word
teqere, meaning to **cover**.

✳ Function

The skin forms a protective covering for the body that, when unbroken, prevents entry of bacteria and other invading organisms. The skin also protects the body from water loss and the damaging effects of ultraviolet light. Other functions include regulation of body temperature and synthesis of vitamin D (Figure 4-1).

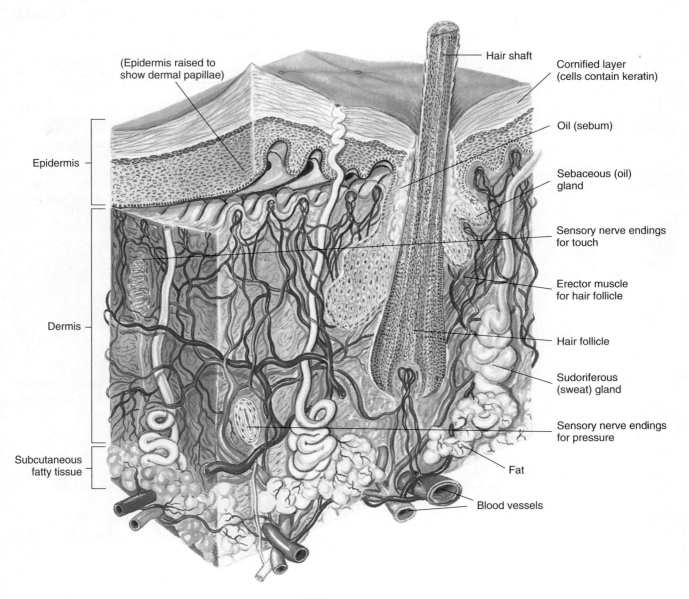

FIGURE 4-1
Structure of the skin.

epi = upon (handwritten margin note)

The Skin

TERM	DEFINITION
epidermis	outer layer of skin
keratin	scleroprotein component of the horny, or corni-fied, layer of the epidermis. It is also contained in the hair and nails.
melanin	color, or pigmentation, of the skin
dermis	inner layer of skin (also called the true skin)
sudoriferous (sweat) glands	tiny, coiled, tubular structures that emerge through pores on the skin's surface and secrete sweat
sebaceous glands	secrete sebum (oil) into the hair follicles where the hair shafts pass through the dermis

Accessory Structures of the Skin

TERM	DEFINITION
hair	compressed, keratinized cells that arise from hair follicles, the sacs that enclose the hair fibers
nails	originate in the epidermis. Nails are found on the upper surface of the ends of the fingers and toes. The white area at the base of the nail is called the **lunula**, or **moon**.

A&P Booster

For more anatomy and physiology, go to evolve.elsevier.com.
Select: **Extra Content**, A & P Booster, Chapter 4.

Refer to p. 10 for your Evolve Access Information.

EXERCISE 1

Match the terms in the first column with the correct definitions in the second column. *To check your answers to the exercises in this chapter, go to Answers, p. 135, at the end of the chapter.*

_____ 1. dermis
_____ 2. epidermis
_____ 3. hair
_____ 4. melanin
_____ 5. nail
_____ 6. sebaceous glands
_____ 7. sudoriferous glands
_____ 8. keratin

a. secrete sweat
b. responsible for skin color
c. true skin
d. outermost layer of the skin
e. component of the horny layer of the epidermis
f. originates in the epidermis
g. composed of compressed, keratinized cells
h. secrete sebum

WORD PARTS

Word parts you need to learn to complete this chapter are listed on the following pages. The exercises at the end of each list will help you learn their definitions and spelling.

 To use electronic flashcards, go to evolve.elsevier.com. Select: Chapter 4, **Flashcards**.

Refer to p. 10 for your Evolve Access Information.

Combining Forms of the Integumentary System

 Use the flashcards accompanying this text or electronic flashcards to assist you in memorizing the word parts for this chapter.

COMBINING FORM	DEFINITION
cutane/o, derm/o, dermat/o	skin
hidr/o	sweat
kerat/o *(NOTE: kerat/o is also used to refer to the cornea of the eye; see Chapter 12.)*	horny tissue, hard
onych/o, ungu/o	nail
seb/o	sebum (oil)
trich/o	hair

 Do not be concerned about which **combining form** to use for **skin** or **nail**. As you continue to study and use medical terms, you will become familiar with common usage of each word part.

EXERCISE FIGURE **A**

Fill in the blanks with combining forms in this diagram of a cross section of the skin. *To check your answers, go to p. 135.*

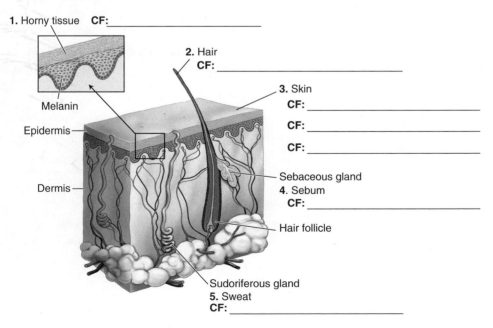

1. Horny tissue **CF:**_____

Melanin

Epidermis

Dermis

2. Hair **CF:**_____

3. Skin **CF:** _____
CF: _____
CF: _____

Sebaceous gland
4. Sebum **CF:** _____

Hair follicle

Sudoriferous gland
5. Sweat **CF:** _____

EXERCISE FIGURE B

Fill in the blanks with combining forms in this cross section of the finger with nail.

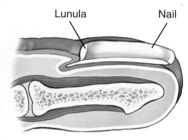

Lunula   Nail

CF: _____

CF: _____

EXERCISE 2

Write the definitions of the following combining forms.

1. hidr/o _____
2. derm/o _____
3. onych/o _____
4. trich/o _____
5. kerat/o _____

6. dermat/o _____
7. seb/o _____
8. ungu/o _____
9. cutane/o _____

EXERCISE 3

Write the combining form for each of the following.

1. hair _____
2. sweat _____
3. nail   a. _____
         b. _____
4. sebum _____

5. skin   a. _____
         b. _____
         c. _____
6. horny tissue, hard _____

Combining Forms Commonly Used with Integumentary System Terms

COMBINING FORM	DEFINITION
aut/o	self
bi/o	life
coni/o	dust
crypt/o	hidden
heter/o	other
myc/o	fungus
necr/o	death (cells, body)
pachy/o	thick
rhytid/o	wrinkles
staphyl/o	grapelike clusters
strept/o	twisted chains
xer/o	dry

 The prefix **bi-**, which means **two**, was presented in Chapter 3. The word root **bi** means **life**.

EXERCISE 4

Write the definitions of the following combining forms.

1. necr/o _____   7. bi/o_____
2. staphyl/o _____   8. heter/o_____
3. crypt/o_____   9. strept/o _____
4. pachy/o _____   10. xer/o_____
5. coni/o_____   11. aut/o_____
6. myc/o_____   12. rhytid/o _____

EXERCISE 5

Write the combining form for each of the following.

1. fungus _____   7. wrinkles_____
2. death (cells, body) _____   8. grapelike clusters _____
3. other _____   9. self _____
4. dry _____   10. hidden _____
5. thick_____   11. dust _____
6. twisted chains _____   12. life _____

Prefixes

PREFIX	DEFINITION
epi-	on, upon, over
intra-	within
para-	beside, beyond, around, abnormal
per-	through
sub-	under, below
trans-	through, across, beyond

EXERCISE 6

Write the definitions of the following prefixes.

1. sub- _____
2. para-_____
3. epi-_____
4. intra- _____
5. per- _____
6. trans- _____

EXERCISE 7

Write the prefix for each of the following.

1. within_____
2. under, below _____
3. on, upon, over _____
4. beside, beyond, around, abnormal _____
5. through _____
6. through, across, beyond_____

✳ Suffixes

SUFFIX	DEFINITION
-a	noun suffix, no meaning
-coccus (pl. -cocci)	berry-shaped (form of bacterium)
-ectomy	excision or surgical removal
-ia	diseased or abnormal state, condition of
-itis	inflammation
-malacia	softening
-opsy	view of, viewing
-phagia	eating or swallowing
-plasty	surgical repair
-rrhea	flow, discharge
-tome	instrument used to cut

Refer to **Appendix A** and **Appendix B** for alphabetical lists of word parts and their meanings.

EXERCISE 8

Match the suffixes in the first column with the correct definitions in the second column.

_____ 1. -coccus
_____ 2. -ectomy
_____ 3. -itis
_____ 4. -malacia
_____ 5. -opsy
_____ 6. -rrhea
_____ 7. -phagia
_____ 8. -plasty
_____ 9. -tome
_____ 10. -ia
_____ 11. -a

a. inflammation
b. surgical repair
c. berry-shaped
d. eating or swallowing
e. excision or surgical removal
f. instrument used to cut
g. thick
h. flow, discharge
i. view of, viewing
j. softening
k. diseased or abnormal state, condition of
l. noun suffix, no meaning

EXERCISE 9

Write the definitions of the following suffixes.

1. -plasty _____

2. -ectomy _____

3. -malacia _____

4. -itis _____

5. -tome _____

6. -phagia _____

7. -rrhea _____

8. -coccus _____

9. -opsy _____

10. -ia _____

11. -a _____

For review and/or assessment, go to evolve.elsevier.com. Select:
Chapter 4, **Activities,** Word Parts
Chapter 4, **Games,**   Name that Word Part

Refer to p. 10 for your Evolve Access Information.

MEDICAL TERMS

The terms you need to learn to complete this chapter are listed on the following pages. The exercises at the end of each list will help you learn each word well enough to add it to your vocabulary.

Disease and Disorder Terms
Built from Word Parts

The following terms are built from word parts you have already learned and can be translated literally to find their meanings. Further explanation of terms beyond the definition of their word parts, if needed, is included in parentheses.

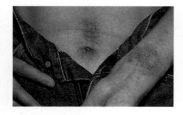

FIGURE 4-2
Contact dermatitis.

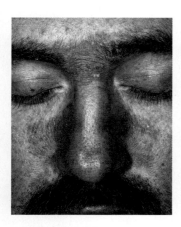

FIGURE 4-3
Seborrheic dermatitis.

TERM	DEFINITION
dermatitis (*der*-ma-TĪ-tis)	inflammation of the skin (Figures 4-2 and 4-3)
dermatoconiosis (*der*-ma-tō-*kō*-nē-Ō-sis)	abnormal condition of the skin caused by dust
dermatofibroma (*der*-ma-tō-fī-BRŌ-ma)	fibrous tumor of the skin
hidradenitis (*hī*-drad-e-NĪ-tis)	inflammation of a sweat gland
leiodermia (*lī*-ō-DER-mē-a)	condition of smooth skin
leukoderma (*lū*-kō-DER-ma)	white skin (white patches caused by depigmentation)
onychocryptosis (*on*-i-kō-krip-TŌ-sis)	abnormal condition of a hidden nail (also called **ingrown nail**)
onychomalacia (*on*-i-kō-ma-LĀ-sha)	softening of the nails
onychomycosis (*on*-i-kō-mī-KŌ-sis)	abnormal condition of a fungus in the nails (Exercise Figure C)
onychophagia (*on*-i-kō-FĀ-ja)	eating the nails (nail biting)
pachyderma (*pak*-i-DER-ma)	thickening of the skin
paronychia (*par*-ō-NIK-ē-a) *(Note: the a from para- has been dropped. The final vowel in a prefix may be dropped when the word to which it is added begins with a vowel.)*	diseased state around the nail (Exercise Figure C)
seborrhea (seb-o-RĒ-a)	discharge of sebum (excessive)
trichomycosis (*trik*-ō-mī-KŌ-sis)	abnormal condition of a fungus in the hair
xeroderma (zē-rō-DER-ma)	dry skin (a mild form of a cutaneous disorder characterized by keratinization and noninflammatory scaling)

EXERCISE FIGURE C

Fill in the blanks to label the diagrams.

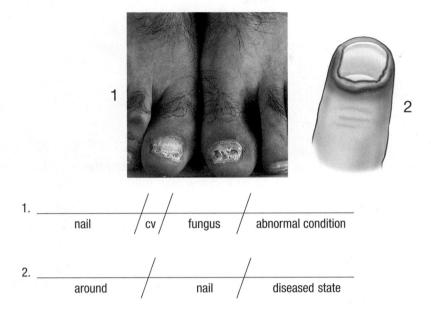

1. _____ / ___ / _____ / _____
   nail   cv   fungus   abnormal condition

2. _____ / _____ / _____
   around   nail   diseased state

EXERCISE 10

Practice saying aloud each of the disease and disorder terms built from word parts.

> (e) To hear the terms, go to evolve.elsevier.com. Select: Chapter 4, **Exercises**, Pronunciation.
>
> Refer to p. 10 for your Evolve Access Information.

☐ Place a check mark in the box when you have completed this exercise.

EXERCISE 11

Analyze and define the following disease and disorder terms built from word parts. If needed, refer to pp. 10–13 to review analyzing and defining techniques.

        WR   CV WR   S

EXAMPLE: onych / o / myc / osis   abnormal condition of a fungus in the nails

           CF

1. dermatoconiosis _____

2. hidradenitis _____

3. dermatitis _____

4. pachyderma _____

5. onychomalacia _____

6. trichomycosis _____

7. dermatofibroma _____

8. paronychia _____

9. onychocryptosis _____

10. seborrhea_____

11. onychophagia _____

12. xeroderma _____

13. leiodermia _____

14. leukoderma _____

EXERCISE 12

Build disease and disorder terms for the following definitions by using the word parts you have learned. If you need help, refer to pp. 12–13 to review word-building techniques.

EXAMPLE: abnormal condition of a fungus in the hair $\dfrac{\text{trich} / \text{o} / \text{myc} / \text{osis}}{\text{WR} / \text{CV} / \text{WR} / \text{S}}$

1. thickening of the skin

   _____ / _____ / _____
      WR   WR   S

2. abnormal condition of a fungus in the nails

   _____ /CV/ _____ / _____
      WR   WR   S

3. discharge of sebum (excessive)

   _____ /CV/ _____
      WR   S

4. inflammation of the skin

   _____ / _____
      WR   S

5. fibrous tumor of the skin

   _____ /CV/ _____ / _____
      WR   WR   S

6. softening of the nails

   _____ /CV/ _____
      WR   S

7. inflammation of a sweat gland

   _____ / _____ / _____
      WR   WR   S

8. abnormal condition of a hidden nail

   _____ /CV/ _____ / _____
      WR   WR   S

9. abnormal condition of the skin caused by dust

   _____ /CV/ _____ / _____
      WR   WR   S

10. eating the nails

    _____ /CV/ _____
       WR   S

11. diseased state around the nail

    _____ / _____ / _____
       P   WR   S

12. dry skin

    _____ /CV/ _____ / _____
       WR   WR   S

13. condition of smooth skin

    _____ /CV/ _____ / _____
       WR   WR   S

14. white skin

    _____ /CV/ _____ / _____
       WR   WR   S

EXERCISE 13

Spell each of the disease and disorder terms built from word parts on p. 100 by having someone dictate them to you.

> To hear and spell the terms, go to evolve.elsevier.com. Select: Chapter 4, **Exercises**, Spelling.
>
> Refer to p. 10 for your Evolve Access Information.
>
> ☐ Place a check mark in the box if you have completed this exercise online.

1. _____   9. _____
2. _____   10. _____
3. _____   11. _____
4. _____   12. _____
5. _____   13. _____
6. _____   14. _____
7. _____   15. _____
8. _____

Disease and Disorder Terms

Not Built from Word Parts

In some of the following terms, you may recognize word parts you have already learned; however, the full meaning of the terms cannot be discerned by the definition of their word parts.

TERM	DEFINITION
abrasion (a-BRĀ-zhun)	scraping away of the skin by mechanical process or injury
abscess (AB-ses)	localized collection of pus
acne (AK-nĕ)	inflammatory disease of the skin involving the sebaceous glands and hair follicles
actinic keratosis (ack-TIN-ik) (ker-a-TŌ-sis)	precancerous skin condition of horny tissue formation that results from excessive exposure to sunlight (Figure 4-4, A). It may evolve into a squamous cell carcinoma.
albinism (AL-bi-niz-um)	congenital hereditary condition characterized by partial or total lack of pigment in the skin, hair, and eyes
basal cell carcinoma (BCC) (BĀ-sal) (sel) (kar-si-NŌ-ma)	epithelial tumor arising from the epidermis. It seldom metastasizes but invades local tissue (see Figure 4-4, C); common in individuals who have had excessive sun exposure.

🏛 **ABSCESS**
is derived from the Latin **ab**, meaning **from**, and **cedo**, meaning **to go**. The tissue dies and goes away, with the pus replacing it.

🏛 **ALBINISM**
Alb is Latin word root meaning **white**. **Leuk** is the Greek word root meaning **white**.

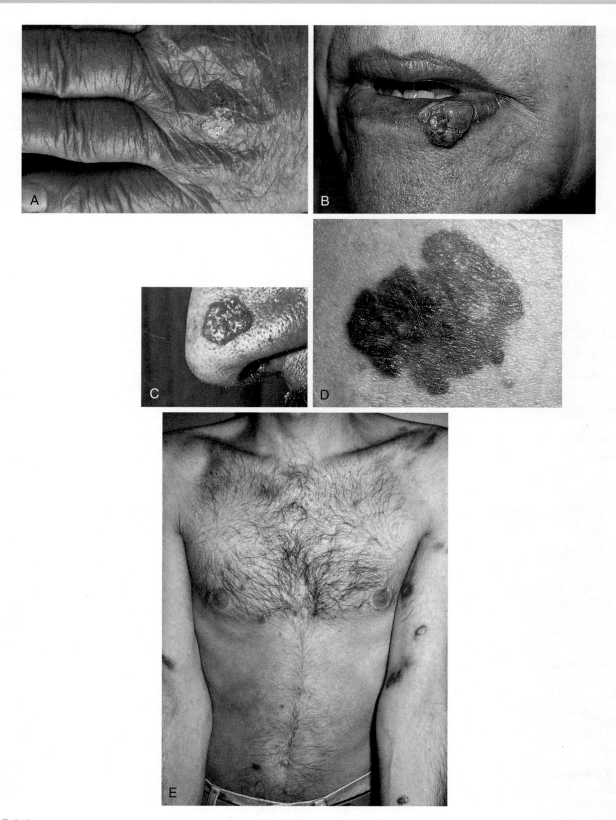

FIGURE 4-4
Percutaneous lesion and cancers of the skin. **A,** Actinic keratosis; **B,** squamous cell carcinoma; **C,** basal cell carcinoma; **D,** melanoma (covered in Chapter 2); **E,** Kaposi sarcoma.

Disease and Disorder Terms—cont'd

Not Built from Word Parts

TERM	DEFINITION
candidiasis (*kan*-di-DĪ-a-sis)	infection of the skin, mouth (also called **thrush**), or vagina caused by the yeast-type fungus *Candida albicans. Candida* is normally present in the mucous membranes; overgrowth causes an infection. Esophageal candidiasis is often seen in patients with AIDS (acquired immunodeficiency syndrome).
carbuncle (KAR-bung-kl)	skin infection composed of a cluster of boils (furuncle, see below) caused by staphylococcal bacteria
cellulitis (*sel*-ū-LĪ-tis)	inflammation of the skin and subcutaneous tissue caused by infection, characterized by redness, swelling, and fever
contusion (kon-TŪ-zhun)	injury with no break in the skin, characterized by pain, swelling, and discoloration (also called a **bruise**)
eczema (EK-ze-ma)	noninfectious, inflammatory skin disease characterized by redness, blisters, scabs, and itching
fissure (FISH-ur)	slit or cracklike sore in the skin
furuncle (FER-ung-kl)	painful skin node caused by staphylococcal bacteria in a hair follicle (also called a **boil**) (Figure 4-5)
gangrene (GANG-grēn)	death of tissue caused by loss of blood supply followed by bacterial invasion (a form of necrosis)
herpes (HER-pēz)	inflammatory skin disease caused by herpes virus characterized by small blisters in clusters. Many types of herpes exist. *Herpes simplex*, for example, causes fever blisters; *herpes zoster*, also called shingles, is characterized by painful skin eruptions that follow nerves inflamed by the virus (see Table 4-1, p. 106).
impetigo (*im*-pe-TĪ-gō)	superficial skin infection characterized by pustules and caused by either staphylococci or streptococci (see Table 4-1, p. 106)
infection (in-FEK-shun)	invasion of pathogens in body tissue. An acute infection may remain localized if the body's defense mechanisms are effective or may persist to become subacute or chronic (see sidebar p. 157). A systemic infection occurs when the pathogen causing a local infection gains access to the vascular or lymphatic system and becomes disseminated throughout the body. (See sepsis, p. 406.)

🏛 **CANDIDA**
comes from the Latin **candidus**, meaning gleaming white; **albicans** is from the Latin verb **albicare**, meaning **to make white**. The growth of the fungus is white, and the infection produces a white discharge.

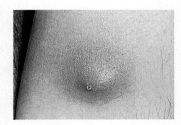

FIGURE 4-5
Furuncle resulting from a Staphylococcus aureus infection.

🏛 **HERPES**
is derived from the Greek **herpo**, meaning to **creep along**. It is descriptive of the course and type of skin lesion.

TYPES OF INFECTION

Infections may be caused by a bacterium, fungus, parasite, or virus. Examples of common skin infections are:

- **Bacterial infections**— carbuncle, cellulitis, furuncle, impetigo, MRSA infection, and paronychia
- **Fungal infections**— candidiasis, tinea, and trichomycosis
- **Parasitic infections**— scabies and pediculosis
- **Viral infections**—fever blister (*herpes simplex*) and shingles (*herpes zoster*)

Table 4-1
Common Skin Disorders

DISORDER	EXAMPLES
Impetigo (Bacterial infection)	
Tinea (fungal infection)	Tinea corporis (also called **ringworm**) Tinea pedis (also called **athlete's foot**)
Scabies (parasitic infection)	Scabies mite
Herpes zoster (also called **shingles**) (viral infection)	

Disease and Disorder Terms—cont'd

Not Built from Word Parts

TERM	DEFINITION
Kaposi sarcoma (KAP-ō-sē) (sar-KŌ-ma)	cancerous condition starting as purple or brown papules on the lower extremities that spreads through the skin to the lymph nodes and internal organs; frequently seen with AIDS (see Figure 4-4, *E*).
laceration (*las*-er-Ā-shun)	torn, ragged-edged wound
lesion (LĒ-zhun)	any visible change in tissue resulting from injury or disease. It is a broad term that includes sores, wounds, ulcers, and tumors.
MRSA infection (mer-SAH) (in-FEK-shun)	invasion of body tissue by methicillin-resistant *Staphylococcus aureus*, a strain of common bacteria that has developed resistance to methicillin and other antibiotics. It can produce skin and soft tissue infections and sometimes bloodstream infections and pneumonia, which can be fatal if not treated. MRSA is quite common in hospitals and long-term care facilities but is increasingly emerging as an important infection in the general population.
pediculosis (pe-*dik*-ū-LŌ-sis)	invasion into the skin and hair by lice
psoriasis (so-RĪ-a-sis)	chronic skin condition producing red lesions covered with silvery scales
rosacea (ro-ZĀ-shē-a)	chronic disorder of the skin that produces erythema, papules, pustules, and broken blood vessels, usually occurring on the central area of the face in people older than 30 years (Figure 4-6) (also called **acne rosacea**)
scabies (SKĀ-bēz)	skin infection caused by the itch mite, characterized by papule eruptions that are caused by the female burrowing into the outer layer of the skin and laying eggs. This condition is accompanied by severe itching (see Table 4-1, p. 106).
scleroderma (*skle*-rō-DER-ma)	disease characterized by chronic hardening (induration) of the connective tissue of the skin and other body organs
squamous cell carcinoma (SqCCA) (SQWĀ-mus) (sel) (*kar*-si-NŌ-ma)	malignant growth that develops from scalelike epithelial tissue. Unlike basal cell carcinoma, there is a significant potential for metastasis. The most frequent cause is chronic exposure to sunlight (see Figure 4-4, *B*).

TYPES OF SKIN LESIONS

Primary lesions are physical changes of the skin of pathological origin. **Secondary lesions** may result from changes in primary lesions or may be caused by injury or infection. **Vascular lesions** are related to blood vessels and include the escape of blood into the tissues (hemorrhage). Examples of types of skin lesions include:

- **Primary lesions**—macule, papule, nodule, wheal, vesicle, pustule, and cyst
- **Secondary lesions**—cicatrix (scar), keloid, and ulcer
- **Vascular lesions**—petechia, purpura, and ecchymosis

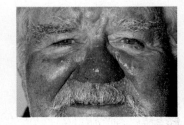

FIGURE 4-6
Rosacea.

CAM TERM

Light therapy is the therapeutic use of ultraviolet, colored, and laser lights to treat skin conditions, including **psoriasis**, **scleroderma**, and **vitiligo**, and seasonal affective disorder, as well as reduce pain and depression. Numerous studies have investigated and found clinical efficacy in the use of a variety of light therapies to rejuvenate damaged skin.

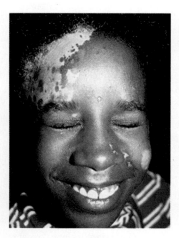

FIGURE 4-7
Vitiligo.

Disease and Disorder Terms—cont'd

Not Built from Word Parts

TERM	DEFINITION
systemic lupus erythematosus (SLE) (sis-TEM-ik) (LŪ-pus) (*e*-ri-*thē*-*ma*-TŌ-sus)	chronic inflammatory disease involving the skin, joints, kidneys, and nervous system. This autoimmune disease is characterized by periods of remission and exacerbations. It also may affect other organs.
tinea (TIN-ē-a)	fungal infection of the skin. The fungi may infect keratin of the skin, hair, and nails. Infections are classified by body regions such as *tinea capitis* (scalp), *tinea corporis* (body), and *tinea pedis* (foot). Tinea in general is also called **ringworm**, and tinea pedis specifically is also called **athlete's foot** (see Table 4-1, p. 106).
urticaria (*ur*-ti-KAR-ē-a)	itchy skin eruption composed of wheals (an individual hive) of varying sizes and shapes. Idiopathic urticaria is sometimes associated with infections and with allergic reactions to food, medicine, or other agents. Urticaria reaction can include swelling of the airways that can be a medical emergency. Other causes include internal disease, physical stimuli, and genetic disorders (also called **hives**) (see Table 4-2, p. 123).
vitiligo (*vit*-i-LĪ-gō)	white patches on the skin caused by the destruction of melanocytes associated with autoimmune disorders (Figure 4-7)

 To watch animations, go to evolve.elsevier.com. Select: Chapter 4, **Animations**, Acne.

Refer to p. 10 for your Evolve Access Information.

EXERCISE 14

Practice saying aloud each of the disease and disorder terms not built from word parts on pp. 103–108.

To hear the terms, go to evolve.elsevier.com. Select: Chapter 4, **Exercises**, Pronunciation.

Refer to p. 10 for your Evolve Access Information.

☐ Place a check mark in the box when you have completed this exercise.

EXERCISE 15

Fill in the blanks with the correct disease and disorder terms.

1. A chronic inflammatory disease affecting the skin, joints, and other organs is

    _____ _____ _____.

2. A(n) _____ is a localized collection of pus.

3. A cracklike sore in the skin is called a(n) _____.

4. The scraping away of the skin by mechanical process or injury is called a(n)

    _____.

5. _____ is a chronic skin condition characterized by red lesions
    covered with silvery scales.

6. An inflammatory skin disease caused by a virus and characterized by small
    blisters in clusters is called _____.

7. _____ is the name given to the invasion of the skin and hair by
    lice.

8. A fungal infection of the skin, also known as *ringworm*, is called

    _____.

9. An injury with no break in the skin and characterized by pain, swelling, and
    discoloration is called a(n) _____.

10. _____ is the name given to tissue death caused by a loss of
    blood supply followed by bacterial invasion.

11. Any visible change in tissue resulting from injury or disease is called a

    _____.

12. _____ _____ is a cancerous condition starting as
    purple or brown papules on the lower extremities.

13. A horny tissue formation that results from excessive exposure to sunlight and is
    precancerous is called _____ _____.

14. A cluster of boils caused by staphylococcal bacteria is a _____.

15. An inflammatory skin disease that involves the oil glands and hair follicles is
    called _____.

16. _____ is the name given to a torn, ragged-edged wound.

17. A painful skin node caused by staphylococcal bacteria in a hair follicle is called
    a(n) _____.

18. A malignant growth that develops from scalelike epithelial tissue is known as

    _____ _____ carcinoma.

19. Inflammation of the skin and subcutaneous tissue caused by infection
    characterized by redness, swelling, and fever is called _____.

20. _____ is the name given to a superficial skin infection
    characterized by pustules and caused by either staphylococci or streptococci.

21. _____ is a noninfectious inflammatory skin disease characterized
    by redness, blisters, scabs, and itching.

22. A skin inflammation caused by the itch mite is called _____.

23. _____ is an itchy skin eruption composed of wheals.

24. An epithelial tumor commonly found on the face of individuals who have had
    excessive sun exposure is _____ _____ carcinoma.

25. _____ is a disease characterized by induration of the connective tissue.

26. _____ is an infection of the mouth, skin, or vagina caused by *Candida albicans*.

27. An invasion of pathogens in body tissue is called _____.

28. _____ is a chronic disorder of the skin on the central area of the face that produces erythema, papules, pustules, and broken blood vessels.

29. A congenital hereditary condition characterized by partial or total lack of pigment in the skin, hair, and eyes is _____.

30. _____ _____ is an invasion of methicillin-resistant *Staphylococcus aureus* in the body tissue.

31. White patches on the skin caused by the destruction of melanocytes is called _____.

EXERCISE 16

Match the words in the first column with their correct definitions in the second column.

_____ 1. abrasion

_____ 2. abscess

_____ 3. acne

_____ 4. actinic keratosis

_____ 5. basal cell carcinoma

_____ 6. carbuncle

_____ 7. cellulitis

_____ 8. contusion

_____ 9. eczema

_____ 10. fissure

_____ 11. furuncle

_____ 12. gangrene

_____ 13. scleroderma

_____ 14. rosacea

_____ 15. MRSA infection

a. death of tissue caused by loss of blood supply and entry of bacteria

b. cracklike sore in the skin

c. cluster of boils

d. chronic induration of connective tissue of the skin and other body organs

e. noninfectious inflammatory skin disease having redness, blisters, scabs, and itching

f. scraped-away skin

g. involves sebaceous glands and hair follicles

h. painful skin node caused by staphylococci in a hair follicle

i. inflammation of skin and subcutaneous tissue with redness, swelling, and fever

j. localized collection of pus

k. injury characterized by pain, swelling, and discoloration

l. precancerous skin condition caused by excessive exposure to sunlight

m. usually occurring in the central area of the face in people older than 30 years

n. epithelial tumor commonly found in individuals who have had excessive sun exposure

o. red lesions with silvery scales

p. potentially serious infection caused by methicillin-resistant *Staphylococcus aureus*

EXERCISE 17

Match the words in the first column with the correct definitions in the second column.

_____ 1. herpes

_____ 2. impetigo

_____ 3. Kaposi sarcoma

_____ 4. laceration

_____ 5. lesion

_____ 6. pediculosis

_____ 7. psoriasis

_____ 8. scabies

_____ 9. squamous cell carcinoma

_____ 10. systemic lupus erythematosus

_____ 11. tinea

_____ 12. urticaria

_____ 13. candidiasis

_____ 14. infection

_____ 15. albinism

_____ 16. vitiligo

a. skin inflammation caused by the itch mite

b. fungal infection of the skin, hair, and nails

c. red lesions covered by silvery scales

d. inflammatory skin disease having clusters of blisters and caused by a virus

e. chronic inflammatory disease involving the skin, joints, kidney, and nervous system

f. cancerous condition that starts as brown or purple papules on the lower extremities

g. composed of wheals

h. torn, ragged-edged wound

i. superficial skin condition having pustules and caused by staphylococci or streptococci

j. characterized by lack of pigment in the skin, hair, and eyes

k. infection of the skin, mouth, or vagina caused by a yeast-type fungus

l. invasion of the hair and skin by lice

m. visible change in tissue resulting from injury or disease

n. malignant growth that develops from scalelike epithelial tissue

o. invasion of body tissue by pathogens

p. cracklike sore in the skin

q. white patches on the skin caused by the destruction of melanocytes

EXERCISE 18

Spell each of the disease and disorder terms not built from word parts on pp. 103–108 by having someone dictate them to you.

> To hear and spell the terms, go to evolve.elsevier.com. Select: Chapter 4, **Exercises**, Spelling.
>
> (e) Refer to p. 10 for your Evolve Access Information.
>
> ☐ Place a check mark in the box if you have completed this exercise online.

1. _____

2. _____

3. _____

4. _____

5. _____

6. _____

7. _____

8. _____

9. _____

10. _____

11. _____

12. _____

13. _____

14. _____

15. _____

16. _____

17. _____   25. _____

18. _____   26. _____

19. _____   27. _____

20. _____   28. _____

21. _____   29. _____

22. _____   30. _____

23. _____   31. _____

24. _____

BIOPSY OF THE SKIN

may be performed by the dermatologist during an office visit. Common techniques include:

- excisional biopsy removes the entire lesion along with a margin of surrounding tissue
- punch biopsy removes a cylindrical portion of tissue with a specifically designed round knife (see Figure 4-8)
- shave biopsy removes a sample of tissue with a cut parallel to the surrounding skin

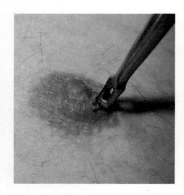

FIGURE 4-8
Punch biopsy.

DERMATOME

also refers to the dermatomic area, the area of skin supplied by a specific sensory nerve root.

Surgical Terms

Built from Word Parts

The following terms are built from word parts you have already learned and can be translated literally to find their meanings. Further explanation of terms beyond the definition of their word parts, if needed, is included in parentheses.

TERM	DEFINITION
biopsy (bx) (BĪ-op-sē)	view of life (the removal of living tissue from the body to be viewed under the microscope) (Figure 4-8)
dermatoautoplasty (*der*-ma-tō-AW-tō-*plas*-tē)	surgical repair using one's own skin (skin graft) (also called **autograft**)
dermatoheteroplasty (*der*-ma-tō-HET-er-ō *plas*-tē)	surgical repair using skin from others (skin graft) (also called **allograft**)
dermatome (DER-ma-tōm) *Note: when two consonants of the same letter come together, one is sometimes dropped.*	instrument used to cut skin (in thin slices for skin grafts)
dermatoplasty (DER-ma-tō-*plas*-tē)	surgical repair of the skin
onychectomy (*on*-i-KEK-to-mē)	excision of a nail
rhytidectomy (*rit*-i-DEK-to-mē)	excision of wrinkles (also called **facelift**)
rhytidoplasty (RIT-i-dō-*plas*-tē)	surgical repair of wrinkles

To watch animations, go to evolve.elsevier.com. Select: Chapter 4, **Animations**, Punch Biopsy

Refer to p. 10 for your Evolve Access Information.

EXERCISE 19

Practice saying aloud each of the surgical terms built from word parts.

> To hear the terms, go to evolve.elsevier.com. Select: Chapter 4, **Exercises**, Pronunciation.
>
> Refer to p. 10 for your Evolve access information.

☐ Place a check mark in the box when you have completed this exercise.

EXERCISE 20

Analyze and define the following surgical terms.

                        WR   CV   S
EXAMPLE: dermat / o / plasty   surgical repair of the skin
                        CF

1. rhytidectomy_____

2. biopsy _____

3. dermatoautoplasty _____

4. onychectomy_____

5. rhytidoplasty_____

6. dermatoheteroplasty_____

7. dermatome _____

EXERCISE 21

Build surgical terms for the following definitions by using the word parts you have learned.

EXAMPLE: surgical repair using one's own skin   dermat /o /aut /o / plasty
                                                      WR /CV/ WR /CV/ S

1. excision of wrinkles   _____
                               WR   /   S

2. view of life (removal of living
   tissue from the body)   _____
                               WR   /   S

3. surgical repair using skin
   from others   _____
                               WR   /CV/ WR   /CV/ S

4. excision of a nail   _____
                               WR   /   S

5. surgical repair of wrinkles _____
                               WR   /CV/   S

6. surgical repair of the skin _____
                               WR   /CV/   S

7. instrument used to cut skin _____
                               WR   /   S

EXERCISE 22

Spell each of the surgical terms built from word parts on p. 112 by having someone dictate them to you.

To hear and spell the terms, go to evolve.elsevier.com. Select: Chapter 4, **Exercises**, Spelling.

Refer to p. 10 for your Evolve Access Information.

☐ Place a check mark in the box if you have completed this exercise online.

1. _____   5. _____

2. _____   6. _____

3. _____   7. _____

4. _____   8. _____

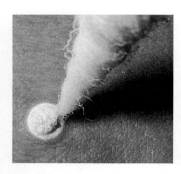

FIGURE 4-9
Cryosurgery performed with a nitrogen-soaked, cotton-tipped applicator.

🏛 **MOHS SURGERY**
allows for complete tumor removal while sparing surrounding normal tissue. It includes removing layers of tissue and examining them for tumor cells. If found, more tissue is removed until the margins are cancer free. It is used to treat skin cancers, especially lesions on the nose and ears, or areas that need tissue sparing. It is named after **Dr. Frederic E. Mohs**, Wisconsin, who first used the concept in 1936. The technique has evolved since that time.

Surgical Terms

Not Built from Word Parts

In some of the following terms, you may recognize word parts you have already learned; however, the full meaning of the terms cannot be discerned by the definition of their word parts.

TERM	DEFINITION
cauterization (*kaw*-tur-ī-ZĀ-shun)	destruction of tissue with a hot or cold instrument, electric current, or caustic substance (also called **cautery**)
cryosurgery (*krī*-ō-SER-jer-ē)	destruction of tissue by using extreme cold, often by using liquid nitrogen (Figure 4-9)
débridement (dā-brēd-MA)	removal of contaminated or dead tissue and foreign matter from an open wound
dermabrasion (*derm*-a-BRĀ-zhun)	procedure to remove skin scars with abrasive material, such as sandpaper
excision (ek-SIZH-en)	removal by cutting
incision (in-SIZH-en)	surgical cut or wound produced by a sharp instrument
incision and drainage (I&D) (in-SIZH-en) and (DRĀ-nij)	surgical cut made to allow the free flow or withdrawal of fluids from a lesion, wound, or cavity
laser surgery (LĀ-zer) (SER-jer-ē)	procedure using an instrument that emits a high-powered beam of light used to cut, burn, vaporize, or destroy tissue
Mohs surgery (mōz) (SER-jer-ē)	technique of microscopically controlled serial excisions of a skin cancer
suturing (SOO-cher-ing)	to stitch edges of a wound surgically (Figure 4-10)

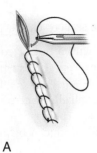
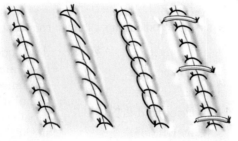

A   B   Intermittent   Continuous   Blanket   Retention
                                 continuous

FIGURE 4-10
A, Suturing; **B,** types of sutures.

EXERCISE 23

Practice saying aloud each of the surgical terms not built from word parts on p. 114.

> To hear the terms, go to evolve.elsevier.com. Select: Chapter 4, **Exercises**, Pronunciation.
>
> Refer to p. 10 for your Evolve Access Information.

☐ Place a check mark in the box when you have completed this exercise.

EXERCISE 24

Fill in the blank with the correct surgical term.

1. _____ _____ is a technique of microscopically controlled serial excisions used for treatment of many skin cancers.

2. A surgical cut or wound produced by a sharp instrument is called a(n)

   _____.

3. Destruction of tissue with a hot or cold instrument, electric current, or caustic substance is called _____.

4. _____ is to stitch the edges of a wound surgically.

5. A surgical cut made to allow the free flow or withdrawal of fluids from a lesion, wound, or cavity is called _____ _____

   _____.

6. _____ is the removal of contaminated or dead tissue and foreign matter from an open wound.

7. Removal by cutting is known as _____.

8. _____ _____ is a procedure using an instrument that emits a high-powered beam of light used to cut, burn, vaporize, or destroy tissue.

9. The destruction of tissue by using extreme cold, often by using liquid nitrogen, is called _____.

10. _____ is a procedure to remove skin scars with abrasive material.

EXERCISE 25

Match the terms in the first column with their correct definitions in the second column.

_____ 1. suturing
_____ 2. dermabrasion
_____ 3. laser surgery
_____ 4. incision and drainage
_____ 5. cauterization
_____ 6. excision
_____ 7. Mohs surgery
_____ 8. débridement
_____ 9. cryosurgery
_____ 10. incision

a. destruction of tissue with a hot or cold instrument, electric current, or caustic substance
b. technique of microscopically controlled serial excisions of a skin cancer
c. surgical cut or wound produced by a sharp instrument
d. surgical cut made to allow the free flow or withdrawal of fluids from a lesion, wound, or cavity
e. removal by cutting
f. removal of contaminated or dead tissue and foreign matter from an open wound
g. procedure using an instrument that emits a high-powered beam of light used to cut, burn, vaporize, or destroy tissue
h. procedure to remove skin scars with abrasive material, such as sandpaper
i. to stitch edges of a wound surgically
j. destruction of tissue by using extreme cold, often by using liquid nitrogen

EXERCISE 26

Spell each of the surgical terms not built from word parts on p. 114 by having someone dictate them to you.

> To hear and spell the terms, go to evolve.elsevier.com. Select: Chapter 4, **Exercises**, Spelling.
>
> Refer to p. 10 for your Evolve Access Information.
>
> ☐ Place a check mark in the box if you have completed this exercise online.

1. _____   6. _____

2. _____   7. _____

3. _____   8. _____

4. _____   9. _____

5. _____   10. _____

Complementary Terms

Built from Word Parts

The following terms are built from word parts you have already learned and can be translated literally to find their meanings. Further explanation of terms beyond the definition of their word parts, if needed, is included in parentheses.

TERM	DEFINITION
dermatologist (*der*-ma-TOL-o-jist)	physician who studies and treats skin (diseases)
dermatology (derm) (der-ma-TOL-o-jē)	study of the skin (a branch of medicine that deals with the diagnosis and treatment of skin diseases)
epidermal (*ep*-i-DER-mal)	pertaining to upon the skin
erythroderma (e-rith-rō-DER-ma)	red skin (abnormal redness of the skin) (Figure 4-11)
hypodermic (*hī*-pō-DER-mik)	pertaining to under the skin (Exercise Figure D)
intradermal (ID) (*in*-tra-DER-mal)	pertaining to within the skin (see Exercise Figure D)
keratogenic (*ker*-a-tō-JEN-ik)	originating in horny tissue
necrosis (ne-KRŌ-sis)	abnormal condition of death (cells and tissue die because of disease)
percutaneous (*per*-kū-TĀ-nē-us)	pertaining to through the skin
staphylococcus (pl. staphylococci) (staph) (*staf*-il-ō-KOK-us) (*staf*-il-ō-KOK-sī)	berry-shaped (bacterium) in grapelike clusters (these bacteria cause many skin diseases) (Exercise Figure E)
streptococcus (pl. streptococci) (strep) (*strep*-tō-KOK-us) (*strep*-tō-KOK-sī)	berry-shaped (bacterium) in twisted chains (see Exercise Figure E)
subcutaneous (subcut) (*sub*-kū-TĀ-nē-us)	pertaining to under the skin (see Exercise Figure D)
transdermal (TD) (trans-DER-mel)	pertaining to through the skin (see Exercise Figure D)
ungual (UNG-gwal)	pertaining to the nail
xanthoderma (*zan*-thō-DER-ma)	yellow skin (also called **jaundice**)

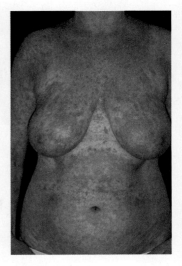

FIGURE 4-11
Exfoliative erythroderma. Erythroderma (red skin) may be caused by drugs, malignancy, psoriasis, and other conditions.

TRANSDERMAL
usually means entering through the skin and refers to the administration of a drug applied to the skin in ointment or patch form. **Percutaneous** usually means performed through the skin, as in the insertion of a needle, catheter, or probe. See **percutaneous endoscopic gastrostomy** highlighted in Chapter 11 (Exercise Figure G).

EXERCISE FIGURE D

Fill in the blanks to build terms, related to the routes of administration pictured below.

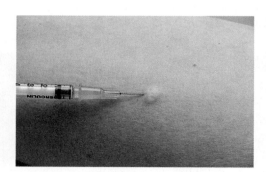

1. _____ / _____ / _____ injection
   within / skin / pertaining to

   Intradermal

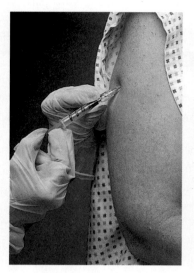

2. *sub* / *cutaneous* injection
   under / skin / pertaining to

   using a *hypodermic* needle
   under / skin / pertaining to

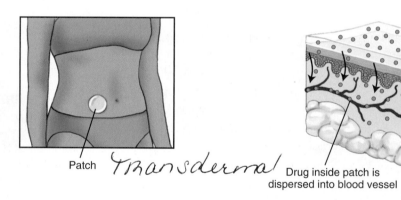

Patch   *Transdermal*   Drug inside patch is
dispersed into blood vessel

Patch
Epidermis
Dermis
Fat

3. _____ / _____ / _____ patch
   through / skin / pertaining to

EXERCISE 27

Practice saying aloud each of the complementary terms built from word parts on p. 117.

> To hear the terms, go to evolve.elsevier.com. Select: Chapter 4, **Exercises**, Pronunciation.
>
> Refer to p. 10 for your Evolve Access Information.

☐ Place a check mark in the box when you have completed this exercise.

EXERCISE 28

Analyze and define the following complementary terms.

	P WR S	
EXAMPLE:	intra / derm / al	pertaining to within the skin

1. ungual _____

2. transdermal _____

3. streptococcus _____

4. hypodermic _____

5. dermatology _____

6. subcutaneous _____

7. staphylococcus _____

8. keratogenic _____

9. dermatologist _____

10. necrosis _____

11. epidermal _____

12. xanthoderma _____

13. erythroderma _____

14. percutaneous _____

EXERCISE 29

Build complementary terms for the integumentary system by using the word parts you have learned.

EXAMPLE: pertaining to under the skin $\dfrac{\text{hypo} / \text{derm} / \text{ic}}{\text{P} / \text{WR} / \text{S}}$

1. study of the skin

  _____
  WR   /CV/   S

2. abnormal condition of death
   (of cells and tissue)

  _____
  WR   /   S

3. pertaining to the nail

  _____
  WR   /   S

4. berry-shaped (bacterium) in
   grapelike clusters (singular)

  _____
  WR   /CV/   S

EXERCISE FIGURE **E**

Fill in the blanks to label the diagrams.

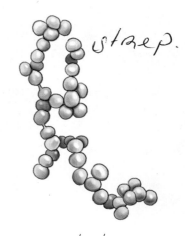

strep.

1. _____ / _____ / _____
   grapelike / cv / berry-shaped
   clusters   (plural)

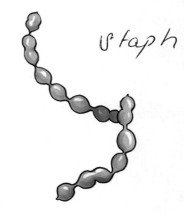

staph

2. _____ / _____ / _____
   twisted / CV / berry-shaped
   chains   (plural)

5. a physician who studies and treats skin (diseases)

_____ /_____/ _____
WR   CV   S

6. pertaining to within the skin

_____ /_____/ _____
P   WR   S

7. pertaining to upon the skin

_____ /_____/ _____
P   WR   S

8. pertaining to under the skin

_____ /_____/ _____
P   WR   S

_____ /_____/ _____
P   WR   S

9. berry-shaped (bacterium) in twisted chains (singular)

_____ /_____/ _____
WR   CV   S

10. originating in the horny tissue

_____ /_____/ _____
WR   CV   S

11. red skin

_____ /____/ _____ /____
WR   CV   WR   S

12. yellow skin

_____ /____/ _____ /____
WR   CV   WR   S

13. pertaining to through the skin

_____ /_____/ _____
P   WR   S

_____ /_____/ _____
P   WR   S

EXERCISE 30

Spell each of the complementary terms built from word parts on p. 117 by having someone dictate them to you.

> To hear and spell the terms, go to evolve.elsevier.com. Select: Chapter 4, **Exercises**, Spelling.
>
> (e) Refer to p. 10 for your Evolve Access Information.
>
> ☐ Place a check mark in the box if you have completed this exercise online.

1. _____   9. _____
2. _____   10. _____
3. _____   11. _____
4. _____   12. _____
5. _____   13. _____
6. _____   14. _____
7. _____   15. _____
8. _____

> For more practice **building medical terms**, go to evolve.elsevier.com. Select:
> Chapter 4, **Activities,** Terms Built from Word Parts
> (e) Chapter 4, **Games,**   Term Storm
>
> Refer to p. 10 for your Evolve Access Information.

Complementary Terms

Not Built from Word Parts

In some of the following terms, you may recognize word parts you have already learned; however, the full meaning of the terms cannot be discerned by the definition of their word parts.

TERM	DEFINITION
alopecia (*al*-ō-PĒ-sha)	loss of hair (Figure 4-12)
bacteria (s. bacterium) (bak-TĒR-ē-a) (bak-TĒR-ē-um)	single-celled microorganisms that reproduce by cell division and may cause infection by invading body tissue
cicatrix (SIK-a-triks)	scar
cyst (sist)	closed sac containing fluid or semisolid material (Table 4-2, p. 123)
cytomegalovirus (CMV) (*sī*-to-MEG-a-lō-*vī*-rus)	herpes-type virus that usually causes disease when the immune system is compromised
diaphoresis (*dī*-a-fo-RĒ-sis)	sweating
ecchymosis (pl. ecchymoses) (*ek*-i-MŌ-sis) (*ek*-i-MŌ-sēz)	escape of blood into the skin (or mucous membrane), causing a small, flat, purple, or blue discoloration, as may occur when blood is withdrawn by a needle and syringe from an arm vein
edema (e-DĒ-ma)	puffy swelling of tissue from the accumulation of fluid
erythema (*er*-i-THĒ-ma)	redness
fungus (pl. fungi) (FUN-gus) (FUN-jī)	organism that feeds by absorbing organic molecules from its surroundings and may cause infection by invading body tissue; single-celled fungi (yeast) reproduce by budding; multicelled fungi (mold) reproduce by spore formation
induration (*in*-dū-RĀ-shun)	abnormal hard spot(s)
jaundice (JAWN-dis)	condition characterized by a yellow tinge to the skin (also called **xanthoderma**)
keloid (KĒ-loyd)	overgrowth of scar tissue (Figure 4-13)
leukoplakia (*lū*-kō-PLĀ-kē-a)	condition characterized by white spots or patches on mucous membrane, which may be precancerous
macule (MAK-ūl)	flat, colored spot on the skin (see Table 4-2, p. 123)

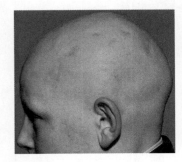

FIGURE 4-12

Alopecia totalis (loss of hair from the scalp) with absence of eyelashes.

🏛 **ALOPECIA**

is derived from the Greek **alopex**, meaning **fox**. One was thought to bald like a mangy fox.

🏛 **DIAPHORESIS**

is derived from Greek **dia**, meaning **through**, and **phoreo**, meaning **carry**. Translated, it means the carrying through of perspiration.

ECCHYMOSIS, PETECHIA, AND PURPURA

are vascular lesions related to blood vessels and the escape of blood into the skin and mucous membrane (hemorrhage). They vary in size, with petechia being the smallest in size, up to .5 cm; purpura being the next largest, up to 1 cm; and ecchymosis being the largest, between 1 and 2 cm.

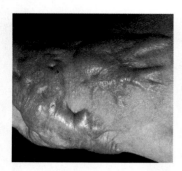

FIGURE 4-13
Burn keloid.

🏛 **PETECHIA**
is originally from the Italian
petechio, meaning **flea bite**.
The small hemorrhagic spot
resembles the mark made by a
flea.

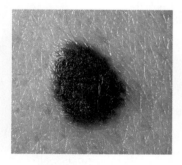

FIGURE 4-14
Nevus (also called *mole*).

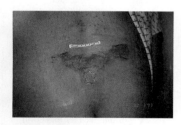

FIGURE 4-15
Stage 2 pressure ulcer (formerly
called ***decubitus ulcer*** or ***bed
sore***).

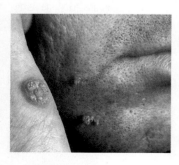

FIGURE 4-16
Verruca (also called *wart*).

Complementary Terms—cont'd

Not Built from Word Parts

TERM	DEFINITION
nevus (pl. nevi) (NĒ-vus) (NĒ-vī)	circumscribed malformation of the skin, usually brown, black, or flesh colored. A congenital nevus is present at birth and is referred to as a birthmark (Figure 4-14) (also called a **mole**).
nodule (NOD-ūl)	small, knotlike mass that can be felt by touch (Table 4-2)
pallor (PAL-or)	paleness
papule (PAP-ūl)	small, solid skin elevation (see Table 4-2)
petechia (pl. petechiae) (pe-TĒ-kē-a) (pe-TĒ-kē-ē)	pinpoint skin hemorrhage
pressure ulcer (decub) (PRESH-ur) (UL-sir)	erosion of the skin caused by prolonged pressure, often occurring in bedridden patients (Figure 4-15) (formerly called **decubitus ulcer** or **bed sore**)
pruritus (prū-RĪ-tus)	itching
purpura (PER-pū-ra)	small hemorrhages in the skin (or mucous membrane), giving a purple-red discoloration; associated with blood disorders or vascular abnormalities
pustule (PUS-tūl)	elevation of skin containing pus (see Table 4-2)
ulcer (UL-ser)	erosion of the skin or mucous membrane (Figures 4-15 and 4-17)
verruca (ver-RŪ-ka)	circumscribed cutaneous elevation caused by a virus (Figure 4-16) (also called **wart**)
vesicle (VES-i-kl)	small elevation of the epidermis containing liquid (see Table 4-2) (also called **blister**)
virus (VĪ-ras)	minute microorganism, much smaller than a bacterium, characterized by a lack of independent metabolism and the ability to replicate only within living host cells; may cause infection by invading body tissue
wheal (hwēl)	transitory, itchy elevation of the skin with a white center and a red surrounding area; a wheal is an individual urticaria (hive) lesion (see Table 4-2)

 To watch animations, go to evolve.elsevier.com. Select: Chapter 4, **Animations**, Pressure Ulcer.
Refer to p. 10 for your Evolve Access Information.

🔍 Refer to **Appendix D** for pharmacology terms related to the integumentary system.

Table 4-2

Common Skin Lesions

LESION	DEFINITION	CUTAWAY SECTIONS	EXAMPLE
Macule	flat, colored spot on the skin		freckle
Papule	small, solid skin elevation		skin tag basal cell carcinoma
Nodule	a small, knotlike mass		lipoma metastatic carcinoma rheumatoid nodule
Wheal	round, itchy elevation of the skin		urticaria (hive)
Vesicle	small elevation of epidermis containing liquid		herpes zoster (shingles) herpes simplex contact dermatitis
Pustule	elevation of the skin containing pus		impetigo acne
Cyst	a closed sac containing fluid or semisolid material		acne

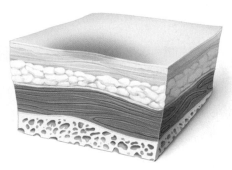

Stage I Nonblanching erythema, skin intact.

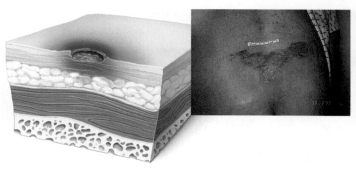

Stage II Partial thickness of skin loss involving the epidermis, dermis or both.

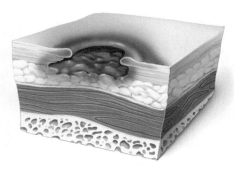

Stage III Full thickness of skin loss involving damage or necrosis to subcutaneous tissue.

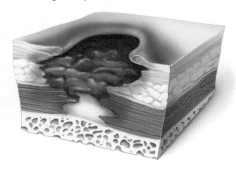

Stage IV Full thickness of skin loss with extensive destruction, tissue necrosis, possible damage to muscle and bone tissue and other supporting structures.

FIGURE 4-17
Stages of pressure ulcer. Stage I, nonblanching erythema, skin intact. **Stage II,** partial thickness of skin loss involving the epidermis, dermis, or both. **Stage III,** full thickness of skin loss involving damage or necrosis to subcutaneous tissue. **Stage IV,** full thickness skin loss with extensive destruction, tissue necrosis, possible damage to muscle and bone tissue and other supporting structures.

DERMATOLOGY, OR GIVE ME A MAN WHO CALLS A SPADE A GEOTOME

I wish the dermatologist
Were less a firm apologist
For all the terminology
That's used in dermatology

Something you or I would deem a
Redness he calls erythema;
If it's blistered, raw and warm he
Has to call it multiforme
Things to him are never simple;
Papule is his word for pimple
What's a macule, clearly stated?
Just a spot that's over-rated!
Over the skin that looks unwell
He chants Latin like a spell;
What he's labeled and obscured
Looks to him as good as cured.

Reprinted with permission from The New England Journal of Medicine, 1977; 297(12):660.

EXERCISE 31

Practice saying aloud each of the complementary terms not built from word parts on pp. 121–122.

> To hear the terms, go to evolve.elsevier.com. Select: Chapter 4, **Exercises**, Pronunciation.
> Refer to p. 10 for your Evolve Access Information.

☐ Place a check mark in the box when you have completed this exercise.

EXERCISE 32

Fill in the blanks with the correct terms.

1. Another name for scar is _____.

2. Sweating is called _____.

3. The medical term for wart is _____.

4. _____ is the name for a flat, colored skin spot.

5. A yellow skin condition is known as _____.

6. The condition of white spots or patches on mucous membrane is called

_____.

7. _____ is a pinpoint hemorrhage of the skin.

8. An erosion of the skin or mucous membrane is called a(n) _____.

9. A(n) _____ is an overgrowth of scar tissue.

10. Another name for paleness is _____.

11. Small, flat, purple or blue skin discoloration caused by hemorrhage, as seen after blood has been withdrawn by needle and syringe, is referred to as

_____.

12. An erosion of the skin caused by prolonged pressure is a(n) _____.

13. A small knotlike mass that can be felt by touch is called a(n) _____.

14. A closed sac containing fluid or semisolid material is called a(n)

_____.

15. Itching is called _____.

16. Another name for redness is _____.

17. Small hemorrhages in the skin, showing a purple-red discoloration and associated with blood disorders or vascular abnormalities, is known as

_____.

18. _____ is another name for mole.

19. Single-celled microorganisms that reproduce by cell division and may cause

infection by invading body tissue are called _____.

20. The term for loss of hair is _____.

21. A small, solid skin elevation is called a(n) _____.

22. A transitory skin elevation with a white center and a red surrounding area is

a(n) _____.

23. A(n) _____ is a skin elevation containing pus.

24. A blister is also called a(n) _____.

25. An organism that feeds by absorbing organic molecules from its surroundings

and may cause infection by invading body tissue is called _____.

26. A(n) _____ is a minute microorganism characterized by a lack of independent metabolism and the ability to replicate only within living host cells; it also may cause infection by invading body tissue.

27. An abnormal hard spot(s) is called _____.

28. _____ is the swelling of tissue.

29. _____ is a herpes-type virus.

EXERCISE 33

Match the words in the first column with their correct definitions in the second column.

_____ 1. pressure ulcer
_____ 2. alopecia
_____ 3. cicatrix
_____ 4. fungus
_____ 5. nodule
_____ 6. bacteria
_____ 7. diaphoresis
_____ 8. cyst
_____ 9. ecchymosis
_____ 10. erythema
_____ 11. jaundice
_____ 12. edema
_____ 13. induration

a. loss of hair
b. small, flat, purple or blue discoloration caused by blood escaping into the skin or mucous membrane
c. yellow color to the skin
d. closed sac containing fluid
e. organism that feeds by absorbing organic molecules from its surroundings and may cause infection by invading body tissue
f. patches
g. sweating
h. swelling of tissue
i. hard spot(s)
j. scar
k. redness
l. single-celled microorganisms that reproduce by cell division and may cause infection by invading body tissue
m. erosion of the skin caused by prolonged pressure
n. small knotlike mass

EXERCISE 34

Match the terms in the first column with their correct definitions in the second column.

_____ 1. keloid
_____ 2. leukoplakia
_____ 3. macule
_____ 4. nevus
_____ 5. pallor
_____ 6. papule
_____ 7. petechiae
_____ 8. pruritus
_____ 9. purpura
_____ 10. pustule
_____ 11. ulcer
_____ 12. verruca
_____ 13. vesicle
_____ 14. wheal
_____ 15. virus
_____ 16. cytomegalovirus

a. mole
b. itching
c. wart
d. condition of white spots or patches on mucous membranes
e. hemorrhages in the skin showing a purple-red color
f. skin elevation containing pus
g. overgrowth of scar tissue
h. small elevation of epidermis containing liquid
i. individual urticaria lesion
j. flat, colored spot on skin
k. small, solid skin elevation
l. paleness
m. minute microorganism characterized by a lack of independent metabolism and the ability to replicate only within living host cells that may cause infection by invading body tissue
n. pinpoint skin hemorrhages
o. erosion of the skin or mucous membrane
p. sweating
q. herpes-type virus

EXERCISE 35

Spell each of the complementary terms not built from word parts on pp. 121–122 by having someone dictate them to you.

To hear and spell the terms, go to evolve.elsevier.com. Select: Chapter 4, **Exercises**, Spelling.

Refer to p. 10 for your Evolve Access Information.

☐ Place a check mark in the box if you have completed this exercise online.

1. _____
2. _____
3. _____
4. _____
5. _____
6. _____
7. _____
8. _____
9. _____
10. _____
11. _____
12. _____
13. _____
14. _____
15. _____
16. _____
17. _____
18. _____
19. _____
20. _____
21. _____
22. _____
23. _____
24. _____
25. _____
26. _____
27. _____
28. _____
29. _____

For review and/or assessment, go to evolve.elsevier.com. Select:
Chapter 4, **Activities**, Terms Not Built from Word Parts
                 Hear It and Type It: Clinical Vignettes
Chapter 4, **Games**,   Term Explorer
                 Termbusters
                 Medical Millionaire

Refer to p. 10 for your Evolve Access Information.

Abbreviations

ABBREVIATION	MEANING
BCC	basal cell carcinoma
bx	biopsy
CMV	cytomegalovirus
CA-MRSA	community-associated MRSA infection
decub	pressure ulcer
derm	dermatology
HA-MRSA	healthcare-associated MRSA infection
I&D	incision and drainage
ID	intradermal
MRSA	methicillin-resistant *Staphylococcus aureus*
SLE	systemic lupus erythematosus
SqCCA	squamous cell carcinoma

Abbreviations—cont'd

ABBREVIATION	MEANING
staph	staphylococcus
strep	streptococcus
subcut	subcutaneous
TD	transdermal

Refer to **Appendix C** for a complete list of abbreviations.

EXERCISE 36

Write the meaning for each of the abbreviations in the following sentences.

1. The most common form of skin cancer is **BCC** _____ _____ _____.

2. Cutaneous **CMV** _____ infections are rarely seen in general medical practice.

3. **SLE** _____ is a chronic relapsing disease, often with long periods of remission.

4. Long-term exposure to sunlight is by far the most frequent cause of **SqCCA** _____ _____ _____.

5. The **bx** _____ results were negative.

6. The medication was administered by **subcut** _____ injection.

7. **Staph** _____ bacterium was cultured from the abscess.

8. The culture confirmed a **strep** _____ infection of the throat.

9. **I&D** _____ _____ _____ is used to treat cutaneous abscesses, such as a furuncle.

10. Hormone replacement therapy is available in **TD** _____ _____ _____ administration.

11. The tuberculin test was administered by an **ID** _____ injection.

12. The patient visited the **derm** _____ clinic for a psoriasis follow-up visit.

13. Débridement may be used to treat a **decub** _____ _____.

14. **MRSA** _____ _____ _____ _____ infections originating in a healthcare setting are called **HA-MRSA** _____ _____ _____ _____, whereas MRSA infections occurring in a person who has not recently been in a healthcare setting is called **CA-MRSA** _____ _____ _____ _____.

For more practice with abbreviations, go to evolve.elsevier.com. Select:
Chapter 4, **Flashcards**
Chapter 4, **Games**, Crossword Puzzle

Refer to p. 10 for your Evolve Access Information.

PRACTICAL APPLICATION

EXERCISE 37 *Interact with Medical Documents*

A. Below is an operative report. Complete the report by writing the medical terms in the blanks that correspond to the numbered definitions on the next page.

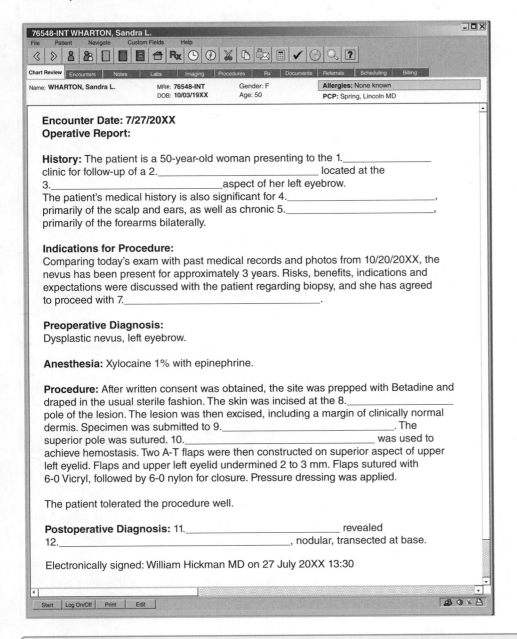

1. study of skin
2. mole
3. pertaining to the middle
4. precancerous skin condition of horny tissue formation
5. noninfectious, inflammatory skin disease with redness, blisters, scabs, and itching
6. changes in tissue resulting from injury or disease
7. removal by cutting
8. pertaining to above
9. study of disease
10. destruction of tissue with a hot or cold instrument, electric current, or caustic substance
11. view of life
12. epithelial tumor arising from epidermis

B. Read the pathology report and answer the questions following it.

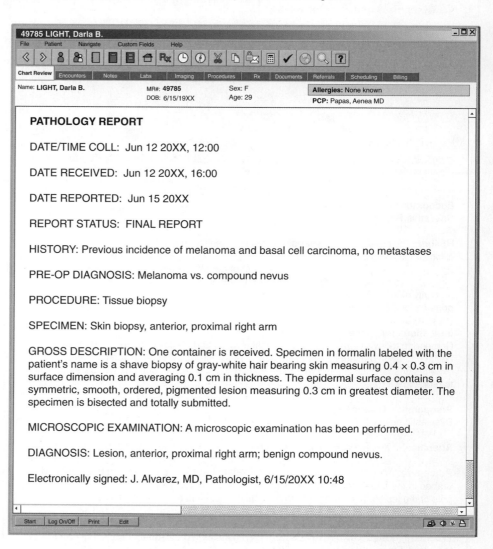

Pathology Report (chart window)

49785 LIGHT, Darla B.

File   Patient   Navigate   Custom Fields   Help

Chart Review | Encounters | Notes | Labs | Imaging | Procedures | Rx | Documents | Referrals | Scheduling | Billing

Name: **LIGHT, Darla B.**   MR#: **49785**   Sex: F   **Allergies:** None known
DOB: 6/15/19XX   Age: 29   **PCP:** Papas, Aenea MD

PATHOLOGY REPORT

DATE/TIME COLL: Jun 12 20XX, 12:00

DATE RECEIVED: Jun 12 20XX, 16:00

DATE REPORTED: Jun 15 20XX

REPORT STATUS: FINAL REPORT

HISTORY: Previous incidence of melanoma and basal cell carcinoma, no metastases

PRE-OP DIAGNOSIS: Melanoma vs. compound nevus

PROCEDURE: Tissue biopsy

SPECIMEN: Skin biopsy, anterior, proximal right arm

GROSS DESCRIPTION: One container is received. Specimen in formalin labeled with the patient's name is a shave biopsy of gray-white hair bearing skin measuring 0.4 × 0.3 cm in surface dimension and averaging 0.1 cm in thickness. The epidermal surface contains a symmetric, smooth, ordered, pigmented lesion measuring 0.3 cm in greatest diameter. The specimen is bisected and totally submitted.

MICROSCOPIC EXAMINATION: A microscopic examination has been performed.

DIAGNOSIS: Lesion, anterior, proximal right arm; benign compound nevus.

Electronically signed: J. Alvarez, MD, Pathologist, 6/15/20XX 10:48

Start | Log On/Off | Print | Edit

---

1. Identify singular and plural forms of medical terms used in the pathology report. Write "p" for plural and "s" for singular next to the terms. Refer to Table 2-5 on p. 49 for plural endings.
   a. melanoma _____
   b. melanomata _____
   c. nevi _____
   d. nevus _____
   e. metastasis _____
   f. metastases _____
   g. biopsy _____
   h. biopsies _____

2. The skin biopsy was obtained from:
   a. near the shoulder on the back of the right arm
   b. near the shoulder on the front of the right arm
   c. near the wrist on the back of the right arm
   d. near the wrist on the front of the right arm

3. Use your medical dictionary to find the meanings of the following terms used in the pathology report:
   a. compound _____
   b. pigmented _____
   c. bisected _____
   d. microscopic _____

EXERCISE 38   *Interpret Medical Terms*

To test your understanding of the terms introduced in this chapter, circle the words that correctly complete the sentences. The italicized words refer to the correct answer.

1. *Berry-shaped bacteria in grapelike clusters* are (**streptococci, staphylococci, pediculosis**).
2. The physician ordered lotions applied to the patient's *skin* to alleviate *dryness*, or (**pachyderma, dermatoconiosis, xeroderma**).
3. The injection given *within the skin* is called a(n) (**intradermal, epidermal, hypodermic**) injection.
4. The diagnosis of *onychomalacia* was given by the physician for (**ingrown nails, nail biting, softening of the nails**).
5. The *pinpoint hemorrhages*, or (**nevi, verrucae, petechiae**), were distributed over the patient's entire body.
6. The primary manifestation of the disease was *sweating*, or (**diaphoresis, ecchymosis, pruritus**).
7. The patient had an *abnormal condition of a fungus in the hair*; therefore the doctor recorded the diagnosis as (**onychocryptosis, trichomycosis, onychomycosis**).
8. The student nurse learned that the medical name for a *blister* was (**verruca, keloid, vesicle**).
9. The patient was to receive a *skin graft from her mother*, so the operation was listed as a (**dermatoplasty, dermatoautoplasty, dermatoheteroplasty**).
10. An *abnormal hard spot* is called (**edema, induration, virus**).
11. Another word for *jaundice* is (**erythroderma, leukoderma, xanthoderma**).
12. *Leiodermia* is a condition of (**striated, smooth, sweaty**) skin.
13. The *localized collection of pus* (**acne, abscess, cyst**) was incised and drained. A culture swab of the wound revealed methicillin-resistant *Staphylococcus aureus*.
14. *A technique of microscopically controlled serial excisions* (**cryosurgery, laser surgery, Mohs surgery**) was used to treat the patient's recurrent squamous cell carcinoma.
15. Antibiotics were not prescribed for the patient who presented with fever blisters, an infection caused by *a minute microorganism characterized by a lack of independent metabolism* (**bacteria, virus, fungus**).
16. *White skin (patches caused by depigmentation)* (**leiodermia, xeroderma, leukoderma**), *congenital, hereditary condition characterized by lack of pigment in skin, hair, and eyes* (**actinic keratosis, albinism, rosacea**), and *white patches on the skin caused by the destruction of melanocytes* (**vitiligo, Kaposi sarcoma, systemic lupus erythematosus**) are all forms of hypomelanosis, a condition characterized by a deficiency of melanin in the tissues.
17. *Small hemorrhages into the tissue, giving the skin a purple-red discoloration* (**pruritus, purpura, papule**) may be caused by blood disorders, vascular abnormalities, or trauma.

EXERCISE 39 — Read Medical Terms in Use

Practice pronunciation of terms by reading aloud the following medical document. Use the pronunciation key following the medical term to assist you in saying the word.

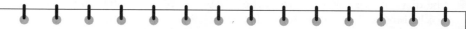

> To hear these terms, go to evolve.elsevier.com.
> Select: Chapter 4, **Exercises**, Read Medical Terms in Use.
>
> Refer to p. 10 for your Evolve Access Information.

Emily visited the **dermatology** (*der*-ma-TOL-o-jē) clinic because of **pruritus** (prū-RĪ-tus) secondary to **dermatitis** (*der*-ma-TĪ-tis) involving her scalp and areas of her elbows and knees. A diagnosis of **psoriasis** (so-RĪ-a-sis) was made. **Eczema** (EK-ze-ma), **scabies** (SKĀ-bēz), and **tinea** (TIN-ē-a) were considered in the differential diagnosis. An emollient cream was prescribed. In addition the patient showed the **dermatologist** (der-ma-TOL-o-jist) the tender, discolored, thickened nail of her right great toe. Emily learned she had **onychomycosis** (*on*-i-kō-mī-KŌ-sis), for which she was given an additional prescription for an oral antifungal drug.

WEB LINK

For more information about diseases and disorders of the integumentary system and current treatments, visit the **American Academy of Dermatology** at *www.aad .org.*

EXERCISE 40 — Comprehend Medical Terms in Use

Test your comprehension of terms in the above medical document by circling the correct answer.

1. Emily sought medical attention because of:
   a. an eroded sore and inflammation of the skin
   b. itching and inflammation of the skin
   c. itching and thickness of the skin
   d. an eroded sore and thickening of the skin
2. T   F, An inflammatory disease of the skin involving sebaceous glands and hair follicles was considered in the differential diagnosis.
3. Emily was given an additional prescription for an abnormal condition of fungus in the:
   a. sudoriferous glands
   b. hair follicles
   c. sebaceous glands
   d. nails

> For a snapshot assessment of your knowledge of integumentary system terms, go to evolve.elsevier.com.
> Select: Chapter 4, **Quick Quizzes**.
>
> Refer to p. 10 for your Evolve Access Information.

CHAPTER REVIEW

ⓔ *Review of Evolve*

Keep a record of online activities you have completed by placing a check mark in the box. You may also record your scores. All activities have been referenced throughout the text.

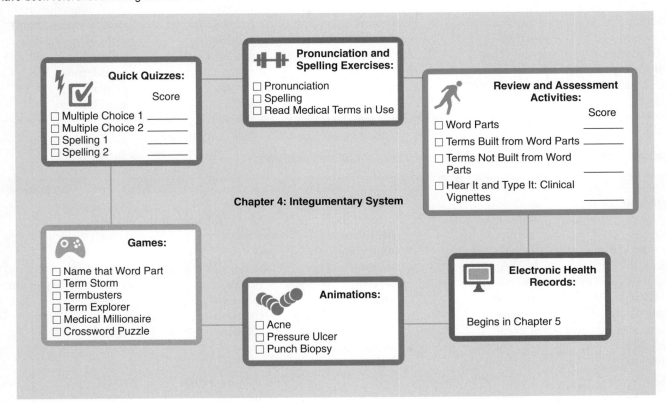

Quick Quizzes:
Score
☐ Multiple Choice 1 _____
☐ Multiple Choice 2 _____
☐ Spelling 1 _____
☐ Spelling 2 _____

Pronunciation and Spelling Exercises:
☐ Pronunciation
☐ Spelling
☐ Read Medical Terms in Use

Review and Assessment Activities:
Score
☐ Word Parts _____
☐ Terms Built from Word Parts _____
☐ Terms Not Built from Word Parts _____
☐ Hear It and Type It: Clinical Vignettes _____

Chapter 4: Integumentary System

Games:
☐ Name that Word Part
☐ Term Storm
☐ Termbusters
☐ Term Explorer
☐ Medical Millionaire
☐ Crossword Puzzle

Animations:
☐ Acne
☐ Pressure Ulcer
☐ Punch Biopsy

Electronic Health Records:
Begins in Chapter 5

Review of Word Parts

Can you define and spell the following word parts?

COMBINING FORMS		PREFIXES	SUFFIXES
aut/o	myc/o	epi-	-a
bi/o	necr/o	intra-	-coccus (*pl.* -cocci)
coni/o	onych/o	para-	-ectomy
crypt/o	pachy/o	per-	-ia
cutane/o	rhytid/o	sub-	-itis
derm/o	seb/o	trans-	-malacia
dermat/o	staphyl/o		-opsy
heter/o	strept/o		-phagia
hidr/o	trich/o		-plasty
kerat/o	ungu/o		-rrhea
	xer/o		-tome

Review of Terms

Can you build, analyze, define, pronounce, and spell the following terms *built from word parts*?

DISEASES AND DISORDERS		SURGICAL	COMPLEMENTARY	
dermatitis	onychomycosis	biopsy (bx)	dermatologist	percutaneous
dermatoconiosis	onychophagia	dermatoautoplasty	dermatology (derm)	staphylococcus (staph)
dermatofibroma	pachyderma	dermatoheteroplasty	epidermal	(*pl.* staphylococci)
hidradenitis	paronychia	dermatome	erythroderma	streptococcus (strep)
leiodermia	seborrhea	dermatoplasty	hypodermic	(*pl.* streptococci)
leukoderma	trichomycosis	onychectomy	intradermal (ID)	subcutaneous (subcut)
onychocryptosis	xeroderma	rhytidectomy	keratogenic	transdermal (TD)
onychomalacia		rhytidoplasty	necrosis	ungual
				xanthoderma

Can you define, pronounce, and spell the following terms *not built from word parts*?

DISEASES AND DISORDERS		SURGICAL	COMPLEMENTARY	
abrasion	infection	cauterization	alopecia	nevus (*pl.* nevi)
abscess	Kaposi sarcoma	cryosurgery	bacteria (*s.* bacterium)	nodule
acne	laceration	débridement	cicatrix	pallor
actinic keratosis	lesion	dermabrasion	cyst	papule
albinism	MRSA infection	excision	cytomegalovirus	petechia (*pl.* petechiae)
basal cell carcinoma	pediculosis	incision	(CMV)	pressure ulcer (decub)
(BCC)	psoriasis	incision and	diaphoresis	pruritus
candidiasis	rosacea	drainage (I&D)	ecchymosis (*pl.*	purpura
carbuncle	scabies	laser surgery	ecchymoses)	pustule
cellulitis	scleroderma	Mohs surgery	edema	ulcer
contusion	squamous cell	suturing	erythema	verruca
eczema	carcinoma (SqCCA)		fungus (*pl.* fungi)	vesicle
fissure	systemic lupus		induration	virus
furuncle	erythematosus		jaundice	wheal
gangrene	(SLE)		keloid	
herpes	tinea		leukoplakia	
impetigo	urticaria		macule	
	vitiligo			

ANSWERS

ANSWERS TO CHAPTER 4 EXERCISES
Exercise Figures

Exercise Figure

A. 1. horny tissue: kerat/o
2. hair: trich/o
3. skin: cutane/o, dermat/o, derm/o
4. sebum: seb/o
5. sweat: hidr/o

Exercise Figure

B. nail: onych/o, ungu/o

Exercise Figure

C. 1. onych/o/myc/osis
2. par/onych/ia

Exercise Figure

D. 1. intra/derm/al
2. sub/cutane/ous, hypo/derm/ic
3. trans/derm/al

Exercise Figure

E. 1. staphyl/o/cocci
2. strept/o/cocci

Exercise 1

1. c   5. f
2. d   6. h
3. g   7. a
4. b   8. e

Exercise 2

1. sweat   6. skin
2. skin   7. sebum (oil)
3. nail   8. nail
4. hair   9. skin
5. horny tissue, hard

Exercise 3

1. trich/o
2. hidr/o
3. a. onych/o
   b. ungu/o
4. seb/o
5. a. derm/o
   b. dermat/o
   c. cutane/o
6. kerat/o

Exercise 4

1. death   7. life
2. grapelike   8. other
   clusters   9. twisted chains
3. hidden   10. dry
4. thick   11. self
5. dust   12. wrinkles
6. fungus

Exercise 5

1. myc/o   7. rhytid/o
2. necr/o   8. staphyl/o
3. heter/o   9. aut/o
4. xer/o   10. crypt/o
5. pachy/o   11. coni/o
6. strept/o   12. bi/o

Exercise 6

1. under, below
2. beside, beyond, around, abnormal
3. on, upon, over
4. within
5. through
6. through, across, beyond

Exercise 7

1. intra-   4. para-
2. sub-   5. per-
3. epi-   6. trans-

Exercise 8

1. c   7. d
2. e   8. b
3. a   9. f
4. j   10. k
5. i   11. l
6. h

Exercise 9

1. surgical repair
2. excision or surgical removal
3. softening
4. inflammation
5. instrument used to cut
6. eating, swallowing
7. flow, discharge
8. berry-shaped
9. view of, viewing
10. diseased or abnormal state, condition of
11. noun suffix, no meaning

Exercise 10

Pronunciation Exercise

Exercise 11

Note: The combining form is identified by the italic and bold print.

1.   WR   CV WR   S
   ***dermat/o*/**coni/osis
          CF
   abnormal condition of the skin caused by dust

2.   WR   WR   S
   hidr/aden/itis
   inflammation of a sweat gland

3.   WR   S
   dermat/itis
   inflammation of the skin

4.   WR   WR   S
   pachy/derm/a
   thickening of the skin

5.   WR CV   S
   ***onych/o*/**malacia
        CF
   softening of the nails

6.   WR CV WR   S
   ***trich/o*/**myc/osis
          CF
   abnormal condition of a fungus in the hair

7.   WR CV WR   S
   ***dermat/o*/**fibr/oma
            CF
   fibrous tumor of the skin

8.   P   WR   S
   par/onych/ia
   diseased state around the nail

9.   WR CV WR   S
   ***onych/o*/**crypt/osis
          CF
   abnormal condition of a hidden nail

10. WR CV S
   ***seb/o*/**rrhea
        CF
   discharge of sebum (excessive)

11.   WR CV   S
   ***onych/o*/**phagia
            CF
   eating the nails, nail biting

12. WR CV WR   S
   ***xer/o*/**derm/a
        CF
   dry skin

13. WR CV WR   S
   ***lei/o*/**derm/ia
        CF
   condition of smooth skin

14. WR CV   WR   S
   ***leuk/o*/**derm/a
        CF
   white skin

Exercise 12

1. pachy/derm/a
2. onych/o/myc/osis

3. seb/o/rrhea
4. dermat/itis
5. dermat/o/fibr/oma
6. onych/o/malacia
7. hidr/aden/itis
8. onych/o/crypt/osis
9. dermat/o/coni/osis
10. onych/o/phagia
11. par/onych/ia
12. xer/o/derm/a
13. lei/o/derm/ia
14. leuk/o/derm/a

Exercise 13
Spelling Exercise; see text p. 103.

Exercise 14
Pronunciation Exercise

Exercise 15
1. systemic lupus erythematosus
2. abscess
3. fissure
4. abrasion
5. psoriasis
6. herpes
7. pediculosis
8. tinea
9. contusion
10. gangrene
11. lesion
12. Kaposi sarcoma
13. actinic keratosis
14. carbuncle
15. acne
16. laceration
17. furuncle
18. squamous cell
19. cellulitis
20. impetigo
21. eczema
22. scabies
23. urticaria
24. basal cell
25. scleroderma
26. candidiasis
27. infection
28. rosacea
29. albinism
30. MRSA infection
31. vitiligo

Exercise 16
1. f		9.	e
2. j		10.	b
3. g		11.	h
4. l		12.	a
5. n		13.	d
6. c		14.	m
7. i		15.	p
8. k			

Exercise 17
1. d		9.	n
2. i		10.	e
3. f		11.	b
4. h		12.	g
5. m		13.	k
6. l		14.	o
7. c		15.	j
8. a		16.	q

Exercise 18
Spelling Exercise; see text p. 111.

Exercise 19
Pronunciation Exercise

Exercise 20
Note: The combining form is identified by the italic and bold print.

1. WR S
   rhytid/ectomy
   excision of wrinkles

2. WR S
   bi/opsy
   view of life (removal of living tissue)

3. WR CV WR CV S
   dermat/o/*aut/o*/plasty
         CF   CF
   surgical repair using one's own skin (for the skin graft)

4. WR S
   onych/ectomy
   excision of a nail

5. WR CV S
   rhytid/o/plasty
        CF
   surgical repair of wrinkles

6. WR CV WR CV S
   dermat/o/*heter/o*/plasty
         CF   CF
   surgical repair using skin from others (for the skin graft)

7. WR S
   derma/tome
   instrument used to cut skin

Exercise 21
1. rhytid/ectomy
2. bi/opsy
3. dermat/o/heter/o/plasty
4. onych/ectomy
5. rhytid/o/plasty
6. dermat/o/plasty
7. derma/tome

Exercise 22
Spelling Exercise; see text p. 114.

Exercise 23
Pronunciation Exercise

Exercise 24
1. Mohs surgery
2. incision
3. cauterization
4. suturing
5. incision and drainage
6. débridement
7. excision
8. laser surgery
9. cryosurgery
10. dermabrasion

Exercise 25
1. i		6.	e
2. h		7.	b
3. g		8.	f
4. d		9.	j
5. a		10.	c

Exercise 26
Spelling Exercise, see text p. 116.

Exercise 27
Pronunciation Exercise

Exercise 28
Note: The combining form is identified by the italic and bold print.

1. WR S
   ungu/al
   pertaining to the nail

2. P WR S
   trans/derm/al
   pertaining to through the skin

3. WR CV S
   strept/o/coccus
        CF
   berry-shaped (bacterium) in twisted chains

4. P WR S
   hypo/derm/ic
   pertaining to under the skin

5. WR CV S
   dermat/o/logy
        CF
   study of the skin

6. P WR S
   sub/cutane/ous
   pertaining to under the skin

7. WR CV S
   staphyl/o/coccus
         CF
   berry-shaped (bacterium) in grapelike clusters

8. WR CV S
   kerat/o/genic
        CF
   originating in horny tissue

9. WR CV S
   ***dermat/o*/logist**
         CF
   physician who studies and treats skin (diseases)

10. WR   S
    necr/osis
    abnormal condition of death (of cells and tissue)

11. P WR S
    epi/derm/al
    pertaining to upon the skin

12. WR CV WR S
    ***xanth/o*/derm/a**
           CF
    yellow skin

13. WR CV WR S
    ***erythr/o*/derm/a**
           CF
    red skin

14. P   WR   S
    per/cutane/ous
    pertaining to through the skin

Exercise 29
1. dermat/o/logy
2. necr/osis
3. ungu/al
4. staphyl/o/coccus
5. dermat/o/logist
6. intra/derm/al
7. epi/derm/al
8. sub/cutane/ous, hypo/derm/ic
9. strept/o/coccus
10. kerat/o/genic
11. erythr/o/derm/a
12. xanth/o/derm/a
13. per/cutane/ous, trans/derm/al

Exercise 30
Spelling Exercise; see text p. 120.

Exercise 31
Pronunciation Exercise

Exercise 32
1. cicatrix
2. diaphoresis
3. verruca
4. macule
5. jaundice
6. leukoplakia
7. petechia
8. ulcer
9. keloid
10. pallor

11. ecchymosis
12. pressure ulcer
13. nodule
14. cyst
15. pruritus
16. erythema
17. purpura
18. nevus
19. bacteria
20. alopecia
21. papule
22. wheal
23. pustule
24. vesicle
25. fungus
26. virus
27. induration
28. edema
29. cytomegalovirus

Exercise 33
1. m	8. d
2. a	9. b
3. j	10. k
4. e	11. c
5. n	12. h
6. l	13. i
7. g	

Exercise 34
1. g	9. e
2. d	10. f
3. j	11. o
4. a	12. c
5. l	13. h
6. k	14. i
7. n	15. m
8. b	16. q

Exercise 35
Spelling Exercise; see text p. 127.

Exercise 36
1. basal cell carcinoma
2. cytomegalovirus
3. systemic lupus erythematosus
4. squamous cell carcinoma
5. biopsy
6. subcutaneous
7. staphylococcus
8. streptococcus
9. incision and drainage
10. transdermal
11. intradermal
12. dermatology
13. pressure ulcer

14. methicillin-resistant *Staphylococcus aureus*, healthcare-associated MRSA infection, community-associated MRSA infection

Exercise 37
A. 1. dermatology
2. nevus
3. medial
4. actinic keratosis
5. eczema
6. lesion
7. excision
8. superior
9. pathology
10. cauterization
11. biopsy
12. basal cell carcinoma

B. 1. a.   s
           b.   p
           c.   p
           d.   s
           e.   s
           f.   p
           g.   s
           h.   p
      2. b
      3. dictionary exercise

Exercise 38
1. staphylococci
2. xeroderma
3. intradermal
4. softening of the nails
5. petechiae
6. diaphoresis
7. trichomycosis
8. vesicle
9. dermatoheteroplasty
10. induration
11. xanthoderma
12. smooth
13. abscess
14. Mohs surgery
15. virus
16. leukoderma, albinism, vitiligo
17. purpura

Exercise 39
Reading Exercise

Exercise 40
1. b
2. *F*, acne is the condition described in the sentence.
3. d

Chapter 5

Respiratory System and Introduction to Diagnostic Procedures and Tests

Outline

Objectives

Upon completion of this chapter you will be able to:

1 Identify organs and structures of the respiratory system.

2 Define and spell word parts related to the respiratory system.

3 Define, pronounce, and spell disease and disorder terms related to the respiratory system.

4 Define, pronounce, and spell surgical terms related to the respiratory system.

5 Define, pronounce, and spell diagnostic terms related to the respiratory system.

6 Define, pronounce, and spell complementary terms related to the respiratory system.

7 Interpret the meaning of abbreviations related to the respiratory system.

8 Interpret, read, and comprehend medical language in simulated medical statements, documents, and electronic health records.

ANATOMY

The respiratory system comprises the nose, pharynx, larynx, trachea, bronchi, and lungs. The upper respiratory tract includes the nose, pharynx, and larynx. The lower respiratory tract includes the trachea, bronchi, and lungs (Figure 5-1).

Function

The function of the respiratory system is the exchange of oxygen (O_2) and carbon dioxide (CO_2) between the atmosphere and body cells. This process is called **respiration** or **breathing**. During **external respiration**, air containing oxygen passes through the respiratory tract, beginning with the nose, pharynx, larynx, trachea, and, finally, bronchi to the lungs (**inhalation** or **inspiration**). There, oxygen passes from the sacs in the lungs, called **alveoli**, to the blood in tiny blood vessels called **capillaries**. At the same time, carbon dioxide passes back from the capillaries to the alveoli and is expelled through the respiratory tract (**exhalation** or **expiration**) (Figure 5-2). During internal respiration, the body cells take on **oxygen** from the blood and simultaneously give back **carbon dioxide**, a waste produced when food and oxygen combine in cells. The carbon dioxide is transported by the blood back to the lungs for exhalation.

RESPIRATION
is also called **breathing** or **ventilation**.

Organs of the Respiratory System

TERM	DEFINITION
nose	lined with mucous membrane and fine hairs; it acts as a filter to moisten and warm the entering air
nasal septum	partition separating the right and left nasal cavities
paranasal sinuses	air cavities within the cranial bones that open into the nasal cavities
pharynx	serves as a food and air passageway. Air enters from the nasal cavities and/or mouth and passes through the pharynx to the larynx. Food enters the pharynx from the mouth and passes into the esophagus; (also called the **throat**).
adenoids	lymphoid tissue located on the posterior wall of the nasal cavity (also called **pharyngeal tonsils**)
tonsils	lymphoid tissue located on the lateral wall at the junction of the oral cavity and oropharynx
larynx	location of the vocal cords. Air enters from the pharynx (also called the **voice box**).
epiglottis	flap of cartilage that automatically covers the opening of the larynx and keeps food from entering the larynx during swallowing
trachea	passageway for air to the bronchi from the larynx; (also called the **windpipe**)
bronchus (*pl.* bronchi)	one of two branches from the trachea that conducts air into the lungs, where it divides and subdivides. The branchings resemble a tree; therefore, they are referred to as a **bronchial tree**.
bronchioles	smallest subdivision of the bronchial tree
alveolus (*pl.* alveoli)	air sacs at the end of the bronchioles. Oxygen and carbon dioxide are exchanged through the alveolar walls and the capillaries (also a term for the socket in the jaw bones into which the teeth fit).

🏛 **ADAM'S APPLE**
is the largest ring of cartilage in the **larynx** and is also known as the thyroid cartilage. The name came from the belief that Adam, realizing he had sinned when he ate the forbidden fruit, was unable to swallow the apple lodged in his throat.

🏛 **BRONCHI**
originated from the Greek **brecho**, meaning **to pour** or **wet**. An ancient belief was that the esophagus carried solid food to the stomach and the bronchi carried liquids.

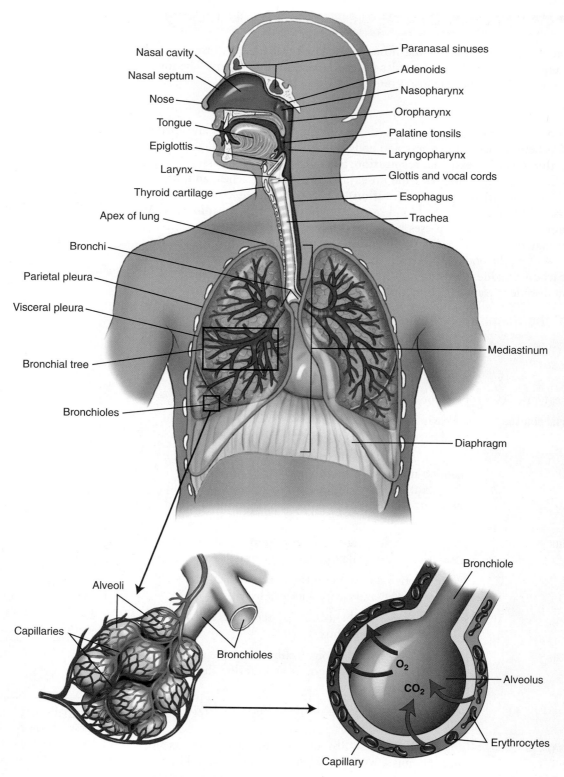

FIGURE 5-1
Organs of the respiratory system.

Organs of the Respiratory System—cont'd

TERM	DEFINITION
lungs	two spongelike organs in the thoracic cavity. The right lung consists of three lobes, and the left lung has two lobes.
pleura	double-folded serous membrane covering each lung (visceral pleura) and lining the thoracic cavity (parietal pleura) with a small space between, called the pleural cavity, which contains serous fluid
diaphragm	muscular partition that separates the thoracic cavity from the abdominal cavity. It aids in the breathing process by contracting and pulling air in, then relaxing and pushing air out.
mediastinum	space between the lungs. It contains the heart, esophagus, trachea, great blood vessels, and other structures.

> **🏛 MEDIASTINUM**
> literally means **to stand in the middle** because it is derived from the Latin **medius**, meaning **middle**, and **stare**, meaning **to stand**.

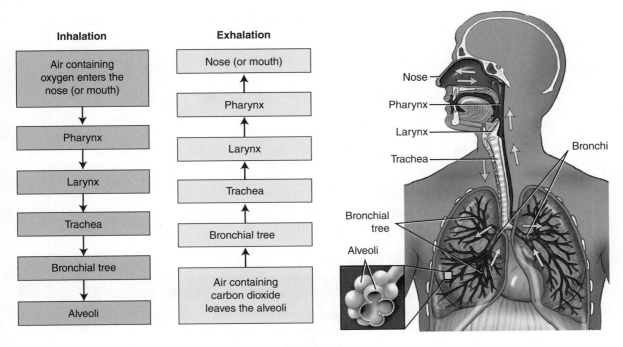

FIGURE 5-2
Flow of air.

A & P Booster
For more anatomy and physiology, go to evolve.elsevier.com.
Select: **Extra Content**, A & P Booster, Chapter 5.

Refer to p. 10 for your Evolve Access Information.

EXERCISE 1

Match the anatomic terms in the first column with the correct definitions in the second column. *To check your answers, go to Answers, p. 201, at the back of this chapter.*

_____ 1. alveoli

_____ 2. bronchi

_____ 3. larynx

_____ 4. lungs

_____ 5. pharynx

_____ 6. pleura

_____ 7. adenoids

_____ 8. trachea

a. tubes carrying air between the trachea and lungs
b. passageway for air to the bronchi from the larynx
c. located in the thoracic cavity
d. membrane covering the lung
e. lymphoid tissue on the posterior wall of the nasal cavity
f. acts as food and air passageway
g. location of the vocal cords
h. air sacs at the end of the bronchioles
i. keeps food out of the trachea and larynx

EXERCISE 2

Fill in the blanks with the correct terms.

1. The partition that separates the right and left nasal cavities is called the

   _____ _____.

2. The _____ is a flap of cartilage that prevents food from entering the larynx.

3. The smallest subdivisions of the bronchial tree are the _____.

4. The _____ serves as a filter to moisten and warm air entering the body.

5. The thoracic cavity is separated from the abdominal cavity by the

   _____.

6. The space between the lungs is called the _____.

7. The lymphoid tissues located on the posterior wall at the junction of the oral cavity and oropharynx is called _____.

 WORD PARTS

Words parts you need to learn to complete this chapter are listed on the following pages. The exercises at the end of each list will help you learn their definitions and spelling.

> Use the flashcards accompanying this text or electronic flashcards to assist you in memorizing the word parts for this chapter.

 To use electronic flashcards, go to evolve.elsevier.com. Select: Chapter 5, **Flashcards**.

Refer to p. 10 for your Evolve Access Information.

Combining Forms of the Respiratory System

COMBINING FORM	DEFINITION
adenoid/o	adenoids
alveol/o	alveolus
bronchi/o, bronch/o	bronchus
diaphragmat/o, phren/o	diaphragm
epiglott/o	epiglottis
laryng/o	larynx
lob/o	lobe
nas/o, rhin/o	nose
pharyng/o	pharynx
pleur/o	pleura
pneum/o, pneumat/o, pneumon/o	lung, air
pulmon/o	lung
sept/o	septum (wall off, fence)
sinus/o	sinus
thorac/o	thorax, chest, chest cavity
tonsill/o _(Note: tonsil has one l, and the combining form has two ls.)_	tonsil
trache/o	trachea

🏛 **LOBE**
literally means **the part that hangs down**, although it comes from the Greek **lobos**, meaning **capsule** or **pod**. This also applies to the lobe of an ear, the liver, or the brain.

🔅 Do not be concerned at this time about which combining form to use for terms such as _lung_ or _nose_ that have more than one combining form. As you continue to study and use medical terms you will become familiar with common usage of each word part.

EXERCISE FIGURE A

Fill in the blanks with combining forms in this diagram of the respiratory system. *To check your answers, go to p. 201.*

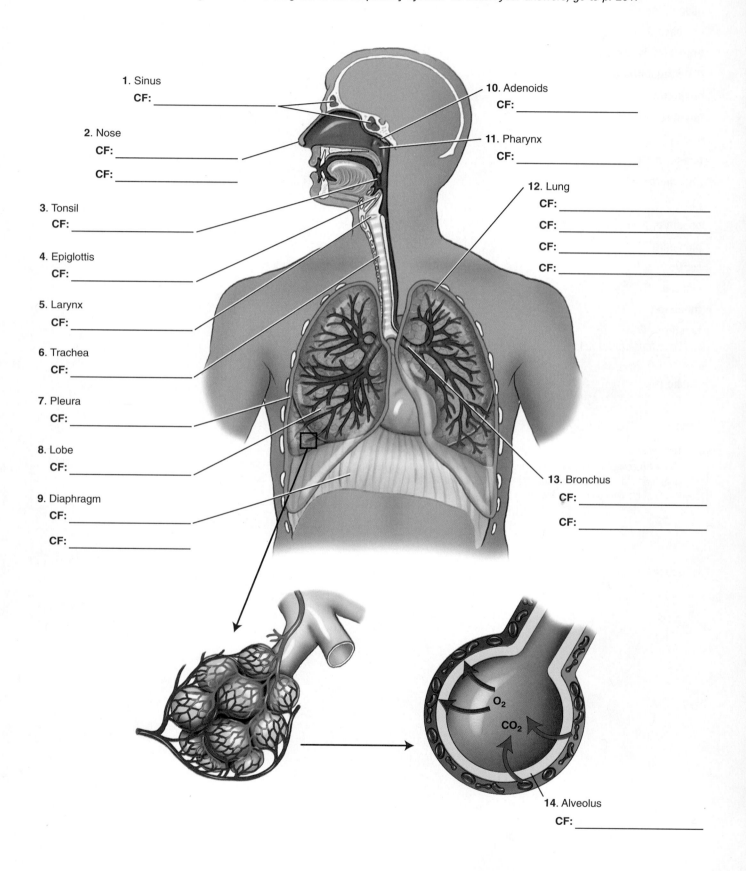

1. Sinus

    CF: _____

2. Nose

    CF: _____

    CF: _____

3. Tonsil

    CF: _____

4. Epiglottis

    CF: _____

5. Larynx

    CF: _____

6. Trachea

    CF: _____

7. Pleura

    CF: _____

8. Lobe

    CF: _____

9. Diaphragm

    CF: _____

    CF: _____

10. Adenoids

    CF: _____

11. Pharynx

    CF: _____

12. Lung

    CF: _____

    CF: _____

    CF: _____

    CF: _____

13. Bronchus

    CF: _____

    CF: _____

O_2

CO_2

14. Alveolus

    CF: _____

EXERCISE 3

Write the definitions of the following combining forms.

1. laryng/o _____
2. bronchi/o, bronch/o _____
3. pleur/o _____
4. pneum/o _____
5. tonsill/o _____
6. pulmon/o _____
7. diaphragmat/o _____
8. trache/o _____
9. alveol/o _____
10. pneumon/o _____
11. thorac/o _____

12. adenoid/o _____
13. pharyng/o _____
14. rhin/o _____
15. sinus/o _____
16. lob/o _____
17. epiglott/o _____
18. pneumat/o _____
19. nas/o _____
20. sept/o _____
21. phren/o _____

EXERCISE 4

Write the combining form for each of the following terms.

1. nose   a. _____
         b. _____
2. larynx _____
3. lung, air   a. _____
             b. _____
             c. _____
4. lung _____
5. tonsil _____
6. trachea _____
7. adenoids _____
8. pleura _____

9. diaphragm   a. _____
             b. _____
10. sinus _____
11. thorax, chest, chest cavity _____
12. alveolus _____
13. pharynx _____
14. bronchus   a. _____
             b. _____
15. lobe _____
16. epiglottis _____
17. septum _____

Combining Forms Commonly Used with Respiratory System Terms

COMBINING FORM	DEFINITION
atel/o	imperfect, incomplete
capn/o	carbon dioxide
hem/o, hemat/o	blood
muc/o	mucus
orth/o	straight
ox/i	oxygen
phon/o	sound, voice
py/o	pus
radi/o	x-rays, ionizing radiation
somn/o	sleep
son/o	sound
spir/o	breathe, breathing
tom/o	to cut, section, or slice

🏛 **OXYGEN**

was discovered in 1774 by Joseph Priestley. In 1775 Antoine-Laurent Lavoisier, a French chemist, noted that all the acids he knew contained oxygen. Because he thought it was an acid producer, he named it using the Greek **oxys**, meaning **sour**, and the suffix **gen**, meaning **to produce**.

EXERCISE 5

Write the definition of the following combining forms.

1. ox/i _____

2. spir/o _____

3. muc/o _____

4. atel/o _____

5. orth/o _____

6. py/o _____

7. hem/o, hemat/o _____

8. somn/o _____

9. capn/o _____

10. phon/o _____

11. son/o _____

12. radi/o _____

13. tom/o _____

EXERCISE 6

Write the combining form for each of the following.

1. breathe, breathing _____

2. oxygen _____

3. imperfect, incomplete _____

4. straight _____

5. pus _____

6. mucus _____

7. blood   a. _____

       b. _____

8. sleep _____

9. sound, voice _____

10. carbon dioxide _____

11. sound _____

12. x-rays, ionizing radiation _____

13. to cut, section, or slice _____

Prefixes

PREFIX	DEFINITION
a-, an- *(Note:* an- *is used when the word root begins with a vowel.)*	absence of, without
endo- *(Note: the prefix* intra-, *introduced in Chapter 4, also means* within.*)*	within
eu-	normal, good
poly-	many, much
tachy-	fast, rapid

EXERCISE 7

Write the definitions of the following prefixes.

1. endo- _____

2. a-, an- _____

3. eu- _____

4. poly- _____

5. tachy- _____

EXERCISE 8

Write the prefix for each of the following.

1. within _____

2. normal, good _____

3. absence of, without   a. _____

                        b. _____

4. many, much _____

5. fast, rapid _____

Suffixes

SUFFIX	DEFINITION
-algia	pain
-ar, -ary, -eal	pertaining to
-cele	hernia or protrusion
-centesis	surgical puncture to aspirate fluid (with a sterile needle)
-ectasis	stretching out, dilatation, expansion
-emia	in the blood
-gram	record, radiographic image
-graph	instrument used to record; record
-graphy	process of recording, radiographic imaging
-meter	instrument used to measure
-metry	measurement
-pexy	surgical fixation, suspension
-pnea	breathing
-rrhagia	rapid flow of blood
-scope	instrument used for visual examination
-scopic	pertaining to visual examination
-scopy	visual examination
-spasm	sudden, involuntary muscle contraction (spasmodic contraction)
-stenosis	constriction or narrowing
-stomy	creation of an artificial opening
-thorax	chest, chest cavity
-tomy	cut into, incision

COMPARING -GRAPH, GRAPHY, -GRAM

-graph is the instrument used to record—the machine—as in **telegraph** or **electrocardiograph**; also means record, as in **radiograph**.

-graphy is the process of recording, the act of setting down or registering a record, as in **photography** or **radiography**.

-gram is the record (picture, radiographic image, or tracing) as in **telegram** or **sonogram**.

Refer to **Appendix A** and **Appendix B** for alphabetical lists of word parts and their meanings.

EXERCISE 9

Match the suffixes in the first column with their correct definitions in the second column.

_____ 1. -algia
_____ 2. -ar, -ary, -eal
_____ 3. -cele
_____ 4. -centesis
_____ 5. -ectasis
_____ 6. -emia
_____ 7. -graphy
_____ 8. -meter
_____ 9. -metry
_____ 10. -scopic
_____ 11. -gram
_____ 12. -graph

a. process of recording, radiographic imaging
b. stretching out, dilatation, expansion
c. surgical puncture to aspirate fluid
d. measurement
e. pertaining to visual examination
f. pertaining to
g. hernia or protrusion
h. instrument used to measure
i. rapid flow of blood
j. instrument used to record; record
k. in the blood
l. pain
m. record, radiographic image

EXERCISE 10

Match the suffixes in the first column with their correct definitions in the second column.

_____	1. -rrhagia	a. cut into, incision
_____	2. -stomy	b. instrument used for visual examination
_____	3. -tomy	c. rapid flow of blood
_____	4. -pexy	d. constriction, narrowing
_____	5. -scope	e. creation of an artificial opening
_____	6. -scopy	f. sudden, involuntary muscle contraction
_____	7. -spasm	g. chest, chest cavity
_____	8. -stenosis	h. surgical fixation, suspension
_____	9. -thorax	i. visual examination
_____	10. -pnea	j. breathing

EXERCISE 11

Write the definitions of the following suffixes.

1. -thorax _____

2. -ar, -ary, -eal _____

3. -stenosis _____

4. -cele _____

5. -stomy _____

6. -pexy _____

7. -meter _____

8. -spasm _____

9. -algia _____

10. -scopy _____

11. -centesis _____

12. -tomy _____

13. -scope _____

14. -rrhagia _____

15. -ectasis _____

16. -graphy _____

17. -metry _____

18. -emia _____

19. -scopic _____

20. -pnea _____

21. -graph _____

22. -gram _____

For review and/or assessment, go to evolve.elsevier.com. Select:
Chapter 5, **Activities,** Word Parts
Chapter 5, **Games,**   Name that Word Part

Refer to p. 10 for your Evolve Access Information.

🏛 **ATELECTASIS**
is derived from the Greek
ateles, meaning **not perfect,**
and **ektasis,** meaning
expansion. It denotes an
incomplete expansion of the
lungs, especially at birth.

MEDICAL TERMS

The terms you need to learn to complete this chapter are listed below and on the following pages. The exercises following each list will help you learn the definition and the spelling of each word.

Disease and Disorder Terms

Built from Word Parts

The following terms are built from word parts you have already learned and can be translated literally to find their meanings. Further explanation of terms beyond the definition of their word parts, if needed, is included in parentheses.

EXERCISE FIGURE B

Fill in the blanks to label the diagram.

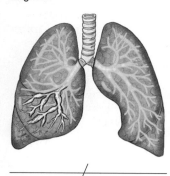

———————— / ————————
  bronchi / dilation

TERM	DEFINITION
adenoiditis (*ad*-e-noyd-Ī-tis)	inflammation of the adenoids
alveolitis (*al*-vē-o-LĪ-tis)	inflammation of the alveoli (pulmonary or dental)
atelectasis (*at*-e-LEK-ta-sis)	incomplete expansion (of the lung or portion of the lung) (Figure 5-3)
bronchiectasis (*bron*-kē-EK-ta-sis)	dilation of the bronchi (Exercise Figure B)
bronchitis (bron-KĪ-tis)	inflammation of the bronchi (Figure 5-4)

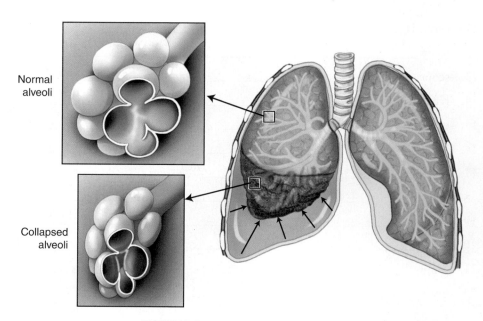

Normal alveoli

Collapsed alveoli

FIGURE 5-3
Atelectasis showing the collapsed alveoli.

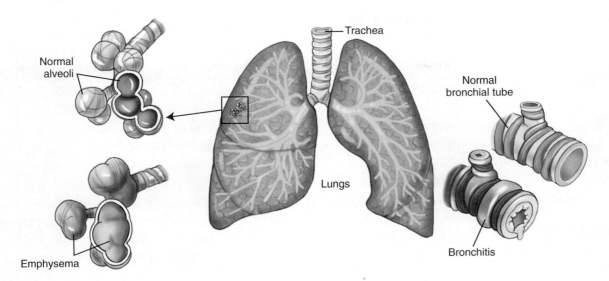

FIGURE 5-4
Emphysema and bronchitis. Chronic bronchitis and emphysema are both components of chronic obstructive pulmonary disease (COPD).

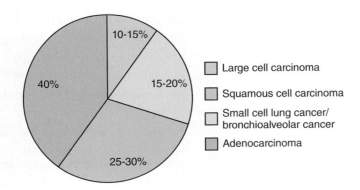

Large cell carcinoma

Squamous cell carcinoma

Small cell lung cancer/
bronchioalveolar cancer

Adenocarcinoma

MESOTHELIOMA

is a rare form of cancer most common in the pleura, the sac covering the lung, and lining the thoracic cavity, and is most often caused by inhalation exposure to asbestos.

Mesothelioma also occurs in the lining of the abdominal cavity and the lining around the heart as well.

FIGURE 5-5
Types of lung cancers. Lung cancer is classified as either small cell or non–small cell carcinoma. The latter is by far the most prevalent and includes adenocarcinoma and squamous cell carcinoma. Lung cancer is one of the most common cancers in the world. It was estimated there would be 226,000 new cases of lung cancer, with 160,000 deaths, in the US in 2012. It is the main cause of death due to cancer for both men and women. Smoking is the most important risk factor for the development of lung cancer. Symptoms include cough, hemoptysis, chest pain, dyspnea, fatigue, and weight loss. Thoracentesis, bronchoscopy, chest radiograph, CT, and PET scanning are used for diagnosis. Treatment includes surgery, chemotherapy, and radiation.

TERM	DEFINITION
bronchogenic carcinoma (bron-kō-JEN-ik) (*kar*-si-NŌ-ma)	cancerous tumor originating in a bronchus (also referred to as **lung cancer**) (Figure 5-5)
bronchopneumonia (*bron*-kō-nū-MŌ-nē-a)	diseased state of the bronchi and lungs (an inflammation of the lungs that begins in the terminal bronchioles)
diaphragmatocele (*dī*-a-frag-MAT-ō-sēl)	hernia of the diaphragm

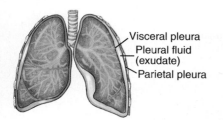

FIGURE 5-6
Pleuritis, also called pleurisy.

Visceral pleura
Pleural fluid (exudate)
Parietal pleura

PNEUMOCONIOSIS

is the general name given for chronic inflammatory disease of the lung caused by excessive inhalation of mineral dust. When the disease is caused by a specific dust, it is named for the dust. For example, the disease caused by **silica dust** is called **silicosis**.

 EXERCISE FIGURE C

Fill in the blanks to label the diagram.

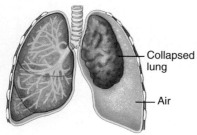

Collapsed lung

Air

1. _____
   air / CV / chest cavity

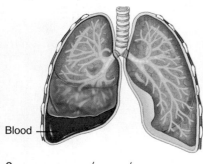

Blood

2. _____
   blood / CV / chest cavity

EPISTAXIS

and rhinorrhagia are both medical terms for **nosebleed**.

Disease and Disorder Terms—cont'd
Built from Word Parts

TERM	DEFINITION
epiglottitis (*ep*-i-glo-TĪ-tis)	inflammation of the epiglottis
hemothorax (*hē*-mō-THOR-aks)	blood in the chest cavity (pleural space) (Exercise Figure C2)
laryngitis (*lar*-in-JĪ-tis)	inflammation of the larynx
laryngotracheobronchitis (LTB) (la-*ring*-gō-*trā*-kē-ō-bron-KĪ-tis)	inflammation of the larynx, trachea, and bronchi (the acute form is called **croup**)
lobar pneumonia (LŌ-bar) (nū-MŌ-nē-a)	pertaining to the lobe(s); diseased state of the lung (infection of one or more lobes of the lung)
nasopharyngitis (*nā*-zō-*far*-in-JĪ-tis)	inflammation of the nose and pharynx
pharyngitis (*far*-in-JĪ-tis)	inflammation of the pharynx
pleuritis (plū-RĪ-tis)	inflammation of the pleura (also called **pleurisy**) (Figure 5-6)
pneumatocele (nū-MAT-ō-sēl)	hernia of the lung (lung tissue protrudes through an opening in the chest)
pneumoconiosis (*nū*-mō-*kō*-nē-Ō-sis)	abnormal condition of dust in the lungs
pneumonia (nū-MŌ-nē-a)	diseased state of the lung (the infection and inflammation are caused by bacteria such as *Pneumococcus, Staphylococcus, Streptococcus,* and *Haemophilus*; viruses; and fungi) (see Figure 5-13, *B*)
pneumonitis (*nū*-mō-NĪ-tis)	inflammation of the lung
pneumothorax (*nū*-mō-THOR-aks)	air in the chest cavity (pleural space), which causes collapse of the lung (often a result of an open chest wound) (Exercise Figure C1)
pulmonary neoplasm (PUL-mō-*nar*-ē) (NĒ-ō-plazm)	pertaining to (in) the lung, new growth (tumor)
pyothorax (*pī*-ō-THOR-aks)	pus in the chest cavity (pleural space) (also called **empyema**)
rhinitis (rī-NĪ-tis)	inflammation of the nose (mucous membranes)
rhinomycosis (*rī*-nō-mī-KŌ-sis)	abnormal condition of fungus in the nose
rhinorrhagia (*rī*-nō-RĀ-ja)	rapid flow of blood from the nose (also called **epistaxis**)
sinusitis (sī-nū-SĪ-tis)	inflammation of the sinuses (Exercise Figure D2)

TERM	DEFINITION
thoracalgia (*thor*-a-KAL-ja)	pain in the chest
tonsillitis (*ton*-sil-Ī-tis)	inflammation of the tonsils
tracheitis (*trā*-kē-Ī-tis)	inflammation of the trachea
tracheostenosis (*trā*-kē-ō-sten-Ō-sis)	narrowing of the trachea

To watch animations, go to evolve.elsevier.com. Select:
Chapter 5, **Animations**, Atelectasis
                            Pneumonia
                            Pneumothorax
                            Hemothorax

Refer to p. 10 for your Evolve access information.

EXERCISE FIGURE D

Fill in the blanks to complete the labeling of the diagram.

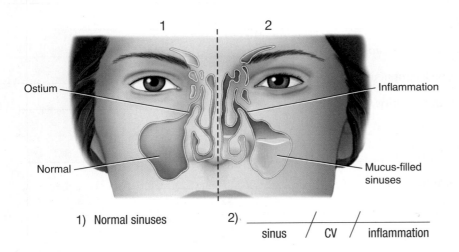

1) Normal sinuses

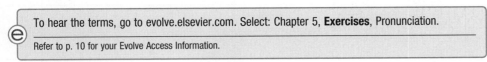

2) _____ / ____ / _____
       sinus   CV   inflammation

EXERCISE 12

Practice saying aloud each of the disease and disorder terms built from word parts on pp. 150–153.

To hear the terms, go to evolve.elsevier.com. Select: Chapter 5, **Exercises**, Pronunciation.

Refer to p. 10 for your Evolve Access Information.

☐ Place a check mark in the box when you have completed this exercise.

CAM TERM

Traditional Chinese medicine (TCM) is an example of a whole medical system, one of NCCAM's five major classifications. TCM is an ancient healing system that uses herbal and nutritional therapy, acupuncture, massage, and therapeutic exercise to balance the Qi (vital energy) within the body to promote wellness and healing for body, mind, and spirit. Studies have demonstrated that a variety of TCM modalities can provide symptomatic relief and improvement in quality of life for patients with **asthma, allergic rhinitis,** and other respiratory ailments.

EXERCISE 13

Analyze and define the following terms.

EXAMPLE: diaphragmat / o / cele   hernia of the diaphragm

1. pleuritis _____

2. nasopharyngitis _____

3. pneumothorax _____

4. sinusitis _____

5. atelectasis _____

6. rhinomycosis _____

7. tracheostenosis _____

8. epiglottitis _____

9. thoracalgia _____

10. pulmonary neoplasm _____

11. bronchiectasis _____

12. tonsillitis _____

13. pneumoconiosis _____

14. bronchopneumonia _____

15. pneumonitis _____

16. laryngitis _____

17. pyothorax _____

18. rhinorrhagia _____

19. bronchitis _____

20. pharyngitis _____

21. tracheitis _____

22. laryngotracheobronchitis _____

23. adenoiditis _____

24. hemothorax _____

25. lobar pneumonia _____

26. rhinitis _____

27. bronchogenic carcinoma _____

28. alveolitis _____

29. pneumonia _____

30. pneumatocele _____

EXERCISE 14

Build disease and disorder terms for the following definitions with the word parts you have learned.

EXAMPLE: inflammation of the tonsils $\dfrac{tonsill}{WR} \Big/ \dfrac{itis}{S}$

1. pain in the chest

$$\overline{}_{WR} \Big/ \overline{}_{S}$$

2. abnormal condition of fungus (infection) in the nose

$$\overline{}_{WR} \Big/ \overline{}_{CV} \Big/ \overline{}_{WR} \Big/ \overline{}_{S}$$

3. pertaining to the lung; new growth (tumor)

$$\overline{}_{WR} \Big/ \overline{}_{S} \qquad \overline{}_{P} \Big/ \overline{}_{S(WR)}$$

4. inflammation of the larynx

$$\overline{}_{WR} \Big/ \overline{}_{S}$$

5. incomplete expansion (of the lung)

$$\overline{}_{WR} \Big/ \overline{}_{S}$$

6. inflammation of the adenoids

$$\overline{}_{WR} \Big/ \overline{}_{S}$$

7. inflammation of the larynx, trachea, and bronchi

$$\overline{}_{WR} \Big/ \overline{}_{CV} \Big/ \overline{}_{WR} \Big/ \overline{}_{CV} \Big/ \overline{}_{WR} \Big/ \overline{}_{S}$$

8. dilation of the bronchi

$$\overline{}_{WR} \Big/ \overline{}_{S}$$

9. inflammation of the pleura

$$\overline{}_{WR} \Big/ \overline{}_{S}$$

10. abnormal condition of dust in the lung

$$\overline{}_{WR} \Big/ \overline{}_{CV} \Big/ \overline{}_{WR} \Big/ \overline{}_{S}$$

11. inflammation of the lung

$$\overline{}_{WR} \Big/ \overline{}_{S}$$

12. inflammation of the sinuses

$$\overline{}_{WR} \Big/ \overline{}_{S}$$

13. narrowing of the trachea

$$\overline{}_{WR} \Big/ \overline{}_{CV} \Big/ \overline{}_{S}$$

14. inflammation of the nose and pharynx

$$\overline{}_{WR} \Big/ \overline{}_{CV} \Big/ \overline{}_{WR} \Big/ \overline{}_{S}$$

15. pus in the chest cavity (pleural space)

$$\overline{}_{WR} \Big/ \overline{}_{CV} \Big/ \overline{}_{S}$$

16. inflammation of the epiglottis

$$\overline{}_{WR} \Big/ \overline{}_{S}$$

17. hernia of the diaphragm

$$\overline{}_{WR} \Big/ \overline{}_{CV} \Big/ \overline{}_{S}$$

18. air in the chest cavity
    (pleural space)

    _____ / _____ / _____
    WR   CV   S

19. diseased state of the bronchi
    and the lungs

    _____ / _____ / _____ / _____
    WR   CV   WR   S

20. rapid flow of blood from the
    nose

    _____ / _____ / _____
    WR   CV   S

21. inflammation of the pharynx

    _____ / _____
    WR   S

22. blood in the chest cavity
    (pleural space)

    _____ / _____ / _____
    WR   CV   S

23. inflammation of the trachea

    _____ / _____
    WR   S

24. inflammation of the bronchi

    _____ / _____
    WR   S

25. pertaining to the lobe(s);
    diseased state of the lung(s)

    _____ / _____   _____ / _____
    WR   S   WR   S

26. inflammation of the nose
    (mucous membranes)

    _____ / _____
    WR   S

27. cancerous tumor originating
    in a bronchus

    _____ / _____ / _____   _____ / _____
    WR   CV   S   WR   S

28. inflammation of the alveoli

    _____ / _____
    WR   S

29. diseased state of the lung

    _____ / _____
    WR   S

30. hernia of the lung

    _____ / _____ / _____
    WR   CV   S

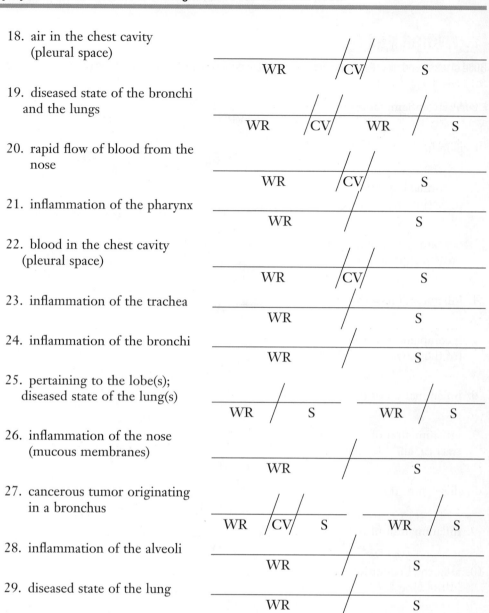

EXERCISE 15

Spell each of the disease and disorder terms built from word parts on pp. 150–153 by having someone dictate them to you.

> To hear and spell the terms, go to evolve.elsevier.com. Select: Chapter 5, **Exercises**, Spelling.
>
> Refer to p. 10 for your Evolve Access Information.
>
> ☐ Place a check mark in the box if you have completed this exercise online.

1. _____
2. _____
3. _____
4. _____
5. _____
6. _____
7. _____
8. _____
9. _____
10. _____
11. _____
12. _____
13. _____
14. _____
15. _____

16. _____
17. _____
18. _____
19. _____
20. _____
21. _____
22. _____
23. _____
24. _____
25. _____
26. _____
27. _____
28. _____
29. _____
30. _____

Disease and Disorder Terms

Not Built from Word Parts

In some of the following terms, you may recognize word parts; however, the terms cannot be translated literally to find their meanings.

TERM	DEFINITION
acute respiratory distress syndrome (ARDS) (a-KŪT) (RES-pi-ra-*tor*-ē) (di-STRES) (SIN-drōm)	respiratory failure as a result of disease or injury. Symptoms include dyspnea, tachypnea, and cyanosis (also called **adult respiratory distress syndrome**).
asthma (AZ-ma)	respiratory disease characterized by coughing, wheezing, and shortness of breath, caused by constriction and inflammation of airways that is reversible between attacks
chronic obstructive pulmonary disease (COPD) (KRON-ik) (ob-STRUK-tiv) (PUL-mō-*nar*-ē) (di-ZĒZ)	a progressive lung disease restricting air flow, which makes breathing difficult. Chronic bronchitis and emphysema are the two main components of COPD. Most COPD is a result of cigarette smoking.

ACUTE RESPIRATORY DISTRESS SYNDROME (ARDS)

is respiratory failure in an adult. In newborns the condition is referred to as **infant respiratory distress syndrome of newborn (IRDS)** or **hyaline membrane disease**.

INSIDIOUS/ACUTE/SUBACUTE/CHRONIC

In reference to disease

Insidious: gradual and subtle onset of disease

Acute: sharp, sudden, short, or severe type of disease

Subacute: between acute and chronic

Chronic: disease that continues for a long time

REACTIVE AIRWAY DISEASE (RAD)

is a general term and not a specific diagnosis. It is used to describe a history of wheezing, coughing, and shortness of breath. In some people RAD may lead to **asthma**.

Disease and Disorder Terms—cont'd

Not Built from Word Parts

TERM	DEFINITION
coccidioidomycosis (kok-*sid*-ē-*oy*-dō-mī-KŌ-sis)	fungal disease affecting the lungs and sometimes other organs of the body (also called **valley fever** or **cocci**)
cor pulmonale (kōr) (*pul*-mō-NAL-ē)	serious cardiac disease associated with chronic lung disorders, such as emphysema
croup (krūp)	condition resulting from acute obstruction of the larynx, characterized by a barking cough, hoarseness, and stridor. It may be caused by viral or bacterial infection, allergy, or foreign body. Occurs mainly in children. (also called **laryngotracheobronchitis**)
cystic fibrosis (CF) (SIS-tik) (fi-BRŌ-sis)	hereditary disorder of the exocrine glands characterized by excess mucus production in the respiratory tract, pancreatic deficiency, and other symptoms
deviated septum (DĒ-vē-*āt*-ed) (SEP-tum)	one part of the nasal cavity is smaller because of malformation or injury of the nasal septum
emphysema (*em*-fi-SĒ-ma)	stretching of lung tissue caused by the alveoli becoming distended and losing elasticity and as a result, the body does not receive enough oxygen (component of COPD) (Figure 5-4)
epistaxis (*ep*-i-STAK-sis)	nosebleed (synonymous with **rhinorrhagia**)
idiopathic pulmonary fibrosis (IPF) (id-ē-ō-PATH-ik) (PUL-mō-*nar*-ē) (fi-BRŌ-sis)	chronic progressive lung disorder characterized by increasing scarring, which ultimately reduces the capacity of the lungs; etiology unknown
influenza (*in*-flū-EN-za)	highly contagious and often severe viral infection of the respiratory tract
obstructive sleep apnea (OSA) (ob-STRUK-tiv) (slēp) (AP-nē-a)	repetitive pharyngeal collapse during sleep, which leads to absence of breathing; can produce daytime drowsiness and elevated blood pressure (Figure 5-7)
pertussis (per-TUS-sis)	highly contagious bacterial infection of the respiratory tract characterized by an acute crowing inspiration, or whoop (also called **whooping cough**)
pleural effusion (PLŪ-ral) (e-FŪ-zhun)	fluid in the pleural space caused by a disease process or trauma
pulmonary edema (PUL-mō-*nar*-ē) (e-DĒ-ma)	fluid accumulation in the alveoli and bronchioles, most often a manifestation of heart failure
pulmonary embolism (PE) (PUL-mō-*nar*-ē) (EM-bo-lizm)	matter foreign to the circulation, carried to the pulmonary artery and its branches, where it blocks circulation to the lungs and can be fatal if of sufficient size or number. Blood clots broken loose from the deep veins of the lower extremities are the most common source of emboli (Figure 5-8).

IDOPATHIC PULMONARY FIBROSIS (IPF)

most often affects adults over the age of 50, the etiology is unknown. Smoking, pollutants, and heredity, may play a role in its genesis. **Symptoms** include exertional **dyspnea** and a **dry cough**. Lung transplant may be indicated in severe cases; there is no cure.

INFLUENZA PANDEMIC

is the sudden outbreak of a flu that becomes very widespread, affecting a region, a continent, or the world. Examples are **H1N1 swine flu** and **H5N1 avian flu**.

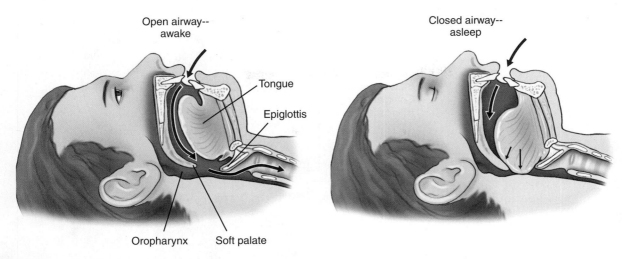

FIGURE 5-7
Obstructive sleep apnea (OSA). During sleep the absence of activity of the pharyngeal muscle structure allows the airway to close. OSA is associated with increased risk for elevated blood pressure, cardiovascular disease, diabetes, and stroke. Obesity is a major risk factor and weight loss can be an effective treatment. **Polysomnography** is used to diagnose OSA. Treatment includes the use of **CPAP (continuous positive airway pressure)** during sleep and **uvulopalatopharyngoplasty (UPPP),** a surgical procedure.

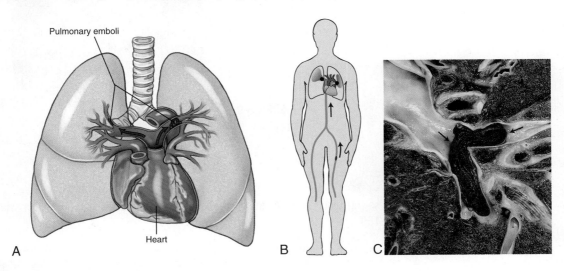

FIGURE 5-8
A, Bilateral pulmonary emboli. **B,** Pulmonary emboli usually originate in the deep veins of the lower extremities. **C,** Necropsy specimen of the lung showing a large embolus.

TERM	DEFINITION
tuberculosis (TB) (tū-*ber*-kū-LŌ-sis)	infectious bacterial disease, most commonly spread by inhalation of small particles and usually affecting the lungs; may spread to other organs
upper respiratory infection (URI) (UP-er) (RES-pi-ra-*tor*-ē) (in-FEK-shun)	infection of the nasal cavity, pharynx, or larynx (commonly called a **cold**) (Figure 5-9)

TUBERCULOSIS (TB)

causes more deaths worldwide than any other infectious disease even though it is preventable and curable. The risk for active TB is higher in HIV-infected persons and drug users. The development of multidrug–resistant TB is becoming a problem in treatment of the disease.

To watch animations, go to evolve.elsevier.com. Select:
Chapter 5, **Animations**, Asthma
Tuberculosis
Pulmonary Embolus

Refer to p. 10 for your Evolve Access Information.

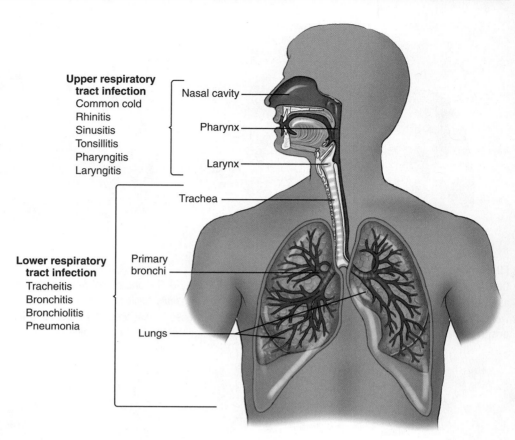

FIGURE 5-9
Upper and lower respiratory tract infections.

EXERCISE 16

Practice saying aloud each of the disease and disorder terms not built from word parts on pp. 157–159.

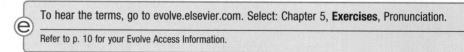

To hear the terms, go to evolve.elsevier.com. Select: Chapter 5, **Exercises**, Pronunciation.

Refer to p. 10 for your Evolve Access Information.

☐ Place a check mark in the box when you have completed this exercise.

EXERCISE 17

Fill in the blanks with the correct terms.

1. A disease characterized by lung tissue stretching that results from the alveoli losing elasticity and becoming distended is called _____.

2. _____ _____ is the name given to the fluid in the pleural space caused by a disease process or a trauma.

3. A cardiac condition that is associated with chronic lung disorders is called _____ _____.

4. A fungal disease affecting the lungs is called _____.

5. _____ _____ is a hereditary disorder characterized by excess mucus production in the respiratory tract.

6. The medical name of a highly contagious respiratory infection commonly referred to as *flu* is _____.

7. Chronic bronchitis and emphysema are two main components of _____ _____ _____ _____.

8. The medical name for the disease characterized by an acute crowing inspiration is _____.

9. _____ is a condition resulting from an acute obstruction of the larynx.

10. A respiratory disease characterized by shortness of breath, wheezing, and coughing is called _____.

11. A condition in which fluid accumulates in the alveoli and bronchioles is _____ _____.

12. A(n) _____ _____ _____ generally refers to an infection involving the nasal cavity, pharynx, or larynx.

13. Foreign matter, such as a blood clot, carried to the pulmonary artery, where it blocks circulation to the lungs, is called a(n) _____ _____.

14. _____ is another name for nosebleed.

15. A chronic progressive lung disorder that ultimately reduces the capacity of the lungs is _____ _____ _____.

16. _____ _____ is one part of the nasal cavity that is smaller than the other because of malformation or injury.

17. The diagnosis for repetitive pharyngeal collapse is _____ _____ _____.

18. An infectious bacterial disease usually affecting the lungs and caused by inhaling infected small particles is _____.

19. _____ _____ _____ _____ is also called adult respiratory distress syndrome.

EXERCISE 18

Match the terms in the first column with the correct definitions in the second column.

_____ 1. asthma	a. alveoli become distended and lose elasticity
_____ 2. chronic obstructive pulmonary disease	b. caused by a virus (commonly called *flu*)
_____ 3. coccidioidomycosis	c. hereditary disorder characterized by excess mucus in the respiratory system
_____ 4. cor pulmonale	d. most often caused by cigarette smoking
_____ 5. croup	e. nosebleed
_____ 6. cystic fibrosis	f. cardiac disease associated with chronic lung disorders
_____ 7. emphysema	g. condition resulting from acute obstruction of the larynx
_____ 8. epistaxis	h. also called *valley fever*
_____ 9. influenza	i. characterized by scarring of the lung
_____ 10. idiopathic pulmonary fibrosis	j. caused by restriction of airways that is reversible between attacks

EXERCISE 19

Match the terms in the first column with the correct definitions in the second column.

_____ 1. pertussis
_____ 2. pleural effusion
_____ 3. pulmonary edema
_____ 4. pulmonary embolism
_____ 5. upper respiratory infection
_____ 6. deviated septum
_____ 7. obstructive sleep apnea
_____ 8. tuberculosis
_____ 9. acute respiratory distress syndrome

a. respiratory failure as a result of disease or injury
b. fluid in the pleural space
c. fluid accumulation in alveoli and bronchioles
d. whooping cough
e. foreign material, carried to the pulmonary artery, where it blocks circulation to the lungs
f. commonly called a cold
g. unequal size of nasal cavities
h. repetitive pharyngeal collapse
i. infectious bacterial disease usually affecting the lungs

EXERCISE 20

Spell each of the disease and disorder terms not built from word parts on pp. 157–159 by having someone dictate them to you.

> To hear and spell the terms, go to evolve.elsevier.com. Select: Chapter 5, **Exercises**, Spelling.
>
> Refer to p. 10 for your Evolve Access Information.
>
> ☐ Place a check mark in the box if you have completed this exercise online.

1. _____
2. _____
3. _____
4. _____
5. _____
6. _____
7. _____
8. _____
9. _____
10. _____

11. _____
12. _____
13. _____
14. _____
15. _____
16. _____
17. _____
18. _____
19. _____

Surgical Terms

Built from Word Parts

The following terms are built from word parts you have already learned and can be translated literally to find their meanings. Further explanation of terms beyond the definition of their word parts, if needed, is included in parentheses.

TERM	DEFINITION
adenoidectomy (*ad*-e-noyd-EK-to-mē)	excision of the adenoids (Exercise Figure E)
adenotome (AD-e-nō-*tōm*) (*Note: the* oid *is missing from the word root* adenoid *in this term.*)	instrument used to cut the adenoids (Exercise Figure E)
bronchoplasty (BRON-kō-*plas*-tē)	surgical repair of a bronchus
laryngectomy (*lār*-in-JEK-to-mē)	excision of the larynx
laryngoplasty (la-RING-gō-*plas*-tē)	surgical repair of the larynx
laryngostomy (*lar*-in-GOS-to-mē)	creation of an artificial opening into the larynx
laryngotracheotomy (la-*ring*-gō-*trā*-kē-OT-o-mē)	incision of the larynx and trachea
lobectomy (lō-BEK-to-mē)	excision of a lobe (of the lung) (Figure 5-10)
pleuropexy (plū-rō-PEK-sē)	surgical fixation of the pleura
pneumonectomy (*nū*-mō-NEK-to-mē)	excision of a lung (see Figure 5-10)
rhinoplasty (RĪ-nō-*plas*-tē)	surgical repair of the nose
septoplasty (SEP-tō-*plas*-tē)	surgical repair of the (nasal) septum
septotomy (sep-TOT-o-mē)	incision of the (nasal) septum
sinusotomy (*sī*-nū-SOT-o-mē)	incision into a sinus
thoracocentesis (*thor*-a-kō-sen-TĒ-sis)	surgical puncture to aspirate fluid from the chest cavity (also called **thoracentesis**) (Exercise Figure F)
thoracotomy (*thor*-a-KOT-o-mē)	incision into the chest cavity (Figure 5-11)
tonsillectomy (*ton*-sil-EK-to-mē)	excision of the tonsils
tracheoplasty (TRĀ-kē-ō-*plas*-tē)	surgical repair of the trachea
tracheostomy (*trā*-kē-OS-to-mē)	creation of an artificial opening into the trachea (Figure 5-12)
tracheotomy (*trā*-kē-OT-o-mē)	incision into the trachea (Figure 5-12)

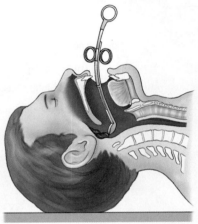

EXERCISE FIGURE E

Fill in the blanks to complete labeling of the diagram.

_____ / _____ performed using
adenoid / excision

a(n) _____ / _____ / _____
adenoid / cv / instrument used to cut

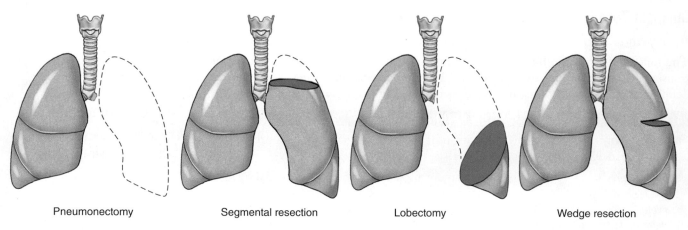

Pneumonectomy   Segmental resection   Lobectomy   Wedge resection

FIGURE 5-10
Types of lung resection. The diagram illustrates the amount of lung tissue removed with each type of surgery.

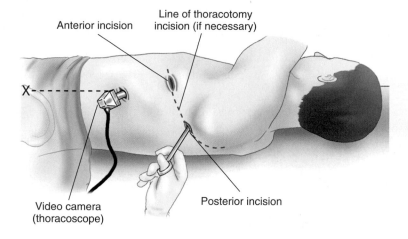

Anterior incision

Line of thoracotomy incision (if necessary)

X

Video camera (thoracoscope)

Posterior incision

FIGURE 5-11
Video-assisted thoracic surgery (VATS) is the use of a **thoracoscope** and video equipment for an endoscopic approach to diagnose and treat thoracic conditions. It replaces the traditional **thoracotomy,** which required a large incision and greater recovery time.

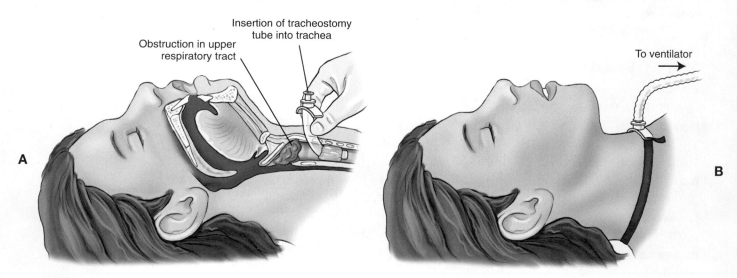

Obstruction in upper respiratory tract

Insertion of tracheostomy tube into trachea

To ventilator

A

B

FIGURE 5-12
A, A tracheotomy is performed to establish an airway when normal breathing is obstructed. **B,** If the opening needs to be maintained, a tube is inserted, creating a tracheostomy. A **tracheostomy** may be temporary, as for prolonged mechanical ventilation to support breathing or it may be permanent, as in airway reconstruction after laryngeal cancer surgery.

EXERCISE FIGURE **F**

Fill in the blanks to complete labeling of the diagram.

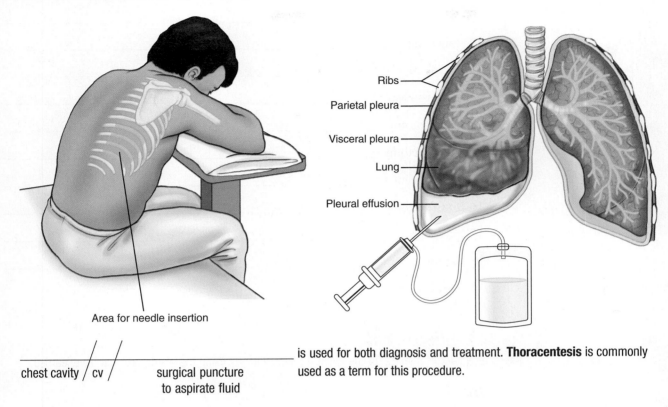

Ribs

Parietal pleura

Visceral pleura

Lung

Pleural effusion

Area for needle insertion

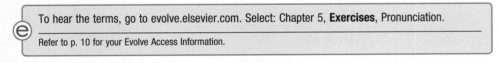

_____ / __ / _____   is used for both diagnosis and treatment. **Thoracentesis** is commonly
chest cavity / cv / surgical puncture   used as a term for this procedure.
to aspirate fluid

EXERCISE **21**

Practice saying aloud each of the surgical terms built from word parts on p. 163.

(e) To hear the terms, go to evolve.elsevier.com. Select: Chapter 5, **Exercises**, Pronunciation.

Refer to p. 10 for your Evolve Access Information.

☐ Place a check mark in the box when you have completed this exercise.

EXERCISE **22**

Analyze and define the following surgical terms.

         WR   S

EXAMPLE: pneumon/ectomy   <u>excision of a lung</u>

1. tracheotomy _____

2. laryngostomy _____

3. adenoidectomy _____

4. rhinoplasty _____

5. adenotome _____

6. tracheostomy _____

7. sinusotomy _____

8. laryngoplasty _____

9. bronchoplasty _____

10. lobectomy _____

11. laryngotracheotomy _____

12. tracheoplasty _____

13. thoracotomy _____

14. laryngectomy _____

15. thoracocentesis _____

16. tonsillectomy _____

17. pleuropexy _____

18. septoplasty _____

19. septotomy _____

EXERCISE 23

Build surgical terms for the following definitions by using the word parts you have learned.

EXAMPLE: surgical fixation of the pleura $\dfrac{pleur}{WR} \Big/ \dfrac{o}{CV} \Big/ \dfrac{pexy}{S}$

1. surgical repair of the trachea _____ WR / CV / S

2. incision of larynx and trachea _____ WR / CV / WR / CV / S

3. instrument used to cut the adenoids _____ WR / CV / S

4. incision into the chest cavity _____ WR / CV / S

5. creation of an artificial opening into the trachea _____ WR / CV / S

6. excision of the tonsils _____ WR / S

7. incision into the trachea _____ WR / CV / S

8. surgical repair of a bronchus _____ WR / CV / S

9. excision of the larynx _____ WR / S

10. surgical repair of the nose _____ WR / CV / S

11. incision into a sinus   _____

                     WR   /CV/   S

12. surgical puncture to aspirate fluid from the chest cavity   _____

                     WR   /CV/   S

13. excision of the adenoids   _____

                     WR   /   S

14. surgical repair of the larynx   _____

                     WR   /CV/   S

15. excision of a lobe (of the lung)   _____

                     WR   /   S

16. creation of an artificial opening into the larynx   _____

                     WR   /CV/   S

17. excision of a lung   _____

                     WR   /   S

18. incision of the septum   _____

                     WR   /CV/   S

19. surgical repair of the septum   _____

                     WR   /CV/   S

EXERCISE 24

Spell each of the surgical terms built from word parts on p. 163 by having someone dictate them to you.

> To hear and spell the terms, go to evolve.elsevier.com. Select: Chapter 5, **Exercises**, Spelling.
>
> Refer to p. 10 for your Evolve Access Information.
>
> ☐ Place a check mark in the box if you have completed this exercise online.

1. _____   11. _____

2. _____   12. _____

3. _____   13. _____

4. _____   14. _____

5. _____   15. _____

6. _____   16. _____

7. _____   17. _____

8. _____   18. _____

9. _____   19. _____

10. _____   20. _____

Table 5-1

Diagnostic Procedures and Tests

Diagnostic procedures and tests are performed for use in the diagnosis, monitoring, and treatment of disease. An overview of the most common types of procedures, **Diagnostic Imaging, Endoscopy,** and **Laboratory Studies follow that will assist you in navigating terms presented in this and subsequent chapters of the text.**

DIAGNOSTIC IMAGING

Diagnostic imaging is a generic term that covers **radiography, computed tomography, nuclear medicine, magnetic resonance imaging,** and **sonography.**

Radiography (x-ray) produces images of internal organs using ionizing radiation produced by an energy source, the x-ray machine (Figure 5-13). Invisible x-rays penetrate solid material such as bone, producing a shadow that can be recorded digitally or on film. The image produced is called a **radiograph**. Radiography is performed to detect **diseases, bone fractures, or other pathology.**

X-RAY FILM/ RADIOGRAPH

are terms used interchangeably; however, they have different meanings. **X-ray film** is the material on which the image is exposed, whereas **radiograph** refers to the processed image. **Radiographic images,** referred to as **x-ray images,** in former editions of this text, can be obtained as hard copy on x-ray film (radiograph) or as digital images stored electronically and viewed on a monitor.

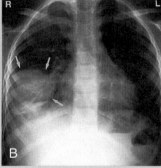
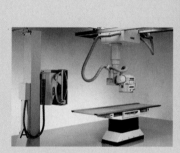

FIGURE 5-13
A, Chest x-ray machine and table. **B,** Chest radiograph revealing pneumonia of the right lung.

X-rays were first discovered in 1895 by Wilhelm Conrad Roentgen in Germany. Because he did not understand the nature of the rays, he named them "x"-rays.

Computed tomography (CT) produces computerized radiographic images (scan) using a complex computer and imaging system (x-rays) to produce a series of sectional (slices) images of body organs or segments (Figure 5-14). The computer can process the data to show images in axial, sagittal, or coronal planes. The density and outline data can be used to show a three-dimensional image. CT is used in **diagnosing tumors, abscesses, cysts, stones, and other conditions.** More radiation is required in CT scanning than radiography.

SCANNING/SCAN

Scanning means to map organs or the body with a sensing device. **Scan** is the image obtained and is often designated by the organ studied, as a **brain scan or liver scan.** Scan is the shortened form for **scintiscan,** an image created by radioisotopes.

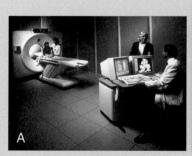
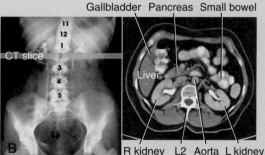

FIGURE 5-14
A, Computed tomography scanner. **B,** An example of CT scan of the abdomen at level of kidneys.

CT scanners were first used in the United States in 1973.

Table 5-1
Diagnostic Procedures and Tests—cont'd

DIAGNOSTIC IMAGING

Magnetic resonance imaging (MRI) produces images by exposing the body to high strength, computer-controlled magnetic fields (Figure 5-15). As the magnetic field changes, the tissues of the body respond in characteristic ways. Very sensitive detectors are used to record the response of the different tissues. Computers are then used to create an image. MRI is preferred over CT to study the brain and spinal cord because it provides better detail of structure. MRI is used in detecting **tumors, bleeding, infection, injury, edema, or obstruction.** Risks of ionizing radiation are avoided by MRI scanning.

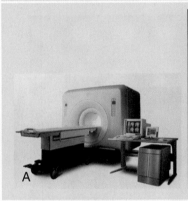
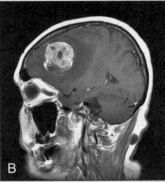

FIGURE 5-15
A, Magnetic resonance scanner. **B,** Sagittal MRI section through the brain showing frontal lobe mass enhanced with contrast medium.

The first MRI scanner was installed in the Unites States in 1981.

Nuclear medicine (NM) produces images (also known as scintiscans, scans, or scintigrams) by administering radioactive material often combined with other materials to cause it to be delivered to the body part of interest (Figure 5-16). The radioactive material and the material to which it is bound, often referred to as a **radiopharmaceutical** or **tracer**, emits energy (usually gamma rays) that is detected by a specialized camera (gamma camera). A computer translates the readings into two-dimensional images (scans) in various shades of grey or color. The most commonly used radiopharmaceutical is **technetium-99m** or **Tc-99m**, although others including **gallium, thallium,** and **iodine** are also used and sometimes appear in the name of the NM test. NM studies are used to detect abnormal function and structure of organs or of various body areas. An **NM lung scan may be performed to detect pulmonary emboli, a bone scan to detect metastatic cancer, or a renal scan to evaluate blood flow to the kidney.** In NM the radioactive source mostly comes from within the body whereas in x-ray and computed tomography the radioactive source is from outside the body. Some NM procedures are done on blood and urine specimens that require no administration of a radioactive source into the body. The risk of radiation is dependent on the dose and radiopharmaceutical used. It can be lower than x-rays studies.

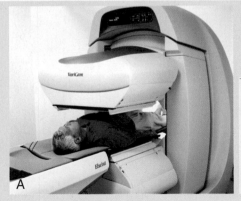
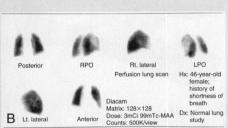

Posterior   RPO   Rt. lateral   LPO
Perfusion lung scan

Lt. lateral   Anterior

Diacam
Matrix: 128×128
Dose: 3mCi 99mTc-MAA
Counts: 500K/view

Hx: 46-year-old female; history of shortness of breath
Dx: Normal lung study

FIGURE 5-16
A, Nuclear medicine scanner. **B,** Lung scan.

By 1970 most body organs could be visualized by NM procedures, and in 1971 Nuclear Medicine was officially recognized by the American Medical Association as a medical specialty.

Table 5-1

Diagnostic Procedures and Tests—cont'd

DIAGNOSTIC IMAGING

Single-photon emission computed tomography (SPECT) is an NM technique that yields three-dimensional computer constructed images (Figure 5-17). SPECT is capable of showing blood flow through an organ and blood-deprived areas of the brain and heart. Using SPECT, the heart can be visualized from several different angles to **assess damage to cardiac tissue following a myocardial infarction (heart attack) or damage to brain tissue caused by a disruption of the normal supply of blood, which often occurs with a stroke.**

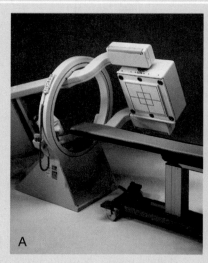
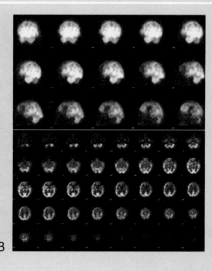

FIGURE 5-17
A, SPECT camera system. **B,** Three dimensional SPECT of brain study showing a patient with left frontal lobe brain infarction. SPECT was developed in 1980.

Positron emission tomography (PET) is a relatively new NM procedure (Figure 5-18). Positron-emitting radioactive material is injected into the body. The positrons are picked up by a ring of detectors positioned around the body. Functional and anatomic abnormalities are demonstrated. The images can be combined with CT images to more precisely show the location of the activity in the body. PET is **used in oncology to assist in diagnosing and staging of cancer and monitoring the effects of treatment. PET is also used in neurology to assist in diagnosing Alzheimer disease.**

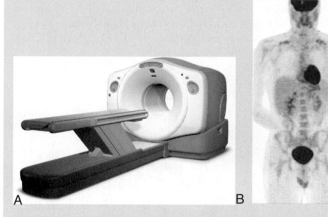

FIGURE 5-18
A, A typical PET/CT scanner. **B,** PET image to evaluate a patient with a history of melanoma. Scan shows physiologic activity no evidence of recurrence. **C,** Image six months later shows metastases throughout the body.

PET began in the 1970s as a research tool. The combination PET/CT scanner was developed in the 1990s.

Table 5-1

Diagnostic Procedures and Tests—cont'd

DIAGNOSTIC IMAGING

Sonography, also referred to as ultrasound, produces scans using high frequency sound waves, which are beyond the range of human hearing (Figure 5-19). A transducer (device that converts energy from one form to another), is passed over the skin of a specific body area. The transducer converts electric energy into high-frequency sound waves, which travel into the body. Some of the sound waves reflect (echo) off the internal structures back to the transducer. The echo is converted by the transducer to electrical impulses, which are tranformed into visual images called sonograms. The composition and layers of different tissue types reflect sound waves differently, allowing an image to emerge. Transducers may also be placed in body cavities (endoscopic) to obtain a sonogram. For example in **transesophageal echocardiography**, the transducer is placed in the esophagus to obtain views of the heart for examining cardiac function and structure. Abdominal sonography may be used to detect **nephrolithiasis (kidney stones) or gall stones (cholelithiasis), and sonography is extensively used to evaluate the fetus during pregnancy.** The risks of ionizing radiation are eliminated by using ultrasound and in typical use, ultrasound is considered relatively harmless. It is also less expensive than MRI, CT, or NM procedures.

ULTRASOUND OR ULTRASONOGRAPHY

are terms also used to describe sonography. Ultra- means "beyond" or "excess." The term ultrasound indicates high frequency sound waves that are beyond audible. The term sonography is used throughout this text.

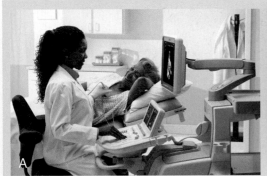
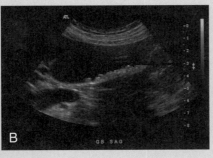
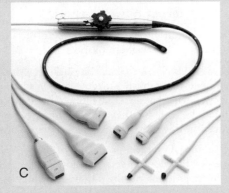

FIGURE 5-19
A, Sonographer performing an ultrasound exam. **B,** Sagittal sonogram showing multiple small gallstones.
C, Ultrasound transducers.

Sonography had its beginning during World War I with the development of sonar. In the 1950s anatomy ultrasound images were seen on a monitor in a series of blips. Digital systems that were introduced in the 1990s provided for images in the digital format that allowed for manipulation, viewing, and storage.

Table 5-1

Diagnostic Procedures and Tests—cont'd

ENDOSCOPY

Endoscopy is a general term for direct observation examination of a hollow body organ or cavity using a tubular instrument with a light source and a viewing lens called an endoscope (Figure 5-20). The original endoscopes were rigid and used for direct observation. Adding lights and lenses to the endoscope allowed visualization of deeper structures. By incorporating fiberoptics and cameras, smaller flexible endoscopes were created allowing the images to be viewed on a monitor. A flexible fiberoptic scope is most often used in gastrointestinal and pulmonary endoscopy. Endoscopic procedures and instruments are named after the body part being visualized. A **bronchoscopy** means **visual examination of the bronchi**, and **bronchoscope** means **instrument used for visual examination of the bronchi**.

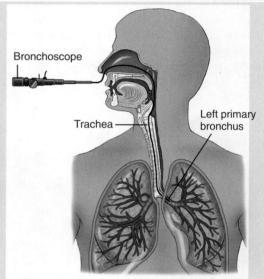

FIGURE 5-20
Bronchoscopy. A bronchoscope is inserted through the nostril, pharynx, larynx, and trachea into the bronchus.

Endoscopy dates back to the time of Hippocrates (460-375 BC) who mentions using a speculum to look into the rectum. By the end of the nineteenth century cystoscopy, proctoscopy, and esophagoscopy were well established.

LABORATORY TESTS

Laboratory tests are performed to establish a diagnosis and/or prognosis, and to monitor and evaluate treatment. Specimens that are studied include blood (most common), urine, stool, sputum, sweat, wound drainage or discharge from body openings, washings, and tissue. Most studies included in this text fall into the following categories:

Hematology studies relate to the physical properties of blood such as the number of blood cells in the specimen or the clotting and bleeding factors. A **white blood cell** (WBC) count is a blood test that measures the number of white blood cells present in a specimen. A **red blood cell** (RBC) count measures the number of red blood cells.

Chemistry studies relate to the study of chemical reactions that occur in the human body and are usually performed on blood or urine specimens. **BUN** (blood urea nitrogen) is a blood test used to measure kidney function. **Urine glucose** is a test performed on a urine specimen, and is used to determine the amount of glucose in the urine.

Microbiology studies identify the microorganisms that cause disease and infection. **Culture and sensitivity** is a common study performed on almost any specimen. The specimen is placed on a medium for growth. If a pathogenic microorganism grows, it is tested for antibiotic sensitivity to determine to which antibiotics, it is susceptible and those to which it is resistant. This information allows the physician to order an antibiotic that will provide the effective treatment.

Urine studies are performed on urine specimens to diagnose and monitor urinary tract disease. They are also used to detect and monitor diseases not related to the kidney such as identifying glucose in the urine, which may indicate diabetes mellitus. A **urinalysis** is the study of urine for color, clarity, degree of acidity or alkalinity, specific gravity, protein, glucose, leukocytes, and bilirubin.

Diagnostic Terms
Built from Word Parts

The following terms are built from word parts you have already learned and can be translated literally to find their meanings. Further explanation of terms beyond the definition of their word parts, if needed, is included in parentheses.

TERM	DEFINITION
ENDOSCOPY	
bronchoscope (BRON-kō-skōp)	instrument used for visual examination of the bronchi (Figure 5-20)
bronchoscopy (bron-KOS-ko-pē)	visual examination of the bronchi (Figure 5-20)
endoscope (EN-dō-skōp)	instrument used for visual examination within (a hollow organ or body cavity). (Endoscopes are used for surgical procedures as well as for viewing.)
endoscopic (*en*-dō-SKOP-ik)	pertaining to visual examination within (a hollow organ or body cavity) (used to describe the practice of performing surgeries that use endoscopes)
endoscopy (en-DOS-ko-pē)	visual examination within (a hollow organ or body cavity)
laryngoscope (la-RING-go-skōp)	instrument used for visual examination of the larynx (Exercise Figure G)

SCOPE

is taken from the Greek **skopein,** which means to **see** or to **view.** It also means **observing for a purpose.** To the ancient Greeks it meant "to look out for, to monitor, or to examine."

Today the following suffixes commonly are used:

- -scope describes the instrument used to view or to examine, such as in the term endoscope.
- -scopy means visual examination, such as in the term endoscopy.
- -scopic means pertaining to visual examination, such as in the term endoscopic.

Endoscopic surgery is performed with the use of endoscopes. Most often the suffixes -**scope, -scopy,** and -**scopic** mean to **examine visually,** and that is the definition given in this text. However, the term **stethoscope** is an **instrument used for listening** to body sounds.

EXERCISE FIGURE G

Fill in the blanks to complete labeling of the diagram.

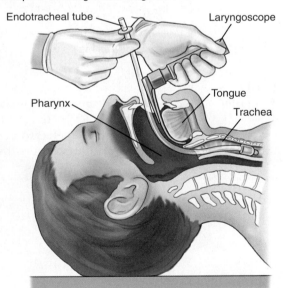

The physician is inserting a(an) _____ / _____ / _____ tube,
within / trachea / pertaining to

using a(an) _____ / _____ / instrument used for visual examination to
larynx / cv

guide the tube into place.

EXERCISE FIGURE **H**

Fill in the blanks to complete labeling of the diagram.

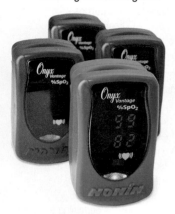

1. Pulse _____ / CV / _____
         oxygen   CV   instrument
                                  used to
                                 measure

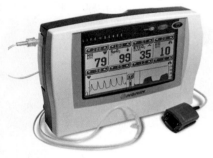

2. _____ / CV / _____
      carbon   CV   instrument used
      dioxide   to measure

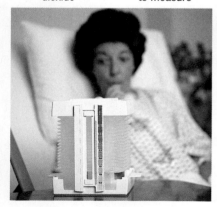

3. _____ / CV / _____
     breathing   CV   instrument used
                           to measure

Diagnostic Terms—cont'd

Built from Word Parts

TERM	DEFINITION
laryngoscopy (*lar*-in-GOS-ko-pē)	visual examination of the larynx
radiograph (RĀ-dē-ō-graph)	record of x-rays (Figure 5-13, *B*)
radiography (rā-dē-OG-rah-fē)	process of recording x-rays
sonogram (SON-ō-gram)	record of sound (Figure 5-19, *B*)
sonography (so-NOG-rah-fē)	process of recording sound (Figure 5-19, *A*)
thoracoscope (tho-RAK-ō-skōp)	instrument used for visual examination of the chest cavity (Figure 5-11)
thoracoscopy (*thor*-a-KOS-ko-pē)	visual examination of the chest cavity
tomography (to-MOG-rah-fē)	process of recording slices (anatomical cross section) (Figure 5-14)
PULMONARY FUNCTION	
capnometer (kap-NOM-e-ter)	instrument used to measure carbon dioxide (levels in expired gas) (Exercise Figure H2)
oximeter (ok-SIM-e-ter) *(Note: the combining vowel is i.)*	instrument used to measure oxygen (saturation in the blood) (Exercise Figure H1)
spirometer (spī-ROM-e-ter)	instrument used to measure breathing (or lung volumes) (Exercise Figure H3)
spirometry (spī-ROM-e-trē)	a measurement of breathing (or lung volumes) (Exercise Figure H3)
SLEEP STUDIES	
polysomnography (PSG) (*pol*-ē-som-NOG-rah-fē)	process of recording many (tests) during sleep (performed to diagnose obstructive sleep apnea [see Figure 5-7]). Tests include **electrocardiography, electromyography, electroencephalography, air flow monitoring,** and **oximetry**.

EXERCISE 25

Practice saying aloud each of the diagnostic terms built from word parts on pp. 173–174.

To hear the terms, go to evolve.elsevier.com. Select: Chapter 5, **Exercises**, Pronunciation.

Refer to p. 10 for your Evolve Access Information.

☐ Place a check mark in the box when you have completed this exercise.

EXERCISE 26

Analyze and define the following diagnostic terms.

        WR   CV   S

EXAMPLE: bronch / o / scopy   visual examination of the bronchi

          CF

1. spirometer _____

2. laryngoscope _____

3. capnometer _____

4. spirometry _____

5. oximeter _____

6. laryngoscopy _____

7. bronchoscope _____

8. thoracoscope _____

9. endoscope _____

10. thoracoscopy _____

11. endoscopic _____

12. endoscopy _____

13. polysomnography _____

14. sonogram _____

15. sonography _____

16. tomography _____

17. radiograph _____

18. radiography _____

EXERCISE 27

Build diagnostic terms that correspond to the following definitions by using the word parts you have learned.

EXAMPLE: instrument used to measure oxygen $\dfrac{ox}{WR} \Big/ \dfrac{i}{CV} \Big/ \dfrac{meter}{S}$

1. visual examination of the larynx

   _____ /CV/ _____
   WR   CV   S

2. instrument used to measure breathing

   _____ /CV/ _____
   WR   CV   S

3. instrument used to measure carbon dioxide

   _____ /CV/ _____
   WR   CV   S

4. instrument used for visual examination of the larynx

   _____ /CV/ _____
   WR   CV   S

5. visual examination of the bronchi

   _____ /CV/ _____
   WR   CV   S

6. measurement of breathing

   _____ /CV/ _____
   WR   CV   S

7. instrument used for visual examination of the bronchi

   _____ /CV/ _____
   WR   CV   S

8. visual examination within (a hollow organ or body cavity)

   _____ / _____
   P   S(WR)

9. instrument used for visual examination of the chest cavity

   _____ /CV/ _____
   WR   CV   S

10. instrument used for visual examination within (a hollow organ or body cavity)

    _____ / _____
    P   S(WR)

11. visual examination of the chest cavity

    _____ /CV/ _____
    WR   CV   S

12. pertaining to visual examination within (a hollow organ or body cavity)

    _____ / _____
    P   S(WR)

13. process of recording of many (tests) during sleep

    _____ / _____ /CV/ _____
    P   WR   CV   S

14. process of recording x-rays

    _____ /CV/ _____
    WR   CV   S

15. record of x-rays

       WR   /CV/   S

16. process of recording sound

       WR   /CV/   S

17. record of sound

       WR   /CV/   S

18. process of recording slices
(anatomical cross sections)

       WR   /CV/   S

EXERCISE 28

Spell each of the diagnostic terms built from word parts on pp. 173–174 by having someone dictate them to you.

> To hear and spell the terms, go to evolve.elsevier.com. Select: Chapter 5, **Exercises**, Spelling.
>
> Refer to p. 10 for your Evolve Access Information.
>
> ☐ Place a check mark in the box if you have completed this exercise online.

1. _____
2. _____
3. _____
4. _____
5. _____
6. _____
7. _____
8. _____
9. _____
10. _____
11. _____
12. _____
13. _____
14. _____
15. _____
16. _____
17. _____
18. _____

Diagnostic Terms

Not Built from Word Parts

In some of the following terms, you may recognize word parts; however, the terms cannot be translated literally to find their meanings.

TERM	DEFINITION
DIAGNOSTIC IMAGING	
chest computed tomography (CT) scan (chest) (kom-PŪ-ted) (tō-MOG-ra-fē) (skan)	computerized radiographic images of the chest performed to diagnose tumors, abscesses, and pleural effusion (see Figure 5-14)
chest radiograph (CXR) (chest) (RĀ-dē-ō-*graf*)	radiographic image of the chest performed to evaluate the lungs and the heart (also called a **chest x-ray**) (see Figure 5-13)

HELICAL COMPUTED TOMOGRAPHY (CT) SCAN

of the chest, also called **spiral CT scan,** is an improvement over standard CT and is the preferred study to identify pulmonary embolism. Images are continually obtained as the patient passes through the gantry, which is part of the scanner. It produces a more concise and faster image, which can be performed with one breath hold.

Diagnostic Terms—cont'd

Not Built from Word Parts

TERM	DEFINITION
ventilation-perfusion scanning (VPS) (*ven*-ti-LĀ-shun) (per-FŪ-zhun)	nuclear medicine procedure performed by inhaling a radionuclide (ventilation) and injecting a radionuclide (perfusion) into an artery followed by imaging to show how well the inhaled air is distributed. Defects in arterial perfusion may indicate pulmonary embolism. (also called **lung scan**) (Figure 5-16)
LABORATORY	
acid-fast bacilli (AFB) smear (AS-id-fast) (bah-SIL-ī) (smēr)	test performed on sputum to determine the presence of acid-fast bacilli, which cause tuberculosis
sputum culture and sensitivity (C&S) (SPŪ-tum) (KUL-cher) (*sen*-si-TIV-i-tē)	test performed on sputum to determine the presence of pathogenic bacteria. Sputum is placed on a medium for growth (culture) and if pathogenic bacteria grow, is then tested for antibiotic sensitivity (sensitivity) identifying which antibiotic will provide the most effective treatment. Used to diagnose pulmonary abscess, bronchitis, and pneumonia.
arterial blood gases (ABGs) (ar-TĒ-rē-al) (blud) (GAS-es)	test performed on arterial blood to determine levels of oxygen (O_2), carbon dioxide (CO_2), and pH (acidity)
peak flow meter (PFM) (pēk) (flō) (MĒ-ter)	portable instrument used to measure how fast air can be pushed out of the lung; used to help monitor asthma and adjust medication accordingly (Figure 5-21)
pulmonary function tests (PFTs) (PUL-mō-*nar*-ē) (FUNK-shun) (tests)	group of tests performed to measure breathing capacity and used to determine external respiratory function; when abnormal, they are useful in distinguishing COPD from asthma

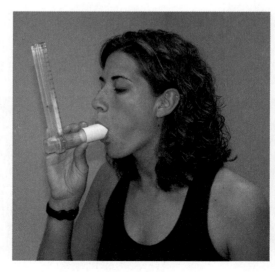

FIGURE 5-21
Peak flow meter.

TERM	DEFINITION
pulse oximetry (puls) (ok-SIM-e-trē)	noninvasive method of measuring oxygen in the blood by using a device that attaches to the fingertip (Exercise Figure H1)
OTHER **auscultation** (*aws*-kul-TĀ-shun)	the act of listening for sounds within the body through a stethoscope; used for assessing and/or diagnosing conditions of the lungs, pleura, heart and abdomen (Figure 5-22).
percussion (per-KUSH-un)	the act of tapping of a body surface with the fingers to determine the density of the part beneath by the sound obtained. A dull sound indicates the presence of fluid in a body space or cavity such as in the pleural space (Figure 5-23).
PPD (purified protein derivative) skin test	test performed on individuals who have recently been exposed to tuberculosis. PPD of the tuberculin bacillus is injected intradermally. Positive tests indicate previous exposure, not necessarily active tuberculosis (also called **TB skin test**).
stethoscope (STETH-ō-skōp)	instrument used to hear internal body sounds; used for performing auscultation and blood pressure measurement (Figure 5-24)

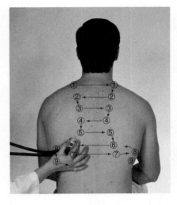

FIGURE 5-22
Auscultation.

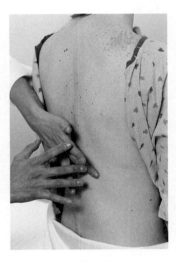

FIGURE 5-23
Percussion.

To watch animations, go to evolve.elsevier.com. Select:
Chapter 5, **Animations**, Pulse Oximetry
                          Endoscopy

Refer to p. 10 for your Evolve Access Information.

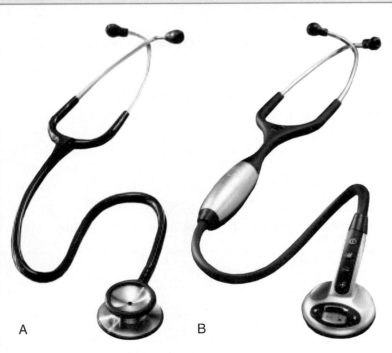

A   B

FIGURE 5-24
Stethoscope types.
A, Acoustic. **B,** Electronic.

EXERCISE 29

Practice saying aloud each of the diagnostic terms not built from word parts on pp. 177–179.

> ℮ To hear the terms, go to evolve.elsevier.com. Select: Chapter 5, **Exercises**, Pronunciation.
>
> Refer to p. 10 for your Evolve Access Information.

☐ Place a check mark in the box when you have completed this exercise.

EXERCISE 30

Fill in the blanks with the correct terms.

1. _____ _____ is a nuclear medicine procedure performed to diagnose pulmonary embolism.

2. Computerized images of the chest, created from a series of sectional images is called a(n) _____ _____ _____ scan.

3. _____ _____ is performed to evaluate the lungs and the heart.

4. The test performed on arterial blood to determine levels of oxygen, carbon dioxide, and pH (acidity) _____ _____ _____.

5. A noninvasive test to measure oxygen in the blood is called _____ _____.

6. A test performed on sputum to diagnose tuberculosis is called _____ _____ _____.

7. _____ is the name of a group of tests performed on breathing capacity to determine external respiratory function or abnormalities.

8. _____ _____ _____ is a test that, when positive, indicates an individual has been exposed to tuberculosis.

9. _____ _____ _____ is used to measure how fast air can be pushed out of the lung.

10. The instrument used to hear internal body sounds is called a(n) _____.

11. An act that involves tapping a body surface with the finger is called _____.

12. The act of listening for sounds within the body through a stethoscope is called _____.

13. A test performed on sputum to determine the presence of pathogenic bacteria is called _____ _____ _____ _____.

EXERCISE 31

Match the terms in the first column with their correct definitions in the second column.

_____ 1. ventilation-perfusion scanning

_____ 2. chest radiograph

_____ 3. chest CT scan

_____ 4. acid-fast bacilli smear

_____ 5. pulse oximetry

_____ 6. arterial blood gases

_____ 7. pulmonary function tests

_____ 8. PPD skin test

_____ 9. auscultation

_____ 10. stethoscope

_____ 11. peak flow meter

_____ 12. percussion

_____ 13. sputum culture and sensitivity

a. computerized images of the chest
b. noninvasive method used to measure oxygen in the blood
c. arterial blood test used to determine levels of oxygen, carbon dioxide, and pH
d. test on sputum for tuberculosis
e. chest x-ray
f. nuclear medicine procedure used to diagnose pulmonary embolism
g. identifies which antibiotic will provide the most effective treatment
h. a group of tests performed to measure breathing capacity
i. instrument to measure pulse waves
j. instrument used for auscultation
k. used to help monitor asthma
l. the act of listening for sounds within the body through a stethoscope
m. the act of tapping a body surface with fingers
n. injected intradermally

EXERCISE 32

Spell each of the diagnostic terms not built from word parts on pp. 177–179 by having someone dictate them to you.

> To hear and spell the terms, go to evolve.elsevier.com. Select: Chapter 5, **Exercises**, Spelling.
>
> (e) Refer to p. 10 for your Evolve Access Information.
>
> ☐ Place a check mark in the box if you have completed this exercise online.

1. _____

2. _____

3. _____

4. _____

5. _____

6. _____

7. _____

8. _____

9. _____

10. _____

11. _____

12. _____

13. _____

Complementary Terms

Built from Word Parts

The following terms are built from word parts you have already learned and can be translated literally to find their meanings. Further explanation of terms beyond the definition of their word parts, if needed, is included in parentheses.

ANOXIA

literally means **without oxygen** or **absence of oxygen.** The term actually denotes an oxygen deficiency in the body tissues.

TERM	DEFINITION
acapnia (a-CAP-nē-a)	condition of absence (less than normal level) of carbon dioxide (in the blood)
alveolar (al-VĒ-ō-lar)	pertaining to the alveolus
anoxia (a-NOK-sē-a)	condition of absence (deficiency) of oxygen
aphonia (ā-FŌ-nē-a)	condition of absence of voice
apnea (AP-nē-a)	absence of breathing
bronchoalveolar (*bron*-kō-al-VĒ-o-lar)	pertaining to the bronchi and alveoli
bronchospasm (BRON-kō-spaz-m)	spasmodic contraction of the bronchi
diaphragmatic (*dī*-a-frag-MAT-ik)	pertaining to the diaphragm (also called **phrenic**)
dysphonia (dis-FŌ-nē-a)	condition of difficult speaking (voice)
dyspnea (DISP-nē-a)	difficult breathing
endotracheal (*en*-dō-TRĀ-kē-al)	pertaining to within the trachea (see Exercise Figure G)
eupnea (ŪP-nē-a)	normal breathing
hypercapnia (*hī*-per-KAP-nē-a)	condition of excessive carbon dioxide (in the blood)
hyperpnea (*hī*-perp-NĒ-a)	excessive breathing
hypocapnia (*hī*-pō-KAP-nē-a)	condition of deficient carbon dioxide (in the blood)
hypopnea (hī-POP-nē-a)	deficient breathing
hypoxemia (*hī*-pok-SĒ-mē-a) *(Note: the o from hypo has been dropped. The final vowel in a prefix may be dropped when the word to which it is added begins with a vowel.)*	deficient oxygen in the blood
hypoxia (hī-POK-sē-a) *(Note: see note for hypoxemia.)*	condition of deficient oxygen (to the tissues)
intrapleural (*in*-tra-PLUR-al)	pertaining to within the pleura (space between the two pleural membranes)

TERM	DEFINITION
laryngeal (lar-IN-jē-al)	pertaining to the larynx
laryngospasm (la-RING-gō-spaz-m)	spasmodic contraction of the larynx
mucoid (MŪ-koyd)	resembling mucus
mucous (MŪ-kus)	pertaining to mucus
nasopharyngeal (nā-zō-fa-RIN-jē-al)	pertaining to the nose and pharynx
orthopnea (or-THOP-nē-a)	able to breathe easier in a straight (upright) position (difficulty breathing in the supine position)
phrenalgia (fre-NAL-ja)	pain in the diaphragm (also called **diaphragmalgia**)
phrenospasm (FREN-ō-spaz-m)	spasm of the diaphragm
pulmonary (PUL-mō-*nar*-ē)	pertaining to the lungs
pulmonologist (*pul*-mon-OL-o-jist)	physician who studies and treats diseases of the lung
pulmonology (*pul*-mon-OL-o-jē)	study of the lung (a branch of medicine dealing with diseases of the lung)
radiologist (rā-dē-OL-o-jist)	physician who specializes in the use of x-rays, ultrasound, and magnetic fields in the diagnosis and treatment of disease
radiology (ra-dē-OL-o-jē)	study of x-rays (a branch of medicine concerned with the use of x-rays, ultrasound, and magnetic fields to diagnose and treat disease)
rhinorrhea (*rī*-nō-RĒ-a)	discharge from the nose (as in a cold)
tachypnea (tak-IP-nē-a)	rapid breathing
thoracic (thō-RAS-ik)	pertaining to the chest

MUCUS

is the noun that describes slimy fluid secreted by the mucous membrane. **Mucous** is the adjective that means pertaining to the mucous membrane. Pronunciation is the same for both terms.

To watch animations, go to evolve.elsevier.com. Select: Chapter 5, **Animations**, Hypoxia.

Refer to p. 10 for your Evolve Access Information.

EXERCISE 33

Practice saying aloud each of the complementary terms built from word parts on these two pages.

To hear the terms, go to evolve.elsevier.com. Select: Chapter 5, **Exercises**, Pronunciation.

Refer to p. 10 for your Evolve Access Information.

☐ Place a check mark in the box when you have completed this exercise.

EXERCISE 34

Analyze and define the following complementary terms.

           P   WR S

EXAMPLE: hyper/capn/ia   condition of excessive carbon dioxide (in the blood)

1. laryngeal _____

2. eupnea _____

3. mucoid _____

4. apnea _____

5. hypoxia _____

6. laryngospasm _____

7. endotracheal _____

8. anoxia _____

9. dysphonia _____

10. bronchoalveolar _____

11. dyspnea _____

12. hypocapnia _____

13. bronchospasm _____

14. orthopnea _____

15. hyperpnea _____

16. acapnia _____

17. hypopnea _____

18. hypoxemia _____

19. aphonia _____

20. rhinorrhea _____

21. thoracic _____

22. mucous _____

23. nasopharyngeal _____

24. diaphragmatic _____

25. intrapleural _____

26. pulmonary _____

27. phrenalgia _____

28. tachypnea _____

29. phrenospasm _____

30. pulmonologist _____

31. pulmonology _____

32. alveolar _____

33. radiology _____

34. radiologist _____

EXERCISE 35

Build the complementary terms for the following definitions by using the word parts you have learned.

EXAMPLE: pertaining to bronchi and alveoli

$$\frac{bronch}{WR} \Big/ \frac{o}{CV} \Big/ \frac{alveol}{WR} \Big/ \frac{ar}{S}$$

1. condition of deficient oxygen

$$\frac{}{P} \Big/ \frac{}{WR} \Big/ \frac{}{S}$$

2. resembling mucus

$$\frac{}{WR} \Big/ \frac{}{S}$$

3. able to breathe easier in a straight (upright) position

$$\frac{}{WR} \Big/ \frac{}{CV} \frac{}{S}$$

4. pertaining to within the trachea

$$\frac{}{P} \Big/ \frac{}{WR} \Big/ \frac{}{S}$$

5. condition of absence of oxygen

$$\frac{}{P} \Big/ \frac{}{WR} \Big/ \frac{}{S}$$

6. difficult breathing

$$\frac{}{P} \Big/ \frac{}{S(WR)}$$

7. pertaining to the larynx

$$\frac{}{WR} \Big/ \frac{}{S}$$

8. condition of excessive carbon dioxide (in the blood)

$$\frac{}{P} \Big/ \frac{}{WR} \Big/ \frac{}{S}$$

9. normal breathing

$$\frac{}{P} \Big/ \frac{}{S(WR)}$$

10. condition of absence of voice

$$\frac{}{P} \Big/ \frac{}{WR} \Big/ \frac{}{S}$$

11. spasmodic contraction of the larynx

$$\frac{}{WR} \Big/ \frac{}{CV} \frac{}{S}$$

12. condition of deficient carbon dioxide (in the blood)

$$\frac{}{P} \Big/ \frac{}{WR} \Big/ \frac{}{S}$$

13. pertaining to the nose and pharynx

$$\frac{}{WR} \Big/ \frac{}{CV} \frac{}{WR} \Big/ \frac{}{S}$$

14. pertaining to the diaphragm

$$\frac{}{WR} \Big/ \frac{}{S}$$

15. condition of absence of breathing

$$\frac{}{P} \Big/ \frac{}{S(WR)}$$

16. deficient oxygen in the blood

$$\frac{}{P} \Big/ \frac{}{WR} \Big/ \frac{}{S}$$

17. excessive breathing

　　　　　　　　　P　　／　　S(WR)

18. spasmodic contraction of
the bronchi

　　　　　　　　　WR　／CV／　S

19. deficient breathing

　　　　　　　　　P　　／　　S(WR)

20. condition of absence of carbon
dioxide (in the blood)

　　　　　　　　　P　／　WR　／　S

21. condition of difficulty in
speaking (voice)

　　　　　　　　　P　／　WR　／　S

22. discharge from the nose

　　　　　　　　　WR　／CV／　S

23. pertaining to mucus

　　　　　　　　　WR　／　S

24. pertaining to the chest

　　　　　　　　　WR　／　S

25. pertaining to within the pleura

　　　　　　　　　P　／　WR　／　S

26. pertaining to the lungs

　　　　　　　　　WR　／　S

27. spasm of the diaphragm

　　　　　　　　　WR　／CV／　S

28. rapid breathing

　　　　　　　　　P　　／　　S(WR)

29. pain in the diaphragm

　　　　　　　　　WR　／　S

30. pertaining to the alveolus

　　　　　　　　　WR　／　S

31. study of the lung

　　　　　　　　　WR　／CV／　S

32. a physician who studies and
treats diseases of the lung

　　　　　　　　　WR　／CV／　S

33. physician who specializes in
the use of x-rays, ultrasound,
and magnetic fields in the
diagnosis and treatment of
disease

　　　　　　　　　WR　／CV／　S

34. study of x-rays (a branch of
medicine concerned with the
use of x-rays, ultrasound, and
magnetic fields to diagnose
and treat disease)

　　　　　　　　　WR　／CV／　S

EXERCISE 36

Spell each of the complementary terms built from word parts on pp. 182–183 by having someone dictate them to you.

> To hear and spell the terms, go to evolve.elsevier.com. Select: Chapter 5, **Exercises**, Spelling.
>
> (e) Refer to p. 10 for your Evolve Access Information.
>
> ☐ Place a check mark in the box if you have completed this exercise online.

1. _____   19. _____
2. _____   20. _____
3. _____   21. _____
4. _____   22. _____
5. _____   23. _____
6. _____   24. _____
7. _____   25. _____
8. _____   26. _____
9. _____   27. _____
10. _____   28. _____
11. _____   29. _____
12. _____   30. _____
13. _____   31. _____
14. _____   32. _____
15. _____   33. _____
16. _____   34. _____
17. _____   35. _____
18. _____

> For review and/or assessment, go to evolve.elsevier.com. Select:
> Chapter 5, **Activities**, Terms Built from Word Parts
> (e) Chapter 5, **Games**,   Term Storm
>
> Refer to p. 10 for your Evolve Access Information.

Complementary Terms

Not Built from Word Parts

In some of the following terms, you may recognize word parts; however, the terms cannot be translated literally to find their meanings.

TERM	DEFINITION
airway (ĂR-wā)	passageway by which air enters and leaves the lungs as well as a mechanical device used to keep the air passageway unobstructed
asphyxia (as-FIK-sē-a)	deprivation of oxygen for tissue use; suffocation

Complementary Terms—cont'd

Not Built from Word Parts

TERM	DEFINITION
aspirate (AS-per-āt)	to withdraw fluid or suction fluid; also to draw foreign material into the respiratory tract
bronchoconstrictor (*bron*-kō-kon-STRIK-tor)	agent causing narrowing of the bronchi
bronchodilator (*bron*-kō-dī-LĀ-tor)	agent causing the bronchi to widen
crackles (KRAK-els)	discontinuous sounds heard primarily with a stethoscope during inspiration that resemble the sound of the rustling of cellophane. Often heard at the base of the lung posteriorly in heart failure, pneumonia, and pulmonary fibrosis. (also called **rales**)
hyperventilation (*hī*-per-*ven*-ti-LĀ-shun)	ventilation of the lungs beyond normal body needs
hypoventilation (*hī*-pō-*ven*-ti-LĀ-shun)	ventilation of the lungs that does not fulfill the body's gas exchange needs
mucopurulent (*mū*-kō-PŪR-ū-lent)	containing both mucus and pus
mucus (MŪ-kus)	slimy fluid secreted by the mucous membranes
nebulizer (NEB-ū-lī-zer)	device that creates a mist used to deliver medication for giving respiratory treatment (Figure 5-25)
nosocomial infection (nos-ō-KŌ-mē-al) (in-FEK-shun)	an infection acquired during hospitalization
paroxysm (PAR-ok-sizm)	periodic, sudden attack
patent (PĀ-tent)	open, the opposite of closed or compromised, thus allowing passage of air, as in patent trachea and bronchi (can be applied to any tubular passageway in the body, as in a patent artery, allowing passage of blood)
rhonchi (RONG-kī)	low-pitched, with a snoring quality, breath sounds heard with a stethoscope suggesting secretions in the large airways
sputum (SPŪ-tum)	mucous secretion from the lungs, bronchi, and trachea expelled through the mouth
stridor (STRĪD-ir)	harsh, high-pitched breath sound heard on inspiration; indicates an acute laryngeal obstruction
ventilator (VEN-ti-*lā*-tor)	mechanical device used to assist with or substitute for breathing (Figure 5-26)

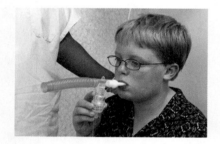

FIGURE 5-25
Nebulizer.

SPUTUM

is derived from the Latin **spuere**, meaning **to spit**. In a 1693 dictionary it is defined as a "secretion thicker than ordinary spittle."

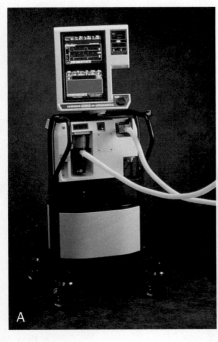
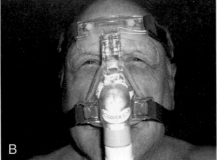

A B

FIGURE 5-26
A, Invasive ventilator. Positive pressure ventilator is applied to the patient's airway through an **endo-tracheal** or **tracheostomy** tube and is used when spontaneous breathing is inadequate to sustain life.
B, CPAP (continuous positive airway pressure) is a noninvasive ventilation device used for patients who can initiate their own breathing and is often used to treat **obstructive sleep apnea**. BiPAP (bilevel positive airway pressure) not shown, is another noninvasive device that delivers two levels of pressure, whereas the CPAP machine delivers a predetermined level of pressure.

 Refer to **Appendix D** for pharmacology terms related to the respiratory system.

EXERCISE 37

Practice saying aloud each of the complementary terms not built from word parts on pp. 187–188.

 To hear the terms, go to evolve.elsevier.com. Select: Chapter 5, **Exercises**, Pronunciation.

Refer to p. 10 for your Evolve Access Information.

☐ Place a check mark in the box when you have completed this exercise.

EXERCISE 38

Fill in the blanks with the correct terms.

1. Another term for ventilation of the lungs beyond normal body needs is

   _____.

2. A device that creates a mist used to deliver medication for giving respiratory treatment is a(n) _____.

3. A(n) _____ is an agent that causes the air passages to widen.

4. A patient who has difficulty breathing can be attached to a mechanical breathing device called a(n) _____.

5. Another term for suffocation is _____.

6. Material made up of mucous secretions from the lungs, bronchi, and trachea, expelled through the mouth, is called _____.

7. To suction or withdraw fluid is to _____.

8. A(n) _____ is a mechanical device that keeps the air passageway unobstructed.

9. Harsh, high pitched, breath sound heard on inspiration is called _____.

10. Low-pitched breath sounds heard with a stethoscope are called _____.

11. Material containing both mucus and pus is referred to as being _____.

12. _____ is the name given to ventilation of the lungs that does not fulfill the body's gas exchange needs.

13. An infection acquired during hospitalization is called _____.

14. The term that applies to a periodic sudden attack is _____.

15. An airway must be kept _____ (open) for the patient to breathe.

16. An agent that causes bronchi to narrow is called a(n) _____.

17. _____ is the name given to the slimy fluid secreted by the mucous membranes.

18. Resembling the sound of rustling cellophane, _____ may be a presenting sign in pneumonia.

EXERCISE 39

Match the terms in the first column with their correct definitions in the second column.

_____ 1. airway
_____ 2. aspirate
_____ 3. bronchoconstrictor
_____ 4. bronchodilator
_____ 5. rhonchi
_____ 6. crackles
_____ 7. hyperventilation
_____ 8. asphyxia
_____ 9. stridor

a. suggesting secretions in the large airways
b. mechanical device used to keep the air passageway unobstructed
c. agent that narrows the bronchi
d. discontinuous sounds heard mainly at the base of the lungs with a stethoscope during inspiration
e. mucus from throat and lungs
f. suffocation
g. ventilation of the lungs beyond normal body needs
h. to draw foreign material into the respiratory tract
i. agent that widens the bronchi
j. indicates acute laryngeal obstruction

EXERCISE 40

Match the terms in the first column with their correct definitions in the second column.

_____ 1. hypoventilation
_____ 2. mucopurulent
_____ 3. mucus
_____ 4. nebulizer
_____ 5. nosocomial
_____ 6. patent
_____ 7. sputum
_____ 8. ventilator
_____ 9. paroxysm

a. open
b. mucous secretion from lungs, bronchi, and trachea, expelled through the mouth
c. respiratory treatment device that sends a mist
d. mechanical breathing device
e. ventilation of the lungs that does not fulfill the body's gas exchange needs
f. periodic, sudden attack
g. agent that widens air passages
h. containing both mucus and pus
i. slimy fluid secreted by mucous membranes
j. hospital-acquired infection

EXERCISE 41

Spell each of the complementary terms not built from word parts on pp. 187–188 by having someone dictate them to you.

To hear and spell the terms, go to evolve.elsevier.com. Select: Chapter 5, **Exercises**, Spelling.

Refer to p. 10 for your Evolve Access Information.

☐ Place a check mark in the box if you have completed this exercise online.

1. _____   10. _____
2. _____   11. _____
3. _____   12. _____
4. _____   13. _____
5. _____   14. _____
6. _____   15. _____
7. _____   16. _____
8. _____   17. _____
9. _____   18. _____

For more practice with medical terms, go to evolve.elsevier.com. Select:
Chapter 5, **Activities**, Terms Not Built from Word Parts
                              Hear It and Type It: Clinical Vignettes
Chapter 5, **Games**,   Term Explorer
                              Termbusters
                              Medical Millionaire

Refer to p. 10 for your Evolve Access Information.

Abbreviations

ABBREVIATION	TERM
ABGs	arterial blood gases
AFB	acid-fast bacilli
ARDS	acute respiratory distress syndrome
C&S	culture and sensitivity
CPAP	continuous positive airway pressure
CF	cystic fibrosis
CO_2	carbon dioxide
COPD	chronic obstructive pulmonary disease
CT	computed tomography
CXR	chest radiograph (chest x-ray)
flu	influenza
IPF	idiopathic pulmonary fibrosis

Abbreviations—cont'd

ABBREVIATION	TERM
LLL	left lower lobe
LTB	laryngotracheobronchitis
LUL	left upper lobe
O₂	oxygen
OSA	obstructive sleep apnea
PE	pulmonary embolism
PFM	peak flow meter
PFTs	pulmonary function tests
PSG	polysomnography
RLL	right lower lobe
RML	right middle lobe
RUL	right upper lobe
SOB	shortness of breath
TB	tuberculosis
URI	upper respiratory infection
VPS	ventilation-perfusion scanning

Refer to **Appendix C** for a complete list of abbreviations.

EXERCISE 42

Write the meaning of the abbreviations in the following sentences.

1. A variety of tests are used to diagnose **COPD** _____

   _____ _____ _____, including

   PFTs _____ _____ _____, **CXR**

   _____ _____, **ABGs** _____ _____

   _____, and chest **CT** _____ _____ scan.

   SOB _____ _____ _____ is often a

   symptom of COPD.

2. **VPS** _____ _____ is very helpful in

   diagnosing **PE**

   _____ _____.

3. The lobes of the left lung are **LUL** _____ _____

   _____ and **LLL** _____ _____

   _____; the lobes of the right lung are **RUL** _____

   _____ _____, **RML** _____ _____

   _____, and **RLL** _____ _____

   _____.

4. **AFB** _____ _____ smear is used to
   support the diagnosis of **TB** _____.
5. **PSG** _____ is used to confirm the diagnosis of
   OSA _____ _____ _____.
6. Respiration is the exchange of O_2 _____ and CO_2 _____
   _____ between the atmosphere and body cells.
7. Measurements obtained from using a **PFM** _____ _____
   _____ can be used to adjust medication for persons with asthma.
8. The etiology of **IPF** _____ _____ _____ is
   unknown.
9. The patient had a persistent cough, hemoptysis, and fever. The chest
   radiograph was compatible with a pulmonary infection. The physician ordered
   a sputum **C&S** _____ _____ _____ to
   determine the presence of pathogenic bacteria.

EXERCISE 43

Write the definition for the following abbreviations.

1. ARDS _____ _____ _____ _____
2. CF _____ _____
3. flu _____
4. LTB _____
5. URI _____ _____ _____
5. CPAP _____ _____ _____

> For practice with abbreviations, go to evolve.elsevier.com. Select:
> Chapter 5, **Flashcards**
> Chapter 5, **Games**, Crossword Puzzle
>
> Refer to p. 10 for your Evolve Access Information.

Common Abbreviations Used in the Respiratory Care Department within a Healthcare Facility	
BiPAP	bilevel positive airway pressure
CPT	chest physiotherapy
DPI	dry powder inhaler
HME	heat/moisture exchanger
IPPB	intermittent positive-pressure breathing
MDI	metered-dose inhaler
NIPPV	noninvasive positive-pressure ventilator
PEP	positive expiratory pressure
SVN	small-volume nebulizer
VAP	ventilator-associated pneumonia

PRACTICAL APPLICATION

EXERCISE 44 *Interact with Medical Documents and Electronic Health Records*

A. Complete the medical report by writing the medical terms in the blanks. Use the list of definitions with the corresponding numbers following it.

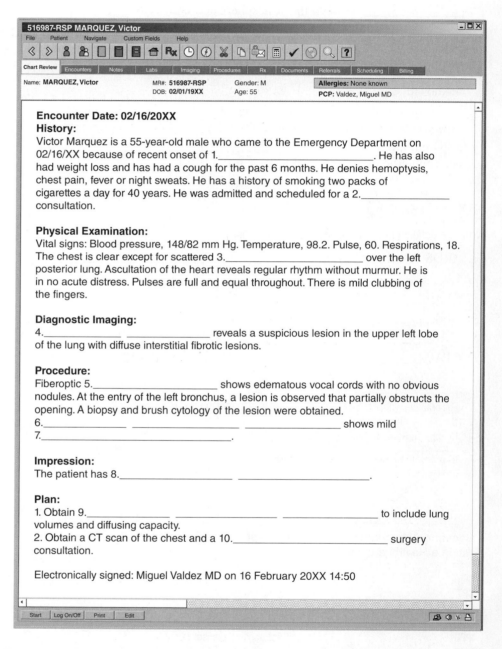

516987-RSP MARQUEZ, Victor

File Patient Navigate Custom Fields Help

Chart Review | Encounters | Notes | Labs | Imaging | Procedures | Rx | Documents | Referrals | Scheduling | Billing

Name: **MARQUEZ, Victor** MR#: **516987-RSP** Gender: M **Allergies:** None known
DOB: **02/01/19XX** Age: 55 **PCP:** Valdez, Miguel MD

Encounter Date: 02/16/20XX
History:
Victor Marquez is a 55-year-old male who came to the Emergency Department on 02/16/XX because of recent onset of 1._____. He has also had weight loss and has had a cough for the past 6 months. He denies hemoptysis, chest pain, fever or night sweats. He has a history of smoking two packs of cigarettes a day for 40 years. He was admitted and scheduled for a 2._____ consultation.

Physical Examination:
Vital signs: Blood pressure, 148/82 mm Hg. Temperature, 98.2. Pulse, 60. Respirations, 18. The chest is clear except for scattered 3._____ over the left posterior lung. Ascultation of the heart reveals regular rhythm without murmur. He is in no acute distress. Pulses are full and equal throughout. There is mild clubbing of the fingers.

Diagnostic Imaging:
4._____ _____ reveals a suspicious lesion in the upper left lobe of the lung with diffuse interstitial fibrotic lesions.

Procedure:
Fiberoptic 5._____ shows edematous vocal cords with no obvious nodules. At the entry of the left bronchus, a lesion is observed that partially obstructs the opening. A biopsy and brush cytology of the lesion were obtained.
6._____ _____ _____ shows mild 7._____.

Impression:
The patient has 8._____ _____.

Plan:
1. Obtain 9._____ _____ _____ to include lung volumes and diffusing capacity.
2. Obtain a CT scan of the chest and a 10._____ surgery consultation.

Electronically signed: Miguel Valdez MD on 16 February 20XX 14:50

Start | Log On/Off | Print | Edit

1. difficult breathing
2. pertaining to the lungs
3. low pitched with a snoring quality breath sounds heard with a stethoscope
4. radiographic image used to evaluate the lungs and heart
5. visual examination of the bronchi
6. test performed on arterial blood to determine the presence of oxygen, carbon dioxide, and other gases
7. deficient oxygen in the blood
8. cancerous tumor originating in the bronchus
9. group of tests performed on breathing
10. pertaining to the chest

B. Read the following diagnostic imaging report of a CT scan of the chest (see Figure 5-13, *B*). Answer the questions following it.

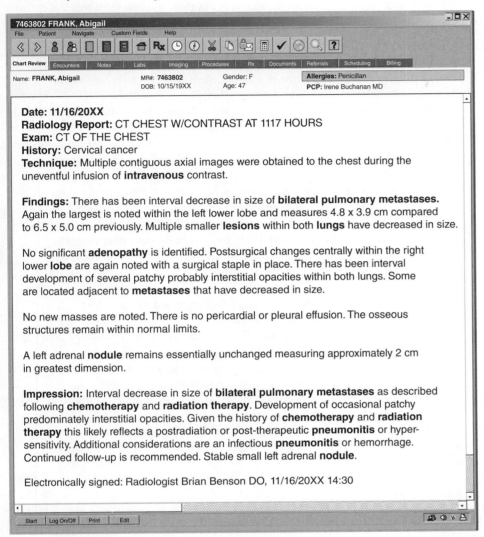

Date: 11/16/20XX
Radiology Report: CT CHEST W/CONTRAST AT 1117 HOURS
Exam: CT OF THE CHEST
History: Cervical cancer
Technique: Multiple contiguous axial images were obtained to the chest during the uneventful infusion of **intravenous** contrast.

Findings: There has been interval decrease in size of **bilateral pulmonary metastases.** Again the largest is noted within the left lower lobe and measures 4.8 x 3.9 cm compared to 6.5 x 5.0 cm previously. Multiple smaller **lesions** within both **lungs** have decreased in size.

No significant **adenopathy** is identified. Postsurgical changes centrally within the right lower **lobe** are again noted with a surgical staple in place. There has been interval development of several patchy probably interstitial opacities within both lungs. Some are located adjacent to **metastases** that have decreased in size.

No new masses are noted. There is no pericardial or pleural effusion. The osseous structures remain within normal limits.

A left adrenal **nodule** remains essentially unchanged measuring approximately 2 cm in greatest dimension.

Impression: Interval decrease in size of **bilateral pulmonary metastases** as described following **chemotherapy** and **radiation therapy**. Development of occasional patchy predominately interstitial opacities. Given the history of **chemotherapy** and **radiation therapy** this likely reflects a postradiation or post-therapeutic **pneumonitis** or hyper-sensitivity. Additional considerations are an infectious **pneumonitis** or hemorrhage. Continued follow-up is recommended. Stable small left adrenal **nodule**.

Electronically signed: Radiologist Brian Benson DO, 11/16/20XX 14:30

1. The diagnostic imaging exam performed uses
   a. combined series of cross-sectional x-rays
   b. ionizing radiation produced by a light source
   c. mathematically constructed images and magnetic fields
   d. radiopharmaceuticals

2. T F Fluid is present in the pleural space.
3. T F Following chemotherapy and radiation, metastases in one lung was decreased.
4. T F The patchy interstitial opacities likely reflect a postradiation or post-therapeutic inflammation of the lung.

C. Complete the **three medical documents** within the electronic health record (EHR) on Evolve.

> Many health care records today are stored and used in an electronic system called **electronic health records (EHRs).** Electronic health records contain a collection of health information of an individual patient. The digitally formatted record can be shared through computer networks with patients, physicians, and other health care providers.

For practice with medical terms using electronic health records, go to evolve.elsevier.com.
Select: Chapter 5, **Electronic Health Records.**

Refer to p. 10 for your Evolve Access Information.

EXERCISE 45 *Interpret Medical Terms*

To test your understanding of the terms introduced in this chapter, circle the words that correctly complete the sentences. The italicized words refer to the correct answer.

1. The patient was admitted to the emergency department with a *severe nosebleed,* or (**rhinomycosis, epistaxis, nasopharyngitis**).
2. The accident caused damage to the *larynx,* necessitating a *surgical repair,* or a (**laryngectomy, laryngostomy, laryngoplasty**).
3. Mr. Prince was *able to breathe easier in an upright position,* so the nurse recorded that he had (**orthopnea, eupnea, dyspnea**).
4. The *test on arterial blood to determine oxygen, carbon dioxide, and pH levels* (**pulse oximetry, pulmonary function tests, arterial blood gases**) indicated that the patient was *deficient in oxygen,* or had (**dysphonia, hypoxia, hypocapnia**).
5. The physician informed the patient that a heart attack was not the cause of the *chest pain,* or (**thoracalgia, pneumothorax, thoracentesis**).
6. The patient reported dizziness brought on by *ventilation of the lungs beyond normal body needs,* or (**hyperventilation, hypoventilation, dysphonia**).
7. The physician wished the patient to have the medication given by *a device that delivers mist,* so he ordered that the treatment be given by (**airway, nebulizer, ventilator**).
8. The patient with *blood in the chest cavity* was diagnosed as having a (**pneumothorax, pleuritis, hemothorax**).
9. After surgery, the patient had a *block in the circulation to the pulmonary artery* or (**pleural effusion, pulmonary edema, pulmonary embolism**).
10. The patient was diagnosed as having *a fungal disease affecting the lung,* or (**obstructive sleep apnea, tuberculosis, coccidioidomycosis**).
11. The physician ordered a *radiographic image of the chest* (**chest radiograph, chest CT scan, bronchoscopy**) because she suspected *an infection acquired during hospitalization,* or (**patent, nosocomial, paroxysm**) pneumonia.
12. The patient received an *intradermal injection* (**AFB, ABGs, PPD skin test**) *to determine if she had been exposed to TB.*
13. The patient was experiencing *rapid breathing* or (**phrenospasm, tachypnea, phrenalgia**).
14. The nurse practitioner heard *discontinuous sounds during respiration that resembled the sound of the rustling of cellophane* (**stridor, rhonchi, crackles**).
15. A radiographer, an employee of the hospital diagnostic imaging department, uses an x-ray machine to create a *record of x-rays* (**sonogram, radiograph, tomograph**), which would be interpreted by a *physician who specializes in the use of x-rays, ultrasound, and magnetic fields in the diagnosis and treatment of disease* (**radiologist, pulmonologist, pathologist**).
16. The physician ordered an *AFB smear,* a (**diagnostic imaging procedure, laboratory test, endoscopy procedure**) to confirm the diagnosis of TB.

EXERCISE 46   *Read Medical Terms in Use*

Practice pronouncing the terms by reading the following medical document. Use the pronunciation key following the medical terms to assist you in saying the word.

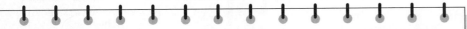

To hear these terms, go to evolve.elsevier.com.
Select: Chapter 5, **Exercises**, Read Medical Terms in Use.

Refer to p. 10 for your Evolve Access Information.

A 24-year-old man visited the emergency department because of **dyspnea** (DISP-nē-a), **hyperpnea** (hī-perp-NĒ-a), **paroxysms** (PAR-ok-sizms) of cough, and the presence of thick, tenacious **mucus** (MŪ-kus). He had a history of **asthma** (AZ-ma) since the age of 12 years. A chest radiograph was negative for **pneumonia** (nū-MŌ-nē-a). **Arterial blood gases** (ar-TĒ-rē-al) (blud) (GAS-es) showed **hypoxemia** (hī-pok-SĒ-mē-a) but no **hypercapnia** (hī-per-KAP-nē-a). **Pulmonary function tests** (PUL-mō-ner-ē) (FUNK-shun) (tests) disclosed bronchoconstriction, which was corrected by a **bronchodilator** (*bron*-kō-dī-LĀ-tor). A **nebulizer** (NEB-ū-lī-zer) was prescribed for treatment. The asthma attack was probably precipitated by an episode of **bronchitis** (bron-KĪ-tis).

WEB LINK

For additional information on diseases of the lung, visit the **American Lung Association** at ***www.lung.org***.

EXERCISE 47   *Comprehend Medical Terms in Use*

Test your comprehension of terms in the previous medical document by answering T for true and F for false.

_____ 1. The patient visited the emergency department because of many symptoms, one of which was sudden, periodic coughing.

_____ 2. Diagnostic procedures were performed to assist with the diagnosis. ABGs showed increased O_2, decreased CO_2, and a normal pH.

_____ 3. An agent that causes the bronchi to widen was used to treat the condition diagnosed with the PFTs.

_____ 4. The asthma attack was precipitated by narrowing of the bronchi.

For a snapshot assessment of your knowledge of the respiratory system terms go to evolve.elsevier.com.
Select: Chapter 5, **Quick Quizzes**.

Refer to p. 10 for your Evolve Access Information.

CHAPTER REVIEW

Review of Evolve

Keep a record of the online activities you have completed by placing a check mark in the box. You may also record your scores. All activities have been referenced throughout the chapter.

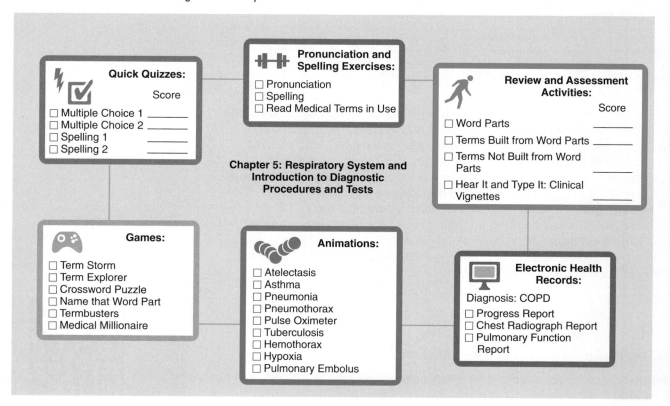

Quick Quizzes:

Score

☐ Multiple Choice 1 _____
☐ Multiple Choice 2 _____
☐ Spelling 1 _____
☐ Spelling 2 _____

Pronunciation and Spelling Exercises:

☐ Pronunciation
☐ Spelling
☐ Read Medical Terms in Use

Review and Assessment Activities:

Score

☐ Word Parts _____
☐ Terms Built from Word Parts _____
☐ Terms Not Built from Word Parts _____
☐ Hear It and Type It: Clinical Vignettes _____

Chapter 5: Respiratory System and Introduction to Diagnostic Procedures and Tests

Games:

☐ Term Storm
☐ Term Explorer
☐ Crossword Puzzle
☐ Name that Word Part
☐ Termbusters
☐ Medical Millionaire

Animations:

☐ Atelectasis
☐ Asthma
☐ Pneumonia
☐ Pneumothorax
☐ Pulse Oximeter
☐ Tuberculosis
☐ Hemothorax
☐ Hypoxia
☐ Pulmonary Embolus

Electronic Health Records:

Diagnosis: COPD

☐ Progress Report
☐ Chest Radiograph Report
☐ Pulmonary Function Report

Review of Word Parts

Can you define and spell the following word parts?

COMBINING FORMS		PREFIXES	SUFFIXES	
adenoid/o	pharyng/o	a-	-algia	-pexy
alveol/o	phon/o	an-	-ar	-pnea
atel/o	phren/o	endo-	-ary	-rrhagia
bronch/o	pleur/o	eu-	-cele	-scope
bronchi/o	pneum/o	poly-	-centesis	-scopic
capn/o	pneumat/o	tachy-	-eal	-scopy
diaphragmat/o	pneumon/o		-ectasis	-spasm
epiglott/o	pulmon/o		-emia	-stenosis
hem/o	py/o		-gram	-stomy
hemat/o	radi/o		-graph	-thorax
laryng/o	rhin/o		-graphy	-tomy
lob/o	sept/o		-meter	
muc/o	sinus/o		-metry	
nas/o	somn/o			
orth/o	son/o			
ox/i	spir/o			
ox/o	thorac/o			
	tom/o			
	tonsill/o			
	trache/o			

Review of Terms

Can you define, pronounce, and spell the following terms *built from word parts?*

DISEASES AND DISORDERS	SURGICAL	DIAGNOSTIC	COMPLEMENTARY
adenoiditis	adenoidectomy	bronchoscope	acapnia
alveolitis	adenotome	bronchoscopy	alveolar
atelectasis	bronchoplasty	capnometer	anoxia
bronchiectasis	laryngectomy	endoscope	aphonia
bronchitis	laryngoplasty	endoscopic	apnea
bronchogenic carcinoma	laryngostomy	endoscopy	bronchoalveolar
bronchopneumonia	laryngotracheotomy	laryngoscope	bronchospasm
diaphragmatocele	lobectomy	laryngoscopy	diaphragmatic
epiglottitis	pleuropexy	oximeter	dysphonia
hemothorax	pneumonectomy	polysomnography (PSG)	dyspnea
laryngitis	rhinoplasty	radiograph	endotracheal
laryngotracheobronchitis (LTB)	septoplasty	radiography	eupnea
lobar pneumonia	septotomy	sonogram	hypercapnia
nasopharyngitis	sinusotomy	sonography	hyperpnea
pharyngitis	thoracocentesis	spirometer	hypocapnia
pleuritis	thoracotomy	spirometry	hypopnea
preumatocele	tonsillectomy	thoracoscope	hypoxemia
pneumoconiosis	tracheoplasty	thoracoscopy	hypoxia
pneumonia	tracheostomy	tomography	intrapleural
pneumonitis	tracheotomy		laryngeal
pneumothorax			laryngospasm
pulmonary neoplasm			mucoid
pyothorax			mucous
rhinitis			nasopharyngeal
rhinomycosis			orthopnea
rhinorrhagia			phrenalgia
sinusitis			phrenospasm
thoracalgia			pulmonary
tonsillitis			pulmonologist
tracheitis			pulmonology
tracheostenosis			radiologist
			radiology
			rhinorrhea
			tachypnea
			thoracic

Can you define, pronounce, and spell the following terms *not built from word parts?*

DISEASES AND DISORDERS	DIAGNOSTIC	COMPLEMENTARY
acute respiratory distress syndrome (ARDS)	acid-fast bacilli (AFB) smear	airway
asthma	arterial blood gases (ABGs)	asphyxia
chronic obstructive pulmonary disease (COPD)	auscultation	aspirate
	chest computed tomography (CT) scan	bronchoconstrictor
coccidioidomycosis	chest radiograph (CXR)	bronchodilator
cor pulmonale	culture and sensitivity (C&S)	crackles
croup	peak flow meter (PFM)	hyperventilation
cystic fibrosis (CF)	percussion	hypoventilation
deviated septum	PPD skin test	mucopurulent
emphysema	pulmonary function tests (PFTs)	mucus
epistaxis	pulse oximetry	nebulizer
idiopathic pulmonary fibrosis (IPF)	sputum culture and sensitivity (C&S)	nosocomial infection
influenza (flu)	stethoscope	paroxysm
obstructive sleep apnea (OSA)	ventilation-perfusion scanning (VPS)	patent
pertussis		rhonchi
pleural effusion		sputum
pulmonary edema		stridor
pulmonary embolism (PE)		ventilator
tuberculosis (TB)		
upper respiratory infection (URI)		

ANSWERS

ANSWERS TO CHAPTER 5 EXERCISES
Exercise Figures

Exercise Figure

A. 1. sinus: sinus/o
2. nose: nas/o, rhin/o
3. tonsil: tonsill/o
4. epiglottis: epiglott/o
5. larynx: laryng/o
6. trachea: trache/o
7. pleura: pleur/o
8. lobe: lob/o
9. diaphragm: diaphragmat/o, phren/o
10. adenoids: adenoid/o
11. pharynx: pharyng/o
12. lung: pneum/o, pneumat/o, pneumon/o, pulmon/o
13. bronchus: bronch/o, bronchi/o
14. alveolus: alveol/o

Exercise Figure

B. bronchi/ectasis

Exercise Figure

C. 1. pneum/o/thorax
2. hem/o/thorax

Exercise Figure

D. sinus/itis

Exercise Figure

E. adenoid/ectomy, aden/o/tome

Exercise Figure

F. thorac/o/centesis

Exercise Figure

G. endo/trache/al, laryng/o/scope

Exercise Figure

H. 1. ox/i/meter
2. capn/o/meter
3. spir/o/meter

Exercise 1
1. h   5. f
2. a   6. d
3. g   7. e
4. c   8. b

Exercise 2
1. nasal septum
2. epiglottis
3. bronchioles
4. nose
5. diaphragm
6. mediastinum
7. tonsils

Exercise 3
1. larynx
2. bronchus
3. pleura
4. lung, air
5. tonsil
6. lung
7. diaphragm
8. trachea
9. alveolus
10. lung, air
11. thorax, chest cavity
12. adenoids
13. pharynx
14. nose
15. sinus
16. lobe
17. epiglottis
18. lung, air
19. nose
20. septum
21. diaphragm

Exercise 4
1. a. nas/o
   b. rhin/o
2. laryng/o
3. a. pneum/o
   b. pneumat/o
   c. pneumon/o
4. pulmon/o
5. tonsill/o
6. trache/o
7. adenoid/o
8. pleur/o
9. a. diaphragmat/o
   b. phren/o
10. sinus/o
11. thorac/o
12. alveol/o
13. pharyng/o
14. a. bronchi/o
    b. bronch/o
15. lob/o
16. epiglott/o
17. sept/o

Exercise 5
1. oxygen
2. breathe, breathing
3. mucus
4. imperfect, incomplete
5. straight

6. pus
7. blood
8. sleep
9. carbon dioxide
10. sound, voice
11. sound
12. x-rays, ionizing radiation
13. to cut, section, or slice

Exercise 6
1. spir/o   8. somn/o
2. ox/i   9. phon/o
3. atel/o   10. capn/o
4. orth/o   11. son/o
5. py/o   12. radi/o
6. muc/o   13. tom/o
7. a. hem/o
   b. hemat/o

Exercise 7
1. within
2. absence of, without
3. normal, good
4. many, much
5. fast, rapid

Exercise 8
1. endo-   4. poly-
2. eu-   5. tachy-
3. a. a-
   b. an-

Exercise 9
1. l   7. a
2. f   8. h
3. g   9. d
4. c   10. e
5. b   11. m
6. k   12. j

Exercise 10
1. c   6. i
2. e   7. f
3. a   8. d
4. h   9. g
5. b   10. j

Exercise 11
1. chest cavity
2. pertaining to
3. constriction, narrowing
4. hernia, protrusion
5. creation of an artificial opening

6. surgical fixation, suspension
7. instrument used to measure
8. sudden, involuntary muscle contraction
9. pain
10. visual examination
11. surgical puncture to aspirate fluid
12. cut into, incision
13. instrument used for visual examination
14. rapid flow of blood
15. stretching out, dilatation, expansion
16. process of recording, radiographic imaging
17. measurement
18. in the blood
19. pertaining to visual examination
20. breathing
21. instrument used to record; record
22. record, radiographic image

Exercise 12
Pronunciation Exercise

Exercise 13
Note: The combining form is identified by italic and bold print.

1. WR   S
   pleur/itis
   inflammation of the pleura

2. WR CV   WR   S
   ***nas/o**/pharyng/itis*
     CF
   inflammation of the nose and pharynx

3.   WR CV   S
   ***pneum/o**/thorax*
        CF
   air in the chest cavity

4. WR   S
   sinus/itis
   inflammation of the sinuses

5. WR   S
   atel/ectasis
   incomplete expansion (or collapsed lung)

6. WR CV WR   S
   ***rhin/o**/myc/osis*
        CF
   abnormal condition of fungus in the nose

7. WR   CV   S
   ***trache/o**/stenosis*
          CF
   narrowing of the trachea

8.   WR   S
   epiglott/itis
   inflammation of the epiglottis

9.   WR   S
   thorac/algia
   pain in the chest

10.   WR   S   P   S(WR)
   pulmon/ary neo/plasm
   pertaining to (in) the lung new growth (tumor)

11.   WR   S
   bronchi/ectasis
   dilation of the bronchi

12.   WR   S
   tonsill/itis
   inflammation of the tonsils

13.   WR CV WR   S
   ***pneum/o**/coni/osis*
          CF
   abnormal condition of dust in the lungs

14.   WR CV   WR   S
   ***bronch/o**/pneumon/ia*
          CF
   diseased state of bronchi and lungs

15.   WR   S
   pneumon/itis
   inflammation of the lung

16.   WR   S
   laryng/itis
   inflammation of the larynx

17. WR CV   S
   ***py/o**/thorax*
        CF
   pus in the chest cavity

18. WR CV   S
   ***rhin/o**/rrhagia*
        CF
   rapid flow of blood from the nose

19.   WR   S
   bronch/itis
   inflammation of the bronchi

20.   WR   S
   pharyng/itis
   inflammation of the pharynx

21.   WR   S
   trache/itis
   inflammation of the trachea

22.   WR CV WR CV WR   S
   ***laryng/o/trache/o**/bronch/itis*
        CF   CF
   inflammation of the larynx, trachea, and bronchi

23.   WR   S
   adenoid/itis
   inflammation of the adenoids

24.   WR CV   S
   ***hem/o**/thorax*
        CF
   blood in the chest cavity (pleural space)

25. WR S   WR   S
   lob/ar pneumon/ia
   pertaining to the lobe, diseased state of a lung

26. WR S
   rhin/itis
   inflammation of the nose

27.   WR CV S   WR   S
   ***bronch/o**/genic carcin/oma*
          CF
   cancerous tumor originating in a bronchus

28. WR   S
   alveol/itis
   inflammation of the alveoli

29.   WR   S
   pneumon/ia
   diseased state of the lung

30. WR   CV S
   ***pneumat/o**/cele*
        CF
   hernia of the lung

Exercise 14
1. thorac/algia
2. rhin/o/myc/osis
3. pulmon/ary neo/plasm
4. laryng/itis
5. atel/ectasis
6. adenoid/itis
7. laryng/o/trache/o/bronch/itis
8. bronchi/ectasis
9. pleur/itis
10. pneum/o/coni/osis
11. pneumon/itis
12. sinus/itis
13. trache/o/stenosis
14. nas/o/pharyng/itis
15. py/o/thorax
16. epiglott/itis
17. diaphragmat/o/cele
18. pneum/o/thorax
19. bronch/o/pneumon/ia
20. rhin/o/rrhagia
21. pharyng/itis
22. hem/o/thorax
23. trache/itis
24. bronch/itis
25. lob/ar pneumon/ia
26. rhin/itis
27. bronch/o/genic carcin/oma
28. alveol/itis
29. pneumon/ia
30. pneumat/o/cele

Exercise 15
Spelling Exercise; see text p. 157.

Exercise 16
Pronunciation Exercise

Exercise 17
1. emphysema
2. pleural effusion
3. cor pulmonale
4. coccidioidomycosis
5. cystic fibrosis
6. influenza
7. chronic obstructive pulmonary disease
8. pertussis
9. croup
10. asthma
11. pulmonary edema
12. upper respiratory infection
13. pulmonary embolism
14. epistaxis
15. idiopathic pulmonary fibrosis
16. deviated septum
17. obstructive sleep apnea
18. tuberculosis
19. acute respiratory distress syndrome

Exercise 18
1. j	6. c
2. d	7. a
3. h	8. e
4. f	9. b
5. g	10. i

Exercise 19
1. d	6. g
2. b	7. h
3. c	8. i
4. e	9. a
5. f	

Exercise 20
Spelling Exercise; see text p. 162.

Exercise 21
Pronunciation Exercise

Exercise 22
Note: The combining form is identified by italic and bold print.
1.   WR CV S
   ***trache/o*/tomy**
          CF
   incision into the trachea

2. WR CV S
   ***laryng/o*/stomy**
              CF
   creation of an artificial opening into the larynx

3.   WR   S
   adenoid/ectomy
   excision of the adenoids

4.   WR CV S
   ***rhin/o*/plasty**
          CF
   surgical repair of the nose

5.   WR CV S
   ***aden/o*/tome**
          CF
   instrument used to cut the adenoids

6.   WR CV S
   ***trache/o*/stomy**
              CF
   creation of an artificial opening into the trachea

7.   WR CV S
   ***sinus/o*/tomy**
             CF
   incision into a sinus

8.   WR CV S
   ***laryng/o*/plasty**
                CF
   surgical repair of the larynx

9.   WR CV S
   ***bronch/o*/plasty**
              CF
   surgical repair of a bronchus

10. WR   S
   lob/ectomy
   excision of a lobe (of the lung)

11.   WR CV WR CV S
   ***laryng/o/trache/o*/tomy**
              CF   CF
   incision of larynx and trachea

12.   WR CV S
   ***trache/o*/plasty**
              CF
   surgical repair of the trachea

13.   WR CV S
   ***thorac/o*/tomy**
              CF
   incision into the chest cavity

14.   WR   S
   laryng/ectomy
   excision of the larynx

15.   WR CV   S
   ***thorac/o*/centesis**
                CF
   surgical puncture to aspirate fluid from the chest cavity

16.   WR   S
   tonsill/ectomy
   excision of the tonsils

17. WR CV S
   ***pleur/o*/pexy**
          CF
   surgical fixation of the pleura

18. WR CV S
   ***sept/o*/plasty**
          CF
   surgical repair of the septum

19. WR CV S
   ***sept/o*/tomy**
          CF
   incision of the septum

Exercise 23
1. trache/o/plasty
2. laryng/o/trache/o/tomy
3. aden/o/tome
4. thorac/o/tomy
5. trache/o/stomy
6. tonsill/ectomy
7. trache/o/tomy
8. bronch/o/plasty
9. laryng/ectomy
10. rhin/o/plasty
11. sinus/o/tomy
12. thorac/o/centesis
13. adenoid/ectomy
14. laryng/o/plasty
15. lob/ectomy
16. laryng/o/stomy
17. pneumon/ectomy
18. sept/o/tomy
19. sept/o/plasty

Exercise 24
Spelling Exercise; see text p. 167.

Exercise 25
Pronunciation Exercise

Exercise 26
Note: The combining form is identified by italic and bold print.
1.   WR CV   S
   ***spir/o*/meter**
          CF
   instrument used to measure breathing

2.   WR CV S
   ***laryng/o*/scope**
              CF
   instrument used for visual examination of the larynx

3.   WR CV S
   ***capn/o*/meter**
          CF
   instrument used to measure carbon dioxide

4. WR CV S
   spir/o/metry
       CF
   measurement of breathing

5. WR CV S
   ox/i/meter
       CF
   instrument used to measure oxygen

6. WR CV S
   laryng/o/scopy
        CF
   visual examination of the larynx

7. WR CV S
   bronch/o/scope
         CF
   instrument used for visual
   examination of the bronchi

8. WR CV S
   thorac/o/scope
         CF
   instrument used for visual
   examination of the chest cavity

9. P S(WR)
   endo/scope
   instrument used for visual
   examination within (a hollow organ
   or body cavity)

10. WR CV S
    thorac/o/scopy
          CF
    visual examination of the chest cavity

11. P S(WR)
    endo/scopic
    pertaining to visual examination
    within (a hollow organ or body
    cavity)

12. P S(WR)
    endo/scopy
    visual examination within (a hollow
    organ or body cavity)

13. P WR CV S
    poly/*somn/o*/graphy
              CF
    process of recording many (tests)
    during sleep

14. WR CV S
    son/o/gram
        CF
    record of sound

15. WR CV S
    son/o/graphy
        CF
    process of recording sound

16. WR CV S
    tom/o/graphy
        CF
    process of recording slices
    (anatomical cross sections)

17. WR CV S
    radi/o/graph
         CF
    record of x-rays

18. WR CV S
    radi/o/graphy
         CF
    process of recording x-rays

Exercise 27

1. laryng/o/scopy
2. spir/o/meter
3. capn/o/meter
4. laryng/o/scope
5. bronch/o/scopy
6. spir/o/metry
7. bronch/o/scope
8. endo/scopy
9. thorac/o/scope
10. endo/scope
11. thorac/o/scopy
12. endo/scopic
13. poly/somn/o/graphy
14. radi/o/graphy
15. radi/o/graph
16. son/o/graphy
17. son/o/gram
18. tom/o/graphy

Exercise 28
Spelling Exercise; see text p. 177.

Exercise 29
Pronunciation Exercise

Exercise 30

1. ventilation-perfusion scanning
2. chest computed tomography
3. chest radiograph
4. arterial blood gases
5. pulse oximetry
6. acid-fast bacilli smear
7. pulmonary function tests
8. PPD skin test
9. peak flow meter
10. stethoscope
11. percussion
12. auscultation
13. sputum culture and sensitivity

Exercise 31
1. f	8. n
2. e	9. l
3. a	10. j
4. d	11. k
5. b	12. m
6. c	13. g
7. h	

Exercise 32
Spelling Exercise; see text p. 181.

Exercise 33
Pronunciation Exercise

Exercise 34
Note: The combining form is identified by italic and bold print.

1. WR S
   laryng/eal
   pertaining to the larynx

2. P S(WR)
   eu/pnea
   normal breathing

3. WR S
   muc/oid
   resembling mucus

4. P S(WR)
   a/pnea
   absence of breathing

5. P WR S
   hyp/ox/ia
   condition of deficient oxygen (to
   tissues)

6. WR CV S
   laryng/o/spasm
         CF
   spasmodic contraction of the larynx

7. P WR S
   endo/trache/al
   pertaining to within the trachea

8. P WR S
   an/ox/ia
   condition of absence of oxygen

9. P WR S
   dys/phon/ia
   condition of difficulty in speaking
   (voice)

10. WR CV WR S
    bronch/o/alveol/ar
          CF
    pertaining to the bronchi and alveoli

11. P S(WR)
    dys/pnea
    difficult breathing

12. P WR S
    hypo/capn/ia
    condition of deficient in carbon
    dioxide (in the blood)

13. WR CV S
    bronch/o/spasm
          CF
    spasmodic contraction of the
    bronchus

14. WR CV S
    orth/o/pnea
        CF
    able to breathe easier in a straight
    (upright) position

15. P S(WR)
    hyper/pnea
    excessive breathing

16. P WR S
    a/capn/ia
    condition of absence of carbon
    dioxide (in the blood)

17. P S(WR)
    hypo/pnea
    deficient breathing

18. P WR S
    hyp/ox/emia
    deficient oxygen in the blood

19. P WR S
    a/phon/ia
    condition of absence of voice

20. WR CV S
    ***rhin/o*/rrhea**
       CF
    discharge from the nose

21. WR S
    thorac/ic
    pertaining to the chest

22. WR S
    muc/ous
    pertaining to mucus

23. WR CV WR S
    ***nas/o*/pharyng/eal**
       CF
    pertaining to the nose and pharynx

24.   WR S
    diaphragmat/ic
    pertaining to the diaphragm

25. P WR S
    intra/pleur/al
    pertaining to within the pleura

26.   WR S
    pulmon/ary
    pertaining to the lungs

27.   WR S
    phren/algia
    pain in the diaphragm

28. P S(WR)
    tachy/pnea
    rapid breathing

29. WR CV S
    ***phren/o*/spasm**
       CF
    spasm of the diaphragm

30.   WR CV S
    ***pulmon/o*/logist**
          CF
    a physician who studies and treats
    diseases of the lung

31. WR CV S
    ***pulmon/o*/logy**
          CF
    study of the lung

32. WR S
    alveol/ar
    pertaining to the alveolus

33. WR CV S
    ***radi/o*/logy**
       CF
    study of x-rays (a branch of medicine
    concerned with the use of x-rays,
    ultrasound, and magnetic fields to
    diagnose and treat disease)

34. W CV S
    ***radi/o*/logist**
       CF
    physician who specializes in the use
    of x-rays, ultrasound, and magnetic
    fields in the diagnosis and treatment
    of disease

Exercise 35

1. hyp/ox/ia
2. muc/oid
3. orth/o/pnea
4. endo/trache/al
5. an/ox/ia
6. dys/pnea
7. laryng/eal
8. hyper/capn/ia
9. eu/pnea
10. a/phon/ia
11. laryng/o/spasm
12. hypo/capn/ia
13. nas/o/pharyng/eal
14. diaphragmat/ic
15. a/pnea
16. hyp/ox/emia
17. hyper/pnea
18. bronch/o/spasm
19. hypo/pnea
20. a/capn/ia
21. dys/phon/ia
22. rhin/o/rrhea
23. muc/ous
24. thorac/ic
25. intra/pleur/al
26. pulmon/ary
27. phren/o/spasm
28. tachy/pnea
29. phren/algia
30. alveol/ar
31. pulmon/o/logy
32. pulmon/o/logist
33. radi/o/logist
34. radi/o/logy

Exercise 36
Spelling Exercise; see text p. 187.

Exercise 37
Pronunciation Exercise

Exercise 38

1. hyperventilation
2. nebulizer
3. bronchodilator
4. ventilator
5. asphyxia
6. sputum
7. aspirate
8. airway
9. stridor
10. rhonchi
11. mucopurulent
12. hypoventilation
13. nosocomial
14. paroxysm
15. patent
16. bronchoconstrictor
17. mucus
18. crackles

Exercise 39

1. b	6. d
2. h	7. g
3. c	8. f
4. i	9. j
5. a	

Exercise 40

1. e	6. a
2. h	7. b
3. i	8. d
4. c	9. f
5. j	

Exercise 41
Spelling Exercise; see text p. 191.

Exercise 42

1. chronic obstructive pulmonary
   disease; pulmonary function
   tests, chest radiograph, arterial
   blood gases, computed
   tomography, shortness of
   breath, chronic obstructive
   pulmonary disease
2. ventilation-perfusion scanning;
   pulmonary embolism
3. left upper lobe; left lower lobe; right
   upper lobe, right middle lobe, right
   lower lobe
4. acid-fast bacilli; tuberculosis
5. polysomnography; obstructive sleep
   apnea
6. oxygen; carbon dioxide
7. peak flow meter
8. idiopathic pulmonary fibrosis
9. culture and sensitivity

Exercise 43

1. acute respiratory distress syndrome
2. cystic fibrosis
3. influenza
4. laryngotracheobronchitis
5. upper respiratory infection
6. continuous positive airway pressure

Exercise 44

A.
1. dyspnea
2. pulmonary
3. rhonchi
4. chest radiograph
5. bronchoscopy
6. arterial blood gases
7. hypoxemia
8. bronchogenic carcinoma
9. pulmonary function tests
10. thoracic

B.
1. 9
2. F
3. F
4. T

C. Online Exercise

Exercise 45

1. epistaxis
2. laryngoplasty
3. orthopnea
4. arterial blood gases, hypoxia
5. thoracalgia
6. hyperventilation
7. nebulizer
8. hemothorax
9. pulmonary embolism
10. coccidioidomycosis
11. chest radiograph, nosocomial
12. PPD skin test
13. tachypnea
14. crackles
15. radiograph, radiologist
16. laboratory test

Exercise 46

Reading Exercise

Exercise 47

1. T
2. F, "hypoxemia" means deficient oxygen in the blood; "hypercapnia" means excessive carbon dioxide in the blood.
3. T
4. F, "bronchitis" means inflammation of the bronchi

Urinary System

Outline

Objectives

Upon completion of this chapter you will be able to:

1 Identify organs and structures of the urinary system.

2 Define and spell word parts related to the urinary system.

3 Define, pronounce, and spell disease and disorder terms related to the urinary system.

4 Define, pronounce, and spell surgical terms related to the urinary system.

5 Define, pronounce, and spell diagnostic terms related to the urinary system.

6 Define, pronounce, and spell complementary terms related to the urinary system.

7 Interpret the meaning of abbreviations related to the urinary system.

8 Interpret, read, and comprehend medical language in simulated medical statements, documents, and electronic health records.

ANATOMY

Organs of the urinary system are the kidneys, ureters, bladder, and urethra (Figures 6-1, 6-2, and 6-3).

Function

The urinary system removes waste material from the body, regulates fluid volume, maintains electrolyte concentration in the body fluid, and assists in blood pressure regulation. The kidneys secrete urine formed from water and waste materials such as urea, potassium chloride, sodium chloride, phosphates, and other elements. Urine is collected in the renal pelvis of the kidney and is transported through the ureters into the bladder, where it is stored until it can be eliminated. Urine passes from the bladder through the urethra and urinary meatus to the outside of the body (Figure 6-4).

Organs of the Urinary System

TERM	DEFINITION
kidneys	two bean-shaped organs located on each side of the vertebral column on the posterior wall of the abdominal cavity behind the parietal peritoneum. Their function is to remove waste products from the blood and to aid in maintaining water and electrolyte balances.
nephron	urine-producing microscopic structure. Approximately 1 million nephrons are located in each kidney.
glomerulus (*pl.* glomeruli)	cluster of capillaries at the entrance of the nephron. The process of filtering the blood, thereby forming urine, begins here.
renal pelvis	funnel-shaped reservoir that collects the urine and passes it to the ureter
hilum	indentation on the medial side of the kidney where the renal artery, vein, and pelvis are located and the ureter leaves the kidney.
ureters	two slender tubes, approximately 10 to 13 inches (26 to 33 cm) long, that receive the urine from the kidneys and carry it to the posterior portion of the bladder
urinary bladder	muscular, hollow organ that temporarily holds the urine. As it fills, the thick, muscular wall becomes thinner, and the organ increases in size.
urethra	lowest part of the urinary tract, through which the urine passes from the urinary bladder to the outside of the body. This narrow tube varies in length by sex. It is approximately 1.5 inches (3.8 cm) long in the female and approximately 8 inches (20 cm) in the male, in whom it is also part of the reproductive system. It carries seminal fluid (semen) at the time of ejaculation.
urinary meatus	opening through which the urine passes to the outside

🏛 **GLOMERULUS**
is derived from the Latin **glomus,** which means **ball of thread.** It was thought that the rounded cluster of capillary loops at the nephron's entrance resembled thread in a ball.

🏛 **BLADDER**
is a derivative of the Anglo-Saxon **blaeddre,** meaning a **blister** or **windbag.**

🏛 **MEATUS**
is derived from the Latin **meare,** meaning **to pass** or **to go.** Other anatomic passages share the same name, such as the auditory meatus.

A & P Booster
For more anatomy and physiology, go to evolve.elsevier.com.
Select: **Extra Content**, A & P Booster, Chapter 6.

Refer to p. 10 for your Evolve Access Information.

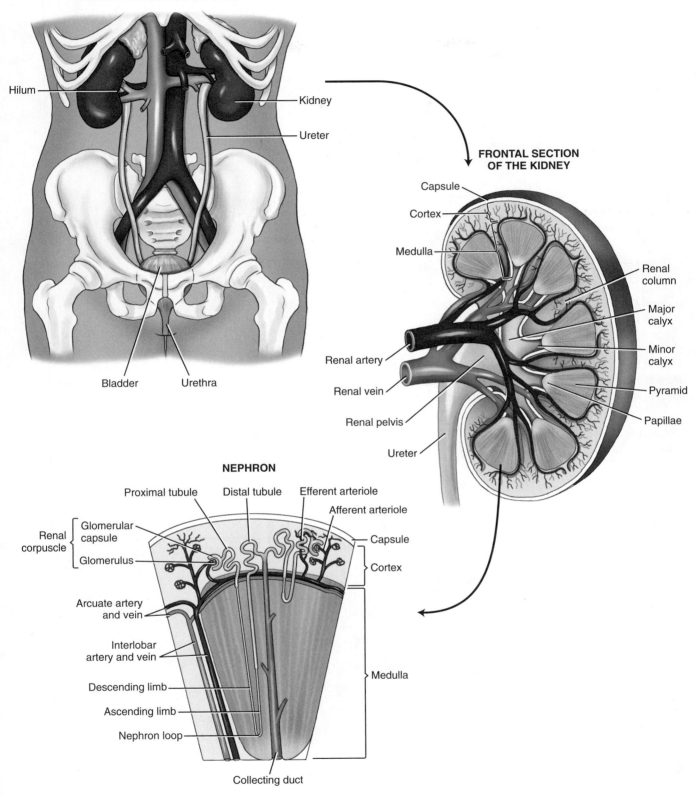

FIGURE 6-1
The urinary system.

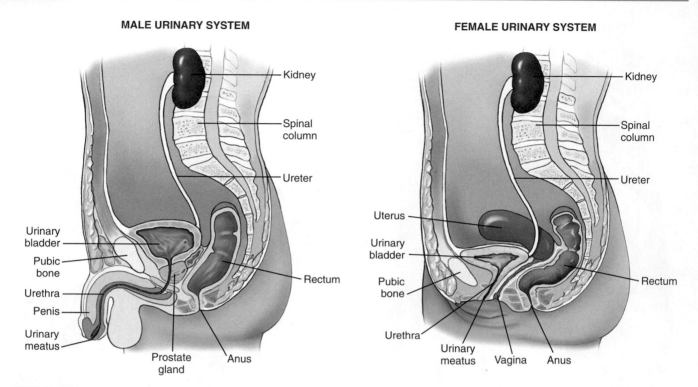

MALE URINARY SYSTEM

Kidney
Spinal column
Ureter
Urinary bladder
Pubic bone
Urethra
Penis
Urinary meatus
Prostate gland
Anus
Rectum

FEMALE URINARY SYSTEM

Kidney
Spinal column
Ureter
Uterus
Urinary bladder
Pubic bone
Urethra
Urinary meatus
Vagina
Anus
Rectum

FIGURE 6-2

Male and female urinary systems, sagittal view. The male urethra is approximately 8 inches (20 cm) in length compared with the female urethra, which is approximately 1.5 inches (3.8 cm) in length.

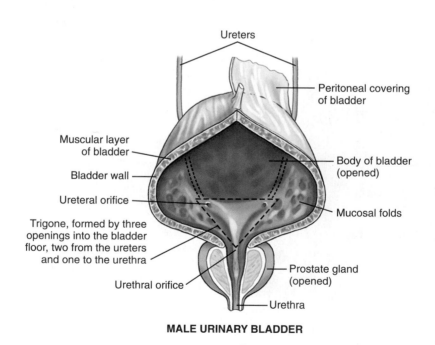

Ureters
Peritoneal covering of bladder
Muscular layer of bladder
Bladder wall
Ureteral orifice
Body of bladder (opened)
Mucosal folds
Trigone, formed by three openings into the bladder floor, two from the ureters and one to the urethra
Urethral orifice
Prostate gland (opened)
Urethra

MALE URINARY BLADDER

FIGURE 6-3

Male urinary bladder.

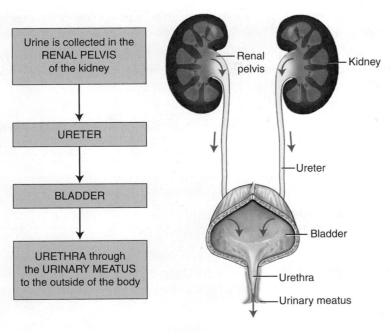

```
┌─────────────────────────┐
│ Urine is collected in the│
│     RENAL PELVIS         │
│     of the kidney        │
└─────────────────────────┘
             │
             ▼
┌─────────────────────────┐
│         URETER           │
└─────────────────────────┘
             │
             ▼
┌─────────────────────────┐
│        BLADDER           │
└─────────────────────────┘
             │
             ▼
┌─────────────────────────┐
│   URETHRA through        │
│  the URINARY MEATUS      │
│ to the outside of the body│
└─────────────────────────┘
```

FIGURE 6-4
Flow of urine.

EXERCISE 1

Match the anatomic terms in the first column with the correct definitions in the second column. *To check your answers to the exercises in this chapter, go to Answers, p. 252, at the end of the chapter.*

_____ 1. kidney(s)
_____ 2. glomerulus
_____ 3. nephron
_____ 4. ureter(s)
_____ 5. urinary bladder
_____ 6. urinary meatus
_____ 7. urethra

a. stores urine
b. outside opening through which the urine passes
c. carries urine from the kidneys to the urinary bladder
d. cluster of capillaries in the kidney where the urine begins to form
e. carries urine from the bladder to the urinary meatus
f. kidney's urine-producing unit
g. organs that remove waste products from the blood

WORD PARTS

Word parts you need to know to complete this chapter are listed on the following pages. The exercises at the end of each list will help you learn their definitions and spellings.

> Use the flashcards accompanying this text or electronic flashcards to assist you in memorizing the word parts for this chapter.

> To use electronic flashcards, go to evolve.elsevier.com. Select: Chapter 6, **Flashcards**.
>
> Refer to p. 10 for your Evolve Access Information.

Combining Forms of the Urinary System

COMBINING FORM	DEFINITION
cyst/o, vesic/o *(Note: these refer to the urinary bladder unless otherwise identified.)*	bladder, sac
glomerul/o	glomerulus
meat/o	meatus (opening)
nephr/o, ren/o	kidney
pyel/o	renal pelvis
ureter/o	ureter
urethr/o	urethra

 PYELOS

is the Greek word for **tub-shaped vessel,** which describes the renal pelvis shape.

EXERCISE FIGURE **A**

Fill in the blanks with combining forms for this diagram of the urinary system. *To check your answers, go to p. 252.*

1. Kidney

CF:_____

CF:_____

Aorta

Inferior vena cava

3. Ureter

CF:_____

4. Bladder

CF:_____

CF:_____

2. Meatus

CF:_____

5. Urethra

CF:_____

EXERCISE FIGURE B

Fill in the blanks with combining forms to label this diagram of the internal kidney structure.

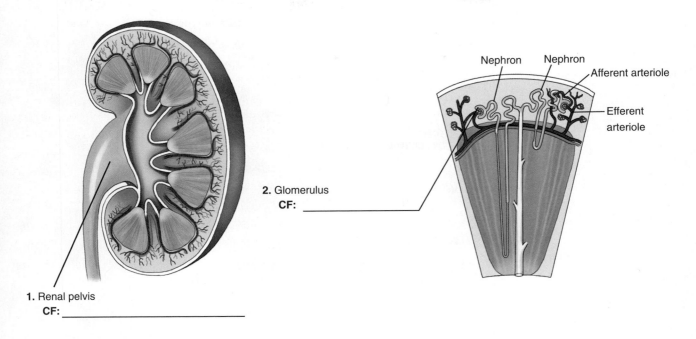

2. Glomerulus
CF: _____

1. Renal pelvis
CF: _____

EXERCISE 2

Write the definitions of the following combining forms.

1. glomerul/o _____
2. vesic/o _____
3. nephr/o _____
4. pyel/o _____
5. ureter/o _____

6. cyst/o _____
7. urethr/o _____
8. ren/o _____
9. meat/o _____

EXERCISE 3

Write the combining form for each of the following terms.

1. kidney   a. _____
             b. _____
2. bladder, sac   a. _____
                   b. _____
3. ureter _____

4. renal pelvis _____
5. glomerulus _____
6. urethra _____
7. meatus _____

Combining Forms Commonly Used with Urinary System Terms

COMBINING FORM	DEFINITION
albumin/o	albumin
azot/o	urea, nitrogen
blast/o	developing cell, germ cell
glyc/o, glycos/o	sugar
hydr/o	water
lith/o	stone, calculus
noct/i *(Note: the combining vowel is i.)*	night
olig/o	scanty, few
urin/o, ur/o	urine, urinary tract

EXERCISE 4

Write the definitions of the following combining forms.

1. hydr/o _____
2. azot/o _____
3. noct/i _____
4. lith/o _____
5. albumin/o _____
6. urin/o _____
7. glyc/o _____
8. blast/o _____
9. olig/o _____
10. ur/o _____
11. glycos/o _____

EXERCISE 5

Write the combining form for each of the following.

1. sugar   a. _____
            b. _____
2. urine, urinary tract   a. _____
                          b. _____
3. water _____
4. developing cell, germ cell _____
5. albumin _____
6. night _____
7. urea, nitrogen _____
8. stone, calculus _____
9. scanty, few _____

Suffixes

SUFFIX	DEFINITION
-iasis, -esis	condition
-lysis	loosening, dissolution, separating
-ptosis	drooping, sagging, prolapse
-rrhaphy	suturing, repairing
-tripsy	surgical crushing
-trophy	nourishment, development
-uria	urine, urination

 Refer to **Appendix A** and **Appendix B** for alphabetized lists of word parts and their meanings.

EXERCISE 6

Match the suffixes in the first column with their correct definitions in the second column.

_____ 1. -iasis, -esis
_____ 2. -lysis
_____ 3. -rrhaphy
_____ 4. -ptosis
_____ 5. -tripsy
_____ 6. -trophy
_____ 7. -uria

a. nourishment, development
b. urine, urination
c. condition
d. surgical crushing
e. suturing, repairing
f. drooping, sagging, prolapse
g. loosening, dissolution, separating

EXERCISE 7

Write the definitions of the following suffixes.

1. -rrhaphy _____

2. -lysis _____

3. -iasis, -esis _____

4. -trophy _____

5. -uria _____

6. -ptosis _____

7. -tripsy _____

For review and/or assessment, go to evolve.elsevier.com. Select:
Chapter 6, **Activities**, Word Parts
Chapter 6, **Games**, Name that Word Part

Refer to p. 10 for your Evolve Access Information.

MEDICAL TERMS

The terms you need to learn to complete this chapter are listed next. The exercises following each list will help you learn the definition and the spelling of each word.

Disease and Disorder Terms

Built from Word Parts

The following terms are built from word parts you have already learned and can be translated literally to find their meanings. Further explanation of terms beyond the definition of their word parts, if needed, is included in parentheses.

TERM	DEFINITION
azotemia (*az*-ō-TĒ-mē-a)	urea in the blood (a toxic condition resulting from disease of the kidney in which waste products are in the blood that are normally excreted by the kidney); (also called **uremia**)
cystitis (sis-TĪ-tis)	inflammation of the bladder (Figure 6-5)
cystocele (SIS-tō-sēl)	protrusion of the bladder
cystolith (SIS-tō-lith)	stone(s) in the bladder (Exercise Figure C)
glomerulonephritis (glō-*mer*-ū-lō-ne-FRĪ-tis)	inflammation of the glomeruli of the kidney
hydronephrosis (*hī*-drō-ne-FRŌ-sis)	abnormal condition of water in the kidney (distention of the renal pelvis with urine because of an obstruction)
nephritis (ne-FRĪ-tis)	inflammation of a kidney
nephroblastoma (*nef*-rō-blas-TŌ-ma)	kidney tumor containing developing (germ) cells (malignant tumor) (also called **Wilms tumor**)
nephrohypertrophy (*nef*-rō-hī-PER-tro-fē) *(Note: the prefix hyper- appears in the middle of this term.)*	excessive development (increase in size) of the kidney
nephrolithiasis (*nef*-rō-lith-Ī-a-sis)	condition of stone(s) in the kidney
nephroma (nef-RŌ-ma)	tumor of the kidney
nephromegaly (*nef*-rō-MEG-a-lē)	enlargement of a kidney
nephroptosis (*nef*-rop-TŌ-sis)	drooping kidney
pyelitis (*pī*-e-LĪ-tis)	inflammation of the renal pelvis
pyelonephritis (*pī*-e-lō-ne-FRĪ-tis)	inflammation of the renal pelvis and the kidney (Figures 6-5, *B*, and Figure 6-6)
ureteritis (ū-*rē*-ter-Ī-tis)	inflammation of a ureter
ureterocele (ū-RĒ-ter-ō-*sēl*)	protrusion of a ureter (distally into the bladder)

UREMIA, ALSO CALLED AZOTEMIA

translated literally is **urine in the blood;** however, the term means **urea** and other waste products **in the blood.**

The term was first used by Pierre Piorry, a French physician (1794-1879). He also created the medical terms **toxin, toxemia,** and **septicemia.**

🏛 **WILMS TUMOR, ALSO CALLED NEPHROBLASTOMA**

is a rare malignancy of the kidney that primarily affects children. Named for German surgeon Dr. Max Wilms who described the disease in 1899, Wilms tumors are generally **unilateral** and can be successfully managed with appropriate surgical and oncology treatment.

NEPHROPTOSIS

is also known as a **floating kidney** and occurs when the kidney is no longer held in place and drops out of its normal position. The kidney is normally held in position by connective and adipose tissue, so it is prone to injury, which may also cause the ureter to twist. Truck drivers and horseback riders are prone to this condition.

TERM	DEFINITION
ureterolithiasis (ū-*rē*-ter-ō-lith-Ī-a-sis)	condition of stone(s) in the ureter
ureterostenosis (ū-*rē*-ter-ō-sten-Ō-sis)	narrowing of the ureter
urethrocystitis (ū-*rē*-thrō-sis-TĪ-tis)	inflammation of the urethra and the bladder

To watch animations, go to evolve.elsevier.com. Select:
Chapter 6, **Animations**, Bladder Infection
CT Scan of Hydronephrosis
Hydronephrosis

Refer to p. 10 for your Evolve Access Information.

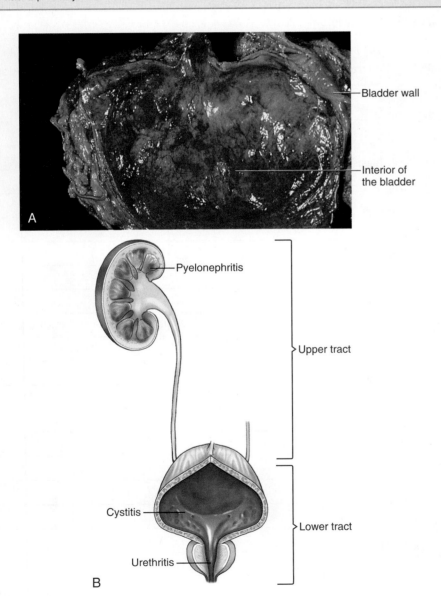

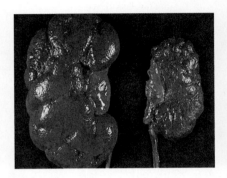

FIGURE 6-6
Kidney on left, chronic pyelone-phritis. *Kidney on right,* normal size with some scarring.

FIGURE 6-5
Urinary tract infection. **A,** Acute cystitis. The swollen and red mucosa demonstrates inflammation. Cystitis is more common in women because the urethra is short, allowing easy access of bacteria to the urinary bladder. **B,** Upper and lower urinary tract infections. If cystitis is not treated promptly, the infection can spread to the kidneys, causing pyelonephritis.

EXERCISE FIGURE **C**

Fill in the blanks to label the diagram.

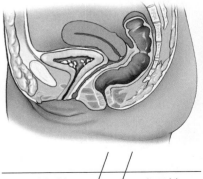

bladder / cv / stone(s)

EXERCISE 8

Practice saying aloud each of the disease and disorder terms built from word parts on pp. 216–217.

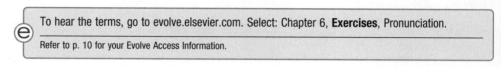

To hear the terms, go to evolve.elsevier.com. Select: Chapter 6, **Exercises**, Pronunciation.

Refer to p. 10 for your Evolve Access Information.

☐ Place a check mark in the box when you have completed this exercise.

EXERCISE 9

Analyze and define the following terms.

EXAMPLE: glomerul / o / nephr / itis   inflammation of the glomeruli of the kidney

1. nephroma _____

2. cystolith _____

3. nephrolithiasis _____

4. azotemia _____

5. nephroptosis _____

6. cystocele _____

7. nephrohypertrophy _____

8. cystitis _____

9. pyelitis _____

10. ureterocele _____

11. hydronephrosis _____

12. nephromegaly _____

13. ureterolithiasis _____

14. pyelonephritis _____

15. ureteritis _____

16. nephritis _____

17. urethrocystitis _____

18. ureterostenosis _____

19. nephroblastoma _____

EXERCISE 10

Build disease and disorder terms for the following definitions with the word parts you have learned.

EXAMPLE: inflammation of the ureter $\dfrac{ureter}{WR} \Big/ \dfrac{itis}{S}$

1. enlargement of the kidney

   _____ WR ___/CV/___ S

2. inflammation of the bladder

   _____ WR ___/___ S

3. excessive development of the kidney

   _____ WR ___/CV/___ P ___/___ S

4. inflammation of the urethra and bladder

   _____ WR ___/CV/___ WR ___/___ S

5. protrusion of the bladder

   _____ WR ___/CV/___ S

6. abnormal condition of water in the kidney

   _____ WR ___/CV/___ WR ___/___ S

7. stone(s) in the bladder

   _____ WR ___/CV/___ WR

8. inflammation of the glomeruli of the kidney

   _____ WR ___/CV/___ WR ___/___ S

9. tumor of the kidney

   _____ WR ___/___ S

10. drooping kidney

    _____ WR ___/CV/___ S

11. inflammation of a kidney

    _____ WR ___/___ S

12. stone(s) in the kidney

    _____ WR ___/CV/___ WR ___/___ S

13. protrusion of a ureter

    _____ WR ___/CV/___ S

14. inflammation of the renal pelvis

    _____ WR ___/___ S

15. urea in the blood

    _____ WR ___/___ S

16. narrowing of the ureter

    _____ WR ___/CV/___ S

17. inflammation of the renal pelvis and the kidney

    _____ WR ___/CV/___ WR ___/___ S

18. stone(s) in the ureter

_____ / / _____ / _____
WR /CV/ WR / S

19. kidney tumor containing developing (germ) cells

_____ / / _____ / _____
WR /CV/ WR / S

EXERCISE 11

Spell each of the disease and disorder terms built from word parts on pp. 216–217. by having someone dictate them to you.

> To hear and spell the terms, go to evolve.elsevier.com. Select: Chapter 6, **Exercises**, Spelling.
>
> Refer to p. 10 for your Evolve Access Information.
>
> ☐ Place a check mark in the box if you have completed this exercise online.

1. _____   11. _____
2. _____   12. _____
3. _____   13. _____
4. _____   14. _____
5. _____   15. _____
6. _____   16. _____
7. _____   17. _____
8. _____   18. _____
9. _____   19. _____
10. _____   20. _____

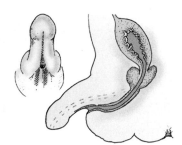

FIGURE 6-7
Hypospadias.

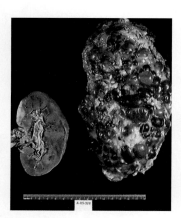

FIGURE 6-8
Kidney on left, Cross-Section of normal kidney. *Kidney on right*, polycystic kidney disease.

Disease and Disorder Terms

Not Built from Word Parts

In some of the following terms, you may recognize word parts you have already learned; however, the full meaning of the terms cannot be discerned by the definition of their word parts.

TERM	DEFINITION
epispadias (*ep*-i-SPĀ-dē-as)	congenital defect in which the urinary meatus is located on the upper surface of the penis
hypospadias (*hī*-pō-SPĀ-dē-as)	congenital defect in which the urinary meatus is located on the underside of the penis; a similar defect can occur in the female (Figure 6-7)
polycystic kidney disease (*pol*-ē-SIS-tik) (KID-nē) (di-ZĒZ)	condition in which the kidney contains many cysts and is enlarged (Figure 6-8)

TERM	DEFINITION
renal calculus (pl. calculi) (RĒ-nal) (KAL-kū-lus) (KAL-kū-lī)	stone in the kidney
renal failure (RĒ-nal) (FĀL-ūr)	loss of kidney function resulting in its inability to remove waste products from the body and maintain electrolyte balance
renal hypertension (RĒ-nal) (*hī*-per-TEN-shun)	elevated blood pressure resulting from kidney disease
urinary retention (Ū-rin-*ār-ē*) (re-TEN-shun)	abnormal accumulation of urine in the bladder because of an inability to urinate
urinary suppression (Ū-rin-*ār-ē*) (sū-PRESH-un)	sudden stoppage of urine formation
urinary tract infection (UTI) (Ū-rin-*ār-ē*) (trakt) (in-FEK-shun)	infection of one or more organs of the urinary tract (see Figure 6-5)

> 🍃 **CAM TERM**
>
> **Biologically based therapies,** one of the National Center for Complementary and Alternative Medicine's (NCCAM) five major classifications of CAM, are therapies that use substances found in nature such as herbs, foods, minerals, and vitamins. Studies suggest that cranberry juice or standardized cranberry extracts in capsules may be effective in reducing the number of recurrent **urinary tract infections** in women.

Table 6-1

Renal Failure

Acute renal failure (ARF) is a sudden and severe reduction in renal function resulting in a collection of metabolic waste in the body. ARF may be caused by excessive bleeding, trauma, obstruction, adverse drug reactions, or severe infection. Prompt treatment can reverse the condition and recovery can occur.

Chronic kidney disease (CKD), unlike ARF, is a progresive, irreversible, loss of renal function, and the onset of uremia. Hypertension, diabetes mellitus, and glomerulonephritis may cause CKD. Dialysis and kidney transplant are used in treating this disease, which was formerly referred to as **chronic renal failure (CRF).**

End-stage renal disease (ESRD) is what chronic renal failure is called when kidney function is too poor to sustain life.

EXERCISE 12

Practice saying aloud each of the disease and disorder terms not built from word parts on these two pages.

> ⓔ To hear the terms, go to evolve.elsevier.com. Select: Chapter 6, **Exercises**, Pronunciation.
>
> Refer to p. 10 for your Evolve Access Information.

☐ Place a check mark in the box when you have completed this exercise.

EXERCISE 13

Fill in the blanks with the correct terms.

1. Stone in the kidney is also called _____ _____.

2. The inability to urinate, which results in an abnormal amount of urine in the bladder, is known as _____ _____.

3. The name given to a condition in which a kidney is enlarged and contains many cysts is _____ _____ _____.

4. The condition in which the urinary meatus is located on the underside of the penis is called _____.

5. Elevated blood pressure resulting from kidney disease is _____ _____.

6. Sudden stoppage of urine formation is referred to as _____ _____.

7. _____ is a condition in which the urinary meatus is located on the upper surface of the penis.

8. Infection of one or more organs of the urinary system is called _____ _____ _____.

9. Loss of kidney function is called _____ _____.

EXERCISE 14

Match the terms in the first column with the correct definitions in the second column.

_____ 1. epispadias
_____ 2. hypospadias
_____ 3. renal calculus
_____ 4. renal hypertension
_____ 5. polycystic kidney disease
_____ 6. urinary retention
_____ 7. urinary suppression
_____ 8. urinary tract infection
_____ 9. renal failure

a. enlarged kidney with many cysts
b. sudden stoppage of urine formation
c. urinary meatus on the upper surface of the penis
d. kidney stone
e. inability to urinate
f. urinary meatus on the underside of the penis
g. infection of one or more organs of the urinary system
h. characterized by elevated blood pressure
i. inability to remove waste products from the body and maintain electrolyte balance
j. excessive amount of urine

EXERCISE 15

Spell each of the disease and disorder terms not built from word parts on pp. 220–221 by having someone dictate them to you.

> To hear and spell the terms, go to evolve.elsevier.com. Select: Chapter 6, **Exercises**, Spelling.
>
> Refer to p. 10 for your Evolve Access Information.
>
> ☐ Place a check mark in the box if you have completed this exercise online.

1. _____
2. _____
3. _____
4. _____
5. _____

6. _____
7. _____
8. _____
9. _____

Surgical Terms

Built from Word Parts

The following terms are built from word parts you have already learned and can be translated literally to find their meanings. Further explanation of terms beyond the definition of their word parts, if needed, is included in parentheses.

TERM	DEFINITION
cystectomy (sis-TEK-to-mē)	excision of the bladder
cystolithotomy (*sis*-tō-li-THOT-o-mē)	incision into the bladder to remove stone(s)
cystorrhaphy (sist-OR-a-fē)	suturing the bladder
cystostomy (sis-TOS-to-mē)	creation of an artificial opening into the bladder (bladder opening brought to the surface of the skin) (Exercise Figure D)
cystotomy, vesicotomy (sis-TOT-o-mē) (*ves*-i-KOT-o-mē)	incision of the bladder
lithotripsy (LITH-ō-trip-sē)	surgical crushing of stone(s) (Exercise Figure E)
meatotomy (*mē*-a-TOT-o-mē)	incision of the meatus (to enlarge it)
nephrectomy (ne-FREK-to-mē)	excision of the kidney
nephrolithotomy (*nef*-rō-li-THOT-o-mē)	incision of the kidney to remove stone(s) (Figure 6-9)
nephrolithotripsy (*nef*-rō-LITH-o-trip-sē)	surgical crushing of stone(s) in the kidney (Figure 6-9)
nephrolysis (ne-FROL-i-sis)	separating the kidney (from other body structures)
nephropexy (NEF-rō-*peks*-ē)	surgical fixation of the kidney

EXERCISE FIGURE **D**

Fill in the blanks to label the diagram.

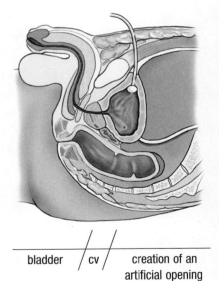

bladder / cv / creation of an artificial opening

Surgical Terms—cont'd

Built from Word Parts

TERM	DEFINITION
nephrostomy (nef-ROS-to-mē)	creation of an artificial opening into the kidney (Exercise Figure F)
pyelolithotomy (pī-el-ō-lith-OT-o-mē)	incision into the renal pelvis to remove stone(s) (Exercise Figure G)
pyeloplasty (PĪ-el-ō-*plas*-tē)	surgical repair of the renal pelvis
ureterectomy (ū-*rē*-ter-EK-to-mē)	excision of the ureter
ureterostomy (ū-*rē*-ter-OS-to-mē)	creation of an artificial opening into the ureter (ureter opening brought to the surface of the skin)
urethroplasty (ū-RĒ-thrō-*plas*-tē)	surgical repair of the urethra
vesicourethral suspension (*ves*-i-kō-ū-RĒ-thral) (*sus*-PEN-shun)	suspension pertaining to the bladder and urethra

To watch animations, go to evolve.elsevier.com.
Select: Chapter 6, **Animations**, Nephrostomy.

Refer to p. 10 for your Evolve Access Information.

STRESS INCONTINENCE

is the involuntary intermittent leakage of urine as a result of pressure, from a cough or a sneeze, on the weakened area around the urethra and bladder. The Marshall-Marchetti Krantz technique, or **vesicourethral suspension** with a midurethral sling is a suspension surgery performed on patients with stress incontinence.

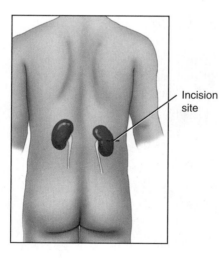
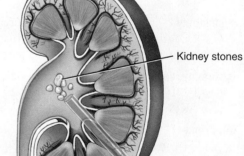

Incision site

Kidney stones

Nephroscope

Stones removed

FIGURE 6-9

Percutaneous nephrolithotomy or percutaneous lithotripsy uses a small incision in the back to remove medium or larger-size kidney stones.

A nephroscope is passed into the kidney through the incision. In a **nephrolithotomy,** the surgeon removes the stone through the nephroscope. In a **nephrolithotripsy,** the stone is broken into fragments by a lithotripter and then removed through the nephroscope.

EXERCISE

Practice saying aloud each of the surgical terms built from word parts on pp. 223–224.

 To hear the terms, go to evolve.elsevier.com. Select: Chapter 6, **Exercises**, Pronunciation.

Refer to p. 10 for your Evolve Access Information.

☐ Place a check mark in the box when you have completed this exercise.

EXERCISE FIGURE **E**

Fill in the blanks to complete the labeling of the diagram.

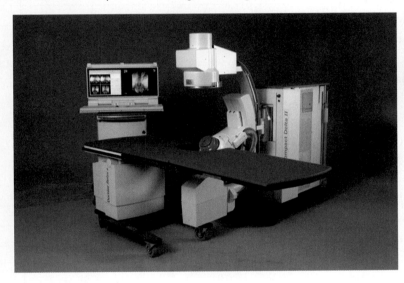

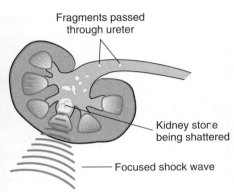

Fragments passed
through ureter

Kidney store
being shattered

Focused shock wave

Extracorporeal shock wave _____ / _____ / _____
                          stone   cv   surgical crushing

ESWL breaks down the kidney stone into fragments by shock waves from outside the body. The broken fragments are eliminated from the body with the passing of urine.

EXERCISE FIGURE **F**

Fill in the blanks to label the diagram.

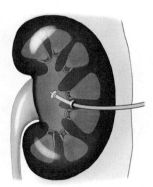

Percutaneous _____ / _____ / _____
              kidney   cv   creation of an
                                  artificial opening

EXERCISE FIGURE **G**

Fill in the blanks to label the diagram.

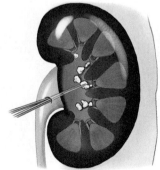

_____ / _____ / _____ / _____ / _____
renal   cv   stone   cv   incision
pelvis

EXERCISE 17

Analyze and define the following surgical terms.

1. vesicotomy _____
2. cystotomy _____
3. nephrostomy _____
4. nephrolysis _____
5. cystectomy _____
6. pyelolithotomy _____
7. nephropexy _____
8. cystolithotomy _____
9. nephrectomy _____
10. ureterectomy _____
11. cystostomy _____
12. pyeloplasty _____
13. cystorrhaphy _____
14. meatotomy _____
15. lithotripsy _____
16. urethroplasty _____
17. vesicourethral (suspension) _____
18. nephrolithotomy _____
19. ureterostomy _____
20. nephrolithotripsy _____

EXERCISE 18

Build surgical terms for the following definitions by using the word parts you have learned.

1. creation of an artificial
   opening into the ureter
   _____
   WR   /CV/   S

2. excision of the kidney
   _____
   WR   /   S

3. incision of the kidney
   to remove stone(s)
   _____
   WR   /CV/   WR   /CV/   S

4. suturing the bladder
   _____
   WR   /CV/   S

5. separating the kidney
   (from other structures)
   _____
   WR   /CV/   S

6. creation of an artificial
   opening into the kidney
   _____
   WR   /CV/   S

7. surgical repair of the urethra
   _____
   WR   /CV/   S

8. excision of the bladder

        WR   /   S

9. incision of the meatus

        WR /CV/ S

10. incision of the bladder

a.   WR /CV/ S

b.   WR /CV/ S

11. surgical repair of the renal pelvis

        WR /CV/ S

12. excision of the ureter

        WR   /   S

13. surgical fixation of the kidney

        WR /CV/ S

14. incision into the bladder to remove stone(s)

   WR /CV/ WR /CV/ S

15. surgical crushing of a stone

        WR /CV/ S

16. suspension pertaining to the bladder and urethra

   WR /CV/ WR / S   (suspension)

17. creation of an artificial opening into the bladder

        WR /CV/ S

18. incision into the renal pelvis to remove stone(s)

   WR /CV/ WR /CV/ WR

19. surgical crushing of stone(s) in the kidney

   WR /CV/ WR /CV/ S

EXERCISE 19

Spell each of the surgical terms built from word parts on pp. 223–224 by having someone dictate them to you.

> To hear and spell the terms, go to evolve.elsevier.com. Select: Chapter 6, **Exercises**, Spelling.
>
> Refer to p. 10 for your Evolve Access Information.
>
> ☐ Place a check mark in the box if you have completed this exercise online.

1. _____
2. _____
3. _____
4. _____
5. _____
6. _____
7. _____
8. _____
9. _____
10. _____

11. _____
12. _____
13. _____
14. _____
15. _____
16. _____
17. _____
18. _____
19. _____
20. _____

Surgical Terms

Not Built from Word Parts

In some of the following terms, you may recognize word parts you have already learned; however, the full meaning of the terms cannot be discerned by the definition of their word parts.

EXTRACORPOREAL means occurring outside the body.

RENAL REPLACEMENT THERAPIES
- Hemodialysis
- Peritoneal dialysis
- Kidney transplant

TERM	DEFINITION
extracorporeal shock wave lithotripsy (ESWL) (*eks*-tra-kor-POR-ē-al) (LITH-ō-*trip*-sē)	noninvasive surgical procedure to crush stone(s) in the kidney or ureter by administration of repeated shockwaves. Stone fragments are eliminated from the body in urine. (also called **shock wave lithotripsy [SWL]**) (see Exercise Figure E).
fulguration (*ful*-gū-RĀ-shun)	destruction of living tissue with an electric spark (a method commonly used to destroy bladder growths) (Figure 6-10)
renal transplant (RĒ-nal) (TRANS-plant)	surgical implantation of a donor kidney into a patient with inadequate renal function (Figure 6-11)

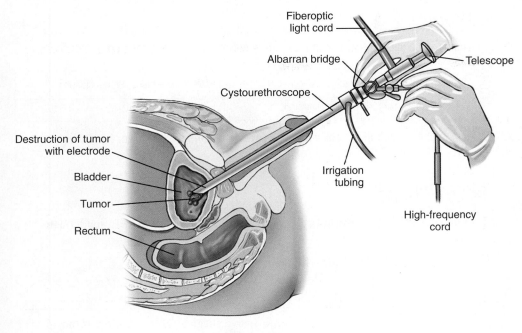

FIGURE 6-10
Bladder fulguration.

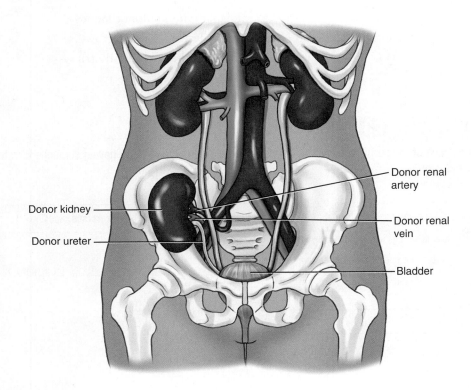

FIGURE 6-11
Renal transplant showing donor kidney and blood vessels in place. Recipient's kidney is not always removed unless it is infected or is a cause of hypertension.

EXERCISE 20

Practice saying aloud each of the surgical terms not built from word parts on p. 228.

> To hear the terms, go to evolve.elsevier.com. Select: Chapter 6, **Exercises**, Pronunciation.
>
> Refer to p. 10 for your Evolve Access Information.

☐ Place a check mark in the box when you have completed this exercise.

EXERCISE 21

1. The surgical implantation of a donor kidney into a patient with inadequate renal function is called _____ _____.

2. The destruction of living tissue with an electric spark is

   _____.

3. _____ _____ _____

   _____ is a noninvasive surgical procedure for removal of kidney or ureteral stones.

EXERCISE 22

Match the terms in the first column with their correct definitions in the second column.

_____ 1. fulguration   a. implantation of a donor kidney

_____ 2. renal transplant   b. used to destroy bladder growths

_____ 3. ESWL   c. also called shock wave lithotripsy

EXERCISE 23

Spell each of the surgical terms not built from word parts on p. 228 by having someone dictate them to you.

> To hear and spell the terms, go to evolve.elsevier.com. Select: Chapter 6, **Exercises**, Spelling.
>
> Refer to p. 10 for your Evolve Access Information.
>
> ☐ Place a check mark in the box if you have completed this exercise online.

1. _____   3. _____

2. _____

Diagnostic Terms
Built from Word Parts

The following terms are built from word parts you have already learned and can be translated literally to find their meanings. Further explanation of terms beyond the definition of their word parts, if needed, is included in parentheses.

TERM	DEFINITION
DIAGNOSTIC IMAGING	
cystogram (SIS-tō-gram)	radiographic image of the bladder (Figure 6-12)
cystography (sis-TOG-ra-fē)	radiographic imaging of the bladder
intravenous urogram (IVU) (*in*-tra-VĒ-nus) (Ū-rō-gram)	radiographic image of the urinary tract (with contrast medium injected intravenously) (also called **intravenous pyelogram [IVP]**)
nephrography (ne-FROG-ra-fē)	radiographic imaging of the kidney
nephrosonography (*nef*-rō-so-NOG-ra-fē)	process of recording the kidney using sound (ultrasonography)
nephrotomogram (*nef*-rō-TŌ-mō-gram)	sectional radiographic image of the kidney (Figure 6-14, *A*)
renogram (RĒ-nō-gram)	radiographic record of the kidney (a nuclear medicine test, used to evaluate kidney function); (also called **renal scan** or **nephrogram**) (see Figure 6-14, *B*)
retrograde urogram (RET-rō-grād) (Ū-rō-gram)	radiographic image of the urinary tract (retrograde means to move in a direction opposite from normal; contrast medium is instilled into the bladder, ureter, or renal pelvis through a urethral catheter. (Exercise Figure H)
voiding cystourethrography (VCUG) (VOID-ing) (*sis*-tō-*ū*-rē-THROG-ro-fē)	radiographic imaging of the bladder and the urethra (Figure 6-15). (Radiopaque contrast media is instilled in the bladder. Radiographic images are taken of the bladder before and during urination.)
ENDOSCOPY	
cystoscope (SIS-tō-skōp)	instrument used for visual examination of the bladder
cystoscopy (sis-TOS-ko-pē)	visual examination of the bladder (Figure 6-16)
nephroscopy (ne-FROS-ko-pē)	visual examination of the kidney (Figure 6-17)
ureteroscopy (*ū*-*rē*-ter-OS-ko-pē)	visual examination of the ureter
urethroscope (*ū*-RĒ-thrō-skōp)	instrument used for visual examination of the urethra

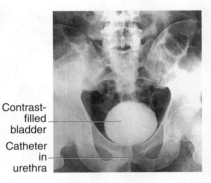

FIGURE 6-12
Cystogram.

Contrast-filled bladder

Catheter in urethra

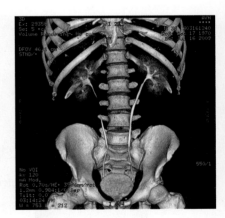

FIGURE 6-13
CT urogram showing three-dimensional, reconstructed view of the kidneys, ureters, and bladder. CT urogram scans are now the primary diagnostic tool for detecting **urinary tract stones** and **perirenal infections**. **Intravenous urograms** may still be used to evaluate an obstructing mass.

To watch animations, go to evolve.elsevier.com. Select: Chapter 6, **Animations**, Cystourethrogram.

Refer to p. 10 for your Evolve Access Information.

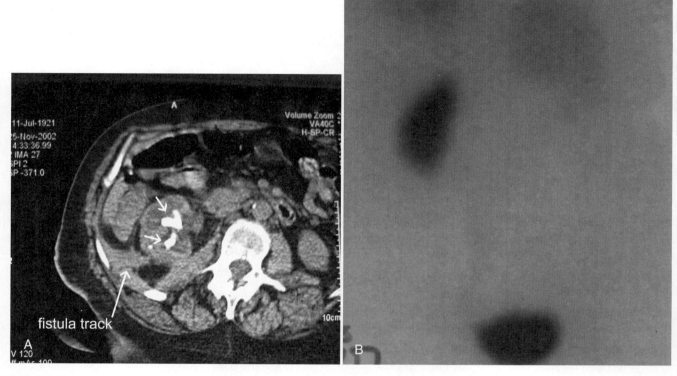

FIGURE 6-14

A, Nephrotomogram. Small arrows point to a large calculus within the renal pelvis. **B,** Renogram. Nuclear medicine image from the same patient, showing no function of the affected kidney.

EXERCISE FIGURE **H**

Fill in the blanks to label the diagram.

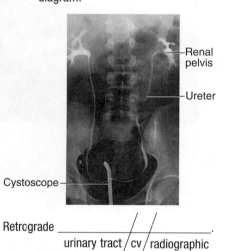

Renal pelvis

Ureter

Cystoscope

Retrograde _____.
    urinary tract / cv / radiographic
                    image.

A urethral catheter is passed by use of a cystoscope, and contrast material is injected to show urinary system structures.

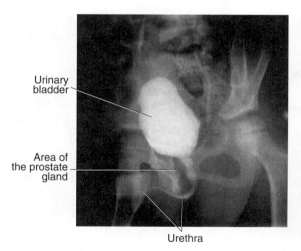

Urinary bladder

Area of the prostate gland

Urethra

FIGURE 6-15

Voiding cystourethrogram, male.

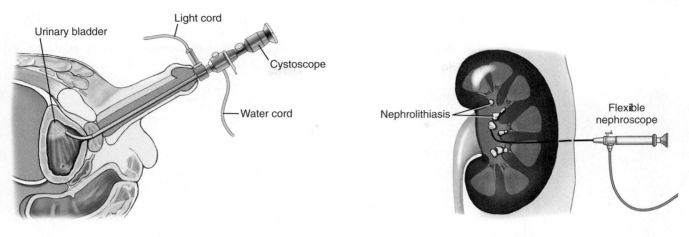

FIGURE 6-16
Cystoscopy.

FIGURE 6-17
Nephroscopy.

EXERCISE 24

Practice saying aloud each of the diagnostic terms built from word parts on p. 231.

> ⓔ To hear the terms, go to evolve.elsevier.com. Select: Chapter 6, **Exercises**, Pronunciation.
>
> Refer to p. 10 for your Evolve Access Information.

☐ Place a check mark in the box when you have completed this exercise.

EXERCISE 25

Analyze and define the following diagnostic terms.

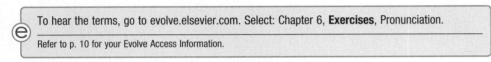

1. (voiding) cystourethrography _____
2. cystography _____
3. urethroscope _____
4. nephrosonography _____
5. cystoscope _____
6. nephrotomogram _____
7. cystogram _____
8. cystoscopy _____
9. nephrography _____
10. (intravenous) urogram _____
11. (retrograde) urogram _____
12. renogram _____
13. nephroscopy _____
14. ureteroscopy _____

EXERCISE 26

Build diagnostic terms that correspond to the following definitions by using the word parts you have learned.

1. visual examination of the bladder

   _____ /___/ _____
   WR   CV   S

2. sectional radiographic image of the kidney

   _____ /___/ _____ /___/ ___
   WR   CV   WR   CV   S

3. radiographic image of the urinary tract (with contrast medium injected intravenously)

   intravenous _____ /___/ _____
                   WR   CV   S

4. instrument used for visual examination of the urethra

   _____ /___/ _____
   WR   CV   S

5. process of radiographic recording the kidney using sound

   _____ /___/ _____ /___/ ___
   WR   CV   WR   CV   S

6. radiographic image of the bladder

   _____ /___/ _____
   WR   CV   S

7. instrument used for visual examination of the bladder

   _____ /___/ _____
   WR   CV   S

8. radiographic imaging of the bladder and the urethra

   voiding _____ /___/ _____ /___/ ___
               WR   CV   WR   CV   S

9. radiographic imaging of the bladder

   _____ /___/ _____
   WR   CV   S

10. (radiographic) record of the kidney, used to evaluate kidney function

    _____ /___/ _____
    WR   CV   S

11. radiographic imaging of the kidney

    _____ /___/ _____
    WR   CV   S

12. radiographic image of the urinary tract (with contrast medium instilled through a catheter in a direction opposite from normal)

    retrograde _____ /___/ _____
                   WR   CV   S

13. visual examination
of the kidney

_____
WR   /CV/   S

14. visual examination of
the ureter

_____
WR   /CV/   S

EXERCISE 27

Spell each of the diagnostic terms built from word parts on p. 231 by having someone dictate them to you.

> To hear and spell the terms, go to evolve.elsevier.com. Select: Chapter 6, **Exercises**, Spelling.
>
> Refer to p. 10 for your Evolve Access Information.
>
> ☐ Place a check mark in the box if you have completed this exercise online.

1. _____   8. _____
2. _____   9. _____
3. _____   10. _____
4. _____   11. _____
5. _____   12. _____
6. _____   13. _____
7. _____   14. _____

Diagnostic Terms

Not Built from Word Parts

In some of the following terms, you may recognize word parts you have already learned; however, the full meaning of the terms cannot be discerned by the definition of their word parts.

TERM	DEFINITION
DIAGNOSTIC IMAGING	
KUB (kidney, ureter, and bladder) (K-Ū-B)	simple radiographic image of the abdomen. It is often used to view the kidneys, ureters, and bladder to determine size, shape, and location. Also used to identify calculi in the kidney, ureters, or bladder, or to diagnose intestinal obstruction; (also called **flat plate of the abdomen**) (Figure 6-18)
LABORATORY	
blood urea nitrogen (BUN) (ū-RĒ-a) (NĪ-trō-jen)	blood test that measures the amount of urea in the blood. An increased BUN detects an abnormality in renal function.

BUN

The abbreviation BUN for blood urea nitrogen is commonly used in the healthcare setting. It is pronounced B-Ū-N and not bŭn.

Diagnostic Terms—cont'd

Not Built from Word Parts

TERM	DEFINITION
creatinine (crē-AT-i-nin)	blood test that measures the amount of creatinine in the blood. An elevated amount may indicate impaired kidney function.
specific gravity (SG) (spe-SIF-ik) (GRAV-i-tē)	test performed on a urine specimen to measure the concentrating or diluting ability of the kidneys
urinalysis (UA) (ū-rin-AL-is-is)	multiple routine tests performed on a urine specimen. Physical examination and chemical analysis of a urine specimen provides screening for blood, glucose, protein, and other substances in the urine and offers a picture of overall health.

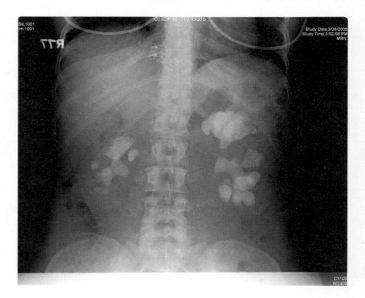

FIGURE 6-18
KUB. Note the bilateral calculi that fill the renal pelvis. Due to the distinctive shape, these are called **staghorn calculi** because of the resemblance to the antlers of a stag.

 To watch animations, go to evolve.elsevier.com. Select:
Chapter 6, **Animations**, Urinalysis Showing Infection.

Refer to p. 10 for your Evolve Access Information.

EXERCISE 28

Practice saying aloud each of the diagnostic terms not built from word parts on pp. 235–236.

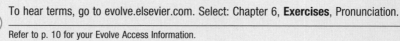 To hear terms, go to evolve.elsevier.com. Select: Chapter 6, **Exercises**, Pronunciation.

Refer to p. 10 for your Evolve Access Information.

☐ Place a check mark in the box when you have completed this exercise.

EXERCISE 29

Fill in the blanks with the correct terms.

1. Radiographic image of the abdomen used to view the kidneys, ureters, and bladder to determine size, shape, and location is called _____.
2. A test performed on a urine specimen to measure concentrating and diluting ability of the kidneys is called _____ _____.
3. _____ _____ _____ measures the amount of urea in the blood.
4. Multiple routine tests performed on a urine specimen are referred to as a(n) _____.
5. _____ is a blood test that measures the amount of creatinine in the blood.

EXERCISE 30

Match the terms in the first column with their correct definitions in the second column.

_____ 1. specific gravity
_____ 2. blood urea nitrogen
_____ 3. urinalysis
_____ 4. KUB
_____ 5. creatinine

a. radiographic image of the kidneys, ureters, and bladder
b. blood test that measures the amount of urea in the blood
c. urine test to measure concentrating or diluting abilities of the kidneys
d. multiple routine tests performed on a urine sample
e. blood test that measures the amount of creatinine in the blood

EXERCISE 31

Spell each of the diagnostic terms not built from word parts on pp. 235–236 by having someone dictate them to you.

To hear and spell the terms, go to evolve.elsevier.com. Select: Chapter 6, **Exercises**, Spelling.

Refer to p. 10 for your Evolve Access Information.

☐ Place a check mark in the box if you have completed this exercise online.

1. _____   4. _____
2. _____   5. _____
3. _____

Complementary Terms

Built from Word Parts

The following terms are built from word parts you have already learned and can be translated literally to find their meanings. Further explanation of terms beyond the definition of their word parts, if needed, is included in parentheses.

TERM	DEFINITION
albuminuria (*al*-bū-min-Ū-rē-a)	albumin in the urine (albumin is an important protein in the blood, but when found in the urine, it indicates a kidney problem)
anuria (an-Ū-rē-a)	absence of urine (failure of the kidney to produce urine)
diuresis (*dī*-ū-RĒ-sis) (*Note: the* a *is dropped from dia- because uresis begins with a vowel.*)	condition of urine passing through (increased excretion of urine)
dysuria (dis-Ū-rē-a)	difficult or painful urination
glycosuria (*glī*-kō-SŪ-rē-a)	sugar (glucose) in the urine
hematuria (*hēm*-a-TŪ-rē-a)	blood in the urine
meatal (mē-Ā-tal)	pertaining to the meatus
nephrologist (ne-FROL-o-jist)	physician who studies and treats diseases of the kidney
nephrology (ne-FROL-o-jē)	study of the kidney (a branch of medicine dealing with diseases of the kidney)
nocturia (nok-TŪ-rē-a)	night urination
oliguria (*ol*-i-GŪ-rē-a)	scanty urine (amount)
polyuria (*pol*-ē-Ū-rē-a)	much (excessive) urine
pyuria (pī-Ū-rē-a)	pus in the urine
urinary (Ū-rin-*ār*-ē)	pertaining to urine
urologist (ū-ROL-o-jist)	physician who studies and treats diseases of the urinary tract
urology (ū-ROL-o-jē)	study of the urinary tract (a branch of medicine dealing with diseases of the male and female urinary systems and the male reproductive system)

DIURETICS

are medications that stimulate **diuresis** and are commonly called "water pills." Diuretics cause a marked increase in the excretion of urine and are used to reduce edema and manage high blood pressure.

UROLOGIST/ NEPHROLOGIST

A **urologist** treats diseases of the male and female urinary system and the male reproductive system both medically and surgically. A **nephrologist** treats kidney diseases and prescribes dialysis therapy.

EXERCISE 32

Practice saying aloud each of the complementary terms built from word parts.

ⓔ To hear terms, go to evolve.elsevier.com. Select: Chapter 6, **Exercises**, Pronunciation.

Refer to p. 10 for your Evolve Access Information.

☐ Place a check mark in the box when you have completed this exercise.

EXERCISE 33

Analyze and define the following complementary terms.

1. nocturia _____
2. urologist _____
3. oliguria _____
4. nephrologist _____
5. hematuria _____
6. urology _____
7. polyuria _____
8. albuminuria _____
9. anuria _____
10. diuresis _____
11. pyuria _____
12. urinary _____
13. glycosuria _____
14. dysuria _____
15. nephrology _____
16. nephrologist _____

EXERCISE 34

Build the complementary terms for the following definitions by using the word parts you have learned.

1. night urination

     _____ / _____
        WR   S

2. scanty urine

     _____ / _____
        WR   S

3. pus in the urine

     _____ / _____
        WR   S

4. physician who studies and
   treats diseases of the
   urinary tract

   —————————— /CV/ —————————
   WR   /CV/   S

5. much (excessive) urine

   —————————— / ——————————
   P   /   S

6. physician who studies and
   treats diseases of the kidney

   —————————— /CV/ —————————
   WR   /CV/   S

7. pertaining to urine

   —————————— / ——————————
   WR   /   S

8. blood in the urine

   —————————— / ——————————
   WR   /   S

9. study of the urinary tract

   —————————— /CV/ —————————
   WR   /CV/   S

10. condition of urine
    passing through
    (increased excretion of urine)

    ———— / ———— / ————
    P   /   WR   /   S

11. absence of urine

    —————————— / ——————————
    P   /   S(WR)

12. sugar in the urine

    —————————— / ——————————
    WR   /   S

13. difficult or painful urination

    —————————— / ——————————
    P   /   S(WR)

14. albumin in the urine

    —————————— / ——————————
    WR   /   S

15. pertaining to the meatus

    —————————— / ——————————
    WR   /   S

16. study of the kidney

    —————————— /CV/ —————————
    WR   /CV/   S

EXERCISE 35

Spell each of the complementary terms built from word parts on p. 238 by having someone dictate them to you.

> ⓔ To hear and spell the terms, go to evolve.elsevier.com. Select: Chapter 6, **Exercises**, Spelling.
>
> Refer to p. 10 for your Evolve Access Information.
>
> ☐ Place a check mark in the box if you have completed this exercise online.

1. _____   9. _____
2. _____   10. _____
3. _____   11. _____
4. _____   12. _____
5. _____   13. _____
6. _____   14. _____
7. _____   15. _____
8. _____   16. _____

> ⓔ For review and/or assessment, go to evolve.elsevier.com. Select:
> Chapter 6, **Activities**, Terms Built from Word Parts
> Chapter 6, **Games**,   Term Storm
>
> Refer to p. 10 for your Evolve Access Information.

Complementary Terms

Not Built from Word Parts

In some of the following terms, you may recognize word parts you have already learned; however, the full meaning of the terms cannot be discerned by the definition of their word parts.

TERM	DEFINITION
catheter (cath) (KATH-e-ter)	flexible, tubelike device, such as a urinary catheter, for withdrawing or instilling fluids
distended (dis-TEN-ded)	stretched out (a bladder is distended when filled with urine)
enuresis (*en*-ū-RĒ-sis)	involuntary urination
hemodialysis (HD) (*hē*-mō-dī-AL-i-sis)	procedure for removing impurities from the blood because of an inability of the kidneys to do so (Figure 6-19)
incontinence (in-KON-ti-nens)	inability to control the bladder and/or bowels
micturate (MIK-tū-rāt)	to urinate or void

🏛 **CATHETER**
is derived from the Greek **katheter,** meaning a **thing let down.** A catheter lets down the urine from the bladder.

ENURESIS

Nocturnal enuresis, or bed-wetting, has been described in early literature and continues to be a problem affecting 15% to 20% of school-aged children. There is no one cause for bed wetting.

Diurnal enuresis is daytime wetting, which may be caused by a small bladder. Various treatments are used to treat diurnal enuresis. Children generally outgrow daytime wetting.

🏛 **MICTURATE**
is derived from the Latin **mictus,** meaning **a making of water.** The noun form of micturate is **micturition.** Note the spelling of each. **Micturition** is often misspelled as **micturation.**

EXERCISE FIGURE

Fill in the blanks to complete labeling of the diagram.

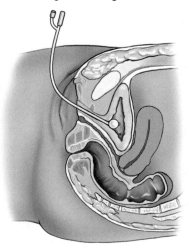

_____ / _____ catheterization
urine / pertaining to

A catheter has been inserted through the urethra and urine has been drained. The balloon on the end of the catheter has been infl ated to hold the catheter in the bladder for a period of time. This type of catheter is called a **retention catheter**; commonly referred to as a **Foley catheter.**

URODYNAMIC STUDIES

examines the process of voiding and tests bladder tone, capacity, and pressure along with urine flow and perineal muscle function. Prostatic hypertrophy, urethral stricture, and advanced prostatic cancer will diminish urine flow rate.

Complementary Terms—cont'd

Not Built from Word Parts

TERM	DEFINITION
peritoneal dialysis (*pār*-i-tō-NĒ-al) (dī-AL-i-sis)	procedure for removing toxic wastes when the kidney is unable to do so; the peritoneal cavity is used as the receptacle for the fluid used in the dialysis (Figure 6-20)
stricture (STRIK-chūr)	abnormal narrowing, such as a urethral stricture
urinal (Ū-rin-al)	receptacle for urine
urinary catheterization (Ū-rin-*ār*-ē) (*kath*-e-*ter*-i-ZĀ-shun)	passage of a catheter into the urinary bladder to withdraw urine (Exercise Figure I)
urodynamics (*ū*-rō-dī-NAM-iks)	pertaining to the force and flow of urine within the urinary tract
void (voyd)	to empty or evacuate waste material, especially urine

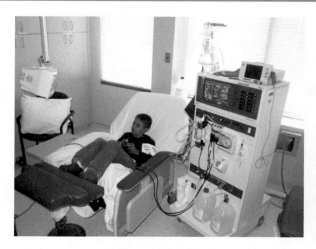

FIGURE 6-19
Hemodialysis.

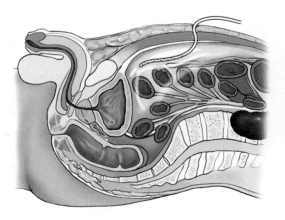

FIGURE 6-20
Peritoneal dialysis. A sterile dialyzing fluid is instilled into the peritoneal cavity by gravity and dwells there for a period of time ordered by the physician. The fluid, containing the nitrogenous wastes and excess water that a healthy kidney normally removes, is drained from the cavity.

EXERCISE 36

Practice saying aloud each of the complementary terms not built from word parts on pp. 241–242.

 To hear terms, go to evolve.elsevier.com. Select: Chapter 6, **Exercises**, Pronunciation.

Refer to p. 10 for your Evolve Access Information.

☐ Place a check mark in the box when you have completed this exercise.

EXERCISE 37

Fill in the blanks with the correct terms.

1. A receptacle for urine is a(n) _____.
2. The procedure for removing impurities from the blood because of the inability of the kidneys to do so is called _____.
3. A _____ bladder is stretched out.
4. A flexible, tubelike device for withdrawing or instilling fluids is a(n) _____.
5. The inability to control the bladder and/or bowels is called _____.
6. The passage of a catheter into the urinary bladder to withdraw urine is a(n) _____ _____.
7. To remove toxic wastes caused by kidney insufficiency by placing dialyzing fluid in the peritoneal cavity is called _____ _____.
8. To void is to _____ _____ _____.
9. An abnormal narrowing is a(n) _____.
10. Involuntary urination is called _____.
11. _____ is another word for void, or urinate.
12. _____ is the name given to the force and flow of urine.

EXERCISE 38

Match the terms in the first column with their correct definitions in the second column.

_____ 1. catheter

_____ 2. urinary catheterization

_____ 3. distended

_____ 4. void

_____ 5. hemodialysis

_____ 6. incontinence

a. to evacuate or empty waste material, especially urine

b. overdevelopment of the kidney

c. inability to control the bladder and/or bowels

d. process for removing impurities from the blood when the kidneys are unable to do so

e. flexible, tubelike device for withdrawing or instilling fluids

f. stretched out

g. passage of a tubelike device into the urinary bladder to remove urine

EXERCISE 39

Match the terms in the first column with their correct definitions in the second column.

_____ 1. micturate

_____ 2. peritoneal dialysis

_____ 3. stricture

_____ 4. urinal

_____ 5. enuresis

_____ 6. urodynamics

a. to urinate or void

b. receptacle for urine

c. force and flow of urine within the urinary tract

d. absence of urine

e. use of peritoneal cavity to hold dialyzing fluid in the removal of toxic wastes

f. involuntary urination

g. narrowing

EXERCISE 40

Spell each of the complementary terms not built from word parts on pp. 241–242 by having someone dictate them to you.

> To hear and spell the terms, go to evolve.elsevier.com. Select: Chapter 6, **Exercises**, Spelling.
>
> Refer to p. 10 for your Evolve Access Information.
>
> ☐ Place a check mark in the box if you have completed this exercise online.

1. _____

2. _____

3. _____

4. _____

5. _____

6. _____

7. _____

8. _____

9. _____

10. _____

11. _____

12. _____

For review and/or assessment, go to evolve.elsevier.com. Select:
Chapter 6, **Activities**, Medical Terms Not Built from Word Parts
                        Hear It and Type It: Clinical Vignettes
 Chapter 6, **Games**,   Term Explorer
                        Termbusters
                        Medical Millionaire

Refer to p. 10 for your Evolve Access Information.

Refer to **Appendix D** for pharmacology terms related to the urinary system.

Abbreviations

ABBREVIATION	DEFINITION
ARF	acute renal failure
BUN	blood urea nitrogen
cath	catheterization, catheter
CKD	chronic kidney disease
ESRD	end-stage renal disease
ESWL	extracorporeal shock wave lithotripsy
HD	hemodialysis
IVP	intravenous pyelogram
IVU	intravenous urogram
OAB	overactive bladder
SG	specific gravity
UA	urinalysis
UTI	urinary tract infection
VCUG	voiding cystourethrogram

EXERCISE 41

1. When imaging is used to diagnose obstructive uropathy, a KUB is usually performed first. An **IVU** _____ _____, also called **IVP** _____ _____, may be used for confirming or excluding obstruction and determining its level and cause. For further examination a **VCUG** _____ _____ may be performed to evaluate the posterior urethra and check for vesicoureteral reflux.

2. **SG** _____ _____ is one of many tests performed on the urine specimen during a **UA** _____. It measures the concentration of particles, including water and electrolytes in the urine.

3. **BUN** _____ _____ _____ is a laboratory test done on a blood sample to determine kidney function.

4. The number, size, and type of stones are important in determining if **ESWL** _____ _____ _____ _____ is the best method for treating renal calculi.

5. Bladder **cath** _____ carries the risk of **UTI** _____ _____ _____.

6. Peritoneal dialysis, **HD** _____, and renal transplant are known as renal replacement therapies.

7. **ARF** _____ _____ _____ is sudden and full recovery can occur with prompt treatment. **CKD** _____ _____ _____ is irreversible and progressive. **ESRD** _____ _____ _____ _____ is when kidney function will not sustain life. A kidney transplant or renal dialysis may be used as treatment.

8. Urge incontinence is another name for **OAB** _____ _____ and involves a sudden, strong need to urinate. As the bladder contracts, leakage of urine occurs.

For more practice with abbreviations, go to evolve.elsevier.com. Select:
Chapter 6, **Flashcards**
Chapter 6, **Games**, Crossword Puzzle

Refer to p. 10 for your Evolve Access Information.

PRACTICAL APPLICATION

EXERCISE 42 *Interact with Medical Documents and Electronic Health Records*

A. Complete the discharge summary report by writing the medical terms in the blanks. Use the list of definitions with the corresponding numbers.

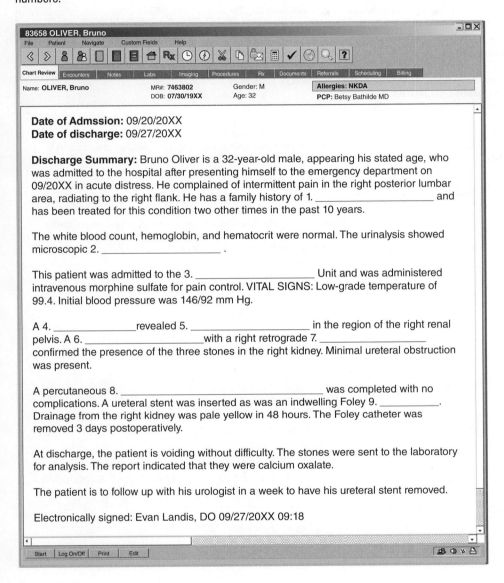

1. condition of stones in the kidney
2. study of the urinary tract
3. blood in the urine
4. radiographic image of the abdomen
5. stones

6. visual examination of the bladder
7. radiographic image of the urinary tract
8. incision into the kidney to remove a stone
9. flexible, tubelike device

EXERCISE 42   *Interact with Medical Documents—cont'd*

B. Read the operative report and answer the questions following it.

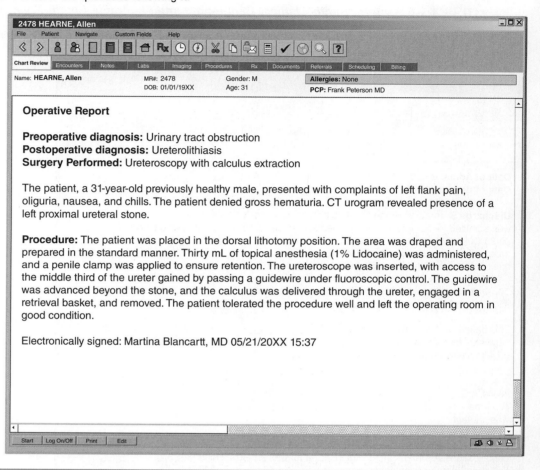

1. The patient presented with a complaint of
   a. difficult or painful urination.
   b. excessive urine.
   c. scanty urine.
   d. pus in the urine.
2. The presence of a ureteral stone was revealed by
   a. radiographic imaging.
   b. magnetic resonance imaging.
   c. ultrasound.
   d. computed tomography.

3. T F More than one stone was removed from the ureter.
4. Ureteroscope and ureteral are terms not included in the chapter. Using your knowledge of the meaning of word parts, define these terms.
   a. ureteral _____
   b. ureteroscope _____

C. Complete the **three medical documents** within the electronic health record (EHR) on Evolve.

Many and maybe most healthcare records today are stored and used in an electronic system called **Electronic Health Records (EHR).** Electronic health records contain a collection of health information of an individual patient; the digitally formatted record can be shared through computer networks with patients, physicians, and other health care providers.

For practice with medical terms using electronic health records, go to evolve.elsevier.com. Select: Chapter 6, **Exercises**, Electronic Health Records.

Refer to p. 10 for your Evolve Access Information.

EXERCISE 43 *Interpret Medical Terms*

To test your understanding of the terms introduced in this chapter, circle the words that correctly complete the sentences. The italicized words refer to the correct answer.

1. The patient was diagnosed with a *drooping kidney*, or (**nephromegaly, nephrohypertrophy, nephroptosis**).
2. The patient's radiographic image showed *stones in the ureter*, or a condition known as (**ureterocele, ureterolithiasis, ureterostenosis**).
3. The patient was scheduled for a right ureteral pelvic junction *ESWL*, a surgical procedure, to (**separate tissue, create an artificial opening, remove a stone**).
4. The physician first suspected diabetes when told of the *excessive amounts of urine voided*, or (**oliguria, polyuria, dysuria**).
5. The physician told the patient with the drooping kidney that it was necessary to *secure the kidney in place* by performing a (**nephropexy, nephrolysis, nephrotripsy**).
6. The patient had a *sudden stoppage of urine formation*, or (**urinary suppression, urinary retention, azotemia**).
7. The patient was scheduled for a *radiographic image of the urinary bladder*, or a (**cystoscopy, cystogram, cystography**).
8. The patient's mother informed the doctor of her son's *involuntary urination*, or (**diuresis, dysuria, enuresis**).
9. The patient was admitted to the hospital for *kidney and ureteral infection*, or (**polycystic kidney disease, urinary retention, urinary tract infection**).
10. *UA* is the abbreviation for (**urine, urinary, urinalysis**).
11. Percutaneous *nephrolithotripsy* is a (**surgical procedure, disease, diagnostic procedure**).

EXERCISE 44 *Read Medical Terms in Use*

Practice pronunciation of the terms by reading the following medical document. Use the pronunciation key following the medical terms to assist you in saying the word.

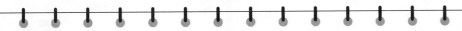

To hear these terms, go to evolve.elsevier.com.
Select: Chapter 6, **Exercises**, Read Medical Terms in Use.

Refer to p. 10 for your Evolve Access Information.

A 76-year-old woman consulted with her primary care physician because of **hematuria** (*hēm*-a-TŪ-rē-a) and **dysuria** (dis-Ū-rē-a). She was referred to a **urologist** (ū-ROL-o-jist). **Urinalysis** (ū-rin-AL-is-is) disclosed 1+ albumin and mild **pyuria** (pī-Ū-rē-a) in addition to the hematuria. A spiral CT scan was obtained. Mild **nephrolithiasis** (*nef*-rō-lith-Ī-a-sis) was observed but no **hydronephrosis** (*hī*-drō-ne-FRŌ-sis). Finally a **cystoscopy** (sis-TOS-ko-pē) was performed, which showed mild **cystitis** (sis-TĪ-tis). A **urinary tract infection** (Ū-rin-*ār*-ē) (trakt) (in-FEK-shun) was diagnosed and the patient responded favorably to antibiotics. The urologist did not advise **lithotripsy** (LITH-ō-trip-sē) for the **renal calculi** (RĒ-nal) (KAL-kū-lī).

EXERCISE 45 *Comprehend Medical Terms in Use*

Test your comprehension of terms in the previous medical document by circling the correct answer.

1. Symptoms that prompted the patient to seek treatment from the urologist were:
   a. scanty urine and painful urination
   b. painful urination and bloody urine
   c. pus and blood in the urine
   d. sugar and blood in the urine

2. The CT image revealed _____ in the kidney.
   a. stones
   b. blood
   c. water
   d. tumors

3. Which of the following was rejected as treatment for kidney stones?
   a. urinalysis
   b. intravenous urogram
   c. cystoscopy
   d. lithotripsy

For a snapshot assessment of your knowledge of the urinary system terms, go to evolve.elsevier.com.
Select: Chapter 6, **Quick Quizzes**.

Refer to p. 10 for your Evolve Access Information.

CHAPTER REVIEW

Review of Evolve

Keep a record of the online activities you have completed by placing a check mark in the box. You may also record your scores. All activities have been referenced throughout the chapter.

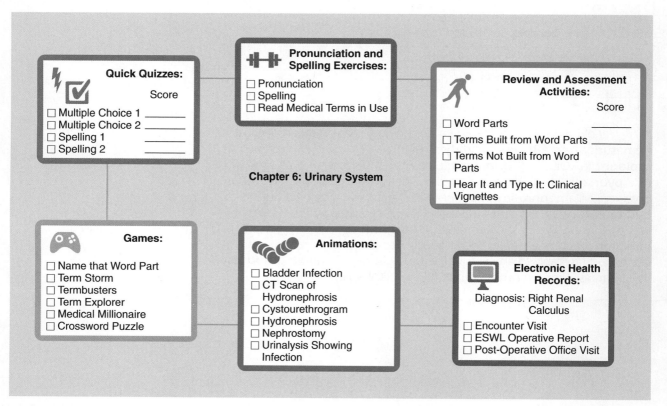

Quick Quizzes:

Score
- [ ] Multiple Choice 1 _____
- [ ] Multiple Choice 2 _____
- [ ] Spelling 1 _____
- [ ] Spelling 2 _____

Pronunciation and Spelling Exercises:
- [ ] Pronunciation
- [ ] Spelling
- [ ] Read Medical Terms in Use

Review and Assessment Activities:

Score
- [ ] Word Parts _____
- [ ] Terms Built from Word Parts _____
- [ ] Terms Not Built from Word Parts _____
- [ ] Hear It and Type It: Clinical Vignettes _____

Chapter 6: Urinary System

Games:
- [ ] Name that Word Part
- [ ] Term Storm
- [ ] Termbusters
- [ ] Term Explorer
- [ ] Medical Millionaire
- [ ] Crossword Puzzle

Animations:
- [ ] Bladder Infection
- [ ] CT Scan of Hydronephrosis
- [ ] Cystourethrogram
- [ ] Hydronephrosis
- [ ] Nephrostomy
- [ ] Urinalysis Showing Infection

Electronic Health Records:

Diagnosis: Right Renal Calculus
- [ ] Encounter Visit
- [ ] ESWL Operative Report
- [ ] Post-Operative Office Visit

Review of Word Parts

Can you define and spell the following word parts?

COMBINING FORMS		SUFFIXES
albumin/o	olig/o	-esis
azot/o	pyel/o	-iasis
blast/o	ren/o	-lysis
cyst/o	ureter/o	-ptosis
glomerul/o	urethr/o	-rrhaphy
glyc/o	ur/o	-tripsy
glycos/o	urin/o	-trophy
hydr/o	vesic/o	-uria
lith/o		
meat/o		
nephr/o		
noct/i		

Review of Terms

Can you define, pronounce, and spell the following terms *built from word parts*?

DISEASES AND DISORDERS	SURGICAL	DIAGNOSTIC	COMPLEMENTARY
azotemia	cystectomy	cystogram	albuminuria
cystitis	cystolithotomy	cystography	anuria
cystocele	cystorrhaphy	cystoscope	diuresis
cystolith	cystostomy	cystoscopy	dysuria
glomerulonephritis	cystotomy	intravenous urogram (IVU)	glycosuria
hydronephrosis	lithotripsy	nephrography	hematuria
nephritis	meatotomy	nephroscopy	meatal
nephroblastoma	nephrectomy	nephrosonography	nephrologist
nephrohypertrophy	nephrolithotomy	nephrotomogram	nephrology
nephrolithiasis	nephrolithotripsy	renogram	nocturia
nephroma	nephrolysis	retrograde urogram	oliguria
nephromegaly	nephropexy	ureteroscopy	polyuria
nephroptosis	nephrostomy	urethroscope	pyuria
pyelitis	pyelolithotomy	voiding cystourethrography	urinary
pyelonephritis	pyeloplasty	(VCUG)	urologist
ureteritis	ureterectomy		urology
ureterocele	ureterostomy		
ureterolithiasis	urethroplasty		
ureterostenosis	vesicourethral suspension		
urethrocystitis	vesicotomy		

Can you define, pronounce, and spell the following terms *not built from word parts*?

DISEASES AND DISORDERS	SURGICAL	DIAGNOSTIC	COMPLEMENTARY
epispadias	extracorporeal shock wave	blood urea nitrogen (BUN)	catheter (cath)
hypospadias	lithotripsy (ESWL)	creatinine	distended
polycystic kidney disease	fulguration	KUB	enuresis
renal calculus (*pl.* calculi)	renal transplant	specific gravity (SG)	hemodialysis (HD)
renal failure		urinalysis (UA)	incontinence
renal hypertension			micturate
urinary retention			peritoneal dialysis
urinary suppression			stricture
urinary tract infection (UTI)			urinal
			urinary catheterization
			urodynamics
			void

ANSWERS

Exercise Figures

Exercise Figure

A. 1. kidney: nephr/o, ren/o
2. meatus: meat/o
3. ureter: ureter/o
4. bladder: cyst/o, vesic/o
5. urethra: urethr/o

Exercise Figure

B. 1. renal pelvis: pyel/o
2. glomerulus: glomerul/o

Exercise Figure

C. cyst/o/lith

Exercise Figure

D. cyst/o/stomy

Exercise Figure

E. lith/o/tripsy

Exercise Figure

F. nephr/o/stomy

Exercise Figure

G. pyel/o/lith/o/tomy

Exercise Figure

H. ur/o/gram

Exercise Figure

I. urin/ary

Exercise 1

1. g
2. d
3. f
4. c
5. a
6. b
7. e

Exercise 2

1. glomerulus
2. bladder, sac
3. kidney
4. renal pelvis
5. ureter
6. bladder, sac
7. urethra
8. kidney
9. meatus

Exercise 3

1. a. nephr/o
   b. ren/o
2. a. cyst/o
   b. vesic/o
3. ureter/o
4. pyel/o
5. glomerul/o
6. urethr/o
7. meat/o

Exercise 4

1. water
2. urea, nitrogen
3. night
4. stone, calculus
5. albumin
6. urine, urinary tract
7. sugar
8. developing cell, germ cell
9. scanty, few
10. urine, urinary tract
11. sugar

Exercise 5

1. a. glyc/o
   b. glycos/o
2. a. urin/o
   b. ur/o
3. hydr/o
4. blast/o
5. albumin/o
6. noct/i
7. azot/o
8. lith/o
9. olig/o

Exercise 6

1. c
2. g
3. e
4. f
5. d
6. a
7. b

Exercise 7

1. suturing, repairing
2. loosening, dissolution, separating
3. condition
4. nourishment, development
5. urine, urination
6. drooping, sagging, prolapse
7. surgical crushing

Exercise 8

Pronunciation Exercise

Exercise 9

Note: The combining form is identified by italic and bold print.

1. WR   S
    nephr/oma
    tumor of the kidney

2. WR CV WR
    ***cyst/o*/lith**
         CF
    stone(s) in the bladder

3. WR CV WR S
    ***nephr/o*/lith/iasis**
          CF
    stone(s) in the kidney

4. WR   S
    azot/emia
    urea in the blood

5. WR CV S
    ***nephr/o*/ptosis**
          CF
    drooping kidney

6. WR CV S
    ***cyst/o*/cele**
         CF
    protrusion of the bladder

7. WR CV P   S
    ***nephr/o*/hyper/trophy**
          CF
    excessive development of the kidney

8. WR S
    cyst/itis
    inflammation of the bladder

9. WR S
    pyel/itis
    inflammation of the renal pelvis

10. WR CV S
    ***ureter/o*/cele**
          CF
    protrusion of a ureter

11. WR CV WR   S
    ***hydr/o*/nephr/osis**
          CF
    abnormal condition of water in the kidney

12. WR CV S
    ***nephr/o*/megaly**
          CF
    enlargement of a kidney

13. WR CV WR S
    ***ureter/o*/lith/iasis**
           CF
    stone(s) in the ureter

14. WR CV WR   S
    ***pyel/o*/nephr/itis**
          CF
    inflammation of the renal pelvis and the kidney

15. WR   S
    ureter/itis
    inflammation of a ureter

16. WR   S
    nephr/itis
    inflammation of a kidney

17. WR CV WR S
    ***urethr/o*/cyst/itis**
            CF
    inflammation of the urethra and bladder

18. WR CV S
    ***ureter/o*/stenosis**
           CF
    narrowing of the ureter

19. WR CV WR   S
    ***nephr/o*/blast/oma**
          CF
    kidney tumor containing developing cells

Exercise 10
1. nephr/o/megaly
2. cyst/itis
3. nephr/o/hyper/trophy
4. urethr/o/cyst/itis
5. cyst/o/cele
6. hydr/o/nephr/osis
7. cyst/o/lith
8. glomerul/o/nephr/itis
9. nephr/oma
10. nephr/o/ptosis
11. nephr/itis
12. nephr/o/lith/iasis
13. ureter/o/cele
14. pyel/itis
15. azot/emia
16. ureter/o/stenosis
17. pyel/o/nephr/itis
18. ureter/o/lith/iasis
19. nephr/o/blast/oma

Exercise 11
Spelling Exercise, see text p. 220.

Exercise 12
Pronunciation Exercise

Exercise 13
1. renal calculus
2. urinary retention
3. polycystic kidney disease
4. hypospadias
5. renal hypertension
6. urinary suppression
7. epispadias
8. urinary tract infection
9. renal failure

Exercise 14
1. c   6. e
2. f   7. b
3. d   8. g
4. h   9. i
5. a

Exercise 15
Spelling Exercise; see text p. 223.

Exercise 16
Pronunciation Exercise

Exercise 17
Note: The combining form is identified by italic and bold print.
1. WR CV S
   vesic/o/tomy
      CF
   incision into the bladder

2. WR CV S
   cyst/o/tomy
     CF
   incison into bladder

3. WR CV S
   nephr/o/stomy
      CF
   creation of an artificial opening into the kidney

4. WR CV S
   nephr/o/lysis
      CF
   separating the kidney

5. WR S
   cyst/ectomy
   excision of the bladder

6. W CV WR CV S
   pyel/o/lith/o/tomy
     CF   CF
   incision into the renal pelvis to remove stone(s)

7. WR CV S
   nephr/o/pexy
      CF
   surgical fixation of the kidney

8. WR CV WR CV S
   cyst/o/lith/o/tomy
     CF   CF
   incision into the bladder to remove stone(s)

9. WR S
   nephr/ectomy
   excision of the kidney

10. WR S
    ureter/ectomy
    excision of the ureter

11. WR CV S
    cyst/o/stomy
      CF
    creation of an artificial opening into the bladder

12. WR CV S
    pyel/o/plasty
      CF
    surgical repair of the renal pelvis

13. WR CV S
    cyst/o/rrhaphy
      CF
    suturing the bladder

14. WR CV S
    meat/o/tomy
      CF
    incision of the meatus

15. WR CV S
    lith/o/tripsy
      CF
    surgical crushing of stone(s)

16. WR CV S
    urethr/o/plasty
      CF
    surgical repair of the urethra

17. WR CV WR S
    vesic/o/urethr/al (suspension)
      CF
    suspension pertaining to the bladder and urethra

18. WR CV WR CV S
    nephr/o/lith/o/tomy
      CF   CF
    incision of the kidney to remove stone(s)

19. WR CV S
    ureter/o/stomy
      CF
    creation of an artificial opening into the ureter

20. WR CV WR CV S
    nephr/o/lith/o/tripsy
      CF   CF
    surgical crushing of stone(s) in the kidney

Exercise 18
1. ureter/o/stomy
2. nephr/ectomy
3. nephr/o/lith/o/tomy
4. cyst/o/rrhaphy
5. nephr/o/lysis
6. nephr/o/stomy
7. urethr/o/plasty
8. cyst/ectomy
9. meat/o/tomy
10. a. cyst/o/tomy
    b. vesic/o/tomy
11. pyel/o/plasty
12. ureter/ectomy
13. nephr/o/pexy
14. cyst/o/lith/o/tomy
15. lith/o/tripsy
16. vesic/o/urethr/al (suspension)
17. cyst/o/stomy
18. pyel/o/lith/o/tomy
19. nephr/o/lith/o/tripsy

Exercise 19
Spelling Exercise; see text p. 228.

Exercise 20
Pronunciation Exercise

Exercise 21
1. renal transplant
2. fulguration
3. extracorporeal shock wave lithotripsy

Exercise 22
1. b   3. c
2. a

Exercise 23
Spelling Exercise; see text p. 230.

Exercise 24
Pronunciation Exercise

Exercise 25
Note: The combining form is identified by italic and bold print.

1. WR CV WR CV S
    (voiding) ***cyst/o/urethr/o*/**graphy
         CF   CF
    radiographic imaging of the bladder and the urethra

2. WR CV   S
    ***cyst/o*/**graphy
         CF
    radiographic imaging of the bladder

3. WR CV S
    ***urethr/o*/**scope
           CF
    instrument used for visual examination of the urethra

4. WR CV WR CV S
    ***nephr/o/son/o*/**graphy
           CF   CF
    process of recording the kidney with sound

5. WR CV S
    ***cyst/o*/**scope
          CF
    instrument used for visual examination of the bladder

6. WR CV WR CV S
    ***nephr/o/tom/o*/**gram
           CF   CF
    sectional radiographic image of the kidney

7. WR CV S
    ***cyst/o*/**gram
          CF
    radiographic image of the bladder

8. WR CV S
    ***cyst/o*/**scopy
          CF
    visual examination of the bladder

9. WR CV S
    ***nephr/o*/**graphy
           CF
    radiographic imaging of the kidney

10. WR CV S
    (intravenous) ***ur/o*/**gram
                       CF
    radiographic image of the urinary tract (with contrast medium injected intravenously)

11. WR CV S
    (retrograde) ***ur/o*/**gram
                      CF
    radiographic image of the urinary tract

12. WR CV S
    ***ren/o*/**gram
          CF
    (graphic) record of the kidney

13. WR   CV S
    ***nephr/o*/**scopy
            CF
    visual examination of the kidney

14. WR CV S
    ***ureter/o*/**scopy
            CF
    visual examination of the ureter

Exercise 26
1. cyst/o/scopy
2. nephr/o/tom/o/gram
3. (intravenous) ur/o/gram
4. urethr/o/scope
5. nephr/o/son/o/graphy
6. cyst/o/gram
7. cyst/o/scope
8. (voiding) cyst/o/urethr/o/graphy
9. cyst/o/graphy
10. ren/o/gram
11. nephr/o/graphy
12. (retrograde) ur/o/gram
13. nephr/o/scopy
14. ureter/o/scopy

Exercise 27
Spelling Exercise; see text p. 235.

Exercise 28
Pronunciation Exercise

Exercise 29
1. KUB
2. specific gravity
3. blood urea nitrogen
4. urinalysis
5. creatinine

Exercise 30
1. c   4. a
2. b   5. e
3. d

Exercise 31
Spelling Exercise; see text p. 237.

Exercise 32
Pronunciation Exercise

Exercise 33
Note: The combining form is identified by italic and bold print.

1. WR   S
    noct/uria
    night urination

2. WR CV S
    ***ur/o*/**logist
         CF
    physician who studies and treats diseases of the urinary tract

3. WR   S
    olig/uria
    condition of scanty urine (amount)

4. WR CV S
    ***nephr/o*/**logist
           CF
    physician who studies and treats diseases of the kidney

5. WR   S
    hemat/uria
    blood in the urine

6. WR CV S
    ***ur/o*/**logy
         CF
    study of the urinary tract

7. P S(WR)
    poly/uria
    much (excessive) urine

8. WR   S
    albumin/uria
    albumin in the urine

9. P S(WR)
    an/uria
    absence of urine

10. P WR S
    di/ur/esis
    condition of urine passing through (increased excretion of urine)

11. WR S
    py/uria
    pus in the urine

12. WR S
    urin/ary
    pertaining to urine

13. WR   S
    glycos/uria
    sugar in the urine

14. P S(WR)
    dys/uria
    difficult or painful urination

15. WR CV S
    ***nephr/o*/**logy
           CF
    study of the kidney

16. WR CV S
    ***nephr/o*/**logist
           CF
    physician who studies and treats diseases of the kidney

Exercise 34
1. noct/uria
2. olig/uria
3. py/uria
4. ur/o/logist
5. poly/uria
6. nephr/o/logist
7. urin/ary
8. hemat/uria
9. ur/o/logy
10. di/ur/esis
11. an/uria
12. glycos/uria
13. dys/uria
14. albumin/uria
15. meat/al
16. nephr/o/logy

Exercise 35
Spelling Exercise; see text p. 241.

Exercise 36
Pronunciation Exercise

Exercise 37
1. urinal
2. hemodialysis
3. distended
4. catheter
5. incontinence
6. urinary catheterization
7. peritoneal dialysis
8. evacuate waste material
9. stricture
10. enuresis

11. micturate
12. urodynamics

Exercise 38
1. e	4. a
2. g	5. d
3. f	6. c

Exercise 39
1. a	4. b
2. e	5. f
3. g	6. c

Exercise 40
Spelling Exercise; see text p. 244.

Exercise 41
1. intravenous urogram; intravenous pyelogram; voiding cystourethrogram
2. specific gravity; urinalysis
3. blood urea nitrogen
4. extracorporeal shock wave lithotripsy
5. catheterization; urinary tract infection
6. hemodialysis
7. acute renal failure, chronic kidney disease, end-stage renal disease.
8. overactive bladder

Exercise 42
A. 1. nephrolithiasis
   2. urology
   3. hematuria
   4. KUB

5. calculi
6. cystoscopy
7. urogram
8. nephrolithotomy
9. catheter

B. 1. c
   2. d
   3. *F*, calculus is singular for stone
   4. a. pertaining to the ureter
      b. instrument used for visual examination of the ureter

C. Online Exercise

Exercise 43
1. nephroptosis
2. ureterolithiasis
3. remove a stone
4. polyuria
5. nephropexy
6. urinary suppression
7. cystogram
8. enuresis
9. urinary tract infection
10. urinalysis
11. surgical procedure

Exercise 44
Reading Exercise

Exercise 45
1. b
2. a
3. d

Outline

Objectives

Upon completion of this chapter you will be able to:

1 Identify organs and structures of the male reproductive system.

2 Define and spell word parts related to the male reproductive system.

3 Define, pronounce, and spell disease and disorder terms related to the male reproductive system.

4 Define, pronounce, and spell surgical terms related to the male reproductive system.

5 Define, pronounce, and spell diagnostic terms related to the male reproductive system.

6 Define, pronounce, and spell complementary terms related to the male reproductive system.

7 Interpret the meaning of abbreviations related to the male reproductive system.

8 Interpret, read, and comprehend medical language in simulated medical statements, documents, and electronic health records.

ANATOMY

The organs of the male reproductive system include the external genitalia, the penis, and scrotum, within which are contained the testes and an initial section of the vas deferens. Internally, the male pelvis includes a major portion of the vas deferens, the seminal vesicles, and the prostate gland. The penis and urethra are shared with the urinary system.

Function

The function of the male reproductive system is to produce, sustain, and transport sperm, the male reproductive germ cells, and to secrete the hormone testosterone (Figures 7-1 and 7-2).

Organs of the Male Reproductive System

TERM	DEFINITION
testis, or testicle (*pl.* testes, or testicles)	primary male sex organs, paired, oval-shaped, and enclosed in a sac called the **scrotum**. The testes produce spermatozoa (sperm cells) and the hormone testosterone.
sperm (spermatozoon, *pl.* spermatozoa)	the microscopic male germ cell, which, when united with the ovum, produces a zygote (fertilized egg) that with subsequent development becomes an embryo (Figures 7-2 and 7-3)
testosterone	the principal male sex hormone. Its chief function is to stimulate the development of the male reproductive organs and secondary sex characteristics such as facial hair.
seminiferous tubules	approximately 900 coiled tubes within the testes in which spermatogenesis occurs

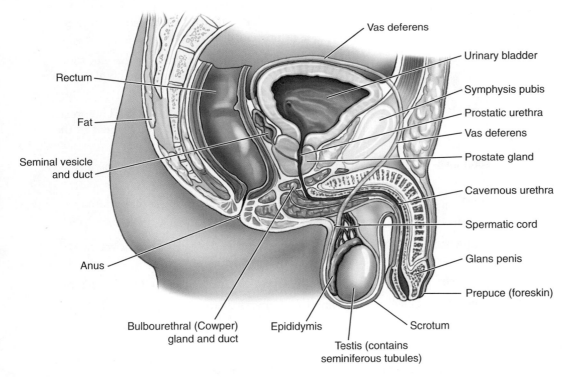

FIGURE 7-1
Male reproductive organs and associated structures.

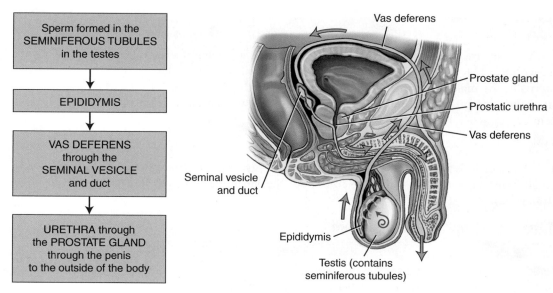

```
┌─────────────────────────┐
│   Sperm formed in the   │
│  SEMINIFEROUS TUBULES   │
│      in the testes      │
└─────────────────────────┘
            │
            ▼
┌─────────────────────────┐
│       EPIDIDYMIS        │
└─────────────────────────┘
            │
            ▼
┌─────────────────────────┐
│      VAS DEFERENS       │
│       through the       │
│     SEMINAL VESICLE     │
│        and duct         │
└─────────────────────────┘
            │
            ▼
┌─────────────────────────┐
│     URETHRA through     │
│   the PROSTATE GLAND    │
│      through the penis  │
│  to the outside of the body │
└─────────────────────────┘
```

FIGURE 7-2
Origination and transportation of sperm.

Organs of the Male Reproductive System—cont'd

TERM	DEFINITION
epididymis	coiled tube atop each of the testes that provides for storage, transit, and maturation of sperm; continuous with the vas deferens
vas deferens, ductus deferens, or seminal duct	duct carrying the sperm from the epididymis to the urethra. The **spermatic cord** encloses each vas deferens with nerves, lymphatics, arteries, and veins. The urethra also connects with the urinary bladder and carries urine outside the body. A circular muscle constricts during intercourse to prevent urination.
seminal vesicles	two main glands located posterior to the base of the bladder that open into the vas deferens. The glands secrete a thick fluid that forms part of the semen.
prostate gland	encircles a proximal section of the urethra. The prostate gland secretes a fluid that aids in the movement of the sperm and ejaculation.
scrotum	sac containing the testes and epididymis, suspended on both sides of and posterior to the penis
penis	male organ of urination and coitus (sexual intercourse)
glans penis	enlarged tip on the end of the penis
prepuce	fold of skin covering the glans penis in uncircumcised males (foreskin of the penis)
semen	composed of sperm, seminal fluids, and other secretions
genitalia (genitals)	reproductive organs (male or female) (also called **gonads**)

🏛 **PROSTATE**
is derived from the Greek **pro**, meaning **before**, and **statis**, meaning **standing** or **sitting**. Anatomically it is the gland standing before the bladder.

ℯ A & P Booster
For more anatomy and physiology, go to evolve.elsevier.com.
Select: **Extra Content**, A & P Booster, Chapter 7.

Refer to p. 10 for your Evolve Access Information.

EXERCISE 1

Match the anatomic terms in the first column with the correct definitions in the second column. *To check your answers to the exercises in this chapter, go to Answers, p. 290, at the end of the chapter.*

_____ 1. epididymis

_____ 2. glans penis

_____ 3. penis

_____ 4. prepuce

_____ 5. prostate gland

_____ 6. scrotum

_____ 7. semen

_____ 8. seminal vesicles

_____ 9. seminiferous tubules

_____ 10. testes

_____ 11. vas deferens

_____ 12. genitalia

_____ 13. sperm

_____ 14. testosterone

a. sac containing testes and epididymis
b. coiled tubes within testes where sperm originate
c. coiled tube atop each testis that provides for storage, transit, and maturation of sperm
d. reproductive organs (male or female)
e. male organ of coitus
f. encircles proximal section of urethra
g. glands that open into the vas deferens
h. primary male sex organs
i. enlarged tip at the end of the penis
j. microscopic male germ cell
k. fold of skin covering the glans penis
l. comprised of sperm and seminal fluid
m. principal male sex hormone
n. duct carrying sperm to the urethra

WORD PARTS

Word parts you need to learn to complete this chapter are listed on the following pages. The exercises at the end of each list help you learn their definitions and spellings.

> Use the flashcards accompanying this text or electronic flashcards to assist you in memorizing the word parts for this chapter.

To use electronic flashcards, go to evolve.elsevier.com.
Select: Chapter 7, **Flashcards**.

Refer to p. 10 for your Evolve Access Information.

Combining Forms of the Male Reproductive System

COMBINING FORM	DEFINITION
balan/o	glans penis
epididym/o	epididymis
orchid/o, orchi/o, orch/o, test/o	testis, testicle
prostat/o	prostate gland
vas/o	vessel, duct
vesicul/o	seminal vesicle

EXERCISE 2

Write the definitions of the following combining forms.

1. test/o _____
2. vas/o _____
3. balan/o _____
4. prostat/o _____
5. orch/o _____

6. vesicul/o _____
7. orchi/o _____
8. epididym/o _____
9. orchid/o _____

EXERCISE FIGURE A

Fill in the blanks with combining forms for this diagram of the male reproductive system. *To check your answers, go to p. 290.*

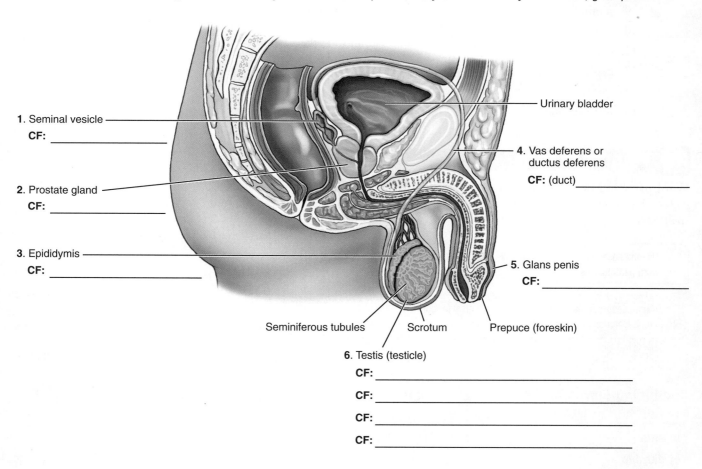

1. Seminal vesicle
   CF: _____

2. Prostate gland
   CF: _____

3. Epididymis
   CF: _____

Urinary bladder

4. Vas deferens or ductus deferens
   CF: (duct) _____

5. Glans penis
   CF: _____

Seminiferous tubules   Scrotum   Prepuce (foreskin)

6. Testis (testicle)
   CF: _____
   CF: _____
   CF: _____
   CF: _____

EXERCISE 3

Write the combining form for each of the following terms.

1. vessel, duct _____
2. prostate gland _____
3. glans penis _____
4. seminal vesicle _____
5. epididymis _____

6. testicle, or testis a. _____
  b. _____
  c. _____
  d. _____

Combining Forms Commonly Used with Male Reproductive System Terms

COMBINING FORM	DEFINITION
andr/o	male
sperm/o, spermat/o	spermatozoon (pl. spermatozoa), sperm (Figure 7-3)

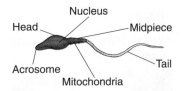

FIGURE 7-3
Spermatozoon, or sperm. In normal ejaculation there may be as many as 300 to 500 million sperm.

EXERCISE 4

Write the definition of the following combining forms.

1. sperm/o _____

2. andr/o _____

3. spermat/o _____

EXERCISE 5

Write the combining form for each of the following.

1. spermatozoon, sperm a. _____

                                  b. _____

2. male _____

Suffix

SUFFIX	DEFINITION
-ism	state of

EXERCISE 6

Write the definition for the suffix.

1. -ism _____

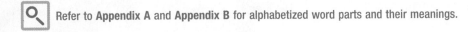

For review and/or assessment, go to evolve.elsevier.com. Select:
Chapter 7, **Activities,** Word Parts
Chapter 7, **Games,**   Name that Word Part

Refer to p. 10 for your Evolve Access Information.

Refer to **Appendix A** and **Appendix B** for alphabetized word parts and their meanings.

EXERCISE FIGURE B

Fill in the blanks with word parts to label the diagram.

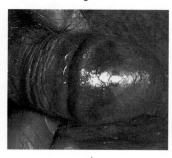

glans penis / inflammation

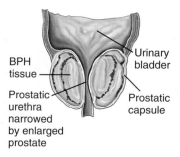

BPH tissue —

Urinary bladder

Prostatic urethra narrowed by enlarged prostate

Prostatic capsule

FIGURE 7-4

Benign prostatic hyperplasia grows inward, causing narrowing of the urethra.

BENIGN PROSTATIC HYPERPLASIA AND BENIGN PROSTATIC HYPERTROPHY

As the male ages, the prostate gland may undergo tissue changes called **prostatic hyperplasia**, which is the abnormal increase in the number of cells. The result is an enlarged prostate gland, referred to as **prostatic hypertrophy**. Benign prostatic hyperplasia is the correct term for the pathologic process, but **benign prostatic hypertrophy** is also currently used to describe this condition. As the gland enlarges, it causes narrowing of the urethra, which interferes with the passage of urine. Symptoms include frequency of urination, nocturia, urinary retention, and incomplete emptying of the bladder.

MEDICAL TERMS

The terms you need to learn to complete this chapter are listed below. The exercises following each list will help you learn the definition and the spelling of each word.

Disease and Disorder Terms
Built from Word Parts

The following terms are built from word parts you have already learned and can be translated literally to find their meanings. Further explanation of terms beyond the definition of their word parts, if needed, is included in parentheses.

TERM	DEFINITION
anorchism (an-OR-kizm)	state of absence of testis (unilateral or bilateral)
balanitis (*bal*-a-NĪ-tis)	inflammation of the glans penis (Exercise Figure B)
balanorrhea (*bal*-a-nō-RĒ-a)	discharge from the glans penis
benign prostatic hyperplasia (BPH) (be-NĪN) (pros-TAT-ik) (*bī*-per-PLĀ-zha)	excessive development pertaining to the prostate gland (nonmalignant enlargement of the prostate gland) (Figure 7-4)
cryptorchidism (krip-TOR-ki-*diz-m*)	state of hidden testes. (During fetal development, testes are located in the abdominal area near the kidneys. Before birth they move down into the scrotal sac. Failure of the testes to descend from the abdominal cavity into the scrotum before birth results in cryptorchidism, or undescended testicles.) (Exercise Figure C)
epididymitis (*ep*-i-*did*-i-MĪ-tis)	inflammation of an epididymis
orchiepididymitis (*or*-kē-*ep*-i-*did*-i-MĪ-tis)	inflammation of the testis and epididymis
orchitis, orchiditis, or testitis (or-KĪ-tis) (or-ki-DĪ-tis) (tes-TĪ-tis)	inflammation of the testis or testicle
prostatitis (pros-ta-TĪ-tis)	inflammation of the prostate gland
prostatocystitis (*pros*-ta-tō-sis-TĪ-tis)	inflammation of the prostate gland and the bladder
prostatolith (pros-TAT-ō-lith)	stone(s) in the prostate gland
prostatorrhea (pros-ta-tō-RĒ-a)	discharge from the prostate gland
prostatovesiculitis (*pros*-ta-tō-ves-*ik*-ū-LĪ-tis)	inflammation of the prostate gland and seminal vesicles

To watch animations, go to evolve.elsevier.com.
Select: Chapter 7, **Animations**, Benign Prostatic Hyperplasia.

Refer to p. 10 for your Evolve Access Information.

EXERCISE 7

Practice saying aloud each of the disease and disorder terms built from word parts.

 To hear the terms, go to evolve.elsevier.com. Select: Chapter 7, **Exercises**, Pronunciation.

Refer to p. 10 for your Evolve Access Information.

☐ Place a check mark in the box when you have completed this exercise.

EXERCISE FIGURE C

Fill in the blanks to label the diagram.

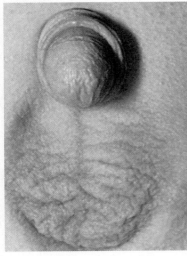

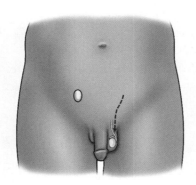

2. The *arrow* shows the path the testis takes in its descent to the scrotal sac before birth

1. _____ / _____ / _____
   hidden / testis / state of

EXERCISE 8

Analyze and define the following disease and disorder terms.

1. prostatolith _____
2. balanitis _____
3. a. orchitis _____
   b. orchiditis _____
   c. testitis _____
4. prostatovesiculitis _____
5. prostatocystitis _____
6. orchiepididymitis _____
7. prostatorrhea _____
8. epididymitis _____
9. (benign) prostatic hyperplasia _____
10. cryptorchidism _____
11. balanorrhea _____
12. prostatitis _____
13. anorchism _____

EXERCISE 9

Build disease and disorder terms for the following definitions with the word parts you have learned.

1. inflammation of the prostate
   gland and urinary bladder

   _____ /___/ _____ /___
   WR   CV   WR   S

2. stone(s) in the prostate gland

   _____ /___/ _____
   WR   CV   WR

3. inflammation of the testis   a. _____ /_____
                                     WR   S

   b. _____ /_____
      WR   S

   c. _____ /_____
      WR   S

4. (a nonmalignant) excessive
   development pertaining to
   the prostate gland

   benign _____ /___   _____ /_____
            WR   S   P   S(WR)

5. state of hidden testes

   _____ /_____ /_____
   WR   WR   S

6. inflammation of the
   prostate gland and seminal
   vesicles

   _____ /___/ _____ /_____
   WR   CV   WR   S

7. state of absence of testis

   _____ /_____ /_____
   P   WR   S

8. inflammation of the prostate
   gland

   _____ /_____
   WR   S

9. inflammation of the testis
   and the epididymis

   _____ /_____ /_____
   WR   WR   S

10. discharge from the glans penis

    _____ /___/ _____
    WR   CV   S

11. inflammation of an epididymis

    _____ /_____
    WR   S

12. inflammation of the glans penis

    _____ /_____
    WR   S

13. discharge from the prostate
    gland

    _____ /___/ _____
    WR   CV   S

EXERCISE 10

Spell each of the disease and disorder terms built from word parts on p. 262 by having someone dictate them to you.

> To hear and spell the terms, go to evolve.elsevier.com. Select: Chapter 7, **Exercises**, Spelling.
>
> Refer to p. 10 for your Evolve Access Information.
>
> ☐ Place a check mark in the box if you have completed this exercise online.

1. _____
2. _____
3. _____
4. _____
5. _____
6. _____
7. _____
8. _____

9. _____
10. _____
11. _____
12. _____
13. _____
14. _____
15. _____

Disease and Disorder Terms
Not Built from Word Parts

In some of the following terms, you may recognize word parts you have already learned; however, the full meaning of the terms cannot be discerned by the definition of their word parts.

TERM	DEFINITION
erectile dysfunction (ED) (e-REK-tĭl) (dis-FUNK-shun)	the inability of the male to attain or maintain an erection sufficient to perform sexual intercourse (formerly called **impotence**)
hydrocele (HĪ-drō-sēl)	scrotal swelling caused by a collection of fluid (Figure 7-5)
phimosis (fĭ-MŌ-sis)	a tightness of the prepuce (foreskin of the penis) that prevents its retraction over the glans penis; it may be congenital or a result of balanitis. Circumcision is the usual treatment (Figure 7-6).
priapism (PRĪ-a-*piz-m*)	persistent abnormal erection of the penis accompanied by pain and tenderness
prostate cancer (PROS-tāt) (KAN-cer)	cancer of the prostate gland, usually occurring in men middle-aged and older (Table 7-1)
spermatocele (SPER-ma-tō-sēl)	scrotal swelling caused by distention of the epididymis containing an abnormal cyst-like collection of fluid and sperm cells
testicular cancer (tes-TIK-ū-ler) (KAN-cer)	cancer of the testicle, usually occurring in men 15 to 35 years of age

ERECTILE DYSFUNCTION (ED)

Oral therapies, such as sildenafil (Viagra), vardenafil (Levitra), and tadalafil (Cialis) are currently first-line treatment for erectile dysfunction and work by relaxing smooth muscle cells and, as such, increasing the flow of blood in the genital area. Second-line treatment includes penile self-injectable drugs and vacuum devices. Surgical implantation of a penile prosthesis is available for men who cannot use or who have not responded to other treatments.

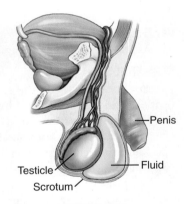

FIGURE 7-5
Hydrocele.

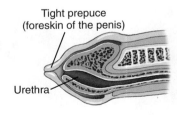

FIGURE 7-6
Phimosis. Cross section of the penis.

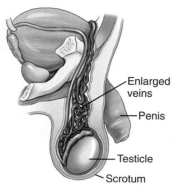

FIGURE 7-7
Varicocele.

Enlarged veins
Penis
Testicle
Scrotum

Disease and Disorder Terms—cont'd
Not Built from Word Parts

TERM	DEFINITION
testicular torsion (tes-TIK-ū-ler) (TOR-shun)	twisting of the spermatic cord causing decreased blood flow to the testis; occurs most often during puberty and often presents with a sudden onset of severe testicular or scrotal pain. Because of lack of blood flow to the testis, it is often considered a surgical emergency.
varicocele (VAR-i-kō-*sēl*)	enlarged veins of the spermatic cord (Figure 7-7)

> To watch animations, go to evolve.elsevier.com. Select: Chapter 7, **Animations**, Testicular Torsion.
>
> Refer to p. 10 for your Evolve Access Information.

Table 7-1
Prostate Cancer

Prostate cancer is the most commonly diagnosed cancer in men and the second most common cause of cancer death among men in the United States. Approximately 95% of all cancers of the prostate are adenocarcinomas, arising from epithelial cells.

DIAGNOSTIC PROCEDURES
1. Digital rectal examination (DRE)
2. Prostate-specific antigen (PSA)
3. Transrectal ultrasound (TRUS)
4. Transrectal ultrasonically guided biopsy
5. Magnetic resonance imaging (MRI) with endorectal surface coil

TREATMENT
Treatment depends on the stage of the prostate cancer, the age of the patient, and choices of treatment by the patient and his physician. Options include the following:
1. **Radical prostatectomy (RP)**, which may be performed by retropubic or perineal routes, laparoscopically, or with the use of robotic-assisted devices
2. **Radiation therapy**, which may be performed with an external beam or with radioactive seeds (brachytherapy)
3. **Bilateral orchidectomy** or **hormonal therapy** to reduce the production of testosterone, which fuels the growth of prostate cancer
4. **Chemotherapy**, treating cancer with drugs
5. **Active Surveillance**, with the intent to pursue active therapy if disease progresses

PROGRESSION OF PROSTATE CANCER

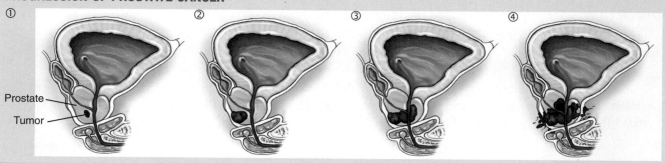

Prostate
Tumor

EXERCISE 11

Practice saying aloud each of the disease and disorder terms not built from word parts on pp. 265–266.

> To hear the terms, go to evolve.elsevier.com. Select: Chapter 7, **Exercises**, Pronunciation.
>
> Refer to p. 10 for your Evolve Access Information.

☐ Place a check mark in the box when you have completed this exercise.

EXERCISE 12

Fill in the blanks with the correct terms.

1. Another way of referring to cancer of the testicle is _____

   _____.

2. A tightness of the prepuce is called _____.

3. The condition of having enlarged veins of the spermatic cord is known

   medically as a(n) _____.

4. A scrotal swelling caused by a collection of fluid is called a(n) _____.

5. Cancer of the prostate gland is called _____

   _____.

6. Inability of the man to attain or maintain an erection is called

   _____ _____.

7. Persistent abnormal erection is called _____.

8. _____ _____ is the twisting of the spermatic

   cord.

9. Scrotal swelling caused by distention of the epididymis containing an abnormal cyst-like collection of fluid and sperm cells is called a(n)

   _____.

EXERCISE 13

Match the terms in the first column with the correct definitions in the second column.

_____ 1. varicocele

_____ 2. phimosis

_____ 3. testicular cancer

_____ 4. erectile dysfunction

_____ 5. hydrocele

_____ 6. prostate cancer

_____ 7. testicular torsion

_____ 8. priapism

_____ 9. spermatocele

a. scrotal swelling caused by a collection of fluid

b. inability to attain or maintain an erection

c. tightness of the prepuce

d. enlarged veins of the spermatic cord

e. cancer of the testicle

f. cancer of the prostate gland

g. stone(s) in the prostate gland

h. persistent abnormal erection

i. twisting of the spermatic cord causing decreased blood flow

j. scrotal swelling caused by distention of the epididymis containing an abnormal cyst-like collection of fluid and sperm cells

EXERCISE 14

Spell each of the disease and disorder terms not built from word parts on pp. 265–266 by having someone dictate them to you.

> To hear and spell the terms, go to evolve.elsevier.com. Select: Chapter 7, **Exercises**, Spelling.
>
> Refer to p. 10 for your Evolve Access Information.
>
> ☐ Place a check mark in the box if you have completed this exercise online.

1. _____   6. _____
2. _____   7. _____
3. _____   8. _____
4. _____   9. _____
5. _____

Surgical Terms
Built from Word Parts

The following terms are built from word parts you have already learned and can be translated literally to find their meanings. Further explanation of terms beyond the definitions of their word parts, if needed, is included in parentheses.

TERM	DEFINITION
balanoplasty (BAL-a-nō-*plas*-tē)	surgical repair of the glans penis
epididymectomy (ep-i-*did*-i-MEK-to-mē)	excision of an epididymis
orchidectomy, orchiectomy (*or*-kid-EK-to-mē), (*or*-kē-EK-to-mē)	excision of the testis (bilateral orchidectomy is called **castration**)
orchidopexy, orchiopexy (OR-kid-ō-pek-sē), (OR-kē-ō-pek-sē)	surgical fixation of a testicle (performed to bring undescended testicle[s] into the scrotum)
orchidotomy, orchiotomy (*or*-kid-OT-o-mē), (*or*-kē-OT-o-mē)	incision into a testis
orchioplasty (OR-kē-ō-*plas*-tē)	surgical repair of a testis
prostatectomy (*pros*-ta-TEK-to-mē)	excision of the prostate gland (Tables 7-1 and 7-2)
prostatocystotomy (*pros*-tat-ō-sis-TOT-o-mē)	incision into the prostate gland and bladder
prostatolithotomy (*pros*-tat-ō-li-THOT-o-mē)	incision into the prostate gland to remove stone(s)
prostatovesiculectomy (*pros*-tat-ō-ves-*ik*-ū-LEK-to-mē)	excision of the prostate gland and seminal vesicles

TERM	DEFINITION
vasectomy (va-SEK-to-mē)	excision of a duct (partial excision of the vas deferens bilaterally, resulting in male sterilization) (Exercise Figure D)
vasovasostomy (*vas*-ō-vā-ZOS-to-mē)	creation of artificial openings between ducts (the severed ends of the vas deferens are reconnected in an attempt to restore fertility in men who have had a vasectomy)
vesiculectomy (ve-*sik*-ū-LEK-to-mē)	excision of the seminal vesicle(s)

EXERCISE 15

Practice saying aloud each of the surgical terms built from word parts on these two pages.

To hear the terms, go to evolve.elsevier.com. Select: Chapter 7, **Exercises**, Pronunciation.

Refer to p. 10 for your Evolve Access Information.

☐ Place a check mark in the box when you have completed this exercise.

EXERCISE 16

Analyze and define the following surgical terms.

1. vasectomy _____
2. prostatocystotomy _____
3. orchidotomy, orchiotomy _____
4. epididymectomy _____
5. orchidopexy, orchiopexy _____
6. prostatovesiculectomy _____
7. orchioplasty _____
8. vesiculectomy _____
9. prostatectomy _____
10. balanoplasty _____
11. vasovasostomy _____
12. orchidectomy, orchiectomy _____
13. prostatolithotomy _____

EXERCISE FIGURE **D**

Fill in the blanks to label the diagram.

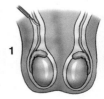
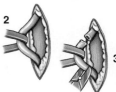
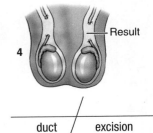

Vas
deferens
Epididymis

Testis

Result

_____ / _____
duct / excision

1. incision is made into the covering of the vas deferens
2. vas deferens is exposed and ligated (tied off)
3. segment of vas deferens is excised
4. vas deferens is repositioned and skin is sutured

EXERCISE 17

Build surgical terms for the following definitions by using the word parts you have learned.

1. excision of the testis
   a. _____ / _____
      WR   S
   b. _____ / _____
      WR   S

2. surgical repair of the glans penis
   _____ / _____ / _____
   WR   CV   S

3. incision into the prostate gland and bladder
   _____ / _____ / _____ / _____ / _____
   WR   CV   WR   CV   S

4. excision of the seminal vesicle(s)
   _____ / _____
   WR   S

5. incision into the prostate gland to remove stone(s)
   _____ / _____ / _____ / _____ / _____
   WR   CV   WR   CV   S

6. incision into a testis
   a. _____ / _____ / _____
      WR   CV   S
   b. _____ / _____ / _____
      WR   CV   S

7. excision of the epididymis
   _____ / _____
   WR   S

8. surgical repair of a testis
   _____ / _____ / _____
   WR   CV   S

9. excision of the prostate gland
   _____ / _____
   WR   S

10. excision of a duct (partial excision of the vas deferens)
    _____ / _____
    WR   S

11. excision of the prostate gland and seminal vesicles
    _____ / _____ / _____ / _____
    WR   CV   WR   S

12. surgical fixation of a testicle
    a. _____ / _____ / _____
       WR   CV   S
    b. _____ / _____ / _____
       WR   CV   S

13. creation of artificial openings between ducts
    _____ / _____ / _____ / _____ / _____
    WR   CV   WR   CV   S

EXERCISE 18

Spell each of the surgical terms built from word parts on pp. 268–269 by having someone dictate them to you.

To hear and spell the terms, go to evolve.elsevier.com. Select: Chapter 7, **Exercises**, Spelling.

Refer to p. 10 for your Evolve Access Information.

☐ Place a check mark in the box if you have completed this exercise online.

1. _____   9. _____
2. _____   10. _____
3. _____   11. _____
4. _____   12. _____
5. _____   13. _____
6. _____   14. _____
7. _____   15. _____
8. _____   16. _____

Surgical Terms
Not Built from Word Parts

In some of the following terms, you may recognize word parts you have already learned; however, the full meaning of the terms cannot be discerned by the definition of their word parts.

TERM	DEFINITION
circumcision (*ser*-kum-SI-zhun)	surgical removal of the prepuce (foreskin); all or part of the foreskin may be removed (Figure 7-8)
hydrocelectomy (*hī*-drō-sē-LEK-to-mē)	surgical removal of a hydrocele
radical prostatectomy (RP) (RAD-i-kel) (*pros*-ta-TEK-to-mē)	excision of the prostate gland with its capsule, seminal vesicles, vas deferens, and sometimes pelvic lymph nodes; performed by a retropubic, perineal, routine laparoscopic approach, or robotic surgery; used to treat prostate cancer (Figure 7-9, B, and Figure 7-10)
suprapubic prostatectomy (*sū*-pra-PŪ-bik) (*pros*-ta-TEK-to-mē)	excision of the prostate gland through an abdominal incision made above the pubic bone and through an incision in the bladder and prostate capsule; used to treat benign prostatic hyperplasia (BPH) (Figure 7-9, A) (also called **suprapubic transvesical prostatectomy**)

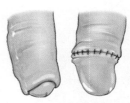

FIGURE 7-8
Circumcision.

Surgical Terms—cont'd
Not Built from Word Parts

TERM	DEFINITION
transurethral incision of the prostate gland (TUIP) (trans-ū-RĒ-thral) (in-SIZH-en) (PROS-tāt)	surgical procedure that widens the urethra by making a few small incisions in the bladder neck and the prostate gland. No prostate tissue is removed. TUIP may be used instead of TURP when the prostate gland is less enlarged (Table 7-2).
transurethral microwave thermotherapy (TUMT) (trans-ū-RĒ-thral) (MĪ-krō-wāv) (*ther*-mō-THER-a-pē)	treatment that eliminates excess tissue present in benign prostatic hyperplasia by using heat generated by microwave (Table 7-2)
transurethral resection of the prostate gland (TURP) (trans-ū-RĒ-thral) (rē-SEK-shun) (PROS-tāt)	surgical removal of pieces of the prostate gland tissue by using an instrument inserted through the urethra. The capsule is left intact; usually performed when the enlarged prostate gland interferes with urination (Table 7-2).

To watch animations, go to evolve.elsevier.com. Select:
Chapter 7, **Animations,** Retropubic Prostatectomy
                      Transurethral Resection of the Prostate Gland

Refer to p. 10 for your Evolve Access Information.

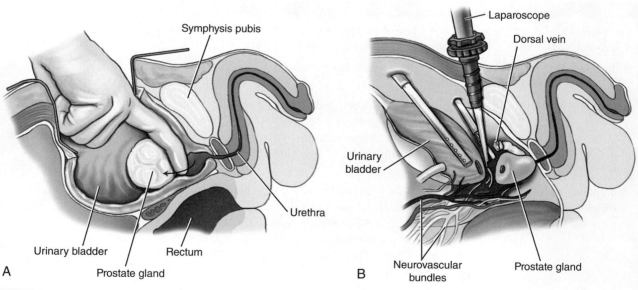

FIGURE 7-9
A, Large incision surgery. In suprapubic prostatectomy, the surgeon approaches the prostate gland through an incision in the urinary bladder and uses a finger to remove the hyperplastic tissue. A similar incision is used for radical retropubic prostatectomy to treat cancer of the prostate. **B,** Small incision surgery. Laparoscopic radical prostatectomy and/or robotic-assisted prostatectomy is a procedure used to treat early stages of prostate cancer.

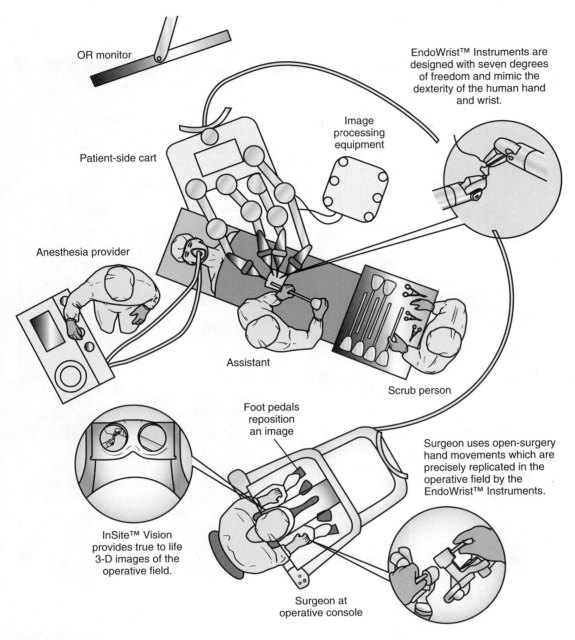

OR monitor

EndoWrist™ Instruments are designed with seven degrees of freedom and mimic the dexterity of the human hand and wrist.

Image processing equipment

Patient-side cart

Anesthesia provider

Assistant

Scrub person

Foot pedals reposition an image

Surgeon uses open-surgery hand movements which are precisely replicated in the operative field by the EndoWrist™ Instruments.

InSite™ Vision provides true to life 3-D images of the operative field.

Surgeon at operative console

FIGURE 7-10

Operating room set-up for robotic-assisted laparoscopic radical prostatectomy (RALRP) with a robotic system. Note the surgeon is performing the procedure at an operative console rather than hands-on surgery.

Table 7-2
Surgical Treatments for Benign Prostatic Hyperplasia

INCISIONAL	THERMOTHERAPY	LASER PROSTATECTOMY
1. Transurethral resection of the prostate gland (TURP) 2. Prostatectomy 3. Transurethral incision of the prostate gland (TUIP)	1. Transurethral microwave thermotherapy (TUMT) 2. Cooled Thermotherapy	1. Transurethral laser incision of the prostate gland (TULIP) 2. Holmium laser enucleation of the prostate gland (HoLEP) 3. Photoselective vaporization of the prostate gland (PVP)

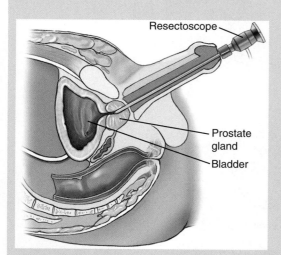

Resectoscope

Prostate gland

Bladder

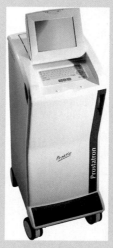

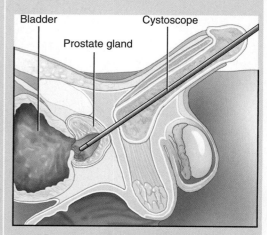

Bladder   Cystoscope

Prostate gland

Transurethral resection of the prostate (TURP) uses a resectoscope inserted through the urethra to the prostate gland. The end of the instrument is equipped to remove pieces of the enlarged prostate gland to relieve bladder outlet obstruction.

Cooled ThermoTherapy device delivers precise microwave energy to heat and destroy prostate tissue while a cooling mechanism protects surrounding tissue.

Photoselective vaporization of the prostate (PVP) uses a laser system operated through a cystoscope inserted through the urethra to the prostate gland. Overgrown prostate tissue is vaporized using heat generated by the laser.

EXERCISE 19

Practice saying aloud each of the surgical terms not built from word parts on pp. 271–272.

 To hear the terms, go to evolve.elsevier.com. Select: Chapter 7, **Exercises**, Pronunciation.

Refer to p. 10 for your Evolve Access Information.

☐ Place a check mark in the box when you have completed this exercise.

EXERCISE 20

Fill in the blanks with the correct term.

1. The surgery performed to remove the prostate gland through the urinary bladder and an abdominal incision is _____ _____.
2. The surgical procedure performed to remove all or part of the prepuce is called a(n) _____.

3. The surgical removal of the prostate gland and surrounding structures, sometimes including pelvic lymph nodes, is called _____ _____.

4. Surgical removal of a hydrocele is _____.

5. _____ _____ _____ is a treatment for benign prostatic hyperplasia that uses heat generated by microwave.

6. A surgical procedure for benign prostatic hyperplasia that widens the urethra by making small incisions is called _____ _____ of the _____ _____.

7. Pieces of prostate gland tissue are removed with an instrument during the surgical procedure called _____ _____ of the _____ _____.

EXERCISE 21

Spell each of the surgical terms not built from word parts on pp. 271–272 by having someone dictate them to you.

> To hear and spell the terms, go to evolve.elsevier.com. Select: Chapter 7, **Exercises**, Spelling.
>
> Refer to p. 10 for your Evolve Access Information.
>
> ☐ Place a check mark in the box if you have completed this exercise online.

1. _____   5. _____

2. _____   6. _____

3. _____   7. _____

4. _____

Diagnostic Terms
Not Built from Word Parts

In some of the following terms, you may recognize word parts you have already learned; however, the full meaning of the terms cannot be discerned by the definition of their word parts.

TERM	DEFINITION
DIAGNOSTIC IMAGING	
transrectal ultrasound (TRUS) (trans-REK-tal) (UL-tra-sound)	ultrasound procedure used to diagnose prostate cancer. Sound waves are sent and received by a transducer probe that is placed into the rectum (Table 7-1).
LABORATORY	
prostate-specific antigen (PSA) (PROS-tāt) (spe-SIF-ik) (AN-ti-jen)	blood test that measures the level of prostate-specific antigen in the blood. Elevated test results may indicate the presence of prostate cancer, urinary or prostatic infection, or excess prostate tissue, as found in benign prostatic hyperplasia or prostatitis (Table 7-1).

Diagnostic Terms—cont'd
Not Built from Word Parts

TERM	DEFINITION
semen analysis (SĒ-men) (a-NAL-i-sis)	microscopic observation of ejaculated semen, revealing the size, structure, and movement of sperm; used to evaluate male infertility and to determine the effectiveness of a vasectomy (also called **sperm count** and **sperm test**).
OTHER **digital rectal examination (DRE)** (DIJ-i-tal) (REK-tal) (eg-*zam*-i-NĀ-shun)	physical examination in which the health care provider inserts a finger into the rectum and palpates the size and shape of the prostate gland through the rectal wall; used to screen for BPH and prostate cancer. BPH usually presents as a uniform, nontender enlargement, whereas cancer usually presents as a stony hard nodule (Table 7-1).

EXERCISE 22

Practice saying aloud each of the diagnostic terms not built from word parts above and on p. 275.

> To hear the terms, go to evolve.elsevier.com. Select: Chapter 7, **Exercises**, Pronunciation.
>
> Refer to p. 10 for your Evolve Access Information.

☐ Place a check mark in the box when you have completed this exercise.

EXERCISE 23

Fill in the blanks with the correct terms.

1. A physical examination in which the healthcare provider palpates for the size and shape of the prostate gland through the rectal wall is called

   _____ _____ _____.

2. A blood test that, when elevated, may indicate the presence of prostate cancer is called _____ _____ _____.

3. A diagnostic ultrasound procedure used to obtain images of the prostate gland is called _____ _____.

4. A laboratory test for microscopic observation of ejaculated semen to evaluate male infertility is called _____ _____.

EXERCISE 24

Spell each of the diagnostic terms not built from word parts above on p. 275 by having someone dictate them to you.

> To hear and spell the terms, go to evolve.elsevier.com. Select: Chapter 7, **Exercises**, Spelling.
>
> Refer to p. 10 for your Evolve Access Information.
>
> ☐ Place a check mark in the box if you have completed this exercise online.

1. _____   3. _____
2. _____   4. _____

Complementary Terms
Built from Word Parts

The following terms are built from word parts you have already learned and can be translated literally to find their meanings. Further explanation of terms beyond the definitions of their word parts, if needed, is included in parentheses.

TERM	DEFINITION
andropathy (an-DROP-a-thē)	disease of the male (specific to the male, such as testitis)
aspermia (a-SPER-mē-a)	condition of without sperm (or semen or ejaculation)
oligospermia (*ol*-i-gō-SPER-mē-a)	condition of scanty sperm (in the semen; may contribute to infertility)
spermatolysis (*sper*-ma-TOL-i-sis)	dissolution (destruction) of sperm

ASPERMIA

condition of without sperm, may indicate the lack of production of spermatozoa, the lack of production of semen, or the lack of ejaculation of semen.

EXERCISE 25

Practice saying aloud each of the complementary terms built from word parts above.

> ⓔ To hear the terms, go to evolve.elsevier.com. Select: Chapter 7, **Exercises**, Pronunciation.
>
> Refer to p. 10 for your Evolve Access Information.

☐ Place a check mark in the box when you have completed this exercise.

EXERCISE 26

Analyze and define the following complementary terms.

1. oligospermia _____
2. andropathy _____
3. spermatolysis _____
4. aspermia _____

EXERCISE 27

Build the complementary terms for the following definitions by using the word parts you have learned.

1. dissolution (destruction) of sperm

   _____ / CV / _____
   WR   CV   S

2. condition of without sperm (or semen or ejaculation)

   _____ / _____ / _____
   P   WR   S

3. disease of the male

   _____ / CV / _____
   WR   CV   S

4. condition of scanty sperm (in the semen)

   _____ / CV / _____ / _____
   WR   CV   WR   S

EXERCISE 28

Spell each of the complementary terms built from word parts on p. 277 by having someone dictate them to you.

To hear and spell the terms, go to evolve.elsevier.com. Select: Chapter 7, **Exercises**, Spelling.

Refer to p. 10 for your Evolve Access Information.

☐ Place a check mark in the box if you have completed this exercise online.

1. _____   3. _____

2. _____   4. _____

For review and/or assessment, go to evolve.elsevier.com. Select:
Chapter 7, **Activities,** Terms Built from Word Parts
Chapter 7, **Games,**   Term Storm

Refer to p. 10 for your Evolve Access Information.

Complementary Terms
Not Built from Word Parts

In some of the following terms, you may recognize word parts you have already learned; however, the full meaning of the terms cannot be discerned by the definition of their word parts.

TERM	DEFINITION
acquired immunodeficiency syndrome (AIDS) (*im*-ū-nō-de-FISH-en-sē) (SIN-drōm)	advanced, chronic immune system suppression caused by human immunodeficiency virus (HIV) infection; manifested by opportunistic infections (such as candidiasis or tuberculosis), neurologic disease (peripheral neuropathy or cognitive motor impairment), and/or secondary neoplasms (Kaposi sarcoma)
artificial insemination (ar-ti-FISH-al) (in-*sem*-i-NĀ-shun)	introduction of semen into the vagina by artificial means
azoospermia (ā-zō-a-SPUR-mē-a)	lack of live sperm in the semen
chlamydia (kla-MID-ē-a)	sexually transmitted disease, caused by the bacterium *C. trachomatis*; sometimes referred to as a **silent STD** because many people are not aware they have the disease. Symptoms that occur when the disease becomes serious are painful urination and discharge from the penis in men and genital itching, vaginal discharge, and bleeding between menstrual periods in women.
coitus (KŌ-i-tus)	sexual intercourse between male and female
condom (KON-dum)	cover for the penis worn during coitus to prevent conception and the spread of sexually transmitted disease

AZOOSPERMIA

the lack of live sperm in the semen, may be:

• **obstructive,** caused by blocked vessels or ducts;

• **nonobstructive,** caused by infection, lack of production of spermatozoa, or retrograde ejaculation where semen travels into the urinary bladder rather than exiting through the urethra.

TERM	DEFINITION
ejaculation (ē-*jak*-ū-LĀ-shun)	ejection of semen from the male urethra
genital herpes (JEN-i-tal) (HER-pēz)	sexually transmitted disease caused by *Herpesvirus hominis type 2* (also called **herpes simplex virus**)
gonorrhea (gon-ō-RĒ-a)	sexually transmitted disease caused by a bacterial organism that inflames the mucous membranes of the genitourinary tract
human immunodeficiency virus (HIV) (*im*-ū-nō-de-FISH-en-sē)	sexually transmitted disease caused by a retrovirus that infects T-helper cells of the immune system; may also be acquired in utero or transmitted through infected blood via needle sharing. Advanced HIV infection progresses to AIDS.
human papillomavirus (HPV) (HŪ-man) (*pap*-i-LŌ-ma-*vī*-rus)	sexually transmitted disease caused by viral infection; there are more than 40 types of HPV that cause benign or cancerous growths in male and female genitals (also called **venereal warts**)
infertility (*in*-fer-TIL-i-tē)	reduced or absent ability to become pregnant; generally defined after one year of frequent, unprotected coitus; may relate to male or female
orgasm (ŌR-gazm)	climax of sexual stimulation
puberty (PŪ-ber-tē)	period when secondary sex characteristics develop and the ability to reproduce sexually begins
sexually transmitted disease (STD) (SEK-shū-al-ē) (TRANS-mi-ted) (di-ZĒZ)	infection spread through sexual contact; STDs affect both males and females, causing damage to reproductive organs and potentially serious health consequences if left untreated (also called **venereal disease [VD]** and **sexually transmitted infection [STI]**)
sterilization (*stār*-i-li-ZĀ-shun)	surgical procedure that renders an individual unable to produce offspring
syphilis (SIF-i-lis)	sexually transmitted disease caused by the bacterium *Treponema pallidum*; may be acquired in utero, or (less often) contracted through direct contact with infected tissue. If untreated, the infection usually progresses through three clinical stages with a latent period. The initial local infection quickly becomes systemic with widespread dissemination of the bacterium (Figure 7-11).
trichomoniasis (*trik*-ō-mō-NĪ-a-sis)	sexually transmitted disease caused by a one-cell organism *Trichomonas*. It infects the genitourinary tract. Men may be asymptomatic or may develop urethritis, an enlarged prostate gland, or epididymitis. Women have vaginal itching, dysuria, and vaginal or urethral discharge.

HUMAN PAPILLOMAVIRUS

is associated as the cause for almost all cervical and anal cancers. Penile, vulvar, vaginal, and throat cancers are also linked to **HPV** infection.

HPV is the most prevalent sexually transmitted disease and vaccines are available to protect men and women from **HPV** infection. (See **HPV vaccine**, Chapter 8, p. 305.)

LIST OF MALE AND FEMALE SEXUALLY TRANSMITTED DISEASES

acquired immunodeficiency syndrome

human immunodeficiency virus infection

syphilis

genital herpes

venereal warts (human papillomavirus)

gonorrhea

chlamydia

trichomoniasis

cytomegalovirus infection

🏛 **VENEREAL**
is derived from **Venus**, the goddess of love. In ancient times it was noted that the disease was part of the misfortunes of love.

🔍 Refer to **Appendix D** for pharmacology terms.

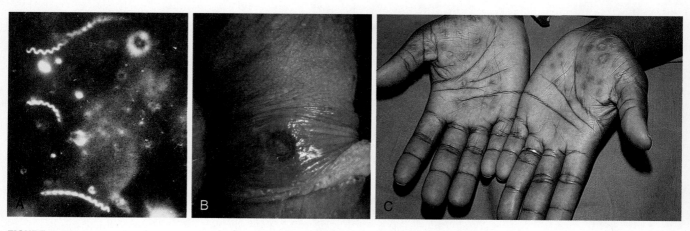

FIGURE 7-11
Syphilis. **A,** *Treponema pallidum*, organism responsible for syphilis viewed microscopically. **B,** Primary syphilis, depicting a syphilitic chancre. **C,** Secondary syphilis, depicting rash on palms of hands.

EXERCISE 29

Practice saying aloud each of the complementary terms not built from word parts on pp. 278–279.

> To hear the terms, go to evolve.elsevier.com. Select: Chapter 7, **Exercises**, Pronunciation.
>
> Refer to p. 10 for your Evolve Access Information.

☐ Place a check mark in the box when you have completed this exercise.

EXERCISE 30

Write the definitions of the following complementary terms.

1. puberty _____
2. orgasm _____
3. gonorrhea _____
4. coitus _____
5. genital herpes _____
6. syphilis _____
7. ejaculation _____
8. sexually transmitted disease _____
9. sterilization _____
10. human papillomavirus _____
11. acquired immunodeficiency syndrome _____
12. trichomoniasis _____
13. artificial insemination _____
14. chlamydia _____
15. condom _____
16. infertility _____
17. human immunodeficiency virus _____
18. azoospermia _____

EXERCISE 31

Match the terms in the first column with their correct definitions in the second column.

_____ 1. coitus
_____ 2. ejaculation
_____ 3. human papillomavirus
_____ 4. genital herpes
_____ 5. gonorrhea
_____ 6. orgasm
_____ 7. condom
_____ 8. azoospermia
_____ 9. infertility

a. climax of sexual stimulation
b. STD caused by *Herpesvirus hominis* type 2
c. ejection of semen
d. lack of live sperm in the semen
e. sexual intercourse between man and woman
f. also called venereal warts
g. STD caused by a bacterium that inflames mucous membranes
h. cover for the penis worn during coitus
i. inability to become pregnant after 1 year of unprotected coitus

EXERCISE 32

Match the terms in the first column with their correct definitions in the second column.

_____ 1. STD
_____ 2. sterilization
_____ 3. syphilis
_____ 4. puberty
_____ 5. AIDS
_____ 6. trichomoniasis
_____ 7. artificial insemination
_____ 8. chlamydia
_____ 9. HIV

a. abbreviation for infections spread through sexual contact
b. advanced, chronic immune system suppression
c. retrovirus that progresses to AIDS
d. STD that usually progresses through three stages
e. introduction of semen into the vagina by artificial means
f. STD caused by a bacterium, *C. trachomatis* (silent STD)
g. surgical procedure rendering an individual unable to produce offspring
h. STD caused by a one-cell organism, *Trichomonas*
i. period when the ability to sexually reproduce begins

EXERCISE 33

Spell each of the complementary terms not built from word parts on pp. 278–279 by having someone dictate them to you.

> To hear and spell the terms, go to evolve.elsevier.com. Select: Chapter 7, **Exercises**, Spelling.
>
> (e) Refer to p. 10 for your Evolve Access Information.
>
> ☐ Place a check mark in the box if you have completed this exercise online.

1. _____   5. _____
2. _____   6. _____
3. _____   7. _____
4. _____   8. _____

9. _____   14. _____

10. _____   15. _____

11. _____   16. _____

12. _____   17. _____

13. _____   18. _____

For review and/or assessment, go to evolve.elsevier.com. Select:
Chapter 7, **Activities**, Terms Not Built from Word Parts
                        Hear It and Type It: Clinical Vignettes
Chapter 7, **Games,**   Term Explorer
                        Termbusters
                        Medical Millionaire

Refer to p. 10 for your Evolve Access Information.

Abbreviations

ABBREVIATION	MEANING
AIDS	acquired immunodeficiency syndrome
BPH	benign prostatic hyperplasia
DRE	digital rectal examination
ED	erectile dysfunction
HIV	human immunodeficiency virus
HPV	human papillomavirus
PSA	prostate-specific antigen
RP	radical prostatectomy
STD	sexually transmitted disease
TRUS	transrectal ultrasound
TUIP	transurethral incision of the prostate
TUMT	transurethral microwave thermotherapy
TURP	transurethral resection of the prostate

Refer to **Appendix C** for a complete list of abbreviations.

EXERCISE 34

Write the meaning of the abbreviations in the following sentences.

1. The physician performed a **DRE** _____
   _____ _____ on the patient to
   assist in diagnosing **BPH**_____ _____
   _____ Surgical treatments
   for BPH include prostatectomy, **TURP** _____
   _____of the _____ gland, **TUMT**
   _____ _____
   _____, and **TUIP** _____
   _____of the _____ gland.

2. **AIDS** _____ _____
   _____is an **STD** _____
   _____ _____. **HIV**
   _____ _____
   _____ is a type of retrovirus that causes AIDS. **HPV**
   _____ _____ is an STD that causes
   female and male venereal warts and is linked to cervical and anal cancers.

3. **PSA** _____
   _____is a laboratory test used to diagnose cancer of the
   prostate.

4. **RP** _____ _____ is a surgical
   procedure to treat prostate cancer.

5. **ED** _____ _____ was formerly
   referred to as impotence.

6. **TRUS** _____ _____, used in the
   diagnosis of prostate cancer, provides imaging of the prostate gland and is used
   as a guide for biopsy of the prostate.

For more practice with abbreviations, go to evolve.elsevier.com. Select:
Chapter 7, **Flashcards**
Chapter 7, **Games**, Crossword Puzzle

Refer to p. 10 for your Evolve Access Information.

PRACTICAL APPLICATION

EXERCISE 35   *Interact with Medical Documents and Electronic Health Records*

A. Complete the emergency department report by writing the medical terms in the blanks. Use the list of definitions with the corresponding numbers.

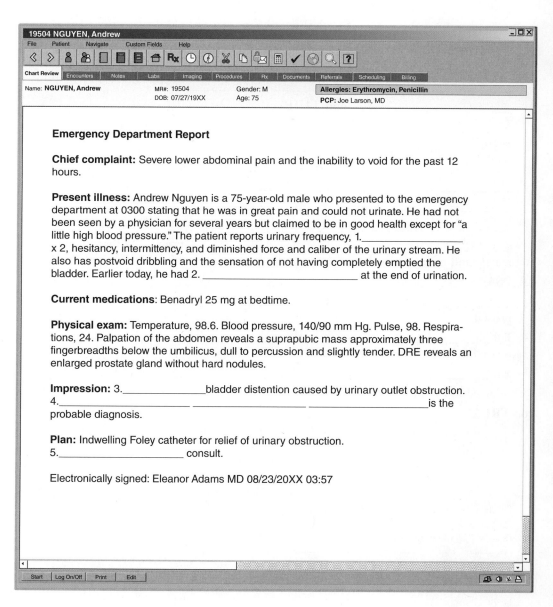

19504 NGUYEN, Andrew

File   Patient   Navigate   Custom Fields   Help

Chart Review | Encounters | Notes | Labs | Imaging | Procedures | Rx | Documents | Referrals | Scheduling | Billing

Name: **NGUYEN, Andrew**   MR#: 19504   Gender: M   **Allergies: Erythromycin, Penicillin**
                            DOB: 07/27/19XX   Age: 75   PCP: Joe Larson, MD

Emergency Department Report

Chief complaint: Severe lower abdominal pain and the inability to void for the past 12 hours.

Present illness: Andrew Nguyen is a 75-year-old male who presented to the emergency department at 0300 stating that he was in great pain and could not urinate. He had not been seen by a physician for several years but claimed to be in good health except for "a little high blood pressure." The patient reports urinary frequency, 1._____ x 2, hesitancy, intermittency, and diminished force and caliber of the urinary stream. He also has postvoid dribbling and the sensation of not having completely emptied the bladder. Earlier today, he had 2. _____ at the end of urination.

Current medications: Benadryl 25 mg at bedtime.

Physical exam: Temperature, 98.6. Blood pressure, 140/90 mm Hg. Pulse, 98. Respirations, 24. Palpation of the abdomen reveals a suprapubic mass approximately three fingerbreadths below the umbilicus, dull to percussion and slightly tender. DRE reveals an enlarged prostate gland without hard nodules.

Impression: 3._____ bladder distention caused by urinary outlet obstruction. 4._____ _____ _____ is the probable diagnosis.

Plan: Indwelling Foley catheter for relief of urinary obstruction. 5._____ consult.

Electronically signed: Eleanor Adams MD 08/23/20XX 03:57

Start | Log On/Off | Print | Edit

1. night urination
2. blood in the urine
3. pertaining to urine

4. nonmalignant excessive development pertaining to the prostate gland (enlargement of the prostate gland)
5. study of the urinary tract

B. Read the letter reviewing a patient's progress and answer the questions following it.

Michigan Oncology Group
44976 East Lincoln
Detroit, MI 97654

January 23, 20XX

Kathryn S. Marcus, MD
Internal Medicine Services
2301 North Brinkley
Detroit, MI 97654

Re: Brindley, Javier
DOB: 08/24/19XX

Dear Dr. Marcus:

It is now three years since this patient had brachytherapy using radioactive seeds for his T2a, Gleason 5 prostate cancer. He continues to experience nocturia and some erectile dysfunction with a prostate obstruction score of 3.

His weight is stable at 209 pounds and blood pressure is 122/82 mm Hg. He has no adenopathy. DRE reveals a smooth prostate with no nodules. There is a slight asymmetry with greater prominence on the right side. The PSA remains 0.1 as of August 20, 20XX.

He is doing well and is likely cured of his cancer. I would like to continue seeing him on a yearly basis with a repeat PSA. He will continue seeing you as needed.

Joseph P. Potter, MD
JPP/bko

---

1. In addition to uncomfortable urination, the patient's symptoms include:
   a. pus in the urine
   b. excessive urine
   c. night urination
   d. blood in the urine
2. Brachytherapy using radioactive seeds was used to treat:
   a. benign prostatic hyperplasia
   b. prostate cancer
   c. erectile dysfunction
3. Which diagnostic test revealed "a smooth prostate"?
   a. transrectal ultrasound
   b. prostate-specific antigen
   c. digital rectal examination
4. Three years after treatment, the patient:
   a. appears to be cancer free
   b. shows disease progression
   c. has been recommended for a radical prostatectomy

C. Complete the **three medical documents** within the electronic health record (EHR) on Evolve.

> Many healthcare records today are stored and used in an electronic system called Electronic Health Records (EHR). Electronic health records contain a collection of health information of an individual patient; the digitally formatted record can be shared through computer networks with patients, physicians, and other health care providers.

> For practice with medical terms using electronic health records, go to evolve.elsevier.com.
> Select: Chapter 7, **Electronic Health Records**.
>
> Refer to p. 10 for your Evolve Access Information.

EXERCISE 36   *Interpret Medical Terms*

To test your understanding of the terms introduced in this chapter, circle the words that correctly complete the sentences. The italicized words refer to the correct answer.

1. A *discharge from the glans penis* is referred to medically as (**balanitis, balanorrhea, balanorrhaphy**).
2. The surgical procedure circumcision is the removal of all or part of the *foreskin*, or (**glans penis, testes, prepuce**).
3. The surgery schedule indicated the patient was to undergo laparoscopic *excision of the prostate gland* (**epididymectomy, prostatectomy, prostatocystotomy**) with robotics.
4. The patient had a diagnosis of (**oligospermia, phimosis, impotence**), or a *narrowing of the opening of the prepuce*.
5. The operation for the surgical fixation of the testicle is (**orchidopexy, orchidotomy, orchioplasty**).
6. A *microscopic observation of ejaculated semen* (**prostate-specific antigen, transrectal ultrasound, semen analysis**) might be ordered after a(n) *excision of a duct (vas deferens)* (**vasovasostomy, vasectomy, varicocele**) to make sure sperm are not present in the semen.
7. The following is a *treatment for benign prostatic hyperplasia using heat* (**transurethral prostatectomy, suprapubic prostatectomy, transurethral microwave thermotherapy**).
8. *State of hidden testicles* (**testitis, anorchism, cryptorchidism**) is an associated risk factor for the development of *cancer of the testicle* (**testicular torsion, testicular cancer, prostate cancer**).
9. Upon diagnosis of an intratesticular mass, a radical inguinal *excision of the testes* (**orchiectomy, prostatectomy, vasectomy**) is recommended as a diagnostic and therapeutic procedure.
10. The term meaning *reduced or absent ability to become pregnant* (**erectile dysfunction, sterilization, infertility**) does not mean complete inability to create offspring as does the term sterility.
11. *Condition of scanty sperm (in semen)* (**aspermia, oligospermia**) and *lack of live sperm in semen* (**azoospermia, spermatolysis**) are terms frequently used in relation to male infertility.

WEB LINK

For more information on a spectrum of topics related to the male reproductive system, visit the National Institutes of Health at www.health.nih.gov and click on Men's Health.

EXERCISE 37   *Read Medical Terms in Use*

Practice pronunciation of the terms by reading the following medical document. Use the pronunciation key following the medical term to assist you in saying the word.

To hear these terms, go to evolve.elsevier.com.
Select: Chapter 7, **Exercises**, Read Medical Terms in Use.

Refer to p. 10 for your Evolve Access Information.

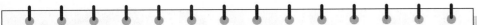

A 62-year-old male was found to have an elevated **prostate-specific antigen** (PROS-tāt) (spe-SIF-ik) (AN-ti-jen) test during a routine physical examination. At the age of 42 years he underwent a **vasectomy** (va-SEK-to-mē). The patient denies having nocturia or any significant change in his urinary stream. **Digital rectal examination** (DIJ-i-tal) (REK-tal) (eg-*zam*-i-NĀ-shun) revealed a mildly enlarged prostate gland with a 1.0 cm stony hard nodule of the right lobe. The urologist performed a **transrectal ultrasound** (trans-REK-tal) (UL-tra-sound) and biopsy. A diagnosis of adenocarcinoma of the prostate was made. The patient elected to undergo a **suprapubic prostatectomy** (sū-pra-PŪ-bik) (*pros*-ta-TEK-to-mē). Urinary incontinence complicated his postoperative course but this lasted for only 3 months. No **erectile dysfunction** (e-REK-tīl) (dis-FUNK-shun) was reported. His prognosis for full recovery should be excellent.

EXERCISE 38   *Comprehend Medical Terms in Use*

Test your comprehension of the terms in the previous medical document by circling the correct answer.

1. Before being diagnosed with cancer of the prostate the patient had surgery for:
   a. sterilization
   b. excision of the seminal vesicle
   c. removal of the prepuce
   d. repair of the glans penis
2. The patient chose which of the following types of treatment for prostate cancer?
   a. radiation
   b. chemotherapy
   c. surgery
   d. hormonal therapy
3. After surgery the patient:
   a. had absence of sperm
   b. had persistent abnormal erection
   c. had a narrowing of the opening of the prepuce of the glans penis
   d. was able to have an erection
4. Using word parts you have already learned, write the definition of terms used in this document from previous chapters.

   a. urin/ary _____

   b. ur/o/logist _____

   c. bi/opsy _____

   d. dia/gno/sis _____

   e. aden/o/carcin/oma _____

For a snapshot assessment of your knowledge of the male reproductive system terms, go to evolve.elsevier.com.
Select: Chapter 7, **Quick Quizzes**.

Refer to p. 10 for your Evolve Access Information.

CHAPTER REVIEW

ⓔ *Review of Evolve*

Keep a record of the online activities you have completed by placing a check mark in the box. You may also record your scores. All activities have been referenced throughout the chapter.

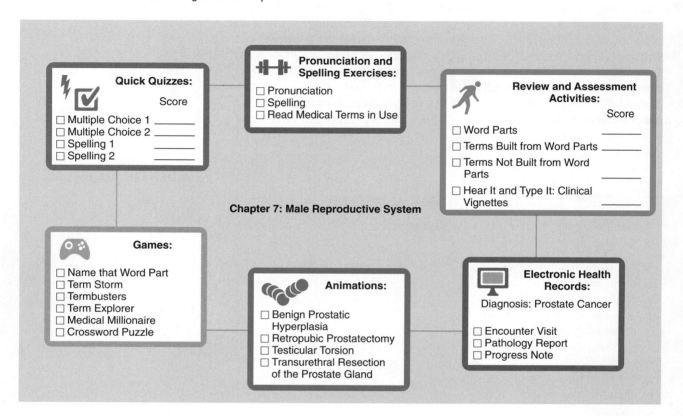

Quick Quizzes:
Score
☐ Multiple Choice 1 _____
☐ Multiple Choice 2 _____
☐ Spelling 1 _____
☐ Spelling 2 _____

Pronunciation and Spelling Exercises:
☐ Pronunciation
☐ Spelling
☐ Read Medical Terms in Use

Review and Assessment Activities:
Score
☐ Word Parts _____
☐ Terms Built from Word Parts _____
☐ Terms Not Built from Word Parts _____
☐ Hear It and Type It: Clinical Vignettes _____

Chapter 7: Male Reproductive System

Games:
☐ Name that Word Part
☐ Term Storm
☐ Termbusters
☐ Term Explorer
☐ Medical Millionaire
☐ Crossword Puzzle

Animations:
☐ Benign Prostatic Hyperplasia
☐ Retropubic Prostatectomy
☐ Testicular Torsion
☐ Transurethral Resection of the Prostate Gland

Electronic Health Records:
Diagnosis: Prostate Cancer

☐ Encounter Visit
☐ Pathology Report
☐ Progress Note

Review of Word Parts

Can you define and spell the following word parts?

COMBINING FORMS		SUFFIX
andr/o	prostat/o	-ism
balan/o	sperm/o	
epididym/o	spermat/o	
orch/o	test/o	
orchi/o	vas/o	
orchid/o	vesicul/o	

Review of Terms

Can you define, pronounce, and spell the following terms *built from word parts*?

DISEASES AND DISORDERS	SURGICAL	COMPLEMENTARY
anorchism	balanoplasty	andropathy
balanitis	epididymectomy	aspermia
balanorrhea	orchidectomy, orchiectomy	oligospermia
benign prostatic hyperplasia (BPH)	orchidopexy, orchiopexy	spermatolysis
cryptorchidism	orchidotomy, orchiotomy	
epididymitis	orchioplasty	
orchiepididymitis	prostatectomy	
orchitis, orchiditis, or testitis	prostatocystotomy	
prostatitis	prostatolithotomy	
prostatocystitis	prostatovesiculectomy	
prostatolith	vasectomy	
prostatorrhea	vasovasostomy	
prostatovesiculitis	vesiculectomy	

Can you define, pronounce, and spell the following terms *not built from word parts*?

DISEASES AND DISORDERS	SURGICAL	DIAGNOSTIC	COMPLEMENTARY
erectile dysfunction (ED)	circumcision	digital rectal examination (DRE)	acquired immunodeficiency syndrome (AIDS)
hydrocele	hydrocelectomy	prostate-specific antigen (PSA)	artificial insemination
phimosis	radical prostatectomy (RP)	semen analysis	azoospermia
priapism	suprapubic prostatectomy	transrectal ultrasound (TRUS)	chlamydia
prostate cancer	transurethral incision of the prostate gland (TUIP)		coitus
spermatocele			condom
testicular cancer	transurethral microwave thermotherapy (TUMT)		ejaculation
testicular torsion			genital herpes
varicocele	transurethral resection of the prostate gland (TURP)		gonorrhea
			human immunodeficiency virus (HIV)
			human papillomavirus (HPV)
			infertility
			orgasm
			puberty
			sexually transmitted disease (STD)
			sterilization
			syphilis
			trichomoniasis

ANSWERS

ANSWERS TO CHAPTER 7 EXERCISES
Exercise Figures

Exercise Figure

A.
1. seminal vesicle: vesicul/o
2. prostate gland: prostat/o
3. epididymis: epididym/o
4. vas deferens or ductus deferens: vas/o
5. glans penis: balan/o
6. testis: orchid/o, orchi/o, orch/o, test/o

Exercise Figure

B. balan/itis

Exercise Figure

C. crypt/orchid/ism

Exercise Figure

D. vas/ectomy

Exercise 1

1. c	8. g
2. i	9. b
3. e	10. h
4. k	11. n
5. f	12. d
6. a	13. j
7. l	14. m

Exercise 2

1. testis, testicle
2. vessel, duct
3. glans penis
4. prostate gland
5. testis, testicle
6. seminal vesicle
7. testis, testicle
8. epididymis
9. testis, testicle

Exercise 3

1. vas/o
2. prostat/o
3. balan/o
4. vesicul/o
5. epididym/o
6. a. orchid/o
   b. orchi/o
   c. orch/o
   d. test/o

Exercise 4

1. spermatozoon, sperm
2. male
3. spermatozoon, sperm

Exercise 5

1. a. sperm/o
   b. spermat/o
2. andr/o

Exercise 6

1. state of

Exercise 7

Pronunciation Exercise

Exercise 8

Note: The combining form is identified by italic and bold print.

1. WR CV WR
    ***prostat/o**/lith*
        CF
    stone(s) in the prostate gland

2. WR S
    balan/itis
    inflammation of the glans penis

3. a. WR S
      orch/itis
   b. WR S
      orchid/itis
   c. WR S
      test/itis
   inflammation of the testis

4. WR CV WR S
    ***prostat/o**/vesicul/itis*
          CF
    inflammation of the prostate gland and seminal vesicles

5. WR CV WR S
    ***prostat/o**/cyst/itis*
          CF
    inflammation of the prostate gland and bladder

6. WR WR S
    orchi/epididym/itis
    inflammation of the testis and epididymis

7. WR CV S
    ***prostat/o**/rrhea*
          CF
    discharge from the prostate gland

8. WR S
    epididym/itis
    inflammation of an epididymis

9.   WR S P S(WR)
    (benign) prostat/ic hyper /plasia
    excessive development pertaining to the prostate gland

10. WR WR S
     crypt/orchid/ism
     state of hidden testes

11. WR CV S
     ***balan/o**/rrhea*
          CF
     discharge from the glans penis

12. WR S
     prostat/itis
     inflammation of the prostate gland

13. P WR S
     an/orch/ism
     state of absence of testis

Exercise 9

1. prostat/o/cyst/itis
2. prostat/o/lith
3. a. orchid/itis
   b. orch/itis
   c. test/itis
4. (benign) prostat/ic hyper/plasia
5. crypt/orchid/ism
6. prostat/o/vesicul/itis
7. an/orch/ism
8. prostat/itis
9. orchi/epididym/itis
10. balan/o/rrhea
11. epididym/itis
12. balan/itis
13. prostat/o/rrhea

Exercise 10

Spelling Exercise; see text p. 265.

Exercise 11

Pronunciation Exercise

Exercise 12

1. testicular cancer
2. phimosis
3. varicocele
4. hydrocele
5. prostate cancer
6. erectile dysfunction
7. priapism
8. testicular torsion
9. spermatocele

Exercise 13

1. d	6. f
2. c	7. i
3. e	8. h
4. b	9. j
5. a	

Exercise 14
Spelling Exercise; see text p. 268.

Exercise 15
Pronunciation Exercise

Exercise 16
Note: The combining form is identified by italic and bold print.
1. WR   S
   vas/ectomy
   excision of a duct
2. WR CV WR CV S
   ***prostat/o/cyst/o*/tomy**
      CF   CF
   incision into the prostate gland and bladder
3. a. WR CV S
   ***orchid/o*/tomy**
      CF
   b. WR CV S
   ***orchi/o*/tomy**
      CF
   incision into a testis
4. WR   S
   epididym/ectomy
   excision of an epididymis
5. a. WR CV S
   ***orchid/o*/pexy**
      CF
   b. WR CV S
   ***orchi/o*/pexy**
      CF
   surgical fixation of a testicle
6. WR CV WR   S
   ***prostat/o*/vesicul/ectomy**
      CF
   excision of the prostate gland and seminal vesicles
7. WR CV S
   ***orchi/o*/plasty**
     CF
   surgical repair of a testis
8. WR   S
   vesicul/ectomy
   excision of the seminal vesicle(s)
9. WR   S
   prostat/ectomy
   excision of the prostate gland
10. WR CV S
    ***balan/o*/plasty**
       CF
    surgical repair of the glans penis
11. WR CV WR CV S
    ***vas/o/vas/o*/stomy**
       CF   CF
    creation of artificial openings between ducts

12. a. WR   S
    orchid/ectomy
    b. WR   S
    orchi/ectomy
    excision of the testis
13. WR CV WR CV S
    ***prostat/o/lith/o*/tomy**
       CF   CF
    incision into the prostate gland to remove stone(s)

Exercise 17
1. a. orchid/ectomy
   b. orchi/ectomy
2. balan/o/plasty
3. prostat/o/cyst/o/tomy
4. vesicul/ectomy
5. prostat/o/lith/o/tomy
6. a. orchid/o/tomy
   b. orchi/o/tomy
7. epididym/ectomy
8. orchi/o/plasty
9. prostat/ectomy
10. vas/ectomy
11. prostat/o/vesicul/ectomy
12. a. orchid/o/pexy
    b. orchi/o/pexy
13. vas/o/vas/o/stomy

Exercise 18
Spelling Exercise; see text p. 271.

Exercise 19
Pronunciation Exercise

Exercise 20
1. suprapubic prostatectomy
2. circumcision
3. radical prostatectomy
4. hydrocelectomy
5. transurethral microwave thermotherapy
6. transurethral incision (of the) prostate gland
7. transurethral resection (of the) prostate gland

Exercise 21
Spelling Exercise; see text p. 275.

Exercise 22
Pronunciation Exercise

Exercise 23
1. digital rectal examination
2. prostate-specific antigen
3. transrectal ultrasound
4. semen analysis

Exercise 24
Spelling Exercise; see text p. 276.

Exercise 25
Pronunciation Exercise

Exercise 26
1. WR CV WR S
   ***olig/o*/sperm/ia**
      CF
   condition of scanty sperm
2. WR CV S
   ***andr/o*/pathy**
      CF
   disease of the male
3. WR CV S
   ***spermat/o*/lysis**
      CF
   dissolution of sperm
4. P WR S
   a/sperm/ia
   condition of without sperm

Exercise 27
1. spermat/o/lysis
2. a/sperm/ia
3. andr/o/pathy
4. olig/o/sperm/ia

Exercise 28
Spelling Exercise; see text p. 278.

Exercise 29
Pronunciation Exercise

Exercise 30
1. period when secondary sex characteristics develop and the ability to sexually reproduce begins
2. climax of sexual stimulation
3. sexually transmitted disease that inflames the mucous membranes of the genitourinary system
4. sexual intercourse between male and female
5. sexually transmitted disease caused by the *herpesvirus hominis* type 2
6. sexually transmitted disease that usually progresses through three clinical stages
7. ejection of semen from the male urethra
8. infection spread through sexual contact
9. surgical procedure rendering an individual unable to produce offspring
10. STD causing growths on the male and female genitalia
11. advanced, chronic immune system suppression caused by HIV infection
12. STD caused by a one-cell organism, *Trichomonas*; it affects the genitourinary tract

13. introduction of semen into the vagina by artificial means
14. STD caused by bacterium, *C. trachomatis*; referred to as silent STD
15. cover for the penis worn during coitus
16. inability to produce offspring
17. retrovirus that progresses to AIDS
18. lack of live sperm in semen

Exercise 31

1. e	6. a
2. c	7. h
3. f	8. d
4. b	9. i
5. g	

Exercise 32

1. a	7. e
2. g	8. f
3. d	9. c
4. i	
5. b	
6. h	

Exercise 33

Spelling Exercise; see text p. 281.

Exercise 34

1. digital rectal examination; benign prostatic hyperplasia; transurethral resection (of the) prostate; transurethral microwave thermotherapy; transurethral incision (of the) prostate
2. acquired immunodeficiency syndrome; sexually transmitted disease; human immunodeficiency virus; human papillomavirus
3. prostate-specific antigen
4. radical prostatectomy
5. erectile dysfunction
6. transrectal ultrasound

Exercise 35

A. 1. nocturia
    2. hematuria
    3. urinary
    4. benign prostatic hyperplasia
    5. urology
B. 1. c
    2. b
    3. c
    4. a
C. Online Exercise

Exercise 36

1. balanorrhea
2. prepuce
3. prostatectomy
4. phimosis
5. orchidopexy
6. semen analysis; vasectomy
7. transurethral microwave thermotherapy
8. cryptorchidism; testicular cancer
9. orchiectomy
10. infertility
11. oligospermia; azoospermia

Exercise 37

Reading Exercise

Exercise 38

1. a
2. c
3. d
4. a. pertaining to urine
   b. physician who studies and treats diseases of the urinary tract
   c. view of life
   d. state of complete knowledge
   e. cancerous tumor of glandular tissue

Female Reproductive System

Outline

Objectives

Upon completion of this chapter you will be able to:

1   Identify organs and structures of the female
    reproductive system.

2   Define and spell word parts related to the
    female reproductive system.

3   Define, pronounce, and spell disease and
    disorder terms related to the female
    reproductive system.

4   Define, pronounce, and spell surgical terms
    related to the female reproductive system.

5   Define, pronounce, and spell diagnostic
    terms related to the female reproductive
    system.

6   Define, pronounce, and spell
    complementary terms related to the female
    reproductive system.

7   Interpret the meaning of abbreviations
    related to the female reproductive system.

8   Interpret, read, and comprehend medical
    language in simulated medical statements,
    documents, and electronic health records.

🔍 ANATOMY

Externally, the female reproductive system consists of the vulva, clitoris, and mammary glands. Internally, this system consists of the vagina, uterus, uterine tubes, and ovaries (Figure 8-1).

Function

The female reproductive system comprises external and internal organs, glands, and structures and is responsible for supporting conception and pregnancy. As the female matures throughout her lifespan, this system develops and changes based on the influence of hormones produced by the ovaries—estrogen and progesterone. These

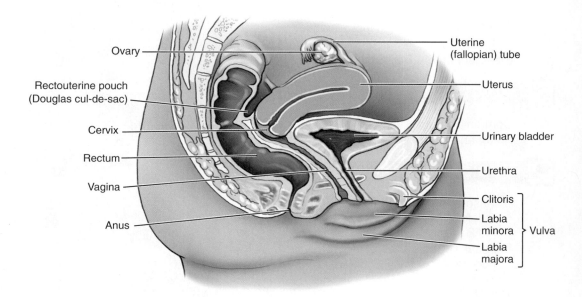

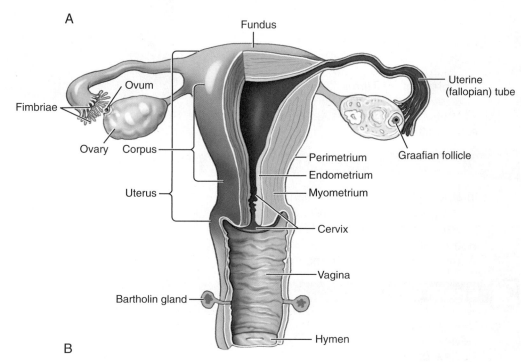

FIGURE 8-1

Female reproductive organs. **A,** Sagittal view. **B,** Frontal view.

hormones are essential for sexual maturation, the menstrual cycle, and pregnancy. Estrogen is also important for the overall health of the female, affecting the structure and function of the integumentary, urinary, cardiac, musculoskeletal, and neurologic systems.

Internal Organs of the Female Reproductive System

TERM	DEFINITION
ovaries	pair of almond-shaped organs located in the pelvic cavity. Egg cells are formed and stored in the ovaries.
ovum (*pl.* ova)	female egg cell
graafian follicles	100,000 microscopic sacs that make up a large portion of the ovaries. Each follicle contains an immature ovum. Normally one graafian follicle develops to maturity monthly between puberty and menopause. It moves to the surface of the ovary and releases the ovum, which passes into the uterine tube.
uterine, or fallopian, tubes	pair of tubes attached to the uterus that provides a passageway for the ovum to move from the ovary to the uterus
fimbria (*pl.* fimbriae)	finger-like projection at the free end of the uterine tube
uterus	pear-sized and pear-shaped muscular organ that lies in the pelvic cavity, except during pregnancy when it enlarges and extends up into the abdominal cavity. Its functions are menstruation, pregnancy, and labor.
endometrium	inner lining of the uterus
myometrium	muscular middle layer of the uterus
perimetrium	outer thin layer that covers the surface of the uterus
corpus, or body	large central portion of the uterus
fundus	rounded upper portion of the uterus
cervix (Cx)	narrow lower portion of the uterus
vagina	a 3-inch (7-8 cm) tube that connects the uterus to the outside of the body
hymen	fold of membrane found near the opening of the vagina
rectouterine pouch	cavity between the posterior wall of the uterus and the anterior wall of the rectum that is closed at the inferior end (also called **Douglas cul-de-sac**)

Glands of the Female Reproductive System

TERM	DEFINITION
Bartholin glands	pair of mucus-producing glands located on each side of the vagina and just above the vaginal opening
mammary glands, or breasts	pair of milk-producing glands of the female. Each breast consists of 15 to 20 divisions, or lobules (Figure 8-2).
mammary papilla	breast nipple
areola	pigmented area around the breast nipple

🏛 **THE GRAAFIAN FOLLICLE** is named for Dutch anatomist Reinier de Graaf, who discovered the sac in 1672.

🏛 **THE FALLOPIAN TUBE** was named in honor of Gabriele Fallopius, 1523-1562, because he described it in his works. Fallopius also gave the **vagina** and the **placenta** their names.

🏛 **BARTHOLIN GLANDS** were described by Caspar Bartholin, a Danish anatomist, in 1675.

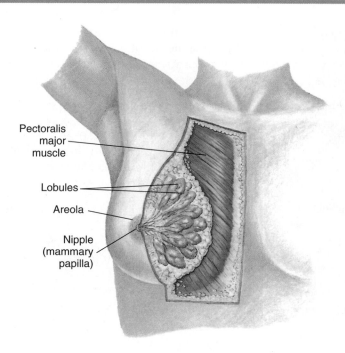

FIGURE 8-2
Female breast.

External Female Reproductive Structures

TERM	DEFINITION
vulva, or external genitalia	two pairs of lips (labia majora and labia minora) that surround the vagina
clitoris	highly erogenous erectile body located anterior to the urethra
perineum	pelvic floor in both the male and female. In females it usually refers to the area between the vaginal opening and the anus.

A & P Booster
For more anatomy and physiology, go to evolve.elsevier.com.
Select: **Extra Content**, A & P Booster, Chapter 2.

Refer to p. 10 for your Evolve Access Information.

EXERCISE 1

Match the definitions in the first column with the anatomic terms in the second column. *To check your answers to the exercises in this chapter, go to Answers, p. 340, at the end of the chapter.*

_____ 1. organs in which egg cells are formed

_____ 2. lower portion of the uterus

_____ 3. lining of the uterus

_____ 4. upper portion of the uterus

_____ 5. pelvic floor

_____ 6. ends of uterine tubes

_____ 7. large central portion of the uterus

_____ 8. layer that covers the uterus

_____ 9. muscle layer of the uterus

a. perimetrium
b. fundus
c. ovaries
d. perineum
e. fimbriae
f. cervix
g. endometrium
h. corpus
i. myometrium
j. ovum

EXERCISE 2

Match the definitions in the first column with the anatomic terms in the second column.

_____ 1. connects the uterus to the outside of the body

_____ 2. mucus-producing glands located on each side of the vagina

_____ 3. breast

_____ 4. female egg cells

_____ 5. external genitals

_____ 6. passageway for ovum

_____ 7. pigmented area around the nipple

_____ 8. microscopic sacs in the ovaries

_____ 9. muscular organ

_____ 10. nipples

_____ 11. rectouterine pouch

a. ovary
b. vagina
c. Bartholin glands
d. mammary gland
e. vulva
f. uterine tube
g. areola
h. Douglas cul-de-sac
i. uterus
j. mammary papillae
k. ova
l. graafian follicles

 WORD PARTS

Word parts you need to learn to complete this chapter are listed on the following pages. The exercises at the end of each list will help you learn their definitions and spellings.

> ☼ Use the flashcards accompanying this text or the electronic flashcards to assist you in memorizing the word parts for this chapter.

> ⓔ To use electronic flashcards, go to evolve.elsevier.com. Select: Chapter 8, **Flashcards**.
>
> Refer to p. 10 for your Evolve Access Information.

Combining Forms of the Female Reproductive System

COMBINING FORM	DEFINITION
arche/o	first, beginning
cervic/o	cervix
colp/o, vagin/o	vagina
culd/o	cul-de-sac
episi/o, vulv/o	vulva
gynec/o, gyn/o	woman
hymen/o	hymen
hyster/o, metr/o, metr/i (Note: the combining vowel i or o may be used with metr/.)	uterus
mamm/o, mast/o	breast
men/o	menstruation
oophor/o	ovary
perine/o	perineum
salping/o	uterine tube (fallopian tube) (Figure 8-3)

> 🏛 **CUL-DE-SAC**
> is a French term meaning "dead-end street." In medical terminology, the combining form *culd/o* is used to describe anatomical structures or cavities that are closed at one end.

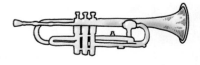

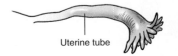

Uterine tube

FIGURE 8-3
Salpinx is derived from the Greek term for trumpet. The term was used for the uterine tubes because of their trumpet-like shape.

EXERCISE FIGURE **A**

Fill in the blanks with combining forms in this diagram of the frontal view of the female reproductive system. *To check your answers, go to p. 340.*

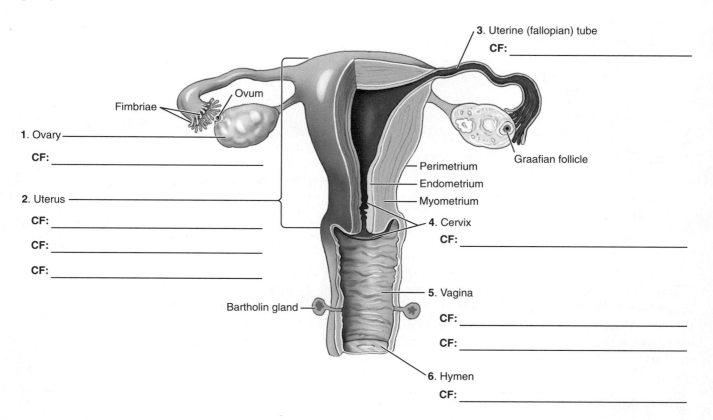

3. Uterine (fallopian) tube
CF: _____

Ovum

Fimbriae

1. Ovary
CF: _____

2. Uterus
CF: _____
CF: _____
CF: _____

Bartholin gland

Perimetrium
Endometrium
Myometrium

Graafian follicle

4. Cervix
CF: _____

5. Vagina
CF: _____
CF: _____

6. Hymen
CF: _____

EXERCISE FIGURE **B**

Fill in the blanks with combining forms in this diagram showing the external reproductive organs.

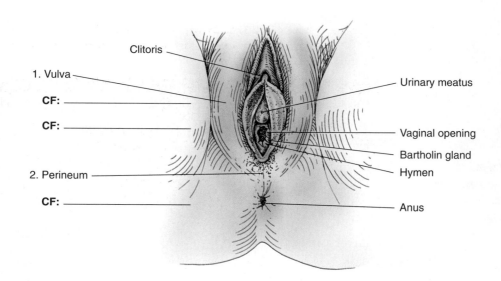

Clitoris

1. Vulva
CF: _____
CF: _____

2. Perineum
CF: _____

Urinary meatus

Vaginal opening

Bartholin gland

Hymen

Anus

EXERCISE 3

Write the definitions of the following combining forms.

1. vagin/o_____
2. oophor/o_____
3. metr/o, metr/i_____
4. gyn/o_____
5. hymen/o_____
6. hyster/o_____
7. men/o_____
8. episi/o_____
9. cervic/o_____
10. colp/o_____
11. gynec/o_____
12. mamm/o_____
13. perine/o_____
14. salping/o_____
15. vulv/o_____
16. mast/o_____
17. arche/o_____
18. culd/o_____

EXERCISE 4

Write the combining form for each of the following terms.

1. vulva   a. _____
             b. _____
2. breast   a. _____
             b. _____
3. menstruation_____
4. ovary _____
5. uterine tube_____
6. perineum_____
7. vagina   a. _____
             b. _____
8. uterus   a. _____
             b. _____
             c. _____
9. woman   a. _____
             b. _____
10. hymen _____
11. cul-de-sac _____
12. cervix _____
13. first, beginning _____

Prefix and Suffixes

PREFIX	DEFINITION
peri-	surrounding (outer)

SUFFIXES	DEFINITION
-atresia	absence of a normal body opening; occlusion; closure
-salpinx *(NOTE: for learning purposes* salpinx *and* atresia *are presented as suffixes.)*	uterine tube (fallopian tube) (Figure 8-3)

🏛 **ATRESIA**

literally means **no perforation or hole.** It is composed of the Greek words **a,** meaning **without,** and **tresis,** meaning **perforation.** The term may be used alone, as in "atresia of the vagina," or combined with other word parts, as in "gynatresia," meaning closure of a part of the female genital tract, usually the vagina.

EXERCISE 5

Write the prefix or suffix for each of the following.

1. uterine tube_____
2. surrounding_____
3. absence of a normal body opening; occlusion; closure _____

EXERCISE 6

Write the definitions of the following prefix and suffixes.

1. -salpinx _____
2. peri- _____
3. -atresia_____

For review and/or assessment, go to evolve.elsevier.com. Select:
Chapter 8, **Activities**, Word Parts
Chapter 8, **Games**,   Name that Word Part

Refer to p. 10 for your Evolve Access Information.

Refer to **Appendix A** and **Appendix B** for alphabetized word parts and their meanings.

💬 MEDICAL TERMS

The terms you need to learn to complete this chapter are listed on the following pages. The exercises following each list will help you learn the definition and spelling of each word.

Disease and Disorder Terms

Built from Word Parts

The following terms are built from word parts you have already learned and can be translated literally to find their meanings. Further explanation of terms beyond the definition of their word parts, if needed, is included in parentheses.

TERM	DEFINITION
amenorrhea (a-*men*-ō-RĒ-a)	absence of menstrual flow
Bartholin adenitis (BAR-tō-lin) (*ad*-e-NĪ-tis)	inflammation of a Bartholin gland (also called **bartholinitis**)
cervicitis (*ser*-vi-SĪ-tis)	inflammation of the cervix (see Figure 8-8)
colpitis, vaginitis (*kol*-PĪ-tis), (*vaj*-i-NĪ-tis)	inflammation of the vagina (see Figure 8-8)
dysmenorrhea (dis-*men*-ō-RĒ-a)	painful menstrual flow
endocervicitis (*en*-dō-*ser*-vi-SĪ-tis)	inflammation of the inner (lining) of the cervix
endometritis (*en*-dō-mē-TRĪ-tis)	inflammation of the inner (lining) of the uterus (endometrium) (see Figure 8-8)

TERM	DEFINITION
hematosalpinx (*hem*-a-tō-SAL-pinks)	blood in the uterine tube
hydrosalpinx (*hī*-drō-SAL-pinks)	water in the uterine tube (see Exercise Figure H, p. 321)
hysteratresia (*his*-ter-a-TRĒ-zha)	closure of the uterus (uterine cavity)
mastitis (*mas*-TĪ-tis)	inflammation of the breast
menometrorrhagia (*men*-ō-*met*-rō-RĀ-jea)	rapid flow of blood from the uterus at menstruation (and between menstrual cycles; increased amount)
menorrhagia (*men*-ō-RĀ-jea)	rapid flow of blood at menstruation (increased amount)
metrorrhagia (*mē*-trō-RĀ-jea)	rapid flow of blood from the uterus (between menstrual cycles)
myometritis (*mī*-o-me-TRĪ-tis)	inflammation of the uterine muscle (myometrium)
oligomenorrhea (*ol*-i-gō-*men*-ō-RĒ-a)	scanty menstrual flow (less often)
oophoritis (*ō*-of-o-RĪ-tis)	inflammation of the ovary
perimetritis (*per*-i-me-TRĪ-tis)	inflammation surrounding the uterus (perimetrium)
pyosalpinx (*pī*-ō-SAL-pinks)	pus in the uterine tube
salpingitis (*sal*-pin-JĪ-tis)	inflammation of the uterine tube (Exercise Figure C and see Figure 8-8, p. 306)
salpingocele (sal-PING-gō-sēl)	hernia of the uterine tube
vulvovaginitis (*vul*-vō-*vaj*-i-NĪ-tis)	inflammation of the vulva and vagina

EXERCISE FIGURE **C**

Fill in the blanks to label the diagram.

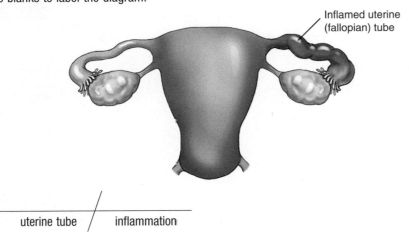

Inflamed uterine
(fallopian) tube

_____ / _____
　uterine tube / inflammation

EXERCISE 7

Practice saying aloud each of the disease and disorder terms built from word parts on pp. 300–301.

 To hear the terms, go to evolve.elsevier.com. Select: Chapter 8, **Exercises**, Pronunciation.

Refer to p. 10 for your Evolve Access Information.

☐ Place a check mark in the box when you have completed this exercise.

EXERCISE 8

Analyze and define the following disease and disorder terms.

1. colpitis _____
2. cervicitis _____
3. hydrosalpinx _____
4. hematosalpinx _____
5. metrorrhagia _____
6. oophoritis _____
7. (Bartholin) adenitis _____
8. vulvovaginitis _____
9. salpingocele _____
10. menometrorrhagia _____
11. amenorrhea _____
12. dysmenorrhea _____
13. mastitis _____
14. perimetritis _____
15. myometritis _____
16. endometritis _____
17. endocervicitis _____
18. pyosalpinx _____
19. hysteratresia _____
20. salpingitis _____
21. vaginitis _____
22. menorrhagia _____
23. oligomenorrhea _____

EXERCISE 9

Build disease and disorder terms for the following definitions with the word parts you have learned.

1. inflammation of the breast

   _____ / _____
   WR   S

2. rapid flow of blood from the
   uterus (between menstrual
   cycles)

   _____ / CV / _____
   WR   S

3. inflammation of the uterine
   tube

   _____ / _____
   WR   S

4. inflammation of the vulva and
   vagina

   _____ / CV / _____ / _____
   WR   WR   S

5. absence of menstrual flow

   _____ / _____ / CV / _____
   P   WR   S

6. inflammation of the cervix

   _____ / _____
   WR   S

7. inflammation of (Bartholin)
   gland   Bartholin _____ / _____
                              WR   S

8. water in the uterine tube

   _____ / CV / _____
   WR   S

9. painful menstrual flow

   _____ / _____ / CV / _____
   P   WR   S

10. blood in the uterine tube

    _____ / CV / _____
    WR   S

11. inflammation of the vagina   a. _____ / _____
                                     WR   S

                                  b. _____ / _____
                                     WR   S

12. rapid flow of blood from the
    uterus at menstruation (and
    between menstrual cycles)

    _____ / CV / _____ / CV / _____
    WR   WR   S

13. inflammation of the ovary

    _____ / _____
    WR   S

14. hernia of the uterine tube

    _____ / CV / _____
    WR   S

15. inflammation surrounding the
    uterus (outer layer)

    _____ / _____ / _____
    P   WR   S

16. inflammation of the inner
    (lining) of the uterus

    _____ / _____ / _____
    P   WR   S

17. inflammation of the inner (lining) of the cervix

_____ / _____ / _____
       P   WR   S

18. inflammation of the uterine muscle

_____ /CV/ _____ / _____
   WR   WR   S

19. pus in the uterine tube

_____ /CV/ _____
   WR   S

20. closure of the uterus (uterine cavity)

_____ / _____
   WR   S

21. scanty menstrual flow (less often)

_____ /CV/ _____ /CV/ _____
   WR   WR   S

22. rapid flow of blood at menstruation (increased amount)

_____ /CV/ _____
   WR   S

EXERCISE 10

Spell each of the disease and disorder terms built from word parts on pp. 300–301 by having someone dictate them to you.

> To hear and spell the terms, go to evolve.elsevier.com. Select: Chapter 8, **Exercises**, Spelling.
>
> ℮ Refer to p. 10 for your Evolve Access Information.
>
> ☐ Place a check mark in the box if you have completed this exercise online.

1. _____
2. _____
3. _____
4. _____
5. _____
6. _____
7. _____
8. _____
9. _____
10. _____
11. _____
12. _____

13. _____
14. _____
15. _____
16. _____
17. _____
18. _____
19. _____
20. _____
21. _____
22. _____
23. _____

Disease and Disorder Terms

Not Built from Word Parts

In some of the following terms, you may recognize word parts you have already learned; however, the full meaning of the terms cannot be discerned by the definition of their word parts.

TERM	DEFINITION
adenomyosis (*ad*-e-nō-mī-Ō-sis)	growth of endometrium into the muscular portion of the uterus
breast cancer (brest) (KAN-cer)	malignant tumor of the breast (Figure 8-4)
cervical cancer (SER-vi-kal) (KAN-cer)	malignant tumor of the cervix, which progresses from cervical dysplasia to carcinoma. Its cause is linked to human papillomavirus (HPV) infection.
endometrial cancer (*en*-dō-MĒ-trē-al) (KAN-cer)	malignant tumor of the endometrium (also called **uterine cancer**) (Figure 8-5)
endometriosis (*en*-dō-*m*ē-trē-Ō-sis)	abnormal condition in which endometrial tissue grows outside of the uterus in various areas in the pelvic cavity, including ovaries, uterine tubes, intestines, and uterus (Figure 8-7)
fibrocystic breast condition (FCC) (*fi*-brō-SIS-tik) (brest) (ken-DISH-en)	disorder characterized by benign cysts in one or both breasts; may cause discomfort (also called **fibrocystic breast disease**)
fibroid tumor (FĪ-broyd) (TŪ-mor)	benign tumor of the uterine muscle (also called **myoma of the uterus** or **leiomyoma**) (Figure 8-6)
ovarian cancer (ō-VAR-ē-an) (KAN-cer)	malignant tumor of the ovary

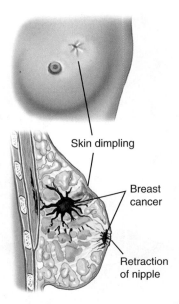

FIGURE 8-4
Clinical signs of breast cancer.

Skin dimpling

Breast cancer

Retraction of nipple

HPV VACCINE

The Food and Drug Administration (FDA) approved a vaccine for human papillomavirus (HPV) in 2006, directly impacting the prevention of **cervical cancer**. The vaccine is highly effective in protecting against a majority of forms of HPV as long as it is administered before a male or female becomes sexually active. Because vaccination is not 100% effective, annual cervical cancer screening (see **Pap smear**, p. 324) is strongly recommended. Refer to Chapter 7, p. 279, for more information on *human papillomavirus*.

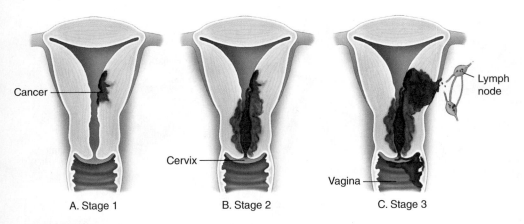

Cancer

Cervix

Vagina

Lymph node

A. Stage 1   B. Stage 2   C. Stage 3

FIGURE 8-5
Endometrial cancer. **A,** Stage 1: Confined to the endometrium. **B,** Stage 2: Spread into support structures of the cervix from the body of the uterus. **C,** Stage 3: Spreads to other organs such as the vagina.

CAM TERM

Massage therapy is the manual manipulation of soft tissue, incorporating stroking, kneading, and percussion motions. Studies have shown that massage therapy is useful as a supportive measure to improve quality of life during cancer treatment by reducing symptoms associated with treatment.

Disease and Disorder Terms—cont'd

Not Built from Word Parts

TERM	DEFINITION
pelvic inflammatory disease (PID) (PEL-vik) (in-FLAM-a-*tor*-ē) (di-ZĒZ)	inflammation of some or all of the female pelvic organs; can be caused by many different pathogens. If untreated, the infection may spread upward from the vagina, involving the uterus, uterine tubes, ovaries, and other pelvic organs. An ascending infection may result in infertility and, in acute cases, fatal septicemia (Figure 8-8).
prolapsed uterus (PRŌ-lapsd) (Ū-ter-us)	downward displacement of the uterus into the vagina (also called **hysteroptosis**) (Exercise Figure D)
toxic shock syndrome (TSS) (TOK-sik) (shok) (SIN-drōm)	severe illness characterized by high fever, rash, vomiting, diarrhea, and myalgia, followed by hypotension and, in severe cases, shock and death; usually affects menstruating women using tampons; caused by *Staphylococcus aureus* and *Streptococcus pyogenes*.
vesicovaginal fistula (*ves*-i-kō-VAJ-i-nal) (FIS-tū-la)	abnormal opening between the bladder and the vagina (Exercise Figure E)

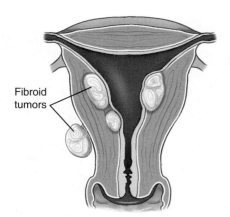

FIGURE 8-6
Fibroid tumors (also called myomas or leiomyomas).

Fibroid tumors

To watch animations, go to evolve.elsevier.com.
Select: Chapter 8, **Animations**, Pelvic Inflammatory Disease.

Refer to p. 10 for your Evolve Access Information.

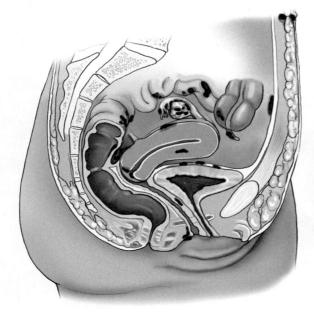

FIGURE 8-7
Endometriosis. Spots indicate common sites of endometrial deposits.

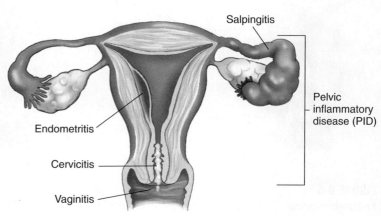

FIGURE 8-8
Ascending infection of the female reproductive system as seen in pelvic inflammatory disease.

Salpingitis

Endometritis

Cervicitis

Vaginitis

Pelvic inflammatory disease (PID)

EXERCISE FIGURE D

Fill in the blanks to complete labeling of the diagram.

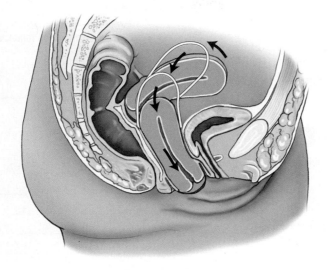

Prolapsed uterus or _____ / ___ / _____
                        uterus   / cv /   prolapse

EXERCISE FIGURE E

Fill in the blanks to complete labeling of the diagram.

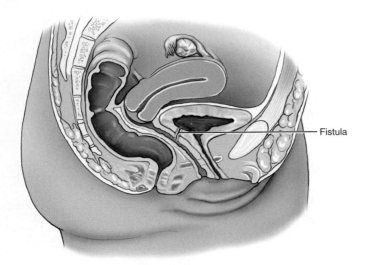

Fistula

A _____ / ___ / _____ / _____ fistula
  bladder   / cv /   vagina   / pertaining to

EXERCISE 11

Practice saying aloud each of the disease and disorder terms not built from word parts on pp. 305–306.

To hear the terms, go to evolve.elsevier.com. Select: Chapter 8, **Exercises**, Pronunciation.

Refer to p. 10 for your Evolve Access Information.

☐ Place a check mark in the box when you have completed this exercise.

EXERCISE 12

Fill in the blanks with the correct definitions.

1. prolapsed uterus _____
2. pelvic inflammatory disease_____
3. vesicovaginal fistula _____
4. fibroid tumor _____
5. endometriosis _____
6. adenomyosis _____
7. toxic shock syndrome_____
8. fibrocystic breast condition_____
9. ovarian cancer_____
10. breast cancer_____
11. cervical cancer _____
12. endometrial cancer_____

EXERCISE 13

Write the term for each of the following.

1. abnormal opening between the bladder and the vagina _____
   _____
2. benign tumor of the uterine muscle_____ _____
3. inflammation of some or all of the female pelvic organs _____
   _____ _____
4. downward displacement of the uterus into the vagina _____
   _____
5. endometrial tissue in the pelvic cavity_____
6. growth of endometrium into the muscular portion of the uterus _____
   _____
7. severe illness usually affects menstruating women using tampons
   _____ _____ _____
8. benign cysts in one or both breasts _____ _____
   _____
9. malignant tumor of the breast _____ _____
10. also called uterine cancer _____ _____
11. malignant tumor of the ovaries _____ _____
12. malignant tumor of the cervix _____ _____

EXERCISE 14

Spell each of the disease and disorder terms not built from word parts on pp. 305–306 by having someone dictate them to you.

> To hear and spell the terms, go to evolve.elsevier.com. Select: Chapter 8, **Exercises**, Spelling.
>
> (e) Refer to p. 10 for your Evolve Access Information.
>
> ☐ Place a check mark in the box if you have completed this exercise online.

1. _____
2. _____
3. _____
4. _____
5. _____
6. _____

7. _____
8. _____
9. _____
10. _____
11. _____
12. _____

Surgical Terms

Built from Word Parts

The following terms are built from word parts you have already learned and can be translated literally to find their meanings. Further explanation of terms beyond the definitions of their word parts, if needed, is included in parentheses.

TERM	DEFINITION
cervicectomy (*ser*-vi-SEK-to-mē)	excision of the cervix
colpoperineorrhaphy (kol-pō-*per*-i-nē-OR-a-fē)	suturing of the vagina and perineum (performed to mend perineal vaginal tears)
colpoplasty (KOL-pō-*plas*-tē)	surgical repair of the vagina
colporrhaphy (kol-POR-a-fē)	suturing of the vagina (wall of the vagina)
culdocentesis (kul-dō-sen-TĒ-sis)	surgical puncture to aspirate fluid from Douglas cu-de-sac (rectouterine pouch) (see Exercise Figure I, p. 322)
episioperineoplasty (e-*piz*-ē-ō-*per*-i-NĒ-o-*plas*-tē)	surgical repair of the vulva and perineum
episiorrhaphy (e-*piz*-ē-OR-a-fē)	suturing of (a tear in) the vulva
hymenectomy (*hī*-men-EK-to-mē)	excision of the hymen
hymenotomy (*hī*-men-OT-o-mē)	incision of the hymen

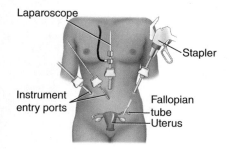

Laparoscope

Stapler

Instrument entry ports

Fallopian tube

Uterus

FIGURE 8-9
Operative setup for laparoscopically assisted vaginal hysterectomy (LAVH). Laparoscopic surgery is performed using a fiberoptic laparoscope, a type of endoscope. The laparoscope is inserted into the abdominopelvic cavity through a tiny incision near the umbilicus, allowing direct observation of the abdominal organs and structures. Three or four additional tiny incisions may be made to accommodate instruments and devices needed to complete the surgery. Laparoscopic surgery results in less trauma and expense to the patient than large-incision **surgery**. Numerous female reproductive system surgeries are performed laparoscopically, including **hysterectomy, hysteropexy, myomectomy, oophorectomy, salpingectomy, salpingostomy,** and **tubal ligation** or **sterilization.** Laparoscopic surgery may also be used to obtain biopsies of female reproductive system organs or to diagnose **endometriosis.**

Surgical Terms—cont'd

Built from Word Parts

TERM	DEFINITION
hysterectomy (*his*-te-REK-to-mē)	excision of the uterus (Table 8-1) (Exercise Figure F) (Figure 8-9)
hysteropexy (HIS-ter-ō-*pek*-sē)	surgical fixation of the uterus
hysterosalpingo-oophorectomy (*his*-ter-ō-sal-*ping*-gō-ō-*of*-o-REK-to-mē)	excision of the uterus, uterine tubes, and ovaries (Table 8-1) (Exercise Figure F)
mammoplasty (MAM-ō-*plas*-tē)	surgical repair of the breast (performed to enlarge or reduce in size, or to reconstruct after removal of a tumor) (Figure 8-10)
mastectomy (mas-TEK-to-mē)	surgical removal of a breast (Table 8-2) (Figure 8-10)
mastopexy (MAS-tō-pek-sē)	surgical fixation of the breast (performed to lift sagging breast tissue or to create symmetry) (Figure 8-10)
oophorectomy (ō-of-o-REK-to-mē)	excision of an ovary
perineorrhaphy (*per*-i-nē-OR-a-fē)	suturing of (a tear in) the perineum
salpingectomy (*sal*-pin-JEK-to-mē)	excision of a uterine tube
salpingo-oophorectomy (sal-*ping*-gō-ō-*of*-o-REK-to-mē)	excision of a uterine tube and ovary (Exercise Figure F)
salpingostomy (*sal*-ping-GOS-to-mē)	creation of an artificial opening in a uterine tube (performed to restore patency)
vulvectomy (vul-VEK-to-mē)	excision of the vulva

Table 8-1

Types of Hysterectomies

Total hysterectomy	Excision of the uterus (abdominal, vaginal, or laparoscopic)
Bilateral hysterosalpingo-oophorectomy	Excision of the uterus, ovaries, and uterine tubes
Radical hysterectomy	Excision of the uterus, ovaries, uterine tubes; lymph nodes, upper portion of the vagina, and the surrounding tissues (abdominal)
Laparoscopically-assisted vaginal hysterectomy	Vaginal excision of the uterus with the use of the laparoscope to view the abdominopelvic cavity.

EXERCISE FIGURE F

Fill in the blanks to label the diagram.

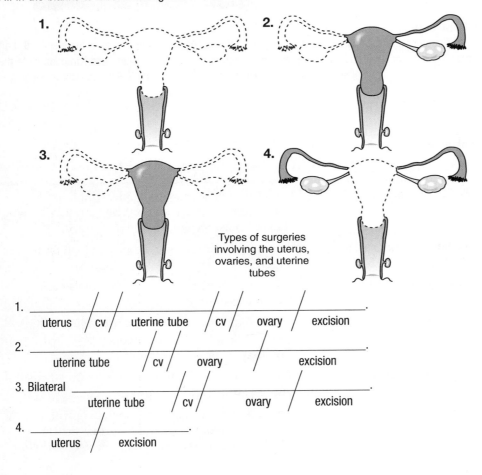

Types of surgeries involving the uterus, ovaries, and uterine tubes

1. _____ / uterus / cv / uterine tube / cv / ovary / excision .

2. _____ / uterine tube / cv / ovary / excision .

3. Bilateral _____ / uterine tube / cv / ovary / excision .

4. _____ / uterus / excision .

TYPES OF MAMMOPLASTY

- **Implant** uses a silicone or saline implant to create a breast.
- **Autologous** uses the patient's own tissue to reconstruct a breast.
- **Flap reconstruction** uses muscle or fat and surrounding tissue that is surgically transferred to the chest to create a breast mound (see Figure 8-10, *B*).

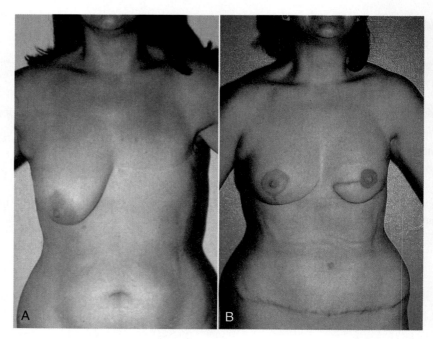

FIGURE 8-10

Breast surgery and reconstruction. **A,** Left breast shows modified radical mastectomy scar. **B,** Left breast shows mammoplasty by TRAM (transverse rectus abdominis muscle) reconstruction (note the extensive lower abdominal scar, repositioned navel, and reconstructed nipple) and right mastopexy.

Table 8-2

Types of Surgeries Performed to Treat Malignant Breast Tumors

Radical mastectomy	Removal of breast tissue, nipple, lymph nodes, and underlying chest wall muscle; also called **Halsted mastectomy** (rarely performed)
Modified radical mastectomy	Removal of breast tissue, nipple, and lymph nodes (Figure 8-10, *A*)
Simple mastectomy	Removal of breast tissue and nipple (also called **total mastectomy**)
Subcutaneous mastectomy	Removal of breast tissue only, preserving the overlying skin, nipple and areola (also called **nipple-sparing mastectomy**)
Segmental mastectomy	Removal of a quadrant, or wedge, of breast tissue (also called **quadrantectomy**)
Lumpectomy	Removal of the cancerous lesion along with a margin of surrounding healthy breast tissue (also called **partial mastectomy** or **breast-conserving surgery**)

EXERCISE 15

Practice saying aloud each of the surgical terms built from word parts on pp. 309–310.

 To hear the terms, go to evolve.elsevier.com. Select: Chapter 8, **Exercises**, Pronunciation.

Refer to p. 10 for your Evolve Access Information.

☐ Place a check mark in the box when you have completed this exercise.

EXERCISE 16

Analyze and define the following surgical terms.

1. colporrhaphy _____
2. colpoplasty _____
3. episiorrhaphy _____
4. hymenotomy _____
5. hysteropexy _____
6. vulvectomy _____
7. perineorrhaphy _____
8. salpingostomy _____
9. salpingo-oophorectomy _____
10. oophorectomy _____
11. mastectomy _____
12. salpingectomy _____
13. cervicectomy _____
14. colpoperineorrhaphy _____
15. episioperineoplasty _____
16. hymenectomy _____
17. hysterosalpingo-oophorectomy _____
18. hysterectomy _____
19. mammoplasty _____
20. mastopexy _____
21. culdocentesis _____

EXERCISE 17

Build surgical terms for the following definitions by using the word parts you have learned.

1. suturing of the vagina

     _____ / CV / _____
       WR   CV   S

2. excision of the cervix

     _____ / _____
       WR   S

3. suturing of the vulva

     _____ / CV / _____
       WR   CV   S

4. surgical repair of the vulva and perineum

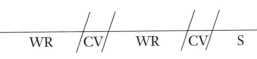

       WR   CV   WR   CV   S

5. surgical repair of the vagina

    WR   /CV/   S

6. suturing of the vagina and
   perineum

    WR /CV/ WR /CV/ S

7. excision of the uterus, ovaries,
   and uterine tubes

  WR /CV/ WR /CV/ WR / S

8. surgical fixation of the uterus

    WR   /CV/   S

9. excision of the hymen

    WR   /   S

10. incision of the hymen

    WR   /CV/   S

11. excision of the uterus

    WR   /   S

12. excision of the ovary

    WR   /   S

13. surgical removal of a breast

    WR   /   S

14. excision of a uterine tube

    WR   /   S

15. suturing of the perineum

    WR   /CV/   S

16. excision of a uterine tube
    and ovary

  WR /CV/ WR / S

17. creation of an artificial
    opening in the uterine tube

    WR   /CV/   S

18. excision of the vulva

    WR   /   S

19. surgical repair of the breast

    WR   /CV/   S

20. surgical fixation of the breast

    WR   /CV/   S

21. surgical puncture to aspirate
    fluid from Douglas cul-de-sac

    WR   /CV/   S

EXERCISE 18

Spell each of the surgical terms built from word parts on pp. 309–310 by having someone dictate them to you.

To hear and spell the terms, go to evolve.elsevier.com. Select: Chapter 8, **Exercises**, Spelling.

Refer to p. 10 for your Evolve Access Information.

☐ Place a check mark in the box if you have completed this exercise online.

1. _____   12. _____
2. _____   13. _____
3. _____   14. _____
4. _____   15. _____
5. _____   16. _____
6. _____   17. _____
7. _____   18. _____
8. _____   19. _____
9. _____   20. _____
10. _____   21. _____
11. _____

Surgical Terms

Not Built from Word Parts

In some of the following terms, you may recognize word parts you have already learned; however, the full meaning of the terms cannot be discerned by the definition of their word parts.

TERM	DEFINITION
anterior and posterior colporrhaphy (A&P repair) (kol-POR-a-fē)	surgical repair of a weakened vaginal wall to correct a cystocele (protrusion of the bladder against the anterior wall of the vagina) and a rectocele (protrusion of the rectum against the posterior wall of the vagina) (Exercise Figure G)
conization (*kon*-i-ZĀ-shun)	surgical removal of a cone-shaped area of the cervix; used in the treatment for noninvasive cervical cancer (also called **cone biopsy**)
dilation and curettage (D&C) (dī-LĀ-shun) (kū-re-TAHZH)	surgical procedure to widen the cervix and scrape the endometrium with an instrument called a *curette*. It is performed to diagnose disease, to correct bleeding, and to empty uterine contents, such as tissue remaining after a miscarriage (Figure 8-11)

Dilation or dilatation are both used in the presentation of dilation and curettage. Dilation is the more common usage and is used in this text.

TYPES OF CONIZATION

- **LEEP** (loop electrosurgical excision procedure) uses a thin electric loop to excise a cone of cervical tissue.
- **Cryosurgery** (also called **cold knife conization**) and laser ablation are also used to treat abnormal cells.

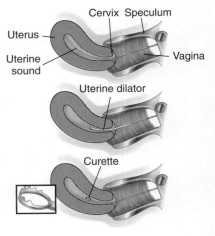

FIGURE 8-11
Dilation and curettage.

Fill in the blanks to complete the labeling of the diagrams.

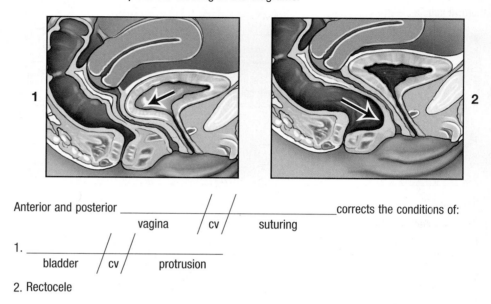

Anterior and posterior _____/__/_____ corrects the conditions of:

                vagina / cv / suturing

1. _____/__/_____

        bladder / cv / protrusion

2. Rectocele

Surgical Terms—cont'd

Not Built from Word Parts

> 🏛 **ABLATION**
>
> is from the Latin **ablatum**, meaning **to carry away.** In surgery **ablation** means **excision or eradication,** especially by cutting with laser or electrical energy.

TERM	DEFINITION
endometrial ablation (*en*-dō-MĒ-trē-al) (ab-LĀ-shun)	procedure to destroy or remove the endometrium by use of laser, electrical, or thermal energy; used to treat abnormal uterine bleeding (Figure 8-12)
laparoscopy or laparoscopic surgery (*lap*-a-ROS-ko-pē) (*lap*-a-rō-SKOP-ik)	visual examination of the abdominopelvic cavity, accomplished by inserting a laparoscope through a tiny incision near the umbilicus. Numerous female reproductive system surgeries are performed with this technique (Figures 8-9, p. 310).
myomectomy (*mī*-ō-MEK-to-mē)	excision of a fibroid tumor (myoma) from the uterus

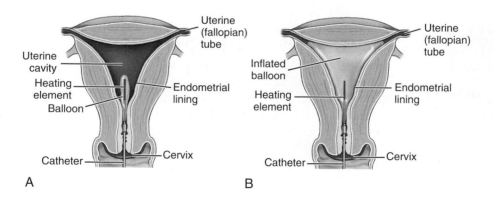

FIGURE 8-12

Endometrial ablation using thermal energy. **A,** The balloon catheter (deflated) is inserted through the cervix into the uterine cavity. **B,** The balloon is inflated with a solution of 5% dextrose and water and heated to 87°C for 8 minutes, ablating the endometrial lining.

TERM	DEFINITION
sentinel lymph node biopsy (SEN-tin-el) (limf) (nōd) (BĪ-op-sē)	injection of blue dye and/or radioactive isotope used to identify the sentinel lymph node(s), the first in the axillary chain and most likely to contain metastasis of breast cancer. The nodes are removed and microscopically examined. If negative, no more nodes are removed (Figure 8-13).
stereotactic breast biopsy (*ster-ē-ō*-TAK-tik) (brest) (BĪ-op-sē)	technique that combines mammography and computer-assisted biopsy to obtain tissue from a breast lesion (Figure 8-14)
tubal ligation (lī-GĀ-shun)	closure of the uterine tubes for sterilization by tying (ligation) (the broader term "tubal sterilization" includes cauterizing the cut ends) (also called **"tying of tubes"**) (Figure 8-15)
uterine artery embolization (UAE) (ū-ter-in) (AR-ter-ē) (*em*-be-li-ZĀ-shun)	minimally invasive procedure used to treat fibroids of the uterus by blocking arteries that supply blood to the fibroids. First, an arteriogram is used to identify the vessels. Once identified, tiny gelatin beads, about the size of grains of sand, are inserted into the vessels to create a blockage. The blockage stops the blood supply to the fibroids causing them to shrink.

TYPES OF BREAST BIOPSY

- **Directed breast biopsy** uses mammography, sonography, or MRI radiographic images to guide a biopsy needle.
- **Surgical breast biopsy** involves making an incision to remove a palpable breast lesion (also called **open** or **incisional biopsy**).
- **Wire localization biopsy** combines both modalities and uses radiographic guidance to place a thin, flexible wire directly into a breast lesion. The lesion is removed surgically with the wire intact.

Deciding on the optimal procedure is based on how a breast lesion is best visualized and the patient's health and preferences.

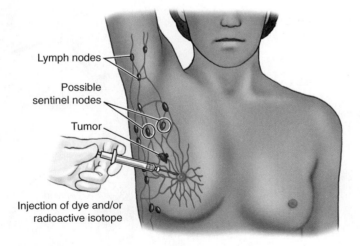

Lymph nodes

Possible sentinel nodes

Tumor

Injection of dye and/or radioactive isotope

🏛 SENTINEL LYMPH NODE BIOPSY was first developed for patients with melanoma. It is now also used to determine metastasis of breast cancer to the lymph nodes. Previously, surgeons would remove 10 to 20 lymph nodes to determine the spread of cancer, often causing lymphedema, which can lead to painful and permanent swelling of the arm. With sentinel lymph node biopsy, if negative, additional lymph nodes are not removed.

FIGURE 8-13

Preparation for sentinel lymph node biopsy. The process of identifying the sentinel node(s) is performed in the nuclear medicine department of radiology. The biopsy is performed in surgery.

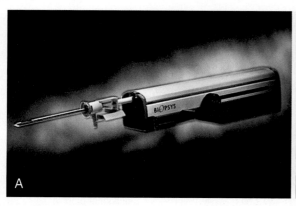
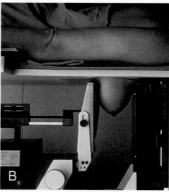
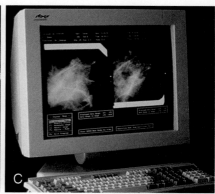

FIGURE 8-14

Stereotactic breast biopsy. Stereotactic breast biopsy is the least invasive method of obtaining tissue to determine if a nonpalpable breast lesion is benign or malignant. Benefits include less pain and scarring, a shorter recovery time, and less expense than conventional surgery. The patient is placed prone on a special table with the breast suspended through an opening. The breast is placed in a mammography machine under the table. A digital mammogram is produced on a computer monitor to identify the exact location of the lesion. The biopsy instrument is guided by a radiologist or surgeon. Tissue obtained from the lesion is examined microscopically. **A,** The Mammotome is used to obtain the specimen for biopsy. **B,** The patient is positioned for stereotactic breast biopsy. **C,** The mammogram appears digitally and is used to determine the placement of the biopsy needle.

TUBAL STERILIZATION

is a form of permanent birth control, preventing pregnancy by cutting or blocking uterine tubes. In **tubal ligation**, which involves surgery, uterine tubes can be:

- cut and tied with surgical gut, cotton, silk, or wire
- cut and cauterized
- closed off with a clip, clamp, ring, or band

In **nonsurgical tubal sterilization**, uterine tubes are blocked by either:

- coils, Essure system
- ablation and plug, Adiana system

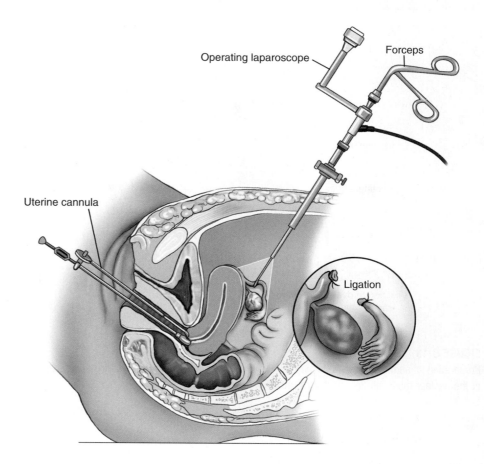

FIGURE 8-15

Laparoscopic tubal sterilization.

EXERCISE 19

Practice saying aloud each of the surgical terms not built from word parts on pp. 315–317.

To hear the terms, go to evolve.elsevier.com. Select: Chapter 8, **Exercises**, Pronunciation.

Refer to p. 10 for your Evolve Access Information.

☐ Place a check mark in the box when you have completed this exercise.

EXERCISE 20

Fill in the blanks with the correct term.

1. A procedure used for sterilization of women is _____

   _____.

2. The surgery used to repair a cystocele and rectocele is a(n) _____

   and _____ _____.

3. D&C is the abbreviation for _____ and _____.

4. _____ _____ _____ is a
   technique used to obtain tissue from a breast lesion.

5. Excision of a fibroid tumor from the uterus is called _____.

6. A procedure to destroy endometrium by laser, electrical, or thermal energy is

   called _____ _____.

7. A procedure used to treat uterine fibroids by blocking the blood supply is

   called _____ _____ _____.

8. Surgical removal of a cone-shaped area of the cervix is called

   _____.

9. A procedure to identify metastasis of breast cancer in the axillary lymph nodes

   for biopsy is called _____ _____

   _____ _____.

10. A surgical procedure performed through a tiny incision near the umbilicus is

    called _____ or _____ _____.

EXERCISE 21

Match the surgical procedures in the first column with the corresponding organs in the second column. You may use the answers in the second column more than once.

_____	1. dilation and curettage	a. uterine tubes
_____	2. laparoscopic surgery for sterilization	b. vagina
_____	3. tubal ligation	c. uterus
_____	4. anterior and posterior colporrhaphy repair	d. ovaries
_____	5. myomectomy	e. vulva
_____	6. stereotactic breast biopsy	f. mammary glands
_____	7. conization	g. lymph nodes
_____	8. endometrial ablation	h. cervix
_____	9. sentinel lymph node biopsy	
_____	10. uterine artery embolization	

EXERCISE 22

Spell each of the surgical terms not built from word parts on pp. 315–317 by having someone dictate them to you.

> e To hear and spell the terms, go to evolve.elsevier.com. Select: Chapter 8, **Exercises**, Spelling.
>
> Refer to p. 10 for your Evolve Access Information.
>
> ☐ Place a check mark in the box if you have completed this exercise online.

1. _____
2. _____
3. _____
4. _____
5. _____

6. _____
7. _____
8. _____
9. _____
10. _____

Diagnostic Terms

Built from Word Parts

The following terms are built from word parts you have already learned and can be translated literally to find their meanings. Further explanation of terms beyond the definitions of their word parts, if needed, is included in parentheses.

TERM	DEFINITION
DIAGNOSTIC IMAGING	
hysterosalpingogram (*his*-ter-ō-*sal*-PING-gō-gram)	radiographic image of the uterus and uterine tubes (after an injection of a contrast agent) (Exercise Figure H)
mammogram (MAM-ō-gram)	radiographic image of the breast (Figure 8-16)
mammography (ma-MOG-ra-fē)	radiographic imaging of the breast (also called **digital mammography** when images are obtained electronically and viewed on a computer) (see Figure 8-16)
sonohysterography (SHG) (*son*-ō-*his*-ter-OG-ra-fē)	process of recording the uterus by use of sound (an ultrasound procedure)
ENDOSCOPY	
colposcope (KOL-pō-skōp)	instrument used for visual examination of the vagina (and cervix)
colposcopy (kol-POS-ko-pē)	visual examination (with a magnified view) of the vagina (and cervix)
culdoscope (KUL-dō-skōp)	instrument used for visual examination of Douglas cul-de-sac (rectouterine pouch)
culdoscopy (kul-DOS-ko-pē)	visual examination of Douglas cul-de-sac (rectouterine pouch) (Exercise Figure I)
hysteroscope (HIS-ter-ō-skōp)	instrument used for visual examination of the uterus (uterine cavity)
hysteroscopy (*his*-ter-OS-ko-pē)	visual examination of the uterus (uterine cavity)

SONOHYSTERO-GRAPHY

is a technique for evaluating the uterine cavity. Saline solution is injected into the uterine cavity, followed by transvaginal sonography. It is used preoperatively to assess polyps, myomas, and adhesions.

> e To watch animations, go to evolve.elsevier.com. Select:
> Chapter 8, **Animations**, Hysteroscopy
> Hysteroscope Insertion
>
> Refer to p. 10 for your Evolve Access Information.

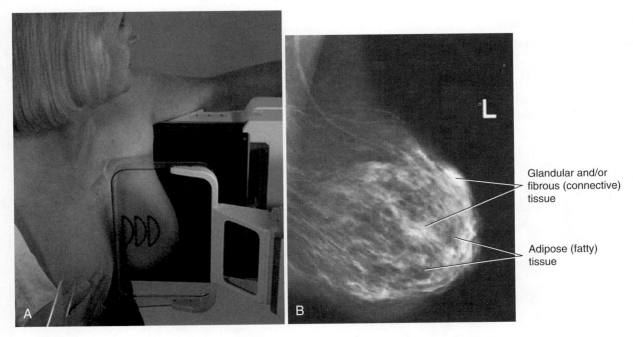

FIGURE 8-16
A, Mammography. **B,** Mammogram.

Glandular and/or
fibrous (connective)
tissue

Adipose (fatty)
tissue

EXERCISE FIGURE **H**

Fill in the blanks to complete the labeling of the diagram.

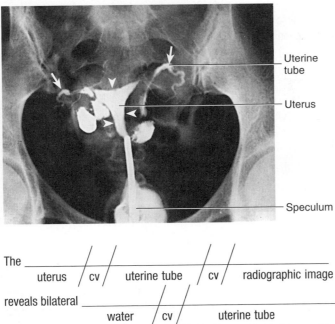

Uterine
tube

Uterus

Speculum

The _____ / cv / _____ / cv / radiographic image
          uterus /   / uterine tube /   /

reveals bilateral _____
                   water / cv /   uterine tube

Liquid contrast medium is injected through the vagina and is used to outline the uterus and uterine tubes before the radiographic image is made. This procedure usually is performed to determine whether obstructions exist in the uterine tubes causing infertility.

EXERCISE FIGURE ▮**I**

Fill in the blanks to complete the labeling of the diagram.

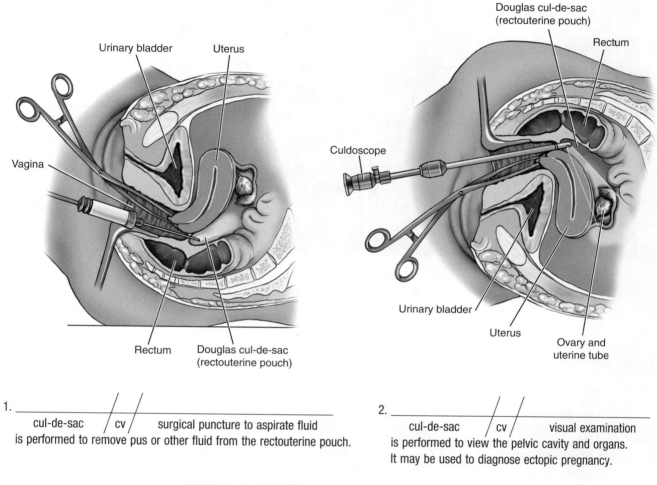

1. _____/_____/_____ _____
       cul-de-sac   cv   surgical puncture to aspirate fluid
      is performed to remove pus or other fluid from the rectouterine pouch.

2. _____/_____/_____ _____
       cul-de-sac   cv   visual examination
      is performed to view the pelvic cavity and organs.
   It may be used to diagnose ectopic pregnancy.

EXERCISE 23

Practice saying aloud each of the diagnostic terms built from word parts on p. 320.

To hear the terms, go to evolve.elsevier.com. Select: Chapter 8, **Exercises**, Pronunciation.

Refer to p. 10 for your Evolve Access Information.

☐ Place a check mark in the box when you have completed this exercise.

EXERCISE 24

Analyze and define the following diagnostic terms.

1. colposcopy_____
2. mammogram_____
3. colposcope_____
4. hysteroscopy_____
5. hysterosalpingogram_____
6. culdoscope_____
7. culdoscopy_____

8. mammography _____

9. hysteroscope _____

10. sonohysterography _____

EXERCISE 25

Build diagnostic terms that correspond to the following definitions by using the word parts you have learned.

1. radiographic image of the uterus and uterine tubes

   _____ / ___ / _____ / ___ / _____
   WR   /CV/   WR   /CV/   S

2. visual examination of the vagina (and cervix)

   _____ / ___ / _____
   WR   /CV/   S

3. instrument used for visual examination of the vagina (and cervix)

   _____ / ___ / _____
   WR   /CV/   S

4. visual examination of the uterus

   _____ / ___ / _____
   WR   /CV/   S

5. radiographic image of the breast

   _____ / ___ / _____
   WR   /CV/   S

6. instrument used for visual examination of Douglas cul-de-sac

   _____ / ___ / _____
   WR   /CV/   S

7. visual examination of Douglas cul-de-sac

   _____ / ___ / _____
   WR   /CV/   S

8. instrument used for visual examination of the uterus

   _____ / ___ / _____
   WR   /CV/   S

9. radiographic imaging of the breast

   _____ / ___ / _____
   WR   /CV/   S

10. process of recording the uterus with sound

    _____ / ___ / _____ / ___ / _____
    WR   /CV/   WR   /CV/   S

EXERCISE 26

Spell each of the diagnostic terms built from word parts on p. 320 by having someone dictate them to you.

> To hear and spell the terms, go to evolve.elsevier.com. Select: Chapter 8, **Exercises**, Spelling.
>
> (e) Refer to p. 10 for your Evolve Access Information.
>
> ☐ Place a check mark in the box if you have completed this exercise online.

1. _____   6. _____
2. _____   7. _____
3. _____   8. _____
4. _____   9. _____
5. _____   10. _____

Diagnostic Terms

Not Built from Word Parts

In some of the following terms, you may recognize word parts you have already learned; however, the full meaning of the terms cannot be discerned by the definition of their word parts.

> **🏛 PAP SMEAR**
>
> is named after Dr. George N. Papanicolaou (1883–1962), a Greek physician practicing in the United States, who developed the cell smear method for the diagnosis of cancer in 1943. The test may be used to sample cells from any organ but is most commonly used on cervical and vaginal secretions. The Pap smear is 95% accurate in detecting cervical carcinoma. In 1966 a liquid-based screening system was approved by the Food and Drug Administration as an alternative for the conventional Pap smear. This system improves detection of squamous intraepithelial lesions.

TERM	DEFINITION
DIAGNOSTIC IMAGING	
transvaginal sonography (TVS) (trans-VAJ-i-nal) (so-NOG-ra-fē)	ultrasound procedure that uses a transducer placed in the vagina to obtain images of the ovaries, uterus, cervix, uterine tubes, and surrounding structures; used to diagnose masses such as ovarian cysts or tumors, to monitor pregnancy, and to evaluate ovulation for the treatment of infertility (Figure 8-17)
LABORATORY	
CA-125 (cancer antigen-125 tumor marker) (C-Ā-125)	blood test used in the detection of ovarian cancer. It is also used to monitor treatment and to determine the extent of the disease.
Pap smear (pap) (smēr)	cytological study of cervical and vaginal secretions used to determine the presence of abnormal or cancerous cells; most commonly used to detect cancers of the cervix (also called **Papanicolaou** [*pap*-a-NIK-kō-lā-oo] **smear** and **Pap test**) (Figure 8-18)

> (e) To watch animations, go to evolve.elsevier.com. Select: Chapter 8, **Animations**, Ovarian Cysts.
>
> Refer to p. 10 for your Evolve Access Information.

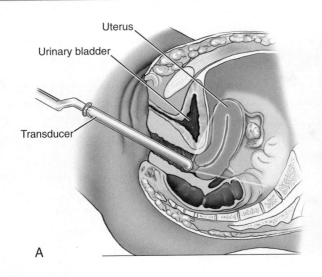

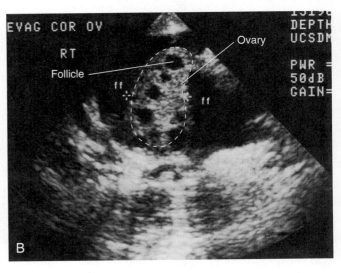

FIGURE 8-17
Transvaginal sonography. A, Transducer placed in the vagina. **B,** Transvaginal coronal image of the right ovary with multiple follicles, showing free fluid surrounding the ovary.

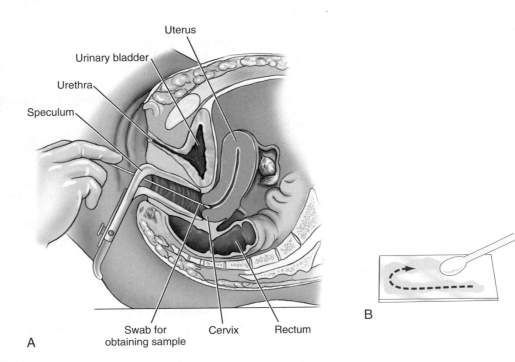

FIGURE 8-18
Pap smear. **A,** Obtaining the specimen. **B,** Transferring the specimen to a glass slide, where it will be stained and studied under a microscope in the laboratory.

EXERCISE 27

Practice saying aloud each of the diagnostic terms not built from word parts.

> e To hear the terms, go to evolve.elsevier.com. Select: Chapter 8, **Exercises**, Pronunciation.
>
> Refer to p. 10 for your Evolve Access Information.

☐ Place a check mark in the box when you have completed this exercise.

EXERCISE 28

Fill in the blanks with the correct definition.

1. Pap smear _____

2. transvaginal sonography _____

3. CA-125 _____

EXERCISE 29

Write the term for each of the following.

1. cytological study of cervical and vaginal secretions _____
   _____

2. blood test used to detect ovarian cancer _____

3. obtains images of the ovaries, uterus, cervix, uterine tubes, and surrounding
   structures _____ _____

EXERCISE 30

Spell each of the disease and disorder terms not built from word parts on p. 324 by having someone dictate them to you.

> To hear and spell the terms, go to evolve.elsevier.com. Select: Chapter 8, **Exercises**, Spelling.
> Refer to p. 10 for your Evolve Access Information.
> ☐ Place a check mark in the box if you have completed this exercise online.

1. _____   3. _____

2. _____

Complementary Terms

Built from Word Parts

The following terms are built from word parts you have already learned and can be translated literally to find their meanings. Further explanation of terms beyond the definition of their word parts, if needed, is included in parentheses.

TERM	DEFINITION
gynecologist (gīn-ek-OL-o-jist)	physician who studies and treats diseases of women (female reproductive system)
gynecology (GYN) (gīn-ek-OL-o-jē)	study of women (a branch of medicine dealing with health and diseases of the female reproductive system)
gynopathic (gīn-ō-PATH-ik)	pertaining to diseases of women
leukorrhea (lū-kō-RĒ-a)	white discharge (from the vagina)

TERM	DEFINITION
mastalgia (mas-TAL-ja)	pain in the breast
mastoptosis (*mas*-top-TŌ-sis)	sagging breast
menarche (me-NAR-kē)	beginning of menstruation (usually occurring between the ages of 11 and 16)
vaginal (VAJ-i-nal)	pertaining to the vagina
vulvovaginal (*vul*-vō-VAJ-i-nal)	pertaining to the vulva and vagina

EXERCISE 31

Practice saying aloud each of the complementary terms built from word parts on these two pages.

> (e) To hear the terms, go to evolve.elsevier.com. Select: Chapter 8, **Exercises**, Pronunciation.
> Refer to p. 10 for your Evolve Access Information.

☐ Place a check mark in the box when you have completed this exercise.

EXERCISE 32

Analyze and define the following complementary terms.

1. gynecologist _____
2. gynecology _____
3. vulvovaginal _____
4. mastalgia _____
5. menarche _____
6. leukorrhea _____
7. gynopathic _____
8. mastoptosis _____
9. vaginal _____

EXERCISE 33

Build complementary terms that correspond to the following definitions by using the word parts you have learned.

1. white discharge (from the vagina)

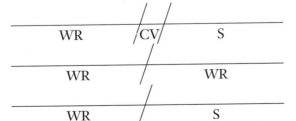

    WR   /CV/   S

2. beginning of menstruation

    WR   /   WR

3. pain in the breast

    WR   /   S

4. pertaining to the vulva and vagina

_____ / _____ / _____ / _____
WR   CV   WR   S

5. a physician who studies and treats diseases of women

_____ / _____ / _____
WR   CV   S

6. study of women (branch of medicine dealing with health and diseases of the female reproductive system)

_____ / _____ / _____
WR   CV   S

7. sagging breast

_____ / _____ / _____
WR   CV   S

8. pertaining to diseases of women

_____ / _____ / _____ / _____
WR   CV   WR   S

9. pertaining to the vagina

_____ / _____
WR   S

EXERCISE 34

Spell each of the complementary terms built from word parts on pp. 326–327 by having someone dictate them to you.

To hear and spell the terms, go to evolve.elsevier.com. Select: Chapter 8, **Exercises**, Spelling.

Refer to p. 10 for your Evolve Access Information.

☐ Place a check mark in the box if you have completed this exercise online.

1. _____   6. _____
2. _____   7. _____
3. _____   8. _____
4. _____   9. _____
5. _____

For review and/or assessment, go to evolve.elsevier.com. Select:
Chapter 8, **Activities,** Terms Built from Word Parts
Chapter 8, **Games,** Term Storm.

Refer to p. 10 for your Evolve Access Information.

Complementary Terms

Not Built from Word Parts

In some of the following terms, you may recognize word parts you have already learned; however, the full meaning of the terms cannot be discerned by the definition of their word parts.

TERM	DEFINITION
contraception (KON-tra-*sep*-shen)	intentional prevention of conception (pregnancy); may also be referred to as **birth control (BC)**
dyspareunia (*dis*-pa-RŪ-nē-a)	difficult or painful intercourse
fistula (FIS-tū-la)	abnormal passageway between two organs or between an internal organ and the body surface
hormone replacement therapy (HRT)	replacement of hormones, estrogen and/or progesterone, to treat symptoms associated with menopause
menopause (MEN-o-pawz)	cessation of menstruation, usually around the ages of 48 to 53 years; may be induced at an earlier age surgically (bilateral oophorectomy) or medically (side effect of chemotherapy treatment)
premenstrual syndrome (PMS) (prē-MEN-stroo-al) (SIN-drom)	syndrome involving physical and emotional symptoms occurring in the 10 days before menstruation. Symptoms include nervous tension, irritability, mastalgia, edema, and headache.
speculum (SPEK-ū-lum)	instrument for opening a body cavity to allow visual inspection (Figure 8-20)

METHODS OF CONTRACEPTION

Numerous contraceptive methods exist, including barrier (condoms), chemical (spermicides), oral pharmaceutical (birth control pill), and device (intrauterine device [IUD]). (See Figure 8-19)

HORMONE REPLACEMENT THERAPY (HRT)

has decreased dramatically since 2002, following release of research data by the Women's Health Initiative, a trial conducted by the National Institutes of Health. This study demonstrated that women taking HRT had a significantly higher incidence of breast cancer, heart disease, and stroke. As a result, current practice recommendations state that menopausal women choosing HRT should take the lowest possible dose for the shortest amount of time.

 Refer to **Appendix D** for pharmacology terms related to the female reproductive system.

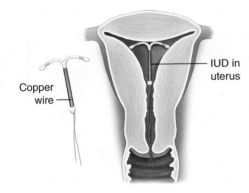

FIGURE 8-19
Intrauterine device (IUD). Inserted through the cervix, this T-shaped device provides long-term contraception by changing the intrauterine environment. IUDs may be made from copper or a spermicide-releasing plastic.

Copper wire

IUD in uterus

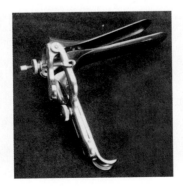

FIGURE 8-20
Vaginal speculum.

EXERCISE 35

Practice saying aloud each of the complementary terms not built from word parts on p. 329.

> (e) To hear the terms, go to evolve.elsevier.com. Select: Chapter 8, **Exercises**, Pronunciation.
>
> Refer to p. 10 for your Evolve Access Information.

☐ Place a check mark in the box when you have completed this exercise.

EXERCISE 36

Write the definitions of the following terms.

1. menopause _____
2. dyspareunia _____
3. fistula _____
4. premenstrual syndrome _____
5. speculum _____
6. hormone replacement therapy _____
7. contraception _____

EXERCISE 37

Write the term for each of the following.

1. abnormal passageway _____
2. painful intercourse _____
3. cessation of menstruation _____
4. syndrome involving physical and emotional symptoms_____
   _____
5. instrument for opening a body cavity _____
6. replacement of hormones to treat symptoms associated with menopause _____ _____ _____
7. intentional prevention of conception _____

EXERCISE 38

Spell each of the complementary terms not built from word parts on p. 329 by having someone dictate them to you.

> To hear and spell the terms, go to evolve.elsevier.com. Select: Chapter 8, **Exercises**, Spelling.
>
> (e) Refer to p. 10 for your Evolve Access Information.
>
> ☐ Place a check mark in the box if you have completed this exercise online.

1. _____   5. _____

2. _____   6. _____

3. _____   7. _____

4. _____

> For review and/or assessment, go to evolve.elsevier.com. Select:
> Chapter 8, **Activities**, Terms Not Built from Word Parts
> (e)   **Games**,   Term Explorer
>   Termbusters
>   Medical Millionaire
>
> Refer to p. 10 for your Evolve Access Information.

Abbreviations

ABBREVIATION	MEANING
A&P repair	anterior and posterior colporrhaphy
BC	birth control
Cx	cervix
D&C	dilation and curettage
FCC	fibrocystic breast condition
GYN	gynecology
HRT	hormone replacement therapy
IUD	intrauterine device
LAVH	laparoscopically assisted vaginal hysterectomy
PID	pelvic inflammatory disease
PMS	premenstrual syndrome
SHG	sonohysterography
TAH/BSO	total abdominal hysterectomy/bilateral salpingo-oophorectomy
TSS	toxic shock syndrome
TVH	total vaginal hysterectomy
TVS	transvaginal sonography
UAE	uterine artery embolization

🔍 Refer to **Appendix C** for a complete list of abbreviations.

EXERCISE 39

Write the meaning for each of the abbreviations in the following sentences.

1. To repair a cystocele and rectocele the patient is scheduled in surgery for an
   A&P repair _____ & _____ _____.

2. Following a **TAH/BSO** _____ _____ _____
   and _____ _____ the gynecologist
   prescribed **HRT** _____ _____ _____ for the
   patient to take for 3 months after surgery.

3. **SHG** _____ and **TVS** _____
   _____ are diagnostic ultrasound procedures used to assist in
   diagnosing diseases and disorders of the female reproductive organs.

4. When performing a **TVH** _____ _____
   _____ the surgeon removes the uterus through the vagina without
   a surgical incision into the abdomen. During a(n) **LAVH** _____
   _____ _____ _____ the surgeon uses a
   fiberoptic laparoscope inserted through a tiny incision near the umbilicus to
   visualize the uterus and guide removal through the vagina.

5. **D&C** _____ & _____ is the dilation of the **Cx**
   _____ and scraping of the endometrium.

6. **FCC** _____ _____ _____ is the most
   common breast problem of women in their 20s.

7. A female patient with probable **PID** _____ _____
   _____ was referred to the **GYN** _____ clinic for
   evaluation and care.

8. The medical management of **PMS** _____ _____
   emphasizes the relief of symptoms.

9. **UAE** _____ _____ _____ offers a minimally
   invasive treatment option for some women with symptomatic fibroid tumors.

10. To provide long-term contraception, the female patient chose to have an **IUD**
    _____ _____ inserted by a gynecologist. While this
    method of **BC** _____ _____ is very effective at
    preventing pregnancy, it does not protect against sexually transmitted infection.

For more practice with abbreviations, go to evolve.elsevier.com. Select:
Chapter 8, **Flashcards**
      Games, Crossword Puzzle

Refer to p. 10 for your Evolve Access Information.

PRACTICAL APPLICATION

EXERCISE 40   *Interact with Medical Documents and Electronic Health Records*

A. Complete the progress note by writing the medical terms in the blanks. Use the list of definitions with the corresponding numbers on the next page.

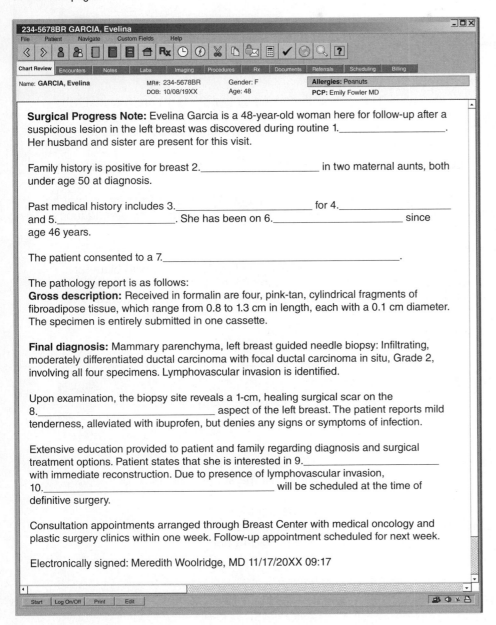

234-5678BR GARCIA, Evelina

File   Patient   Navigate   Custom Fields   Help

Chart Review | Encounters | Notes | Labs | Imaging | Procedures | Rx | Documents | Referrals | Scheduling | Billing

Name: **GARCIA, Evelina**   MR#: 234-5678BR   Gender: F   **Allergies:** Peanuts
                             DOB: 10/08/19XX   Age: 48   **PCP:** Emily Fowler MD

Surgical Progress Note: Evelina Garcia is a 48-year-old woman here for follow-up after a suspicious lesion in the left breast was discovered during routine 1._____.
Her husband and sister are present for this visit.

Family history is positive for breast 2._____ in two maternal aunts, both under age 50 at diagnosis.

Past medical history includes 3._____ for 4._____ and 5._____. She has been on 6._____ since age 46 years.

The patient consented to a 7._____.

The pathology report is as follows:
Gross description: Received in formalin are four, pink-tan, cylindrical fragments of fibroadipose tissue, which range from 0.8 to 1.3 cm in length, each with a 0.1 cm diameter. The specimen is entirely submitted in one cassette.

Final diagnosis: Mammary parenchyma, left breast guided needle biopsy: Infiltrating, moderately differentiated ductal carcinoma with focal ductal carcinoma in situ, Grade 2, involving all four specimens. Lymphovascular invasion is identified.

Upon examination, the biopsy site reveals a 1-cm, healing surgical scar on the 8._____ aspect of the left breast. The patient reports mild tenderness, alleviated with ibuprofen, but denies any signs or symptoms of infection.

Extensive education provided to patient and family regarding diagnosis and surgical treatment options. Patient states that she is interested in 9._____ with immediate reconstruction. Due to presence of lymphovascular invasion, 10._____ will be scheduled at the time of definitive surgery.

Consultation appointments arranged through Breast Center with medical oncology and plastic surgery clinics within one week. Follow-up appointment scheduled for next week.

Electronically signed: Meredith Woolridge, MD 11/17/20XX 09:17

Start | Log On/Off | Print | Edit

1. radiographic imaging of the breast
2. cancerous tumor
3. excision of the uterus
4. growth of endometrium into the muscular portion of the uterus
5. abnormal condition in which endometrial tissue occurs in various areas of the pelvic cavity
6. abbreviation for replacement of hormones to treat menopause
7. combines mammography and computer-assisted biopsy to obtain tissue from a breast lesion
8. pertaining to the middle and to (one) side
9. surgical removal of a breast
10. an injection of blue dye and/or radioactive isotope used to identify the first in the axillary chain and most likely to contain metastasis of breast cancer

B. Read the chart note and answer the questions following it.

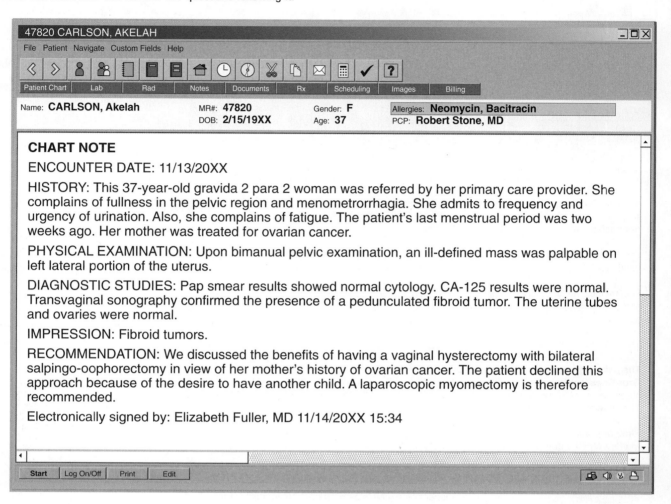

47820 CARLSON, AKELAH

File Patient Navigate Custom Fields Help

Patient Chart | Lab | Rad | Notes | Documents | Rx | Scheduling | Images | Billing

Name: **CARLSON, Akelah**   MR#: **47820**   Gender: **F**   Allergies: **Neomycin, Bacitracin**
DOB: **2/15/19XX**   Age: **37**   PCP: **Robert Stone, MD**

CHART NOTE

ENCOUNTER DATE: 11/13/20XX

HISTORY: This 37-year-old gravida 2 para 2 woman was referred by her primary care provider. She complains of fullness in the pelvic region and menometrorrhagia. She admits to frequency and urgency of urination. Also, she complains of fatigue. The patient's last menstrual period was two weeks ago. Her mother was treated for ovarian cancer.

PHYSICAL EXAMINATION: Upon bimanual pelvic examination, an ill-defined mass was palpable on left lateral portion of the uterus.

DIAGNOSTIC STUDIES: Pap smear results showed normal cytology. CA-125 results were normal. Transvaginal sonography confirmed the presence of a pedunculated fibroid tumor. The uterine tubes and ovaries were normal.

IMPRESSION: Fibroid tumors.

RECOMMENDATION: We discussed the benefits of having a vaginal hysterectomy with bilateral salpingo-oophorectomy in view of her mother's history of ovarian cancer. The patient declined this approach because of the desire to have another child. A laparoscopic myomectomy is therefore recommended.

Electronically signed by: Elizabeth Fuller, MD 11/14/20XX 15:34

Start | Log On/Off | Print | Edit

1. The patient's symptoms include:
   a. absence of menstrual flow
   b. scanty menstrual flow
   c. increased amount of menstrual flow during menses and bleeding between periods
   d. painful menstruation
2. The CA-125 diagnostic study was used to detect the presence of:
   a. ovarian cancer
   b. cervical cancer
   c. endometrial cancer
   d. endometriosis

3. The recommended procedure, a myomectomy, will entail the surgical excision of:
   a. a breast
   b. the uterus
   c. ovarian cancer
   d. a fibroid tumor

C. Complete the **three medical documents** within the electronic health record (EHR) on Evolve.

> Many healthcare records today are stored and used in an electronic system called Electronic Health Records (EHR). Electronic health records contain a collection of health information of an individual patient; the digitally formatted record can be shared through computer networks with patients, physicians, and other health care providers.

> For practice with medical terms using electronic health records, go to evolve.elsevier.com. Select: Chapter 8, **Electronic Health Records**.
>
> Refer to p. 10 for **your** Evolve Access Information.

EXERCISE 41   *Interpret Medical Terms*

To test your understanding of the terms introduced in this chapter, circle the words that correctly complete the sentences. The italicized words refer to the correct answer.

1. The patient was diagnosed as having *painful menstrual flow,* or (**oligomenorrhea, dysmenorrhea, amenorrhea**).
2. *Inflammation of the inner lining of the uterus* is (**endocervicitis, endometritis, endometriosis**).
3. The patient is scheduled in surgery for a *salpingectomy,* which is the excision of the (**uterine tube, ovary, uterus**).
4. An *episiorrhaphy* is a (**suture of the vulva, discharge from the vulva, rapid discharge from the vulva**).
5. A *surgical procedure to reduce breast size* is called reduction (**mammogram, mammography, mammoplasty**).
6. A *hysterosalpingo-oophorectomy* is the excision of the (**uterus, uterine tubes, and ovaries; uterus, ovaries, and cervix; uterus, uterine tubes, and vagina**).
7. *Blood in the uterine tube* is called (**hematosalpinx, hydrosalpinx, pyosalpinx**).
8. *Endometrial tissue occurring in various areas of the pelvic cavity* is called (**adenomyosis, endometriosis, hysteratresia**).
9. The doctor requested a (**hysteroscope, colposcope, speculum**) *to open the vagina for visual examination.*
10. A severe illness *that may affect menstruating women after using tampons is* (**TVS, TSS, TVH**).
11. Cryosurgery, laser ablation, and LEEP are *surgical procedures performed to remove a cone-shaped area of the cervix* called (**colporrhaphy, conization, myomectomy**).

🛜 WEB LINK

For more information on a spectrum of topics related to breast health and the female reproductive system, visit the National Institutes of Health at *www.nlm,nih,gov/ medlineplus/womenhealth. html* and click on Women's Health.

Practice pronunciation of the terms by reading the following information on cancers of the female reproductive system. Use the pronunciation key following the medical terms to assist you in saying the words.

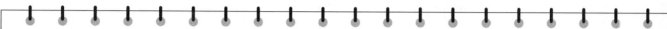

To hear these terms, go to evolve.elsevier.com.
Select: Chapter 8, **Exercises**, Read Medical Terms in Use.

Refer to p. 10 for your Evolve Access Information.

CANCERS OF THE FEMALE REPRODUCTIVE SYSTEM

Breast Cancer

The breast is the most common site of cancer in women. More than 80% of **breast cancer** (brest) (KAN-cer) is infiltrating ductal cancer (IDC), which originates in the mammary ducts. The rate of growth depends on hormonal influences. As long as the cancer remains in the duct, it is considered noninvasive and is called *ductal carcinoma in situ (DCIS)*.

    Mammography (ma-MOG-ra-fē) is the most common method used for diagnosing cancer of the breast. Confirmation is done with a biopsy obtained by conventional surgery or guided breast biopsy, such as **stereotactic breast biopsy** (ster-ē-ō-TAK-tik) (brest) (BĪ-op-sē). Treatment may include lumpectomy, **mastectomy** (mas-TEK-to-mē), chemotherapy, radiation therapy, and hormonal therapy.

Cervical Cancer

In many regions of the world **cervical cancer** (SER-vi-kal) (KAN-cer) is the leading cause of death in women. Cervical cancer resembles and results from a sexually transmitted disease, a feature that distinguishes it from other cancers. Abnormal **vaginal** (VAJ-i-nal) bleeding is the most common symptom. **Pap smear** followed by **colposcopy** (kol-POS-ko-pē) biopsy is used to diagnose this disease. Surgical treatment options are **conization** (*kon*-i-ZĀ-shun), such as LEEP, and **hysterectomy** (his-te-REK-to-mē). Chemotherapy and radiation therapy may also be used. A vaccine for human papillomavirus is now available and can be used for the prevention of cervical cancer.

Endometrial Cancer

Currently 75% of women diagnosed with **endometrial cancer** (en-dō-MĒ-trē-al) (KAN-cer) are postmenopausal. Inappropriate bleeding is the only warning sign; hence early diagnosis is common. Pelvic examination, Pap smear, and endometrial sampling are used to diagnose this disease. Treatment is **hysterosalpingo-oophorectomy** (*his*-ter-ō-sal-ping-gō-ō-*of*-o-REK-to-mē), which may be followed by chemotherapy and radiation therapy. **Laparoscopic** (lap-a-RŌ-skop-ik) -assisted **vaginal hysterectomy** (VAJ-i-nal) (*his*-te-REK-to-mē) may also be used.

Ovarian Cancer

Ovarian cancer (ō-VAR-ē-an) (KAN-cer) is the ninth most common form of cancer in women, yet it is the most challenging to diagnose and causes more deaths than any other cancer of the female reproductive system. Early symptoms are often absent or associated with other problems; thus early diagnosis is uncommon. Early symptoms include abdominal discomfort and bloating; later stages include abdominal or pelvic pain and urinary or menstrual irregularities. **CA-125** and **transvaginal sonography** (trans-VAJ-i-nal) (so-NOG-ra-fē) are used in diagnosing this disease. Treatment is total abdominal **hysterectomy** (*his*-te-REK-to-mē) and bilateral **salpingo-oophorectomy** (sal-ping-gō-ō-*of*-o-REK-to-mē) and removal of as much additional involved tissue as possible, including lymph nodes in the pelvic area. Chemotherapy is usually prescribed following surgery.

EXERCISE 43 *Comprehend Medical Terms in Use*

Test your comprehension of the terms in the previous box by circling the correct answer.

1. Which of the following diagnostic tests would the physician use to diagnose ovarian cancer?
   a. colposcopy biopsy
   b. transvaginal sonography
   c. Pap smear
   d. mammography
2. T   F Surgery is a treatment option for breast, cervical, endometrial, and ovarian cancer.
3. T   F Excision of the uterus, uterine tubes, and ovaries is an accepted surgical treatment for both endometrial and ovarian cancer.
4. A vaccine is now available and can be used for prevention of cancer of the:
   a. ovary
   b. breast
   c. uterine tube
   d. cervix

> For a snapshot assessment of your knowledge of female reproductive system terms go to evolve.
> elsevier.com.
> Select: Chapter 8, **Quick Quizzes**.
>
> Refer to p. 10 for your Evolve Access Information.

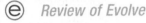

CHAPTER REVIEW

Review of Evolve

Keep a record of the online activities you have completed by placing a check mark in the box. You may also record your scores. All activities have been referenced throughout the chapter.

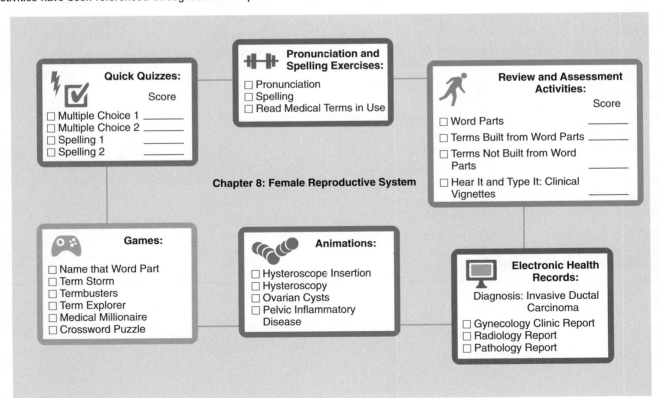

Quick Quizzes:

Score
- [ ] Multiple Choice 1 _____
- [ ] Multiple Choice 2 _____
- [ ] Spelling 1 _____
- [ ] Spelling 2 _____

Pronunciation and Spelling Exercises:
- [ ] Pronunciation
- [ ] Spelling
- [ ] Read Medical Terms in Use

Review and Assessment Activities:

Score
- [ ] Word Parts _____
- [ ] Terms Built from Word Parts _____
- [ ] Terms Not Built from Word Parts _____
- [ ] Hear It and Type It: Clinical Vignettes _____

Chapter 8: Female Reproductive System

Games:
- [ ] Name that Word Part
- [ ] Term Storm
- [ ] Termbusters
- [ ] Term Explorer
- [ ] Medical Millionaire
- [ ] Crossword Puzzle

Animations:
- [ ] Hysteroscope Insertion
- [ ] Hysteroscopy
- [ ] Ovarian Cysts
- [ ] Pelvic Inflammatory Disease

Electronic Health Records:

Diagnosis: Invasive Ductal Carcinoma
- [ ] Gynecology Clinic Report
- [ ] Radiology Report
- [ ] Pathology Report

Review of Word Parts

Can you define and spell the following word parts?

COMBINING FORMS		PREFIX	SUFFIXES
arche/o	men/o	peri-	-atresia
cervic/o	metr/i		-salpinx
colp/o	metr/o		
culd/o	oophor/o		
episi/o	perine/o		
gyn/o	salping/o		
gynec/o	vagin/o		
hymen/o	vulv/o		
hyster/o			
mamm/o			
mast/o			

Review of Terms

Can you build, analyze, define, pronounce, and spell the following terms *built from word parts*?

DISEASES AND DISORDERS	SURGICAL	DIAGNOSTIC	COMPLEMENTARY
amenorrhea	cervicectomy	colposcope	gynecologist
Bartholin adenitis	colpoperineorrhaphy	colposcopy	gynecology (GYN)
cervicitis	colpoplasty	culdoscope	gynopathic
colpitis	colporrhaphy	culdoscopy	leukorrhea
dysmenorrhea	culdocentesis	hysterosalpingogram	mastalgia
endocervicitis	episioperineoplasty	hysteroscope	mastoptosis
endometritis	episiorrhaphy	hysteroscopy	menarche
hematosalpinx	hymenectomy	mammogram	vaginal
hydrosalpinx	hymenotomy	mammography	vulvovaginal
hysteratresia	hysterectomy	sonohysterography (SHG)	
mastitis	hysteropexy		
menometrorrhagia	hysterosalpingo-oophorectomy		
menorrhagia	mammoplasty		
metrorrhagia	mastectomy		
myometritis	mastopexy		
oligomenorrhea	oophorectomy		
oophoritis	perineorrhaphy		
perimetritis	salpingectomy		
pyosalpinx	salpingo-oophorectomy		
salpingitis	salpingostomy		
salpingocele	vulvectomy		
vaginitis			
vulvovaginitis			

Can you define, pronounce, and spell the following terms *not built from word parts*?

DISEASES AND DISORDERS	SURGICAL	DIAGNOSTIC	COMPLEMENTARY
adenomyosis	anterior and posterior	CA-125	contraception
breast cancer	colporrhaphy (A&P repair)	Pap smear	dyspareunia
cervical cancer	conization	transvaginal	fistula
endometrial cancer	dilation and curettage (D&C)	sonography (TVS)	hormone replacement
endometriosis	endometrial ablation		therapy (HRT)
fibrocystic breast condition	laparoscopy		menopause
(FCC)	myomectomy		premenstrual syndrome
fibroid tumor	sentinel lymph node biopsy		(PMS)
ovarian cancer	stereotactic breast biopsy		speculum
pelvic inflammatory disease	tubal ligation		
(PID)	uterine artery embolization		
prolapsed uterus	(UAE)		
toxic shock syndrome (TSS)			
vesicovaginal fistula			

ANSWERS

Exercise Figures

Exercise Figure

A.
1. ovary: oophor/o
2. uterus: hyster/o, metr/o, metr/i
3. uterine (fallopian) tube: salping/o
4. cervix: cervic/o
5. vagina: colp/o, vagin/o
6. hymen: hymen/o

Exercise Figure

B.
1. vulva: episi/o, vulv/o
2. perineum: perine/o

Exercise Figure

C. salping/itis

Exercise Figure

D. hyster/o/ptosis

Exercise Figure

E. vesic/o/vagin/al

Exercise Figure

F.
1. hyster/o/salping/o/-oophor/ectomy
2. salping/o/-oophor/ectomy
3. (bilateral) salping/o/-oophor/ectomy
4. hyster/ectomy

Exercise Figure

G. colp/o/rrhaphy, cyst/o/cele

Exercise Figure

H.
1. hyster/o/salping/o/gram
2. hydr/o/salpinx

Exercise Figure

I.
1. culd/o/centesis
2. culd/o/scopy

Exercise 1

1.	c	6.	e
2.	f	7.	h
3.	g	8.	a
4.	b	9.	i
5.	d		

Exercise 2

1.	b	7.	g
2.	c	8.	l
3.	d	9.	i
4.	k	10.	j
5.	e	11.	h
6.	f		

Exercise 3
1. vagina
2. ovary
3. uterus
4. woman
5. hymen
6. uterus
7. menstruation
8. vulva
9. cervix
10. vagina
11. woman
12. breast
13. perineum
14. uterine tube
15. vulva
16. breast
17. first, beginning
18. cul-de-sac

Exercise 4
1. a. episi/o
   b. vulv/o
2. a. mamm/o
   b. mast/o
3. men/o
4. oophor/o
5. salping/o
6. perine/o
7. a. vagin/o
   b. colp/o
8. a. metr/o
   b. metr/i
   c. hyster/o
9. a. gynec/o
   b. gyn/o
10. hymen/o
11. culd/o
12. cervic/o
13. arche/o

Exercise 5
1. -salpinx
2. peri-
3. -atresia

Exercise 6
1. uterine tube
2. surrounding
3. absence of a normal body opening, occlusion, closure

Exercise 7
Pronunciation Exercise

Exercise 8
Note: The combining form is identified by italic and bold print.

1. WR S
   colp/itis
   inflammation of the vagina

2. WR S
   cervic/itis
   inflammation of the cervix

3. WR CV S
   hydr/o/salpinx
       CF
   water in the uterine tube

4. WR CV S
   hemat/o/salpinx
       CF
   blood in the uterine tube

5. WR CV S
   metr/o/rrhagia
       CF
   rapid flow of blood from the uterus (between menstrual cycles)

6. WR S
   oophor/itis
   inflammation of the ovary

7.   WR   S
   (Bartholin) aden/itis
   inflammation of (Bartholin) gland

8. WR CV WR S
   vulv/o/vagin/itis
       CF
   inflammation of the vulva and vagina

9. WR CV S
   salping/o/cele
        CF
   hernia of the uterine tube

10. WR CV WR CV S
    men/o/metr/o/rrhagia
        CF   CF
    rapid flow of blood from the uterus at menstruation (and between menstrual cycles)

11. P WR CV S
    a/**men/o**/rrhea
         CF
    absence of menstrual flow

12. P   WR CV S
    dys/**men/o**/rrhea
            CF
    painful menstrual flow

13. WR S
    mast/itis
    inflammation of the breast

14. P WR S
    peri/metr/itis
    inflammation surrounding the uterus (outer layer)

15. WR CV WR S
    my/o/metr/itis
       CF
    inflammation of the uterine muscle

16.   P   WR S
    endo/metr/itis
    inflammation of the inner (lining) of
    the uterus

17.   P   WR S
    endo/cervic/itis
    inflammation of the inner (lining) of
    the cervix

18. WR CV S
    py/o/salpinx
       CF
    pus in the uterine tube

19. WR   S
    hyster/atresia
    closure of the uterus (uterine cavity)

20.   WR   S
    salping/itis
    inflammation of the uterine tube

21.   WR S
    vagin/itis
    inflammation of the vagina

22. WR CV   S
    men/o/rrhagia
        CF
    rapid flow of blood at menstruation
    (increased amount)

23. WR CV WR CV S
    olig/o/men/o/rrhea
        CF   CF
    scanty menstrual flow (less often)

Exercise 9
1. mast/itis
2. metr/o/rrhagia
3. salping/itis
4. vulv/o/vagin/itis
5. a/men/o/rrhea
6. cervic/itis
7. (Bartholin) aden/itis
8. hydr/o/salpinx
9. dys/men/o/rrhea
10. hemat/o/salpinx
11. a. colp/itis
    b. vagin/itis
12. men/o/metr/o/rrhagia
13. oophor/itis
14. salping/o/cele
15. peri/metr/itis
16. endo/metr/itis
17. endo/cervic/itis
18. my/o/metr/itis
19. py/o/salpinx
20. hyster/atresia
21. olig/o/men/o/rrhea
22. men/o/rrhagia

Exercise 10
Spelling Exercise; see text p. 304.

Exercise 11
Pronunciation Exercise

Exercise 12
1. downward displacement of the
   uterus into the vagina
2. inflammation of some or all of the
   female pelvic organs
3. abnormal opening between the
   bladder and vagina
4. benign fibroid tumor of the uterine
   muscle
5. abnormal condition in which
   endometrial tissue grows in various
   areas of the pelvic cavity
6. growth of endometrium into the
   muscular portion of the uterus
7. a severe illness characterized by high
   fever, vomiting, diarrhea, and
   myalgia
8. disorder characterized by benign
   cysts in one or more breasts
9. malignant tumor of the ovary
10. malignant tumor of the breast
11. malignant tumor of the cervix
12. malignant tumor of the
    endometrium

Exercise 13
1. vesicovaginal fistula
2. fibroid tumor
3. pelvic inflammatory disease
4. prolapsed uterus
5. endometriosis
6. adenomyosis
7. toxic shock syndrome
8. fibrocystic breast condition
9. breast cancer
10. endometrial cancer
11. ovarian cancer
12. cervical cancer

Exercise 14
Spelling Exercise; see text p. 309.

Exercise 15
Pronunciation Exercise

Exercise 16
*Note: The combining form is identified by
italic and bold print.*
1. WR CV S
    colp/o/rrhaphy
       CF
    suturing of the vagina

2. WR CV S
    colp/o/plasty
       CF
    surgical repair of the vagina

3. WR CV   S
    episi/o/rrhaphy
        CF
    suturing of the vulva (tear)

4. WR CV S
    hymen/o/tomy
        CF
    incision of the hymen

5. WR CV S
    hyster/o/pexy
        CF
    surgical fixation of the uterus

6. WR   S
    vulv/ectomy
    excision of the vulva

7. WR CV   S
    perine/o/rrhaphy
        CF
    suturing of the perineum (tear)

8. WR CV S
    salping/o/stomy
        CF
    creation of an artificial opening in
    the uterine tube

9. WR CV WR   S
    salping/o/-oophor/ectomy
        CF
    excision of a uterine tube and ovary

10. WR   S
    oophor/ectomy
    excision of an ovary

11. WR   S
    mast/ectomy
    surgical removal of a breast

12. WR   S
    salping/ectomy
    excision of a uterine tube

13. WR   S
    cervic/ectomy
    excision of the cervix

14. WR CV WR CV S
    colp/o/perine/o/rrhaphy
        CF   CF
    suturing of the vagina and perineum

15. WR CV WR CV S
    episi/o/perine/o/plasty
        CF   CF
    surgical repair of the vulva and
    perineum

16. WR   S
    hymen/ectomy
    excision of the hymen

17.   WR CV WR CV   WR   S
hyster/o/salping/o/-oophor/ectomy
         CF   CF
excision of the uterus, uterine tubes,
and ovaries

18.   WR   S
hyster/ectomy
excision of the uterus

19.   WR CV S
*mamm/o/*plasty
         CF
surgical repair of the breast

20. WR CV S
*mast/o/*pexy
        CF
surgical fixation of the breast

21. WR CV   S
*culd/o/*centesis
         CF
surgical puncture to aspirate fluid
from the Douglas cul-de-sac

Exercise 17

1. colp/o/rrhaphy
2. cervic/ectomy
3. episi/o/rrhaphy
4. episi/o/perine/o/plasty
5. colp/o/plasty
6. colp/o/perine/o/rrhaphy
7. hyster/o/salping/o/-oophor/ectomy
8. hyster/o/pexy
9. hymen/ectomy
10. hymen/o/tomy
11. hyster/ectomy
12. oophor/ectomy
13. mast/ectomy
14. salping/ectomy
15. perine/o/rrhaphy
16. salping/o/-oophor/ectomy
17. salping/o/stomy
18. vulv/ectomy
19. mamm/o/plasty
20. mast/o/pexy
21. culd/o/centesis

Exercise 18
Spelling Exercise; see text p. 315.

Exercise 19
Pronunciation Exercise

Exercise 20

1. tubal ligation
2. anterior and posterior colporrhaphy
3. dilation and curettage
4. stereotactic breast biopsy
5. myomectomy
6. endometrial ablation
7. uterine artery embolization

8. conization
9. sentinel lymph node biopsy
10. laparoscopy or laparoscopic surgery

Exercise 21

1. c	6. f
2. a	7. h
3. a	8. c
4. b	9. g
5. c	10. c

Exercise 22
Spelling Exercise; see text p. 320.

Exercise 23
Pronunciation Exercise

Exercise 24
*Note: The combining form is identified by
italic and bold print.*

1. WR CV S
*colp/o/*scopy
         CF
visual examination of the vagina

2. WR CV S
*mamm/o/*gram
          CF
radiographic image of the breast

3. WR CV S
*colp/o/*scope
         CF
instrument used for visual
examination of the vagina

4. WR CV S
*hyster/o/*scopy
          CF
visual examination of the uterus

5. WR CV WR CV S
*hyster/o/salping/o/*gram
         CF   CF
radiographic image of the uterus and
uterine tubes

6. WR CV S
*culd/o/*scope
         CF
instrument used for visual
examination of the Douglas
cul-de-sac

7. WR CV S
*culd/o/*scopy
         CF
visual examination of the Douglas
cul-de-sac

8. WR CV S
*mamm/o/*graphy
          CF
radiographic imaging of the breast

9. WR CV S
*hyster/o/*scope
          CF
instrument used for visual
examination of the uterus

10. WR CV WR CV   S
*son/o/hyster/o/*graphy
       CF   CF
process of recording the uterus with
sound

Exercise 25

1. hyster/o/salping/o/gram
2. colp/o/scopy
3. colp/o/scope
4. hyster/o/scopy
5. mamm/o/gram
6. culd/o/scope
7. culd/o/scopy
8. hyster/o/scope
9. mamm/o/graphy
10. son/o/hyster/o/graphy

Exercise 26
Spelling Exercise; see text p. 324.

Exercise 27
Pronunciation Exercise

Exercise 28

1. cytological study of cervical and
vaginal secretions used to determine
the presence of abnormal or
cancerous cells
2. ultrasound procedure that obtains
images of the ovaries, uterus, cervix,
and uterine tubes
3. blood test used to detect and
monitor treatment of ovarian cancer

Exercise 29

1. Pap smear
2. CA-125
3. transvaginal sonography

Exercise 30
Spelling Exercise; see text p. 326.

Exercise 31
Pronunciation Exercise

Exercise 32
*Note: The combining form is identified by
italic and bold print.*

1. WR CV S
*gynec/o/*logist
          CF
physician who studies and treats
(diseases of) women

2. WR CV S
   ***gynec/o*/logy**
      CF
   study of women (branch of medicine dealing with health and diseases of the female reproductive system)

3. WR CV WR S
   ***vulv/o*/vagin/al**
      CF
   pertaining to the vulva and vagina

4. WR   S
   mast/algia
   pain in the breast

5. WR   WR
   men/arche
   beginning of menstruation

6. WR CV S
   ***leuk/o*/rrhea**
      CF
   white discharge (from the vagina)

7. WR CV WR S
   ***gyn/o*/path/ic**
      CF
   pertaining to diseases of women

8. WR CV S
   ***mast/o*/ptosis**
      CF
   sagging breast

9. WR   S
   vagin/al
   pertaining to the vagina

Exercise 33
1. leuk/o/rrhea
2. men/arche
3. mast/algia
4. vulv/o/vagin/al
5. gynec/o/logist
6. gynec/o/logy
7. mast/o/ptosis
8. gyn/o/path/ic
9. vagin/al

Exercise 34
Spelling Exercise; see text p. 328.

Exercise 35
Pronunciation Exercise

Exercise 36
1. cessation of menstruation
2. difficult or painful intercourse
3. abnormal passageway between two organs or between an internal organ and the body surface
4. syndrome involving physical and emotional symptoms occurring during the 10 days before menstruation
5. instrument for opening a body cavity to allow for visual inspection
6. replacement of hormones to treat symptoms associated with menopause
7. intentional prevention of conception

Exercise 37
1. fistula
2. dyspareunia
3. menopause
4. premenstrual syndrome
5. speculum
6. hormone replacement therapy
7. contraception

Exercise 38
Spelling Exercise; see text p. 331.

Exercise 39
1. anterior and posterior colporrhaphy
2. total abdominal hysterectomy and bilateral salpingo-oophorectomy; hormone replacement therapy
3. sonohysterography and transvaginal sonography
4. total vaginal hysterectomy; laparoscopically assisted vaginal hysterectomy
5. dilation and curettage; cervix
6. fibrocystic breast condition

7. pelvic inflammatory disease; gynecology
8. premenstrual syndrome
9. uterine artery embolization
10. intrauterine device; birth control

Exercise 40
A.
1. mammography
2. carcinoma
3. hysterectomy
4. adenomyosis
5. endometriosis
6. HRT
7. stereotactic breast biopsy
8. mediolateral
9. mastectomy
10. sentinel lymph node biopsy

Exercise 40
B.
1. c
2. a
3. d

C. Online Exercise

Exercise 41
1. dysmenorrhea
2. endometritis
3. uterine tube
4. suture of the vulva
5. mammoplasty
6. uterus, uterine tubes, and ovaries
7. hematosalpinx
8. endometriosis
9. speculum
10. TSS
11. conization

Exercise 42
Reading Exercise

Exercise 43
1. b
2. *T*
3. *T*
4. d

Obstetrics and Neonatology

Outline

Objectives

Upon completion of this chapter you will be able to:

1 Identify organs and structures relating to pregnancy.

2 Define and spell word parts related to obstetrics and neonatology.

3 Define, pronounce, and spell disease and disorder terms related to obstetrics and neonatology.

4 Define, pronounce, and spell surgical and diagnostic terms related to obstetrics.

5 Define, pronounce, and spell complementary terms related to obstetrics and neonatology.

6 Interpret the meaning of abbreviations related to obstetrics and neonatology.

7 Interpret, read, and comprehend medical language in simulated medical statements, documents, and electronic health records.

ANATOMY

Obstetrics is the branch of medicine that deals with childbirth and the care of the mother before, during, and after birth. **Neonatology** is the branch of medicine that deals with the diagnosis and treatment of disorders of the newborn.

Terms Relating to Pregnancy

TERM	DEFINITION
gamete	mature germ cell, either sperm (male) or ovum (female)
ovulation	expulsion of a mature ovum from an ovary (Figure 9-1, *A*)
conception, or fertilization	beginning of pregnancy, when the sperm enters the ovum. Fertilization normally occurs in the uterine tubes (Figure 9-1, *A*).
zygote	cell formed by the union of the sperm and the ovum
embryo	unborn offspring in the stage of development from implantation of the zygote to the end of the eighth week of pregnancy. This period is characterized by rapid growth of the embryo.
fetus	unborn offspring from the beginning of the ninth week of pregnancy until birth (Figure 9-2)
gestation, pregnancy	development of a new individual from conception to birth
gestation period	duration of pregnancy; normally 38 to 42 weeks, which can be divided into three equal periods, called *trimesters*
implantation	embedding of the zygote in the uterine lining. The process normally begins about 7 days after fertilization and continues for several days (see Figure 9-1, *A*).
placenta, or afterbirth	a structure that grows on the wall of the uterus during pregnancy and allows for nourishment of the unborn child (see Figure 9-1, *B*)
amniotic, or amnionic, sac	membranous bag that surrounds the fetus before delivery (also called **bag of waters**) (see Figure 9-1, *B*)
chorion	outermost layer of the fetal membrane
amnion	innermost layer of the fetal membrane
amniotic, or amnionic, fluid	fluid within the amniotic sac, which surrounds the fetus

SKIN CHANGES THAT OCCUR THROUGHOUT PREGNANCY

- **striae gravidarum**: "stretch marks" occurring on the abdomen, breast, buttocks, and thighs from weakening of elastic tissues
- **linea nigra**: dark medial line extending from the pubis upward
- **chloasma**: hyperpigmentation of blotchy brown macules usually evenly distributed over the cheeks and forehead

---

A & P Booster

For students desiring more anatomy and physiology, go to evolve.elsevier.com.
Select: **Extra Content**, A & P Booster, Chapter 9.

Refer to p. 10 for your Evolve Access Information.

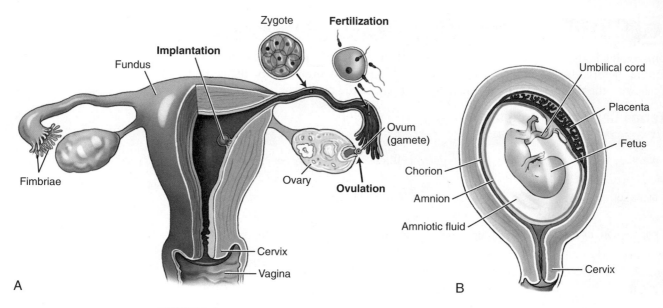

FIGURE 9-1
A, Ovulation, fertilization, and implantation. **B,** Development of the fetus.

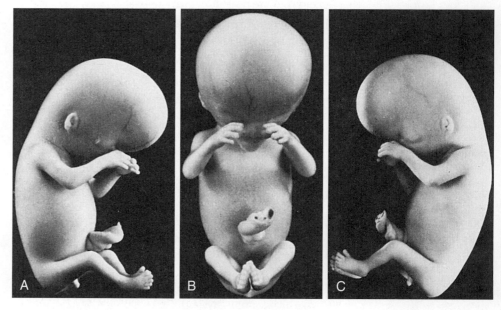

FIGURE 9-2
Human male fetus at 68 days (1.85 inches, 47 mm). **A,** Right. **B,** Frontal. **C,** Left.

EXERCISE 1

Fill in the blanks with the correct terms. *To check your answers to the exercises in this chapter, go to Answers, p. 380, at the end of the chapter.*

1. The expulsion of a mature ovum, or _____, from an ovary is called _____. When the male gamete enters the female gamete, _____ occurs, and a(n) _____ is formed. This marks the beginning of the _____ period.

2. Once the zygote is implanted, it becomes a(n) _____ until the end of the eighth week of gestation. The unborn offspring from the beginning of the ninth week until birth is called a(n) _____.

3. The fetus is surrounded by a(n) _____ sac, which has an outermost layer, called the _____, and an innermost layer, called the _____. This sac contains the _____ fluid that surrounds the fetus.

WORD PARTS

Combining Forms of Obstetrics and Neonatology

Word parts you need to learn to complete this chapter are listed on the following pages. The exercises at the end of each list will help you learn their definitions and spelling.

> ☼ Use the flashcards accompanying this text or electronic flashcards to assist you in memorizing the word parts for this chapter.

> ℮ To use electronic flashcards, go to evolve.elsevier.com. Select: Chapter 9, **Flashcards**.
>
> Refer to p. 10 for your Evolve Access Information.

COMBINING FORM	DEFINITION
amni/o, amnion/o	amnion, amniotic fluid
chori/o	chorion
embry/o	embryo, to be full (Figure 9-3)
fet/o, fet/i *(NOTE: both* i *and* o *may be used as combining vowels with* fet/*)*	fetus, unborn child
gravid/o	pregnancy
lact/o	milk
nat/o	birth
omphal/o	umbilicus, navel
par/o, part/o	bear, give birth to, labor, childbirth
puerper/o	childbirth

Em + bruo = embyro

in + 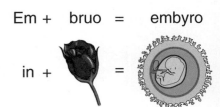 =

FIGURE 9-3
Embryo comes from the Greek ***em,*** meaning "in," plus ***bruo,*** meaning "to bud" or "to shoot."

> 🏛 **PUERPER**
> is made up of two Latin word roots: **puer,** meaning **child,** and **per,** meaning **through.**

EXERCISE FIGURE **A**

Fill in the blanks with combining forms in this diagram of fetal development. *To check your answers, go to p. 380.*

1. Umbilicus

CF: _____

2. Fetus

CF: _____

CF: _____

Umbilical cord

Placenta

3. Amnion

CF: _____

Amniotic fluid

CF: _____

4. Chorion

CF: _____

EXERCISE **2**

Write the definitions of the following combining forms.

1. fet/o, fet/i _____
2. lact/o _____
3. par/o, part/o _____
4. omphal/o _____
5. amni/o, amnion/o _____
6. puerper/o _____
7. gravid/o _____
8. nat/o _____
9. chori/o _____
10. embry/o _____

EXERCISE **3**

Write the combining form for each of the following terms.

1. milk _____
2. fetus   a._____
         b. _____
3. chorion _____
4. amnion, amniotic fluid

   a. _____
   b. _____
5. childbirth _____
6. bear, give birth to, labor, childbirth

   a. _____
   b. _____

7. pregnancy _____

8. embryo _____

9. birth_____

10. umbilicus, navel _____

Combining Forms Commonly Used in Obstetrics and Neonatology

COMBINING FORM	DEFINITION
cephal/o	head
esophag/o	esophagus (tube leading from the throat to the stomach) (see Figure 11-1)
pelv/o, pelv/i (Note: both i and o may be used as the combining vowel with pelv/)	pelvic bone, pelvis (see Chapter 14, Exercise Figure A and Exercise Figure B)
prim/i (Note: the combining vowel is i.)	first
pseud/o	false
pylor/o	pylorus (pyloric sphincter) (see Figure 11-2)
terat/o	malformations

TERAT/O

is translated literally as **monster**; however, in terms containing terat/o relating to obstetrics, terat/o refers to malformations or abnormal development.

EXERCISE 4

Write the definition of the following combining forms.

1. prim/i_____

2. pylor/o_____

3. cephal/o_____

4. esophag/o _____

5. pseud/o _____

6. pelv/o, pelv/i_____

7. terat/o _____

EXERCISE 5

Write the combining form for each of the following.

1. head _____

2. pylorus_____

3. false _____

4. esophagus _____

5. first_____

6. malformations_____

7. pelvic bone, pelvis   a. _____

                                   b._____

Prefixes

PREFIX	DEFINITION
ante-, pre-	before
micro-	small
multi-	many
nulli-	none
post-	after

EXERCISE 6

Write the definitions of the following prefixes.

1. post-_____

2. multi-_____

3. nulli- _____

4. micro- _____

5. ante-_____

6. pre- _____

EXERCISE 7

Write the prefix for each of the following definitions.

1. none_____

2. small_____

3. many _____

4. before   a. _____

    b. _____

5. after _____

Suffixes

SUFFIX	DEFINITION
-amnios	amnion, amniotic fluid
-cyesis	pregnancy
-e	noun suffix, no meaning
-is	noun suffix, no meaning
-rrhexis	rupture
-tocia	birth, labor
-um	noun suffix, no meaning
-us	noun suffix, no meaning

-RRHEXIS

is the last of the four **-rrh** suffixes to be learned. The other three introduced in earlier chapters are:

-rrhea—flow or discharge

-rrhagia—rapid flow (of blood)

-rrhaphy—suturing, repairing

 The noun suffix **-a**, introduced in Chapter 4, also has no meaning.

 Refer to **Appendix A** and **Appendix B** for alphabetized word parts and their meanings.

EXERCISE 8

Write the definitions of the following suffixes.

1. -rrhexis _____

2. -tocia _____

3. -cyesis _____

4. -amnios _____

EXERCISE 9

Write the suffix for each of the following definitions.

1. birth, labor _____

2. rupture_____

3. pregnancy _____

4. amnion, amniotic fluid_____

For review and/or assessment, go to evolve.elsevier.com. Select:
Chapter 9, **Activities**, Word Parts
Chapter 9, **Games**,   Name that Word Part

Refer to p. 10 for your Evolve Access Information.

EXERCISE 10

Write the noun suffixes introduced in this chapter that have no meaning.

1. _____

2. _____

3. _____

4. _____

MEDICAL TERMS

The terms you need to learn to complete this chapter are listed next. The exercises following each list will help you learn the definition and the spelling of each word.

Obstetric Disease and Disorder Terms

Built from Word Parts

The following terms are built from word parts you have already learned and can be translated literally to find their meanings. Further explanation of terms beyond the definition of their word parts, if needed, is included in parentheses.

DYSTOCIA

Difficult labor, or labor that is abnormally long or dysfunctional, occurs in approximately 10% of all births. Causes for **dystocia** may be from maternal factors such as ineffective uterine contractions, or abnormal pelvic shape; or from fetal causes such as large size or abnormal birth presentation. Cultural factors and support systems also may contribute to dystocia.

TERM	DEFINITION
amnionitis (*am*-nē-ō-NĪ-tis)	inflammation of the amnion
chorioamnionitis (*kor*-ē-ō-*am*-nē-ō-NĪ-tis)	inflammation of the chorion and amnion
choriocarcinoma (*kor*-ē-ō-*kar*-si-NŌ-ma)	cancerous tumor of the chorion
dystocia (dis-TŌ-sha)	difficult labor
hysterorrhexis (*his*-ter-ō-REK-sis)	rupture of the uterus
oligohydramnios (*ol*-i-gō-hī-DRAM-nē-os)	scanty amnion water (less than the normal amount of amniotic fluid; 500 mL or less)
polyhydramnios (*pol*-ē-hī-DRAM-nē-os)	much amnion water (more than the normal amount of amniotic fluid; 2000 mL or more) (also called **hydramnios**)

 CAM TERM

Acupressure is the ancient practice of applying finger pressure to specific acapoints on the body to preserve and restore health. Studies suggest that acupressure on specific acupoints may reduce the duration and severity of pain during labor, as well as relieve nausea during pregnancy.

To watch animations, go to evolve.elsevier.com. Select:
Chapter 9, **Animations**, Dystocia Delivery
                        Chorioamnionitis

Refer to p. 10 for your Evolve Access Information.

EXERCISE 11

Practice saying aloud each of the obstetric disease and disorder terms built from word parts above.

To hear the terms, go to evolve.elsevier.com. Select: Chapter 9, **Exercises**, Pronunciation.

Refer to p. 10 for your Evolve access information.

☐ Place a check mark in the box when you have completed this exercise.

EXERCISE 12

Analyze and define the following disease and disorder terms.

1. chorioamnionitis_____
2. choriocarcinoma_____
3. dystocia _____
4. amnionitis _____
5. hysterorrhexis_____
6. oligohydramnios_____
7. polyhydramnios _____

EXERCISE 13

Build disease and disorder terms for the following definitions by using the word parts you have learned.

1. cancerous tumor of the chorion

    WR   / CV /   WR   /   S

2. inflammation of the amnion

    WR   /   S

3. inflammation of the chorion and amnion

    WR   / CV /   WR   /   S

4. difficult labor

    P   /   S(WR)

5. rupture of the uterus

    WR   / CV /   S

6. scanty amnion water (less than normal amniotic fluid)

    WR   / CV /   WR   /   S

7. much amnion water (more than normal amniotic fluid)

    P   /   WR   /   S

EXERCISE 14

Spell each of the obstetric disease and disorder terms built from word parts on p. 352 by having someone dictate them to you.

> To hear and spell the terms, go to evolve.elsevier.com. Select: Chapter 9, **Exercises**, Spelling.
>
> Refer to p. 10 for your Evolve Access Information.
>
> ☐ Place a check mark in the box if you have completed this exercise online.

1. _____   5. _____

2. _____   6. _____

3. _____   7. _____

4. _____

Obstetric Disease and Disorder Terms

Not Built from Word Parts

In some of the following terms you may recognize word parts you have already learned; however, the full meaning of the terms cannot be discerned by the definition of their word parts.

TERM	DEFINITION
abortion (AB) (a-BŌR-shun)	termination of pregnancy by the expulsion from the uterus of an embryo or fetus before viability, usually before 20 weeks of gestation

TYPES OF ABORTION

Spontaneous abortion is the termination of pregnancy that occurs naturally. It is commonly referred to as *miscarriage*.

Induced abortion is the intentional termination of pregnancy by surgical or medical intervention.

Therapeutic abortion is an induced abortion performed because of health risks to the mother or for fetal disease.

Elective abortion is an induced abortion performed at the request of the woman.

Obstetric Disease and Disorder Terms—cont'd

Not Built from Word Parts

TERM	DEFINITION
abruptio placentae (ab-RUP-shē-ō) (pla-SEN-tē)	premature separation of the placenta from the uterine wall (Figure 9-5, *A*)
eclampsia (e-KLAMP-sē-a)	severe complication and progression of preeclampsia characterized by convulsion (see *preeclampsia* on the next page). Eclampsia is a potentially life-threatening disorder.
ectopic pregnancy (ek-TOP-ik) (PREG-nan-sē)	pregnancy occurring outside the uterus, commonly in the uterine tubes (Figure 9-4)
placenta previa (pla-SEN-ta) (PRĒ-vē-a)	abnormally low implantation of the placenta on the uterine wall completely or partially covering the cervix. (Dilation of the cervix can cause separation of the placenta from the uterine wall, resulting in bleeding. With severe hemorrhage, a cesarean section may be necessary to save the mother's life.) (Figure 9-5, *B*)

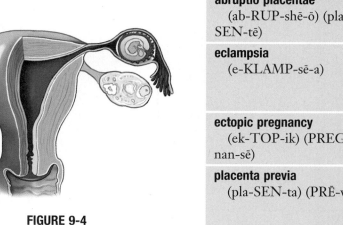

FIGURE 9-4
Ectopic pregnancy.

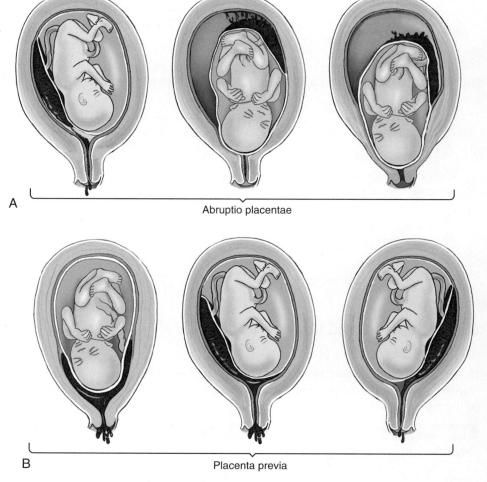

A — Abruptio placentae

B — Placenta previa

FIGURE 9-5
Various presentations of abruptio placentae **(A)** and placenta previa **(B)**.

TERM	DEFINITION
preeclampsia (prē-ē-KLAMP-sē-a)	abnormal condition encountered during pregnancy or shortly after delivery characterized by high blood pressure, edema, and proteinuria, but with no convulsions. The cause is unknown; if not successfully treated, the condition can progress to eclampsia. Eclampsia is the third most common cause of maternal death in the United States after hemorrhage and infection.

To watch animations, go to evolve.elsevier.com. Select:
Chapter 9, **Animations**, Abruptio Placentae
                    Ectopic Pregnancy
                    Placenta Previa

Refer to p. 10 for your Evolve Access Information.

EXERCISE 15

Practice saying aloud each of the obstetric disease and disorder terms not built from word parts on pp. 353–355.

To hear the terms, go to evolve.elsevier.com. Select: Chapter 9, **Exercises**, Pronunciation.

Refer to p. 10 for your Evolve Access Information.

☐ Place a check mark in the box when you have completed this exercise.

EXERCISE 16

Write the definitions of the following terms.

1. abruptio placentae _____
2. abortion _____
3. placenta previa _____
4. eclampsia _____
5. ectopic pregnancy _____
6. preeclampsia _____

EXERCISE 17

Write the term for each of the following definitions.

1. premature separation of the placenta from the uterine wall _____

2. severe complication and progression of preeclampsia _____

3. termination of pregnancy by the expulsion from the uterus of an embryo or fetus _____

4. pregnancy occurring outside the uterus _____

5. abnormally low implantation of the placenta on the uterine wall _____

6. characterized by high blood pressure, edema, and proteinuria, but with no convulsions _____

EXERCISE 18

Spell each of the obstetric disease and disorder terms not built from word parts on pp. 353–355 by having someone dictate them to you.

To hear and spell the terms, go to evolve.elsevier.com. Select: Chapter 9, **Exercises**, Spelling.

Refer to p. 10 for your Evolve Access Information.

☐ Place a check mark in the box if you have completed this exercise online.

1. _____   4. _____

2. _____   5. _____

3. _____   6. _____

Neonatology Disease and Disorder Terms

Built from Word Parts

The following terms are built from word parts you have already learned and can be translated literally to find their meanings. Further explanation of terms beyond the definition of their word parts, if needed, is included in parentheses.

TERM	DEFINITION
microcephalus (*mī*-krō-SEF-a-lus)	(fetus with a very) small head
omphalitis (*om*-fa-LĬ-tis)	inflammation of the umbilicus
omphalocele (OM-fal-ō-*sēl*)	herniation at the umbilicus (a part of the intestine protrudes through the abdominal wall at birth) (Exercise Figure B)
pyloric stenosis (pī-LOR-ik) (ste-NŌ-sis)	narrowing pertaining to the pyloric sphincter. (Congenital pyloric stenosis occurs in 1 of every 200 newborns.)
tracheoesophageal fistula (*trā*-kē-ō-ē-*sof*-a-jĒ-al) (FIS-tū-la)	abnormal passageway pertaining to the trachea and esophagus (between the trachea and esophagus)

EXERCISE 19

Practice saying aloud each of the neonatology disease and disorder terms built from word parts above.

To hear the terms, go to evolve.elsevier.com. Select: Chapter 9, **Exercises**, Pronunciation.

Refer to p. 10 for your Evolve Access Information.

☐ Place a check mark in the box when you have completed this exercise.

EXERCISE FIGURE B

Fill in the blanks to label the diagram.

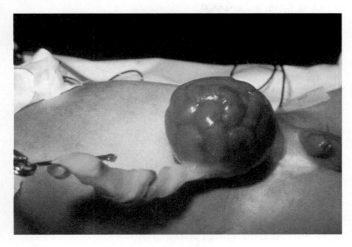

_____ / cv / _____

umbilicus / cv / herniation

EXERCISE 20

Analyze and define the following disease and disorder terms.

1. pyloric (stenosis)_____
2. omphalocele _____
3. omphalitis _____
4. microcephalus_____
5. tracheoesophageal (fistula) _____

EXERCISE 21

Build disease and disorder terms for the following definitions by using the word parts you have learned.

1. hernia at the umbilicus

     _____ / CV / _____
     WR   /CV/   S

2. (fetus with a very) small head

     _____ / _____ / _____
     P   WR   S

3. (narrowing) pertaining to the pyloric sphincter

     _____ / _____ stenosis
     WR   S

4. abnormal passageway pertaining to the trachea and the esophagus (between the trachea and esophagus)

     _____ /CV/ _____ / _____ fistula
     WR   /CV/   WR   S

5. inflammation of the umbilicus

     _____ / _____
     WR   S

EXERCISE 22

Spell each of the neonatology disease and disorder terms built from word parts on p. 356 by having someone dictate them to you.

> To hear and spell the terms, go to evolve.elsevier.com. Select: Chapter 9, **Exercises**, Spelling.
>
> ⓔ Refer to p. 10 for your Evolve Access Information.
>
> ☐ Place a check mark in the box if you have completed this exercise online.

1. _____   4. _____

2. _____   5. _____

3. _____

Neonatology Disease and Disorder Terms

Not Built from Word Parts

In some of the following terms you may recognize word parts you have already learned; however, the full meaning of the terms cannot be discerned by the definition of their word parts.

TERM	DEFINITION
cleft lip or palate (kleft) (lip) (PAL-at)	congenital split of the lip or roof of the mouth, one or both deformities may be present (*cleft* indicates a fissure) (Figure 9-7)
Down syndrome (down) (SIN-drōm)	genetic condition caused by a chromosomal abnormality characterized by varying degrees of intelligence, developmental, and physical disorders or defects (also called **Trisomy** 21) (Figure 9-6)

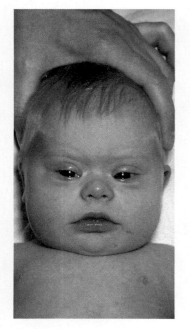

FIGURE 9-6
Neonate with Down syndrome.

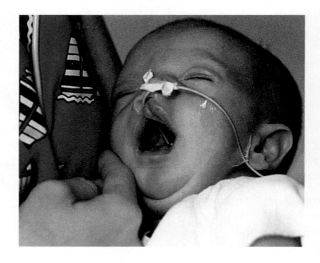

FIGURE 9-7
Unilateral cleft lip. Note the nasogastric feeding tube in place. Neonates born with a cleft lip, palate, or both may require assistive feeding due to an impaired ability to suck.

TERM	DEFINITION
erythroblastosis fetalis (e-*rith*-rō-blas-TŌ-sis) (fē-TAL-is)	condition of the newborn characterized by hemolysis of the erythrocytes. The condition is usually caused by incompatibility of the infant's and mother's blood, occurring when the mother's blood is Rh negative and the infant's blood is Rh positive.
esophageal atresia (e-*sof*-a-JĒ-al) (a-TRĒ-zha)	congenital absence of part of the esophagus. Food cannot pass from the baby's mouth to the stomach (Figure 9-8).
fetal alcohol syndrome (FAS) (FĒ-tal) (AL-kō-hol) (SIN-drōm)	condition caused by excessive alcohol consumption by the mother during pregnancy. Various birth defects may be present, including central nervous system dysfunction and malformations of the skull and face.
gastroschisis (gas-TROS-ki-sis)	congenital fissure of the abdominal wall not at the umbilicus. Enterocele, protrusion of the intestine, is usually present (Figure 9-9).
respiratory distress syndrome (RDS) (RES-pi-ra-*tōr*-ē) (di-STRESS) (SIN-drōm)	respiratory complication in the newborn, especially in premature infants. In premature infants RDS is caused by normal immaturity of the respiratory system resulting in compromised respiration (formerly called **hyaline membrane disease**).
spina bifida (SPĪ-na) (BIF-i-da)	congenital defect in the vertebral column caused by the failure of the vertebral arch to close. If the meninges protrude through the opening the condition is called meningocele. Protrusion of both the meninges and spinal cord is called meningomyelocele. Both terms are covered in Chapter 15 (Figure 9-10).

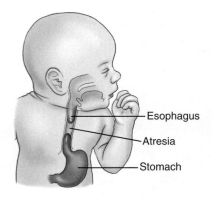

FIGURE 9-8
Esophageal atresia.

BIRTHMARKS

are benign discolorations in the neonate's skin. Common birthmarks include **Congenital dermal melanocytosis**, which are bluish-black areas of hyperpigmentation often found on the lower back or buttocks of darker-skinned neonates, and **hemangiomas**, which are various benign vascular tumors or stains that cause reddish discoloration and/or malformations of the skin surface.

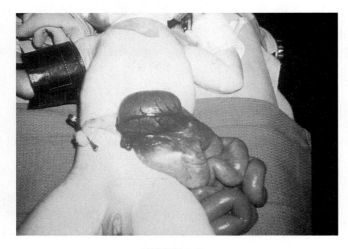

FIGURE 9-9
Gastroschisis.

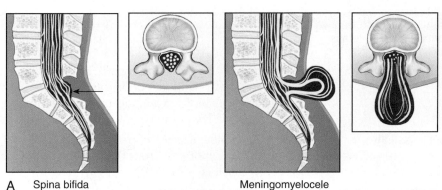

A   Spina bifida   Meningomyelocele

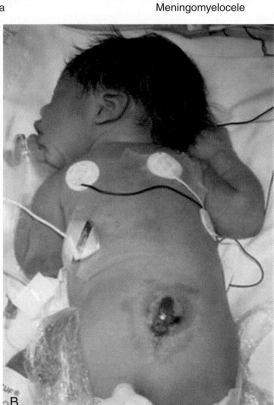

B

FIGURE 9-10
A, Drawings of spina bifida and meningomyelocele. **B,** Photograph of meningomyelocele.

EXERCISE 23

Practice saying aloud each of the neonatology disease and disorder terms not built from word parts found on pp. 358–359.

To hear the terms, go to evolve.elsevier.com. Select: Chapter 9, **Exercises,** Pronunciation.

Refer to p. 10 for your Evolve Access Information.

☐ Place a check mark in the box when you have completed this exercise.

EXERCISE 24

Match the terms in the first column with their correct definitions in the second column.

_____ 1. Down syndrome

_____ 2. cleft lip or palate

_____ 3. spina bifida

_____ 4. erythroblastosis fetalis

_____ 5. fetal alcohol syndrome

_____ 6. respiratory distress syndrome

_____ 7. esophageal atresia

_____ 8. gastroschisis

a. defect of the vertebral column

b. respiratory complication of neonates

c. split of the lip or roof of the mouth

d. caused by incompatibility of the infant's and the mother's blood

e. congenital fissure of the abdominal wall

f. genetic condition caused by chromosomal abnormality

g. congenital absence of part of the esophagus

h. causes various birth defects, including central nervous system dysfunction

EXERCISE 25

Spell each of the neonatal disease and disorder terms not built from word parts on pp. 358–359 by having someone dictate them to you.

> To hear and spell the terms, go to evolve.elsevier.com. Select: Chapter 9, **Exercises**, Spelling.
>
> Refer to p. 10 for your Evolve Access Information.
>
> ☐ Place a check mark in the box if you have completed this exercise online.

1. _____

2. _____

3. _____

4. _____

5. _____

6. _____

7. _____

8. _____

Obstetric Surgical Terms

Built from Word Parts

The following terms are built from word parts you have already learned and can be translated literally to find their meanings. Further explanation of terms beyond the definition of their word parts, if needed, is included in parentheses.

TERM	DEFINITION
amniotomy (_am_-nē-OT-o-mē)	incision into the amnion (rupture of the fetal membrane to induce labor; a special hook is generally used to make the incision)
episiotomy (e-_piz_-ē-OT-o-mē)	incision into the vulva (perineum) (sometimes performed during delivery to prevent a traumatic tear of the vulva) (also called **perineotomy**) (Figure 9-11)

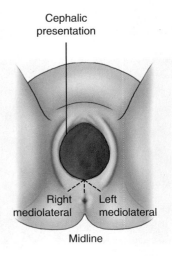

Cephalic presentation

Right mediolateral   Left mediolateral

Midline

FIGURE 9-11
Episiotomies.

Obstetric Diagnostic Terms
Built from Word Parts

TERM	DEFINITION
DIAGNOSTIC IMAGING	
pelvic sonography (PEL-vik) (so-NOG-ra-fē)	pertaining to the pelvis, process of recording sound (pelvic ultrasound is used extensively to evaluate the fetus and pregnancy) (also called **pelvic ultrasonography, pelvic ultrasound,** and **obstetric ultrasonography**) (Figure 9-12)
OTHER	
amniocentesis (*am*-nē-ō-sen-TĒ-sis)	surgical puncture to aspirate amniotic fluid (the needle is inserted through the abdominal and uterine walls, using ultrasound to guide the needle. The fluid is used for the assessment of fetal health and maturity to aid in diagnosing fetal abnormalities.) (Figure 9-13).
amnioscope (AM-nē-ō-*skōp*)	instrument used for visual examination of the amniotic fluid (and the fetus)
amnioscopy (*am*-nē-OS-ko-pē)	visual examination of amniotic fluid (and the fetus)

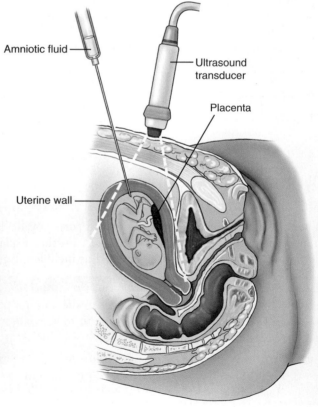

Amniotic fluid

Ultrasound transducer

Placenta

Uterine wall

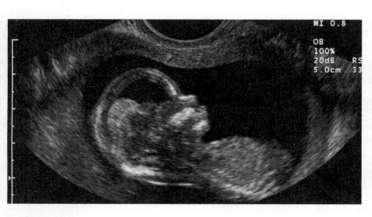

FIGURE 9-12
Pelvic sonography image showing a fetal profile. Some specific uses are to: (1) diagnose early abnormal pregnancy, (2) determine the age of the fetus, (3) measure fetal growth, and (4) determine fetal position.

FIGURE 9-13
Amniocentesis. Ultrasound is used to guide the needle through the abdominal and uterine walls.

EXERCISE 26

Practice saying aloud each of the obstetric surgical and diagnostic terms built from word parts on pp. 361–362.

 To hear the terms, go to evolve.elsevier.com. Select: Chapter 9, **Exercises**, Pronunciation.

Refer to p. 10 for your Evolve Access Information.

☐ Place a check mark in the box when you have completed this exercise.

EXERCISE 27

Analyze and define the following obstetric surgical and diagnostic terms.

1. episiotomy _____

2. amniotomy _____

3. amnioscope _____

4. pelvic sonography _____

5. amniocentesis _____

6. amnioscopy _____

EXERCISE 28

Build obstetric surgical and diagnostic terms for the following definitions by using the word parts you have learned.

1. incision into the amnion

   _____ / ____ / _____
   WR   CV   S

2. incision into the vulva

   _____ / ____ / _____
   WR   CV   S

3. visual examination of the amniotic fluid (and fetus)

   _____ / ____ / _____
   WR   CV   S

4. surgical puncture to aspirate amniotic fluid

   _____ / ____ / _____
   WR   CV   S

5. instrument used for visual examination of the amniotic fluid (and fetus)

   _____ / ____ / _____
   WR   CV   S

6. pertaining to the pelvis, process of recording sound

   _____ / _____
   WR   S

   _____ / ____ / _____
   WR   CV   S

EXERCISE 29

Spell each of the obstetric surgical and diagnostic terms built from word parts on pp. 361–362 by having someone dictate them to you.

> To hear and spell the terms, go to evolve.elsevier.com. Select: Chapter 9, **Exercises**, Spelling.
>
> Refer to p. 10 for your Evolve Access Information.
>
> ☐ Place a check mark in the box if you have completed this exercise online.

1. _____   4. _____
2. _____   5. _____
3. _____   6. _____

Obstetric and Neonatal Complementary Terms

Built from Word Parts

The following terms are built from word parts you have already learned and can be translated literally to find their meanings. Further explanation of terms beyond the definition of their word parts, if needed, is included in parentheses.

TERM	DEFINITION
amniochorial (am-nē-ō-KOR-ē-al)	pertaining to the amnion and chorion
amniorrhea (am-nē-ō-RĒ-a)	discharge (escape) of amniotic fluid
amniorrhexis (am-nē-ō-REK-sis)	rupture of the amnion
antepartum (an-tē-PAR-tum)	before childbirth (reference to the mother)
embryogenic (em-brē-ō-JEN-ik)	producing an embryo
embryoid (EM-brē-oyd)	resembling an embryo
fetal (FĒ-tal)	pertaining to the fetus
gravida (GRAV-i-da)	pregnant (woman); (a woman who is or has been pregnant, regardless of pregnancy outcome)
gravidopuerperal (grav-i-dō-pū-ER-per-al)	pertaining to pregnancy and childbirth (from delivery until reproductive organs return to normal)
intrapartum (in-tra-PAR-tum)	within (during) labor and childbirth
lactic (LAK-tik)	pertaining to milk
lactogenic (lak-tō-JEN-ik)	producing milk (by stimulation)
lactorrhea (lak-tō-RĒ-a)	(spontaneous) discharge of milk

TERM	DEFINITION
multigravida (*mul*-ti-GRAV-i-da)	many pregnancies (a woman who has been pregnant two or more times)
multipara (multip) (mul-TIP-a-ra)	many births (a woman who has given birth to two or more viable offspring)
natal (NĀ-tal)	pertaining to birth
neonate (NĒ-ō-nāt)	new birth (an infant from birth to 4 weeks of age) (synonymous with **newborn [NB]**) (Exercise Figure C)
neonatologist (nē-ō-nā-TOL-o-jist)	physician who studies and treats disorders of the newborn
neonatology (nē-ō-nā-TOL-o-jē)	study of the newborn (branch of medicine that deals with diagnosis and treatment of disorders in newborns)
nulligravida (*nul*-li-GRAV-i-da)	no pregnancies (a woman who has never been pregnant)
nullipara (nu-LIP-a-ra)	no births (a woman who has not given birth to a viable offspring)
para (PAR-a)	birth (a woman who has given birth to an offspring after the point of viability—20 weeks, whether the fetus is alive or stillborn) (Figure 9-14)
postnatal (pōst-NĀ-tal)	pertaining to after birth (reference to the newborn)
postpartum (pōst-PAR-tum)	after childbirth (reference to the mother)
prenatal (prē-NĀ-tal)	pertaining to before birth (reference to the newborn)

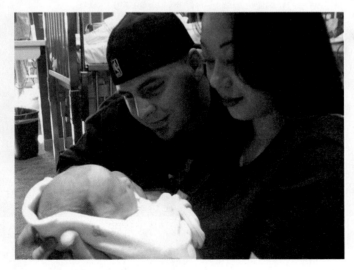

FIGURE 9-14
New mother **(para)** and father hold their **neonate.**

Obstetric and Neonatal Complementary Terms—cont'd

Built from Word Parts

TERM	DEFINITION
primigravida (prī-mi-GRAV-i-da)	first pregnancy (a woman in her first pregnancy)
primipara (primip) (*prī*-MIP-a-ra)	first birth (a woman who has given birth to an offspring after the point of viability—20 weeks)
pseudocyesis (*sū*-dō-sī-Ē-sis)	false pregnancy (a woman who believes she is pregnant—this may be a psychological condition or related to underlying pathology, such as a uterine tumor)
puerpera (pū-ER-per-a)	childbirth (a woman who has just given birth)
puerperal (pū-ER-per-al)	pertaining to (immediately after) childbirth
teratogen (TER-a-tō-jen)	(any agent) producing malformations (in the developing embryo). Teratogens include chemical agents such as drugs, alcohol, viruses, x-rays, and environmental factors.
teratogenic (*ter*-a-tō-JEN-ik)	producing malformations (in the developing embryo)
teratology (*ter*-a-TOL-o-jē)	study of malformations (usually in regard to malformations caused by teratogens on the developing embryo)

APGAR SCORE

Developed in 1952 by Virginia Apgar, MD, the Apgar score provides a basic framework for rapid neonatal assessment by health care providers at 1 minute and 5 minutes after birth. Five vital criteria (**heart rate, respiration, muscle tone, response to stimulation,** and **color**) are assessed and scored on a 0 to 2 scale. The score is totaled, with a 5-minute Apgar score of 7 to 10 considered normal. The Apgar score is used only for quickly reporting a neonate's status and does not predict future health outcomes.

EXERCISE FIGURE **C**

Fill in the blanks to label the diagram.

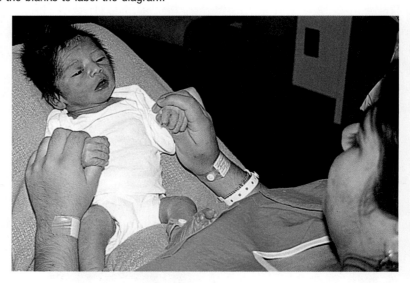

_____ / _____ / e
new / birth /

Terms Relating to Mother and Newborn

	BEFORE BIRTH	AFTER BIRTH
Mother	antepartum	postpartum
Newborn	prenatal	postnatal

Comparing Terms with gravid/o and par/o

GRAVID/O—PREGNANCY	PAR/O—BIRTH
nulli/gravid/a—no pregnancies	nulli/par/a—no births
primi/gravid/a—first pregnancy	primi/par/a—first birth
multi/gravid/a—many pregnancies	multi/par/a—many births

EXERCISE 30

Practice saying aloud each of the complementary terms built from word parts on pp. 364–366.

> To hear the terms, go to evolve.elsevier.com. Select: Chapter 9, **Exercises**, Pronunciation.
>
> Refer to p. 10 for your Evolve Access Information.

☐ Place a check mark in the box when you have completed this exercise.

EXERCISE 31

Analyze and define the following obstetric and neonatal complementary terms.

1. puerpera _____
2. amniorrhexis _____
3. antepartum _____
4. pseudocyesis _____
5. prenatal _____
6. lactic _____
7. lactorrhea _____
8. amniorrhea _____
9. multipara _____
10. embryogenic _____
11. embryoid _____
12. fetal _____
13. gravida _____
14. amniochorial _____
15. multigravida _____
16. lactogenic _____
17. natal _____
18. gravidopuerperal _____
19. neonatology _____
20. nullipara _____
21. para _____
22. primigravida _____
23. postpartum _____

24. neonate _____
25. primipara_____
26. puerperal _____
27. nulligravida _____
28. intrapartum _____
29. teratogen _____
30. postnatal _____
31. teratology _____
32. neonatologist _____
33. teratogenic _____

EXERCISE 32

Build the complementary terms for the following definitions by using the word parts you have learned.

1. pertaining to the amnion and chorion

_____ / ___ / _____ / ___
WR   CV   WR   S

2. before childbirth (reference to the mother)

_____ / _____ / ___
P   WR   S

3. producing an embryo

_____ / ___ / ___
WR   CV   S

4. pertaining to the fetus

_____ / ___
WR   S

5. pertaining to before birth (reference to the newborn)

_____ / _____ / ___
P   WR   S

6. pertaining to milk

_____ / ___
WR   S

7. (spontaneous) discharge of milk

_____ / ___ / ___
WR   CV   S

8. discharge (escape) of amniotic fluid

_____ / ___ / ___
WR   CV   S

9. false pregnancy

_____ / ___ / ___
WR   CV   S

10. producing milk (by stimulation)

_____ / ___ / ___
WR   CV   S

11. rupture of the amnion

_____ / ___ / ___
WR   CV   S

12. resembling an embryo

_____ / ___
WR   S

13. pregnant (woman)

_____ / ___
WR   S

14. pertaining to pregnancy and childbirth

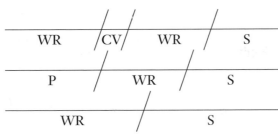

_____ / _____ / _____ / _____
WR   CV   WR   S

15. many births

_____ / _____ / _____
P   WR   S

16. pertaining to birth

_____ / _____
WR   S

17. new birth (an infant from birth to 4 weeks of age)

_____ / _____ / _____
P   WR   S

18. study of the newborn

_____ / _____ / _____ / _____
P   WR   CV   S

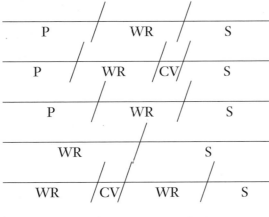

19. no births

_____ / _____ / _____
P   WR   S

20. birth

_____ / _____
WR   S

21. first pregnancy

_____ / _____ / _____ / _____
WR   CV   WR   S

22. after childbirth (reference to the mother)

_____ / _____ / _____
P   WR   S

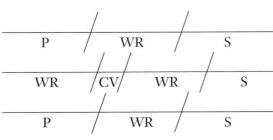

23. first birth

_____ / _____ / _____ / _____
WR   CV   WR   S

24. many pregnancies

_____ / _____ / _____
P   WR   S

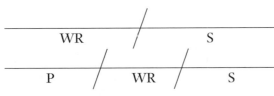

25. pertaining to (immediately after) childbirth

_____ / _____
WR   S

26. no pregnancies

_____ / _____ / _____
P   WR   S

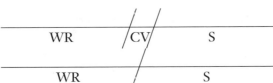

27. (any agent) producing malformations

_____ / _____ / _____
WR   CV   S

28. childbirth

_____ / _____
WR   S

29. within (during) labor and childbirth

_____ / _____ / _____
P   WR   S

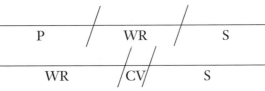

30. producing malformations

_____ / _____ / _____
WR   CV   S

31. physician who studies and treats disorders of the newborn

_____ / _____ / _____ / _____
P   WR   CV   S

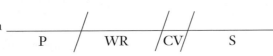

32. pertaining to after birth (reference to the newborn)

_____ / _____ / _____
P   WR   S

33. study of malformations

_____ / _____ / _____
WR   CV   S

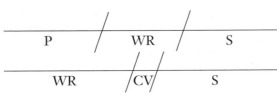

EXERCISE 33

Spell each of the complementary terms built from word parts on pp. 364–366 by having someone dictate them to you.

> To hear and spell the terms, go to evolve.elsevier.com. Select: Chapter 9, **Exercises**, Spelling.
>
> Refer to p. 10 for your Evolve Access Information.
>
> ☐ Place a check mark in the box if you have completed this exercise online.

1. _____
2. _____
3. _____
4. _____
5. _____
6. _____
7. _____
8. _____
9. _____
10. _____
11. _____
12. _____
13. _____
14. _____
15. _____
16. _____
17. _____

18. _____
19. _____
20. _____
21. _____
22. _____
23. _____
24. _____
25. _____
26. _____
27. _____
28. _____
29. _____
30. _____
31. _____
32. _____
33. _____

> For review and/or assessment, go to evolve.elsevier.com. Select:
> Chapter 9, **Activities**, Terms Built from Word Parts
> Chapter 9, **Games**, Term Storm
>
> Refer to p. 10 for your Evolve Access Information.

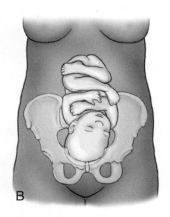

Breech presentation

Cephalic presentation

FIGURE 9-15
A, Breech presentation.
B, Cephalic presentation.

Obstetric and Neonatal Complementary Terms

Not Built from Word Parts

In some of the following terms you may recognize word parts you have already learned; however, the full meaning of the terms cannot be discerned by the definition of their word parts.

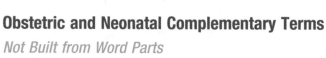

TERM	DEFINITION
breech presentation (brēch)	birth position in which the buttocks, feet, or knees emerge first (Figure 9-15, *A*)
cephalic presentation (se-FAL-ik)	birth position in which any part of the head emerges first. It is the most common presentation (Figure 9-14, *B*).

TERM	DEFINITION
cesarean section (CS, C-section) (se-ZĂR-ē-an) (SEK-shun)	birth of a fetus through an incision in the mother's abdomen and uterus (may also be spelled **caesarean**)
colostrum (k-LOS-trem)	thin, milky fluid secreted by the breast during pregnancy and during the first days after birth before lactation begins
congenital anomaly (kon-JEN-i-tal) (a-NOM-a-lē)	abnormality present at birth; often discovered before birth by sonography and/ or amniocentesis
in vitro fertilization (IVF) (in VĒ-trō) (*fer*-ti-li-ZĀ-shun)	method of fertilizing human ova outside the body and placing the zygote into the uterus; used when infertility is present (Figure 9-16)
lactation (lak-TĀ-shun)	secretion of milk
lochia (LŌ-kē-a)	vaginal discharge after childbirth
meconium (me-KŌ-nē-um)	first stool of the newborn (greenish-black)
midwife (MID-wīf)	individual who practices midwifery
midwifery (MID-wif-rē)	practice of assisting in childbirth
obstetrician (*ob*-ste-TRISH-an)	physician who specializes in obstetrics
obstetrics (OB) (ob-STET-riks)	medical specialty dealing with pregnancy, childbirth, and puerperium
parturition (*par*-tū-RISH-un)	act of giving birth
premature infant (PRĔ-ma-tur) (IN-fent)	infant born before completing 37 weeks of gestation (also called **preterm infant**)
puerperium (*pū*-er-PĒ-rē-um)	period from delivery until the reproductive organs return to normal (approximately 6 weeks)
quickening (KWIK-en-ing)	first feeling of movement of the fetus in utero by the pregnant woman. It usually occurs between 16 and 20 weeks of gestation.
stillborn (STIL-born)	born dead

To watch animations, go to evolve.elsevier.com. Select:
Chapter 9, **Animations**, Breech Presentation Exam
    Breech Delivery, Arms
    Breech Delivery, Face

Refer to p. 10 for your Evolve Access Information.

Refer to **Appendix D** for pharmacology terms related to obstetrics and neonatology.

🏛 CESAREAN SECTION (C-SECTION)
The origin of this term has no relation to the birth of Julius Caesar, as is commonly believed. One suggested etymology is that from 715 to 672 bc it was Roman law that the operation be performed on dying women in the last few months of pregnancy in the hope of saving the child. At that time the operation was called a **caeso matris utero**, which means **the cutting of the mother's uterus.**

MANAGING INFERTILITY
is a condition estimated by the CDC to affect approximately 12% of the U.S. reproductive-age population that has many options for management. These options include medications to stimulate ova production and procedures to provide artificial insemination. **Techniques** that artificially combine **both** ova and sperm are referred to as **assisted reproductive technology (ART).**

COMPARE MIDWIFE & DOULA
Midwives practice midwifery supervise pregnancy, labor, delivery, and puerperium. They assist with delivery independently, care for the newborn, and obtain medical assistance as necessary. A **midwife** may or may not be a registered nurse. Education, certification, and licensure vary by state and country. A **doula** (DOO-la) is a trained birth attendant who provides continual physical and emotional support to the laboring woman. **Doulas** provide a complementary role to the obstetric health care team.

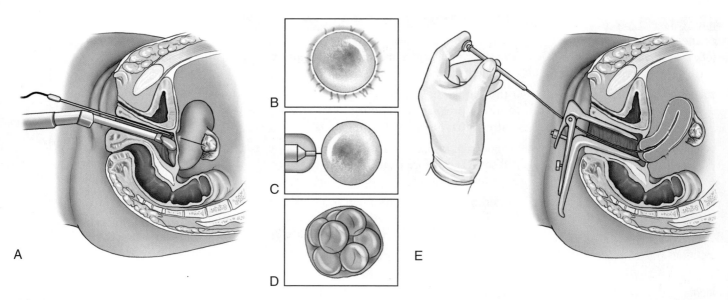

FIGURE 9-16

In vitro fertilization (IVF). After ovarian stimulation, ova are retrieved from the ovary by ultrasound-guided transvaginal needle aspiration **(A)**. The ova are fertilized outside the body in a dish with spermatozoa obtained from semen **(B).** A technique using a single sperm called intracytoplasmic sperm injection may also be used **(C).** After 48 hours the fertilized ova (zygotes) **(D)** are injected into the uterus for implantation **(E).** The first pregnancy after in vitro fertilization was reported more than 3 decades ago. Since then **assisted reproductive technology (ART)** has achieved hundreds of thousands of pregnancies worldwide.

EXERCISE 34

Practice saying aloud each of the complementary terms not built from word parts on pp. 370–371.

 To hear the terms, go to evolve.elsevier.com. Select: Chapter 9, **Exercises**, Pronunciation.

Refer to p. 10 for your Evolve Access Information.

☐ Place a check mark in the box when you have completed this exercise.

EXERCISE 35

Match the definitions in the first column with the correct terms in the second column.

_____ 1. vaginal discharge	a. lochia
_____ 2. medical specialty dealing with pregnancy and childbirth	b. obstetrician
	c. premature infant
_____ 3. abnormality present at birth	d. meconium
_____ 4. period after delivery	e. obstetrics
_____ 5. giving birth	f. parturition
_____ 6. physician specializing in obstetrics	g. puerperium
_____ 7. buttocks, feet, or knees first	h. cesarean section
_____ 8. first stool	i. congenital anomaly
_____ 9. born before completing 37 weeks of gestation	j. breech presentation
_____ 10. birth through an abdominal and uterine incision	

EXERCISE 36

Match the definitions in the first column with the correct terms in the second column.

_____ 1. assisting in childbirth

_____ 2. one who assists in childbirth

_____ 3. secretion of milk

_____ 4. head first

_____ 5. born dead

_____ 6. movement of the fetus

_____ 7. secreted before lactation

_____ 8. method of fertilizing ova outside the body

a. quickening
b. lactation
c. cephalic presentation
d. colostrum
e. midwife
f. stillborn
g. in vitro fertilization
h. midwifery

EXERCISE 37

Write the definitions of the following terms.

1. meconium _____

2. obstetrics _____

3. premature infant_____

4. lochia _____

5. puerperium _____

6. parturition_____

7. obstetrician _____

8. congenital anomaly _____

9. breech presentation _____

10. cesarean section _____

11. quickening_____

12. lactation_____

13. cephalic presentation _____

14. colostrum _____

15. midwife _____

16. stillborn _____

17. midwifery _____

18. in vitro fertilization _____

EXERCISE 38

Spell each of the complementary terms not built from word parts on pp. 370–371 by having someone dictate them to you.

To hear and spell the terms, go to evolve.elsevier.com. Select: Chapter 9, **Exercises**, Spelling.

(e) Refer to p. 10 for your Evolve Access Information.

☐ Place a check mark in the box if you have completed this exercise online.

1. _____   6. _____

2. _____   7. _____

3. _____   8. _____

4. _____   9. _____

5. _____   10. _____

11. _____   15. _____
12. _____   16. _____
13. _____   17. _____
14. _____   18. _____

For review and/or assessment, go to evolve.elsevier.com. Select:
Chapter 9, **Activities**, Terms Not Built from Word Parts
                      Hear It and Type It: Clinical Vignettes
Chapter 9, **Games**,   Term Explorer
                      Termbusters
                      Medical Millionaire

Refer to p. 10 for your Evolve Access Information.

Abbreviations

ABBREVIATION	MEANING
AB	abortion
CS, C-section	cesarean section
DOB	date of birth
EDD	expected (estimated) date of delivery
FAS	fetal alcohol syndrome
IVF	in vitro fertilization
LMP	last menstrual period
multip	multipara
NB	newborn
OB	obstetrics
primip	primipara
RDS	respiratory distress syndrome
VBAC	vaginal birth after cesarean section

Refer to **Appendix C** for a complete list of abbreviations.

EXERCISE 39

Write the definition of the following abbreviations.

1. OB _____

2. EDD _____ _____ of _____

3. LMP _____ _____ _____

4. DOB _____ _____ _____

5. NB _____

6. multip _____

7. C/S, C-section _____ _____

8. VBAC _____ _____ _____ _____ _____

9. RDS _____ _____ _____

10. primip _____

11. FAS _____ _____ _____

12. IVF _____ _____ _____

13. AB _____

For more practice with abbreviations, go to evolve.elsevier.com. Select:
Chapter 9, **Flashcards**
Chapter 9, **Games**, Crossword Puzzle

Refer to p. 10 for your Evolve Access Information.

PRACTICAL APPLICATION

EXERCISE 40   *Interact with Medical Documents and Electronic Health Records*

A. Complete the progress note by writing the medical terms in the blanks. Use the list of definitions with the corresponding numbers.

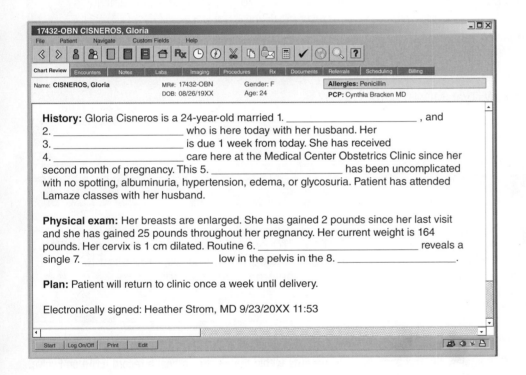

17432-OBN CISNEROS, Gloria

File   Patient   Navigate   Custom Fields   Help

Chart Review   Encounters   Notes   Labs   Imaging   Procedures   Rx   Documents   Referrals   Scheduling   Billing

Name: **CISNEROS, Gloria**   MR#: 17432-OBN   Gender: F   **Allergies:** Penicillin
DOB: 08/26/19XX   Age: 24   **PCP:** Cynthia Bracken MD

History: Gloria Cisneros is a 24-year-old married 1. _____ , and
2. _____ who is here today with her husband. Her
3. _____ is due 1 week from today. She has received
4. _____ care here at the Medical Center Obstetrics Clinic since her
second month of pregnancy. This 5. _____ has been uncomplicated
with no spotting, albuminuria, hypertension, edema, or glycosuria. Patient has attended
Lamaze classes with her husband.

Physical exam: Her breasts are enlarged. She has gained 2 pounds since her last visit
and she has gained 25 pounds throughout her pregnancy. Her current weight is 164
pounds. Her cervix is 1 cm dilated. Routine 6. _____ reveals a
single 7. _____ low in the pelvis in the 8. _____ .

Plan: Patient will return to clinic once a week until delivery.

Electronically signed: Heather Strom, MD 9/23/20XX 11:53

Start   Log On/Off   Print   Edit

LAMAZE

is a method of psychophysical
preparation for childbirth started
in the 1950s by a French
obstetrician, Fernand Lamaze.
The method requires classes
and practice before and
coaching during labor and
delivery.

1. pregnant (woman)
2. birth
3. abbreviation for expected delivery date
4. pertaining to before birth (reference to the newborn)
5. development of a new individual from conception to birth

6. pertaining to the pelvis, process of recording sound
7. unborn offspring from the ninth week of pregnancy
8. birth position in which any part of the head emerges first

B. Read the following radiology report and answer the questions following it.

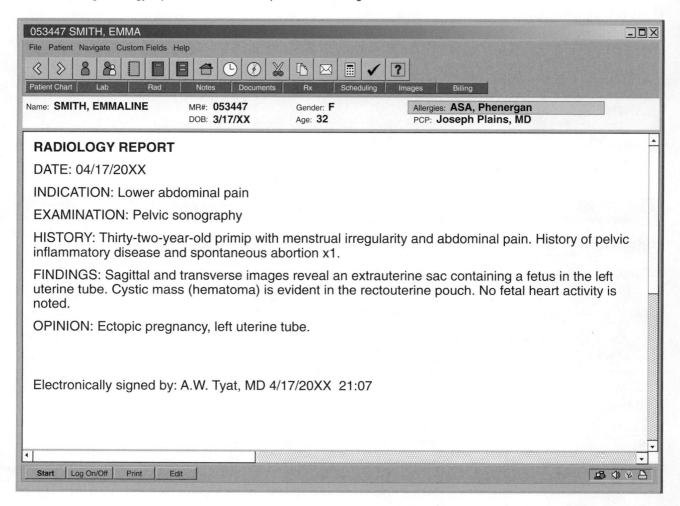

053447 SMITH, EMMA

File Patient Navigate Custom Fields Help

| Patient Chart | Lab | Rad | Notes | Documents | Rx | Scheduling | Images | Billing |

Name: **SMITH, EMMALINE** MR#: **053447** Gender: **F** Allergies: **ASA, Phenergan**
DOB: **3/17/XX** Age: **32** PCP: **Joseph Plains, MD**

RADIOLOGY REPORT

DATE: 04/17/20XX

INDICATION: Lower abdominal pain

EXAMINATION: Pelvic sonography

HISTORY: Thirty-two-year-old primip with menstrual irregularity and abdominal pain. History of pelvic inflammatory disease and spontaneous abortion x1.

FINDINGS: Sagittal and transverse images reveal an extrauterine sac containing a fetus in the left uterine tube. Cystic mass (hematoma) is evident in the rectouterine pouch. No fetal heart activity is noted.

OPINION: Ectopic pregnancy, left uterine tube.

Electronically signed by: A.W. Tyat, MD 4/17/20XX 21:07

Start Log On/Off Print Edit

---

1. The patient has:
   a. been pregnant two or more times
   b. given birth to two or more viable offspring
   c. borne one viable offspring
   d. never been pregnant

2. T F The patient has experienced one abortion
3. T F Radiographic images were used to determine the findings.

C. Complete the **three medical documents** within the electronic health record (EHR) on Evolve.

> Many healthcare records today are stored and used in an electronic system called **Electronic Health Records (EHR).** Electronic health records contain a collection of health information of an individual patient; the digitally formatted record can be shared through computer networks with patients, physicians, and other health care providers.

For practice with medical terms using electronic health records, go to evolve.elsevier.com. Select: Chapter 9, **Electronic Health Records**.

Refer to p. 10 for your Evolve Access Information.

EXERCISE 41 *Interpret Medical Terms*

To test your understanding of the terms introduced in this chapter, circle the words that correctly complete the sentences. The italicized words refer to the correct answer.

1. The premature infant was diagnosed as having *respiratory distress syndrome*, a disease of the (**umbilicus, erythrocytes, lungs**).
2. Because of inadequate uterine contractions, the patient was experiencing *difficult labor*, or (**dysphasia, dystocia, dysuria**).
3. Down syndrome was diagnosed prenatally by laboratory analysis of *amniotic fluid aspirated by surgical puncture*, or (**amniocentesis, amnioscopy, amnioscope**).
4. The word that means *before childbirth* (reference to the mother) is (**intrapartum, antepartum, postpartum**).
5. *Nulligravida* is a woman who (**has never been pregnant, has not given birth**).
6. *Multipara* is a woman who has (**given birth to two or more viable offspring, been pregnant two or more times**).
7. *Primigravida* is a woman (**in her first pregnancy, who has given birth to one child**).
8. The word that means the *act of giving birth* is (**parturition, puerperium, gravidopuerperal**).
9. *Rupture of the uterus* is called (**hysterorrhaphy, hysterorrhexis, hysteroptosis**).
10. Alcohol is (**quickening, colostrum, teratogenic**) when it *produces malformations* resulting in fetal alcohol syndrome.

EXERCISE 42 *Read Medical Terms in Use*

Practice pronunciation of the terms by reading the following medical document. Use the pronunciation key following the medical term to assist you in saying the words.

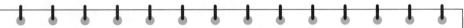

Josephine Alcotts is a 34-year-old **gravida** (GRAV-i-da) 2 **para** (PAR-a) 1 woman. Her LMP was April 20, 20XX. The EDD is January 25, 20XX. The **obstetrician** (*ob*-ste-TRISH-an) prescribed folic acid to prevent **spina bifida** (SPĪ-na) (BIF-i-da). The patient's first pregnancy was complicated by **preeclampsia** (prē-ē-KLAMP-sē-a) and a **breech** (brēch) **presentation,** which required a **cesarean section** (se-ZĀR-ē-an) (SEK-shun). **Pelvic sonography** (PEL-vik) (so-NOG-ra-fē) showed a single female fetus with normal development. She went on to deliver a healthy baby by VBAC 3 days before her expected delivery date.

EXERCISE 43 *Comprehend Medical Terms in Use*

Test your comprehension of terms in the above medical document by circling the correct answer.

1. T F Josephine Alcotts has been pregnant twice and has given birth once.
2. The obstetrician prescribed folic acid to prevent congenital:
   a. split of the lip and roof of the mouth
   b. mental retardation
   c. absence of part of the esophagus
   d. defect of the vertebral column
3. During her first pregnancy the patient had:
   a. abnormally low implantation of the placenta on the uterine wall
   b. high blood pressure, edema, and proteinuria
   c. premature separation of the placenta from the uterine wall
   d. convulsions and coma
4. T F The fetal presentation of the patient's first pregnancy was cephalic.

WEB LINK

For more information about obstetrics, visit The American College of Obstetricians and Gynecologists at **www.acog.org/**. Additional information regarding assistive reproductive technology (ART) can be found at the Centers for Disease Control and Prevention website at **www.cdc.gov/ART/**.

To hear these terms, go to evolve.elsevier.com. Select: Chapter 9, **Exercises**, Read Medical Terms in Use.

Refer to p. 10 for your Evolve Access Information.

For a snapshot assessment of your knowledge of Obstetrics and Neonatology terms, go to evolve.elsevier.com. Select: Chapter 9, **Quick Quizzes**.

Refer to p. 10 for your Evolve Access Information.

CHAPTER REVIEW

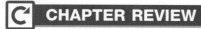 *Review Of Evolve*

Keep a record of the online activities you have completed by placing a check mark in the box. You may also record your scores. All activities have been referenced throughout the chapter.

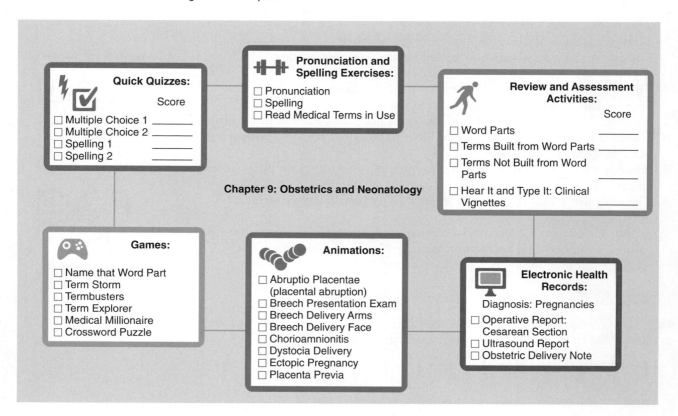

Quick Quizzes:

Score
- ☐ Multiple Choice 1 _____
- ☐ Multiple Choice 2 _____
- ☐ Spelling 1 _____
- ☐ Spelling 2 _____

Pronunciation and Spelling Exercises:
- ☐ Pronunciation
- ☐ Spelling
- ☐ Read Medical Terms in Use

Review and Assessment Activities:

Score
- ☐ Word Parts _____
- ☐ Terms Built from Word Parts _____
- ☐ Terms Not Built from Word Parts _____
- ☐ Hear It and Type It: Clinical Vignettes _____

Chapter 9: Obstetrics and Neonatology

Games:
- ☐ Name that Word Part
- ☐ Term Storm
- ☐ Termbusters
- ☐ Term Explorer
- ☐ Medical Millionaire
- ☐ Crossword Puzzle

Animations:
- ☐ Abruptio Placentae (placental abruption)
- ☐ Breech Presentation Exam
- ☐ Breech Delivery Arms
- ☐ Breech Delivery Face
- ☐ Chorioamnionitis
- ☐ Dystocia Delivery
- ☐ Ectopic Pregnancy
- ☐ Placenta Previa

Electronic Health Records:

Diagnosis: Pregnancies
- ☐ Operative Report: Cesarean Section
- ☐ Ultrasound Report
- ☐ Obstetric Delivery Note

Review of Word Parts

Can you define and spell the following word parts?

COMBINING FORMS		PREFIXES	SUFFIXES
amni/o	lact/o	ante-	-amnios
amnion/o	nat/o	micro-	-cyesis
cephal/o	omphal/o	multi-	-e
chori/o	par/o	nulli-	-is
embry/o	part/o	post-	-rrhexis
esophag/o	pelv/i	pre-	-tocia
fet/i	pelv/o		-um
fet/o	prim/i		-us
gravid/o	pseud/o		
	puerper/o		
	pylor/o		
	terat/o		

Review of Terms

Can you build, analyze, define, pronounce, and spell the following terms *built from word parts*?

DISEASES AND DISORDERS (OBSTETRICS)	DISEASES AND DISORDERS (NEONATOLOGY)	SURGICAL (OBSTETRICS)	DIAGNOSTIC (OBSTETRICS)	COMPLEMENTARY (OBSTETRICS AND NEONATOLOGY)	
amnionitis	microcephalus	amniotomy	amniocentesis	amniochorial	multigravida
chorioamnionitis	omphalitis	episiotomy	amnioscope	amniorrhea	multipara (multip)
choriocarcinoma	omphalocele		amnioscopy	amniorrhexis	natal
dystocia	pyloric stenosis		pelvic sonography	antepartum	neonate
hysterorrhexis	tracheoesophageal			embryogenic	neonatologist
oligohydramnios	fistula			embryoid	neonatology
polyhydramnios				fetal	nulligravida
				gravida	nullipara
				gravidopuerperal	para
				intrapartum	postnatal
				lactic	postpartum
				lactogenic	prenatal
				lactorrhea	primigravida
					primipara (primip)
					pseudocyesis
					puerpera
					puerperal
					teratogen
					teratogenic
					teratology

Can you define, pronounce, and spell the following terms *not built from word parts*?

DISEASES AND DISORDERS (OBSTETRICS)	DISEASES AND DISORDERS (NEONATOLOGY)	COMPLEMENTARY (OBSTETRICS AND NEONATOLOGY)
abortion (AB)	cleft lip or palate	breech presentation
abruptio placentae	Down syndrome	cephalic presentation
eclampsia	erythroblastosis fetalis	cesarean section (CS, C-section)
ectopic pregnancy	esophageal atresia	colostrum
placenta previa	fetal alcohol syndrome (FAS)	congenital anomaly
preeclampsia	gastroschisis	in vitro fertilization (IVF)
	respiratory distress syndrome (RDS)	lactation
	spina bifida	lochia
		meconium
		midwife
		midwifery
		obstetrician
		obstetrics (OB)
		parturition
		premature infant
		puerperium
		quickening
		stillborn

ANSWERS

ANSWERS TO CHAPTER 9 EXERCISES
Exercise Figures

Exercise Figure

A.
1. umbilicus: omphal/o
2. fetus: fet/o, fet/i
3. amnion, amniotic fluid: amni/o, amnion/o
4. chorion: chori/o

Exercise Figure

B. omphal/o/cele

Exercise Figure

C. neo/nat/e

Exercise 1
1. gamete; ovulation; fertilization; zygote; gestation
2. embryo; fetus
3. amniotic; chorion; amnion; amniotic

Exercise 2
1. fetus, unborn child
2. milk
3. bear, give birth to, labor, childbirth
4. umbilicus, navel
5. amnion, amniotic fluid
6. childbirth
7. pregnancy
8. birth
9. chorion
10. embryo, to be full

Exercise 3
1. lact/o
2. a. fet/o, b. fet/i
3. chori/o
4. a. amni/o, b. amnion/o
5. puerper/o
6. a. par/o, b. part/o
7. gravid/o
8. embry/o
9. nat/o
10. omphal/o

Exercise 4
1. first
2. pylorus
3. head
4. esophagus
5. false
6. pelvic bone, pelvis
7. malformations

Exercise 5
1. cephal/o
2. pylor/o

Exercise 6
1. after
2. many
3. none
4. small
5. before
6. before

Exercise 7
1. nulli-
2. micro-
3. multi-
4. a. ante-
   b. pre-
5. post-

Exercise 8
1. rupture
2. birth, labor
3. pregnancy
4. amnion, amniotic fluid

Exercise 9
1. -tocia
2. -rrhexis
3. -cyesis
4. -amnios

Exercise 10
1. -e
2. -is
3. -us
4. -um

Answers may be in any order.

Exercise 11
Pronunciation Exercise

Exercise 12
Note: The combining form is identified by italic and bold print.

1.   WR CV WR   S
   chori/o*/amnion/itis*
         CF
   inflammation of the chorion and amnion

2.   WR CV WR   S
   chori/o*/carcin/oma*
         CF
   cancerous tumor of the chorion

3.   P   S(WR)
   dys/tocia
   difficult labor

4.   WR   S
   amnion/itis
   inflammation of the amnion

5.   WR CV   S
   hyster/o*/rrhexis*
         CF
   rupture of the uterus

6.   WR CV WR   S
   olig/o*/hydr/amnios*
         CF
   scanty amnion water (less than the normal amount of amniotic fluid)

7.   P   WR   S
   poly/hydr/amnios
   much amnion water (more than the normal amount of amniotic fluid)

Exercise 13
1. chori/o/carcin/oma
2. amnion/itis
3. chori/o/amnion/itis
4. dys/tocia
5. hyster/o/rrhexis
6. olig/o/hydr/amnios
7. poly/hydr/amnios

Exercise 14
Spelling Exercise; see text p. 353.

Exercise 15
Pronunciation Exercise

Exercise 16
1. premature separation of the placenta from the uterine wall
2. termination of pregnancy by the expulsion from the uterus of an embryo or fetus
3. abnormally low implantation of the placenta on the uterine wall
4. severe complication and progression of preeclampsia
5. pregnancy occurring outside the uterus
6. abnormal condition, encountered during pregnancy or shortly after delivery, of high blood pressure, edema, and proteinuria

Exercise 17
1. abruptio placentae
2. eclampsia
3. abortion
4. ectopic pregnancy
5. placenta previa
6. preeclampsia

Exercise 18
Spelling Exercise; see text p. 356.

Exercise 19
Pronunciation Exercise

Exercise 20
Note: The combining form is identified by italic and bold print.

1. WR   S
   pylor/ic (stenosis)
   narrowing pertaining to the pyloric sphincter

2. WR   CV   S
   omphal/o/cele
      CF
   hernia at the umbilicus

3. WR   S
   omphal/itis
   inflammation of the umbilicus

4. P   WR   S
   micro/cephal/us (fetus with a very) small head

5. WR   CV   WR   S
   trache/o/esophag/eal (fistula)
      CF
   abnormal passageway pertaining to the trachea and the esophagus (between the trachea and esophagus)

Exercise 21
1. omphal/o/cele
2. micro/cephal/us
3. pylor/ic (stenosis)
4. trache/o/esophag/eal (fistula)
5. omphal/itis

Exercise 22
Spelling Exercise; see text p. 358.

Exercise 23
Pronunciation Exercise

Exercise 24
1. f   5. h
2. c   6. b
3. a   7. g
4. d   8. e

Exercise 25
Spelling Exercise; see text p. 361.

Exercise 26
Pronunciation Exercise

Exercise 27
Note: The combining form is identified by italic and bold print.

1. WR   CV   S
   episi/o/tomy
      CF
   incision into the vulva (perineum)

2. WR   CV   S
   amni/o/tomy
      CF
   incision into the amnion (rupture of the fetal membrane to induce labor)

3. WR   CV   S
   amni/o/scope
      CF
   instrument used for visual examination of amniotic fluid (and fetus)

4. WR   S   WR   CV   S
   pelv/ic ***son/o***/graphy
            CF
   pertaining to the pelvis, process of recording sound

5. WR   CV   S
   amni/o/centesis
      CF
   surgical puncture to aspirate amniotic fluid

6. WR   CV   S
   amni/o/scopy
      CF
   visual examination of amniotic fluid (and fetus)

Exercise 28
1. amni/o/tomy
2. episi/o/tomy
3. amni/o/scopy
4. amni/o/centesis
5. amni/o/scope
6. pelv/ic son/o/graphy

Exercise 29
Spelling Exercise; see text p. 364.

Exercise 30
Pronunciation Exercise

Exercise 31
Note: The combining form is identified by italic and bold print.

1. WR   S
   puerper/a
   childbirth

2. WR   CV   S
   amni/o/rrhexis
      CF
   rupture of the amnion

3. P   WR   S
   ante/part/um
   before childbirth

4. WR   CV   S
   pseud/o/cyesis
      CF
   false pregnancy

5. P   WR   S
   pre/nat/al
   pertaining to before birth

6. WR   S
   lact/ic
   pertaining to milk

7. WR   CV   S
   lact/o/rrhea
      CF
   (spontaneous) discharge of milk

8. WR   CV   S
   amni/o/rrhea
      CF
   discharge (escape) of amniotic fluid

9. P   WR   S
   multi/par/a
   many births

10. WR   CV   S
    embry/o/genic
       CF
    producing an embryo

11. WR   S
    embry/oid
    resembling an embryo

12. WR   S
    fet/al
    pertaining to the fetus

13. WR   S
    gravid/a
    pregnant (woman)

14. WR   CV   WR   S
    amni/o/chori/al
       CF
    pertaining to the amnion and chorion

15. P   WR   S
    multi/gravid/a
    many pregnancies

16. WR   CV   S
    lact/o/genic
       CF
    producing milk (by stimulation)

17. WR   S
    nat/al
    pertaining to birth

18. WR   CV   WR   S
    gravid/o/puerper/al
       CF
    pertaining to pregnancy and childbirth

19. P   WR   CV   S
    neo/***nat/o***/logy
            CF
    study of the newborn

20. P WR S
    nulli/par/a
    no births

21. WR S
    par/a
    birth

22. WR CV WR S
    prim/i/gravid/a
        CF
    first pregnancy

23. P WR S
    post/part/um
    after childbirth

24. P WR S
    neo/nat/e
    new birth (an infant from birth to 4
    weeks of age, synonymous with
    newborn)

25. WR CV WR S
    prim/i/par/a
        CF
    first birth

26. WR   S
    puerper/al
    pertaining to (immediately after)
    childbirth

27. P WR S
    nulli/gravid/a
    no pregnancies

28. P WR S
    intra/part/um
    within (during) labor and childbirth

29. WR CV S
    terat/o/gen
        CF
    any agent producing malformations
    (in the developing embryo)

30. P WR S
    post/nat/al
    pertaining to after birth

31. WR CV S
    terat/o/logy
        CF
    study of malformations (in the
    developing embryo)

32. P WR CV S
    neo/**nat/o**/logist
            CF
    physician who studies and treats
    disorders of the newborn

33. WR CV S
    terat/o/genic
        CF
    producing malformations

Exercise 32
1. amni/o/chori/al
2. ante/part/um

3. embry/o/genic
4. fet/al
5. pre/nat/al
6. lact/ic
7. lact/o/rrhea
8. amni/o/rrhea
9. pseud/o/cyesis
10. lact/o/genic
11. amni/o/rrhexis
12. embry/oid
13. gravid/a
14. gravid/o/puerper/al
15. multi/par/a
16. nat/al
17. neo/nat/e
18. neo/nat/o/logy
19. nulli/par/a
20. par/a
21. prim/i/gravid/a
22. post/part/um
23. prim/i/par/a
24. multi/gravid/a
25. puerper/al
26. nulli/gravid/a
27. terat/o/gen
28. puerper/a
29. intra/part/um
30. terat/o/genic
31. neo/nat/o/logist
32. post/nat/al
33. terat/o/logy

Exercise 33
Spelling Exercise; see text p. 370.

Exercise 34
Pronunciation Exercise

Exercise 35
1. a		6. b	
2. e		7. j	
3. i		8. d	
4. g		9. c	
5. f		10. h	

Exercise 36
1. h		5. f	
2. e		6. a	
3. b		7. d	
4. c		8. g	

Exercise 37
1. first stool of the newborn
2. medical specialty dealing with
   pregnancy, childbirth, and
   puerperium
3. infant born before completing 37
   weeks of gestation

4. vaginal discharge after childbirth
5. period after delivery until the
   reproductive organs return to
   normal
6. act of giving birth
7. physician who specializes in
   obstetrics
8. abnormality present at birth
9. birth position in which the buttocks,
   feet, or knees emerge first
10. birth of a fetus through an incision
    in the mother's abdomen and
    uterus
11. first feeling of movement of the
    fetus in utero by the pregnant
    woman
12. secretion of milk
13. birth position in which any part of
    the head emerges first
14. fluid secreted by the breast during
    pregnancy and after birth until
    lactation begins
15. individual who practices
    midwifery
16. born dead
17. practice of assisting in childbirth
18. method of fertilizing human ova
    outside the body

Exercise 38
Spelling Exercise; see text pp. 373–374.

Exercise 39
1. obstetrics
2. expected (estimated) date of
   delivery
3. last menstrual period
4. date of birth
5. newborn
6. multipara
7. cesarean section
8. vaginal birth after cesarean
   section
9. respiratory distress syndrome
10. primapara
11. fetal alcohol syndrome
12. in vitro fertilization
13. abortion

Exercise 40
A.
1. gravida	6. pelvic
2. para	sonography
3. EDD	7. fetus
4. prenatal	8. cephalic
5. gestation	presentation

B.
1. c
2. T
3. F, sonography was used
C. Online Exercise

Exercise 41
1. lungs
2. dystocia
3. amniocentesis
4. antepartum
5. has never been pregnant
6. given birth to two or more viable offspring
7. in her first pregnancy
8. parturition
9. hysterorrhexis
10. teratogenic

Exercise 42
Reading Exercise

Exercise 43
1. *T*
2. d
3. b
4. *F,* the fetal presentation was breech.

Chapter 10

Cardiovascular, Immune, Lymphatic Systems and Blood

Objectives

Upon completion of this chapter you will be able to:

1 Identify the organs and structures of the cardiovascular and lymphatic systems and blood and the function of the immune system.

2 Define and spell word parts related to the cardiovascular and lymphatic systems and blood.

3 Define, pronounce, and spell disease and disorder terms related to the cardiovascular and lymphatic systems and blood.

4 Define, pronounce, and spell surgical terms related to the cardiovascular and lymphatic systems and blood.

5 Define, pronounce, and spell diagnostic terms related to the cardiovascular system and blood.

6 Define, pronounce, and spell complementary terms related to the cardiovascular, immune systems, and blood.

7 Interpret the meaning of abbreviations presented in the chapter.

8 Interpret, read, and comprehend medical language in simulated medical statements, documents, and electronic health records.

ANATOMY

At first glance this may seem like an overabundance of material to cover in one chapter. It is a lot of material, but as you will see **the systems have interactive functions, and learning the terms for these systems at the same time is beneficial**.

The functions are interactive in many ways. The lymphatic and immune systems support each other by providing an immune response to invading microorganisms and foreign substances. The lymphatic system and blood share macrophages and lymphocytes. Lymph is drained into large veins of the cardiovascular system, and the cardiovascular system is responsible for circulating blood throughout the body.

Cardiovascular System

The cardiovascular system consists of the heart and a closed network of blood vessels composed of arteries, capillaries, and veins (Figure 10-1).

Function

The heart functions as two pumps operating simultaneously. The right side of the heart pumps blood to the lungs while the left side pumps blood to the rest of the body. The exchange of gases, nutrients, and waste between the blood and body tissue

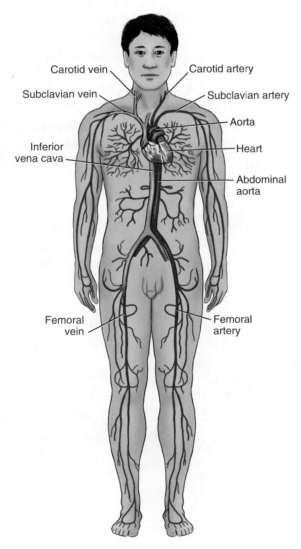

FIGURE 10-1
Cardiovascular system.

takes place in the capillaries. The blood carrying carbon dioxide and waste is carried from the tissues through veins to organs of excretion. Additionally, the cardiovascular system serves a critical role in the body's ability to regulate temperature.

Structures of the Cardiovascular System

TERM	DEFINITION
heart	muscular cone-shaped organ the size of a fist, located behind the sternum (breast bone) and between the lungs. The pumping action of the heart circulates blood throughout the body (Figure 10-2). The heart consists of two smaller upper chambers, the **right atrium** and the **left atrium** (*pl.* **atria**), and two larger lower chambers, the **right ventricle** and the **left ventricle** (*pl.* **ventricles**). The right atrium receives blood returning from the body through the veins and contracts to fill the right ventricle, which then pumps blood to the lungs. The left atrium receives blood from the lungs and contracts to fill the left ventricle, which then contracts to pump blood from the heart through the arteries to body tissues. The **atrial septum** separates the atria and the **ventricular septum** separates the ventricles.
atrioventricular valves	consist of the **tricuspid** and **mitral** valves, which lie between the right atrium and the right ventricle and the left atrium and left ventricle, respectively. Valves of the heart keep blood flowing in one direction.
semilunar valves	**pulmonary** and **aortic** valves located between the right ventricle and the pulmonary artery and between the left ventricle and the aorta, respectively.

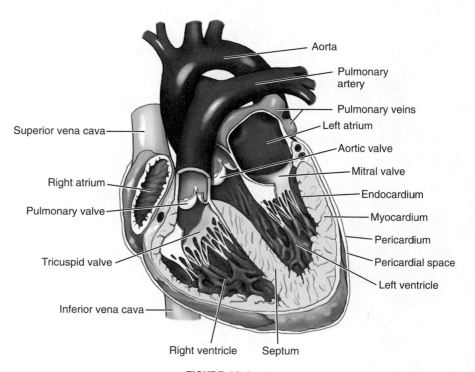

FIGURE 10-2
Interior of the heart.

TERM	DEFINITION
pericardium	two-layer sac surrounding the heart, consisting of an external fibrous and an internal serous layer. The serous layer secretes a fluid that facilitates movement of the heart called pericardial fluid. This fluid is held in the pericardial space between the two serous layers; the external layer is called the fibrous pericardium and the inner layer covering the heart is called epicardium.
three layers of the heart	
epicardium	covers the heart
myocardium	middle, thick, muscular layer
endocardium	inner lining of the heart
blood vessels	tubelike structures that carry blood throughout the body (Figure 10-3)
arteries	blood vessels that carry blood away from the heart. All arteries, with the exception of the pulmonary artery, carry oxygen and other nutrients from the heart to the body cells. The **pulmonary artery**, in contrast, carries carbon dioxide and other waste products from the heart to the lungs.
arterioles	smallest arteries
aorta	largest artery in the body, originating at the left ventricle and descending through the thorax and abdomen
veins	blood vessels that carry blood back to the heart. All veins, with the exception of the pulmonary veins, carry blood containing carbon dioxide and other waste products. The pulmonary veins carry oxygenated blood from the lungs to the heart.
venules	smallest veins

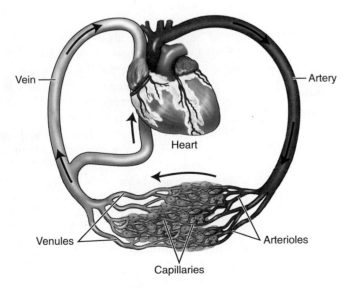

FIGURE 10-3
Types of blood vessels.

Structures of the Cardiovascular System—cont'd

TERM	DEFINITION
venae cavae	largest veins in the body. The **inferior vena cava** carries blood to the heart from body parts below the diaphragm, and the **superior vena cava** returns the blood to the heart from the upper part of the body.
capillaries	microscopic blood vessels that connect arterioles with venules. Materials are passed between the blood and tissue through the capillary walls.

EXERCISE 1

Match the anatomic terms for the cardiovascular system in the first column with the correct definitions in the second column. *To check your answers to the exercises in this chapter, go to Answers, p. 450, at the end of the chapter.*

_____ 1. aorta

_____ 2. arteries

_____ 3. arterioles

_____ 4. atria

_____ 5. mitral valve

_____ 6. capillaries

_____ 7. endocardium

_____ 8. heart

_____ 9. atrioventricular valves

a. lies between the left atrium and left ventricle
b. pumps blood throughout the body
c. smallest arteries
d. inner lining of the heart
e. largest artery in the body
f. connect arterioles with venules
g. blood vessels that carry blood away from the heart
h. upper chambers of the heart
i. tricuspid and mitral valves

EXERCISE 2

Match the anatomic terms for the cardiovascular system in the first column with the correct definitions in the second column.

_____ 1. myocardium

_____ 2. pericardium

_____ 3. semilunar valves

_____ 4. atrial septum

_____ 5. tricuspid valve

_____ 6. veins

_____ 7. ventricles

_____ 8. venules

_____ 9. vena cava

a. carries blood back to the heart
b. two-layer sac that facilitates movement of the heart
c. smallest veins
d. separates the atria
e. lower chambers of the heart
f. largest vein in the body
g. located between the right ventricle and the pulmonary artery and between the left ventricle and the aorta
h. carries oxygenated blood away from the heart
i. located between the right atrium and the right ventricle
j. muscular layer of the heart

Blood

Function

The primary function of blood is to maintain internal balance in the body. Activities of the blood include transportation of nutrients, waste, oxygen, carbon dioxide, and hormones; protection provided by certain cells that protect the body against microorganisms; and regulation by controlling body temperature and maintaining fluid and electrolyte balance.

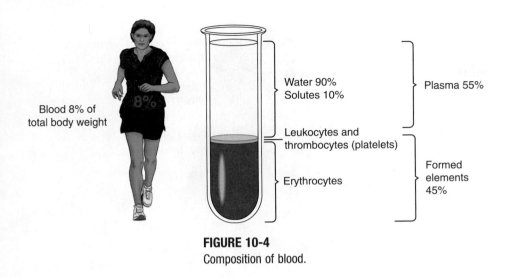

FIGURE 10-4
Composition of blood.

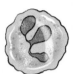
Neutrophil

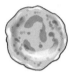
Eosinophil

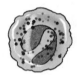
Basophil

Lymphocyte

Monocyte

FIGURE 10-5
Types of leukocytes. Each leukocyte plays a different role in providing immune responses to pathogens, foreign agents, allergies, and abnormal body cells.

Composition of Blood

TERM	DEFINITION
blood	fluid circulated through the heart, arteries, capillaries, and veins; composed of **plasma** and **formed elements**, such as erythrocytes, leukocytes, and thrombocytes (platelets) (Figure 10-4)
plasma	clear, straw-colored, liquid portion of blood in which cells are suspended. Plasma is approximately 90% water and comprises approximately 55% of the total blood volume.
cells (formed elements)	
erythrocytes	red blood cells that carry oxygen. Erythrocytes develop in bone marrow.
leukocytes	white blood cells that combat infection and respond to inflammation. There are five types of white blood cells (Figure 10-5).
platelets (thrombocytes)	one of the formed elements in the blood that is responsible for aiding in the clotting process
serum	clear, watery fluid portion of the blood that remains after a clot has formed

Lymphatic System

The lymphatic system consists of lymph transported through lymphatic vessels, lymph nodes, the spleen, and thymus gland (Figure 10-6).

Function

Three functions of the lymphatic system are to return excessive tissue fluid to the blood, absorb fats and fat-soluble vitamins from the small intestine and transport them to the blood, and provide defense against infection.

Collected extracellular fluid called lymph travels away from body tissue toward the heart and is drained into the cardiovascular system through ducts in the upper chest. Breathing and muscle action help propel lymph through the vessels.

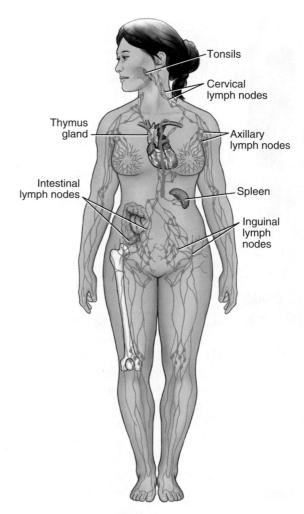

FIGURE 10-6
Lymphatic system.

Structures of the Lymphatic System

TERM	DEFINITION
lymph	transparent, colorless, tissue fluid; contains **lymphocytes** and **monocytes** and flows in a one-way direction to the heart
lymphatic vessels	transports lymph from body tissues to a large vein in the chest. The vessels begin as capillaries spread throughout the body then merge into larger tubes that eventually become ducts in the chest. They provide a one-way flow for lymph, which enters through veins into the circulatory system.
lymph nodes	small, spherical bodies composed of lymphoid tissue. They may be singular or grouped together along the path of the lymph vessels. The nodes filter lymph to keep substances such as bacteria and other foreign agents from entering the blood. They also produce lymphocytes.

TERM	DEFINITION
spleen	located in the left side of the abdominal cavity between the stomach and the diaphragm. In adulthood, the spleen is the largest lymphatic organ in the body. Blood, rather than lymph, flows through the spleen. Blood is cleansed of microorganisms in the spleen. The spleen stores blood and destroys worn out red blood cells.
thymus gland	one of the primary lymphatic organs, it is located anterior to the ascending aorta and posterior to the sternum between the lungs. It plays an important role in the development of the body's immune system, particularly from infancy to puberty. Around puberty the thymus gland atrophies so that most of the gland is connective tissue.

EXERCISE 3

Fill in the blanks with anatomic terms for blood and the lymphatic systems.

The function of the blood is to maintain internal balance in the body. The liquid
portion of blood is called (1) _____, in which (2) _____,
(3) _____, and (4) _____ are suspended.
(5) _____aid in clotting blood; (6) _____ is the clear
liquid that remains after a clot is formed. The lymphatic system provides
defense against infection. The lymphatic system is composed of the fluid
(7) _____; small spherical bodies (8) _____
_____, vessels for transporting lymph, the (9) _____,
which is the largest lymphatic organ; and the (10) _____ gland.

Immune System

The immune system does not have its own organs and structures. Its function depends on organs and structures of other body systems, including the spleen, liver, intestinal tract, lymph nodes, and bone marrow.

Function

The immune system protects the body against pathogens (bacteria, fungi, and viruses), foreign agents that cause allergic reactions (e.g., peanuts) or toxins (e.g., insect bites), and abnormal body cells (e.g., cancer).

It has three lines of defense; the first is the prevention of foreign substances from entering the body. Unbroken skin and mucous membranes act as mechanical barriers. Ear wax and saliva act as chemical barriers.

If the first line of defense is penetrated by microorganisms, a second line of defense continues to battle disease. Second-line defenses include inflammation and fever plus phagocytosis, a process in which some of the white blood cells destroy the invading microorganisms. Also activated are protective proteins such as interferons, which fight viruses, and natural killer (NK) cells, which are effective against microorganisms and cancer cells (Figure 10-7).

Specific immunity, the third line of defense, provides protection against specific pathogens, such as the polio virus, by forming specific antibodies to fight against the infectious agent.

A & P Booster
For more anatomy and physiology, go to evolve.elsevier.com.
Select: **Extra Content**, A & P Booster, Chapter 10.

Refer to p. 10 for your Evolve Access Information.

HARMFUL AGENTS

LINES OF DEFENSE

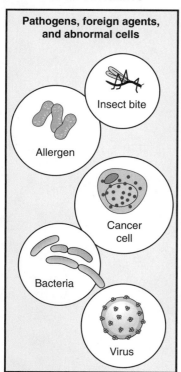

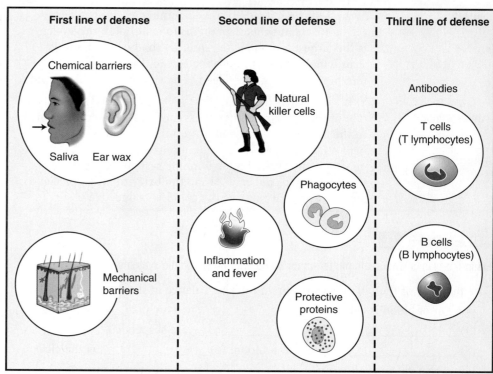

FIGURE 10-7

Three lines of defense provided by the immune system to protect the body against pathogens, foreign agents, and cancer.

EXERCISE 4

Complete the following exercise for the immune system.

1. The function of the immune system is to_____

   _____ .

2. List five organs and structures from other body systems used by the immune system to carry out its function.

   a._____

   b._____

   c._____

   d._____

   e._____

3. The three lines of defense used by the immune system are:

   a._____

   b._____

   c._____

WORD PARTS

Word parts you need to learn to complete this chapter are listed on the following pages. The exercises at the end of each list will help you learn their definitions and spellings.

> Use the flashcards accompanying this text or electronic flashcards to assist you in memorizing the word parts for this chapter.

> To use the electronic flashcards, go to evolve.elsevier.com.
> Select: Chapter 10, **Flashcards**.
>
> Refer to p. 10 for your Evolve Access Information.

Combining Forms of the Cardiovascular and Lymphatic Systems and Blood

COMBINING FORM	DEFINITION
angi/o	vessel (usually refers to blood vessel)
aort/o	aorta
arteri/o	artery
atri/o	atrium
cardi/o	heart
lymph/o	lymph, lymph tissue
lymphaden/o	lymph node
myel/o (NOTE: myel/o also means spinal cord; see Chapter 15)	bone marrow
phleb/o, ven/o	vein
plasm/o	plasma
splen/o (NOTE: only one e in the word root for spleen)	spleen
thym/o	thymus gland
valv/o, valvul/o	valve
ventricul/o	ventricle

🏛 **VITAL AIR**
It was believed in ancient times that **arteries** carried air. Vital air, or pneuma, did not allow blood in the arteries. A cut in an artery allowed vital air to escape and blood to replace it. The Greek arteria, meaning windpipe, was given for this reason.

🏛 **VENTRICLE**
Is derived from the Latin venter, meaning "little belly". It was first applied to the belly and then to the stomach. Later it was extended to mean any small cavity in an organ or body. Modern clinical usage refers to the ventricles located in the heart or brain.

> *lymphaden/o*
> In Chapter 2, the combining form aden/o was defined as **gland**. When used in reference to the lymphatic system, lymphaden/o refers to collection of lymphatic tissue and is called a lymph **node** rather than lymph gland.

Fill in the blanks with combining forms in this diagram of a cutaway section of the heart. *To check your answers, go to p. 450.*

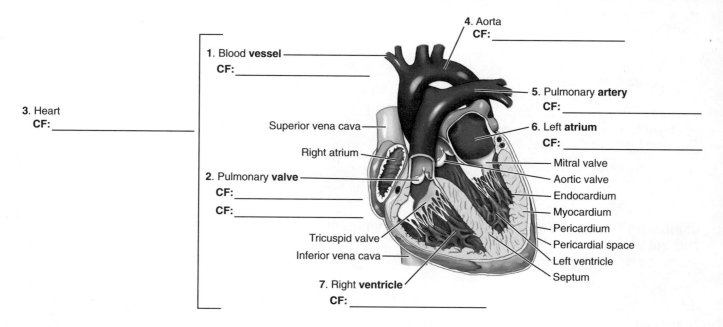

4. Aorta
   CF:_____

1. Blood **vessel**
   CF:_____

5. Pulmonary **artery**
   CF:_____

3. Heart
   CF:_____

Superior vena cava

6. Left **atrium**
   CF:_____

Right atrium

Mitral valve

2. Pulmonary **valve**
   CF:_____
   CF:_____

Aortic valve

Endocardium

Myocardium

Pericardium

Tricuspid valve

Pericardial space

Inferior vena cava

Left ventricle

Septum

7. Right **ventricle**
   CF:_____

EXERCISE 5

Write the definitions of the following combining forms.

1. cardi/o _____

9. thym/o _____

2. atri/o _____

10. phleb/o _____

3. plasm/o _____

11. ventricul/o _____

4. angi/o _____

12. arteri/o _____

5. ven/o _____

13. valvul/o _____

6. aort/o _____

14. lymph/o _____

7. valv/o _____

15. lymphaden/o _____

8. splen/o _____

16. myel/o _____

EXERCISE 6

Write the combining form for each of the following terms.

1. artery _____

2. vein   a. _____

         b. _____

3. heart_____

4. atrium _____

5. ventricle_____

6. lymph, lymph
   tissue _____

7. aorta_____

8. vessel (usually
   blood vessel) _____

9. valve a. _____

         b. _____

10. spleen_____

11. plasma _____

12. thymus gland _____

13. lymph node_____

14. bone marrow_____

Combining Forms Commonly Used with the Cardiovascular and Lymphatic Systems and Blood Terms

COMBINING FORM	DEFINITION
ather/o	yellowish, fatty plaque
ech/o	sound
electr/o	electricity, electrical activity
isch/o	deficiency, blockage
therm/o	heat
thromb/o	clot

EXERCISE 7

Write the definition of the following combining forms.

1. ech/o _____

2. thromb/o_____

3. isch/o _____

4. therm/o _____

5. ather/o_____

6. electr/o _____

EXERCISE 8

Write the combining form for each of the following.

1. clot_____

2. sound _____

3. deficiency, blockage _____

4. yellowish, fatty plaque _____

5. heat _____

6. electricity, electrical
   activity _____

Prefixes

PREFIX	DEFINITION
brady-	slow
pan-	all, total

Suffixes

SUFFIX	DEFINITION
-ac	pertaining to
-apheresis	removal
-penia	abnormal reduction in number
-poiesis	formation
-sclerosis	hardening

Refer to **Appendix A** and **Appendix B** for alphabetical lists of word parts and their meanings.

EXERCISE 9

Write the definitions of the following prefixes and suffixes.

1. brady- _____
2. pan- _____
3. -penia_____
4. -sclerosis _____
5. -apheresis _____
6. -poiesis_____
7. -ac _____

EXERCISE 10

Write the suffix or prefix for each of the following.

1. formation_____   5. abnormal reduction in number____
2. pertaining to _____   6. slow _____
3. hardening _____   7. removal _____
4. all, total _____

For review and/or assessment, go to evolve.elsevier.com. Select:
Chapter 10, **Activities,** Word Parts
Chapter 10, **Games,** Name that Word Part

Refer to p. 10 for your Evolve Access Information.

MEDICAL TERMS

The terms you need to learn to complete this chapter are listed below. The exercises following each list will help you learn the definition and the spelling of each word.

Disease and Disorder Terms

Built from Word Parts

The following terms are built from word parts you have already learned and can be translated literally to find their meanings. Further explanation of terms beyond the definition of their word parts, if needed, is included in parentheses.

TERM	DEFINITION
CARDIOVASCULAR SYSTEM	
angioma (an-jē-Ō-ma)	tumor composed of blood vessels
angiostenosis (*an*-jē-ō-ste-NŌ-sis)	narrowing of a blood vessel
aortic stenosis (ā-OR-tik) (ste-NŌ-sis)	narrowing, pertaining to aorta (narrowing of the aortic valve) (Figure 10-8)
arteriosclerosis (ar-*tēr*-ē-ō-skle-RŌ-sis)	hardening of the arteries
atherosclerosis (*ath*-er-ō-skle-RŌ-sis)	hardening of fatty plaque (deposited on the arterial wall) (Exercise Figure B2)
bradycardia (*brad*-ē-KAR-dē-a) (*NOTE: the* i *in cardi/o has been dropped*)	condition of a slow heart (rate less than 60 beats per minute)
cardiomegaly (*kar*-dē-ō-MEG-a-lē)	enlargement of the heart
cardiomyopathy (*kar*-dē-ō-mī-OP-a-thē)	disease of the heart muscle
endocarditis (*en*-dō-kar-DĪ-tis)	inflammation of the inner (lining) of the heart (particularly heart valves)
myocarditis (*mī*-ō-kar-DĪ-tis)	inflammation of the muscle of the heart
pericarditis (*per*-i-kar-DĪ-tis)	inflammation of the sac surrounding the heart (see Figure 10-13)
phlebitis (fle-BĪ-tis)	inflammation of a vein
polyarteritis (*pol*-ē-*ar*-te-RĪ-tis) (*NOTE: the* i *in arteri/o has been dropped*)	inflammation of many (sites in the) arteries
tachycardia (*tak*-i-KAR-dē-a) (*NOTE: the* i *in cardi/o has been dropped*)	condition of a rapid heart (rate of more than 100 beats per min)
thrombophlebitis (*throm*-bō-fle-BĪ-tis)	inflammation of a vein associated with a (blood) clot
valvulitis (*val*-vū-LĪ-tis)	inflammation of a valve (of the heart)

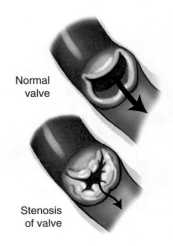

FIGURE 10-8
Aortic stenosis.

EXERCISE FIGURE B

Fill in the blanks to label the diagram.

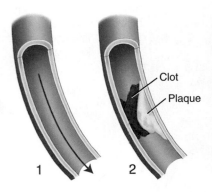

1. Healthy artery with smooth blood flow.

2. Blocked artery due to:

_____ / _____
(blood) clot / abnormal condition

and _____

_____ / _____ / _____
fatty plaque / CV / hardening

Fill in the blanks to complete labeling of the diagram.

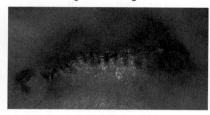

Post-surgical site displaying swelling and

formation of a _____ /_____
 blood / tumor

MULTIPLE MYELOMA

in the United States comprises approximately 6% of all blood malignancies. It most often occurs after age 65. Most patients are asymptomatic until the disease is advanced. **Symptoms and signs** are varied and may include **bone pain** and fractures, **infections, weight loss, anemia, and fatigue.** Treatments include **chemotherapy** and **stem cell transplantation.**

EMBOLUS/ THROMBUS

An **embolus** circulates in the bloodstream until it becomes lodged in a vessel, whereas a **thrombus** is attached to the interior wall of a vessel. When a **thrombus** breaks away and circulates in the bloodstream, it becomes known as an **embolus.**

Disease and Disorder Terms—cont'd

Built from Word Parts

TERM	DEFINITION
BLOOD	
erythrocytopenia (e-rith-rō-sī-tō-PĒ-nē-a)	abnormal reduction of red (blood) cells (this term is synonymous with **anemia**)
hematoma (hē-ma-TŌ-ma)	tumor of blood (collection of blood resulting from a broken blood vessel) (Exercise Figure C)
leukocytopenia (lū-kō-sī-tō-PĒ-nē-a)	abnormal reduction of white (blood) cells (also called **leukopenia**)
multiple myeloma (MUL-te-pl) (mī-e-LŌ-ma)	tumors of the bone marrow
pancytopenia (pan-sī-tō-PĒ-nē-a)	abnormal reduction of all (blood) cells
thrombocytopenia (throm-bō-sī-tō-PĒ-nē-a)	abnormal reduction of (blood) clotting cells
thrombosis (throm-BŌ-sis)	abnormal condition of a (blood) clot (Exercise Figure B)
thrombus (THROM-bus)	(blood) clot (attached to the interior wall of an artery or vein)
LYMPHATIC SYSTEM	
lymphadenitis (lim-fad-e-NĪ-tis)	inflammation of lymph nodes
lymphadenopathy (lim-fad-e-NOP-a-thē)	disease of lymph nodes (characterized by abnormal enlargement of the lymph nodes associated with an infection or malignancy)
lymphoma (lim-FŌ-ma)	tumor of lymphatic tissue (malignant)
splenomegaly (splē-nō-MEG-a-lē)	enlargement of the spleen
thymoma (thī-MŌ-ma)	tumor of the thymus gland

To watch animations, go to evolve.elsevier.com. Select: Chapter 10, **Animations,** Deep Vein Thrombosis.

Refer to p. 10 for your Evolve Access Information.

EXERCISE 11

Practice saying aloud each of the disease and disorder terms built from word parts on pp. 397–398.

To hear the terms, go to evolve.elsevier.com. Select: Chapter 10, **Exercises,** Pronunciation.

Refer to p. 10 for your Evolve Access Information.

☐ Place a check mark in the box when you have completed this exercise.

EXERCISE 12

Analyze and define the following terms.

1. endocarditis _____

2. bradycardia _____

3. cardiomegaly _____

4. arteriosclerosis _____

5. valvulitis _____

6. (multiple) myeloma _____

7. tachycardia _____

8. angiostenosis _____

9. thrombus _____

10. pericarditis _____

11. aortic stenosis _____

12. thrombosis _____

13. atherosclerosis _____

14. myocarditis _____

15. angioma _____

16. thymoma _____

17. lymphoma _____

18. lymphadenitis _____

19. splenomegaly _____

20. hematoma _____

21. polyarteritis _____

22. cardiomyopathy _____

23. lymphadenopathy _____

24. thrombophlebitis _____

25. phlebitis _____

26. pancytopenia _____

27. erythrocytopenia _____

28. leukocytopenia _____

29. thrombocytopenia _____

EXERCISE 13

Build disease and disorder terms for the following definitions by using the word parts you have learned.

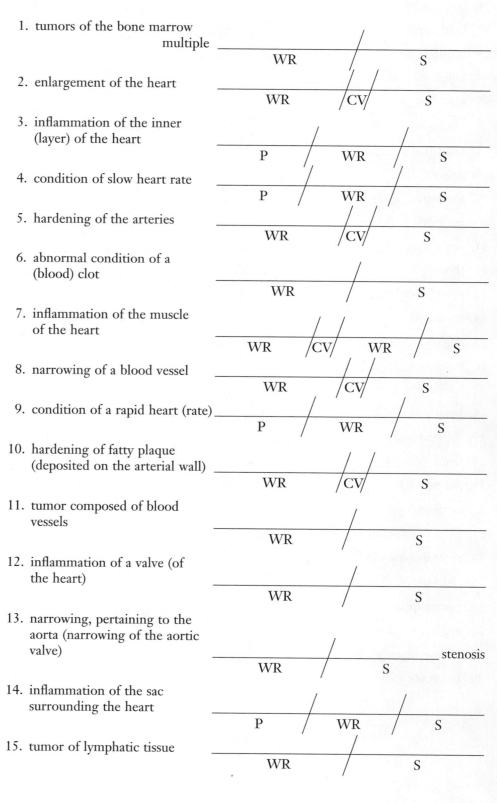

1. tumors of the bone marrow
   multiple _____/_____
              WR   /   S

2. enlargement of the heart
   _____/___/_____
      WR   /CV/   S

3. inflammation of the inner
   (layer) of the heart
   _____/___/_____/_____
      P   /   WR   /   S

4. condition of slow heart rate
   _____/___/_____/_____
      P   /   WR   /   S

5. hardening of the arteries
   _____/___/_____
      WR   /CV/   S

6. abnormal condition of a
   (blood) clot
   _____/_____
      WR   /   S

7. inflammation of the muscle
   of the heart
   _____/___/_____/_____
      WR   /CV/   WR   /   S

8. narrowing of a blood vessel
   _____/___/_____
      WR   /CV/   S

9. condition of a rapid heart (rate) _____/_____/_____
                                        P   /   WR   /   S

10. hardening of fatty plaque
    (deposited on the arterial wall)
    _____/___/_____
       WR   /CV/   S

11. tumor composed of blood
    vessels
    _____/_____
       WR   /   S

12. inflammation of a valve (of
    the heart)
    _____/_____
       WR   /   S

13. narrowing, pertaining to the
    aorta (narrowing of the aortic
    valve)
    _____/_____ stenosis
       WR   /   S

14. inflammation of the sac
    surrounding the heart
    _____/___/_____/_____
       P   /   WR   /   S

15. tumor of lymphatic tissue
    _____/_____
       WR   /   S

16. tumor of the thymus gland

_____ / _____
WR   S

17. enlargement of the spleen

_____ /CV/ _____
WR   CV   S

18. tumor (collection) of blood

_____ / _____
WR   S

19. inflammation of lymph nodes

_____ / _____
WR   S

20. disease of the heart muscle

_____ /CV/ _____ /CV/ _____
WR   CV   WR   CV   S

21. inflammation of many (sites in the) arteries

_____ / _____ / _____
P   WR   S

22. disease of lymph nodes

_____ /CV/ _____
WR   CV   S

23. inflammation of a vein associated with a clot

_____ /CV/ _____ / _____
WR   CV   WR   S

24. inflammation of a vein

_____ / _____
WR   S

25. (blood) clot

_____ / _____
WR   S

26. abnormal reduction of all (blood) cells

_____ / _____ /CV/ _____
P   WR   CV   S

27. abnormal reduction of red (blood) cells

_____ /CV/ _____ /CV/ _____
WR   CV   WR   CV   S

28. abnormal reduction of white (blood) cells

_____ /CV/ _____ /CV/ _____
WR   CV   WR   CV   S

29. abnormal reduction of (blood) clotting cells

_____ /CV/ _____ /CV/ _____
WR   CV   WR   CV   S

EXERCISE 14

Spell each of the disease and disorder terms built from word parts on pp. 397–398 by having someone dictate them to you.

> To hear and spell the terms, go to evolve.elsevier.com. Select: Chapter 10, **Exercises**, Spelling.
>
> Refer to p. 10 for your Evolve Access Information.
>
> ☐ Place a check mark in the box if you have completed this exercise online.

1. _____   16. _____
2. _____   17. _____
3. _____   18. _____
4. _____   19. _____
5. _____   20. _____
6. _____   21. _____
7. _____   22. _____
8. _____   23. _____
9. _____   24. _____
10. _____   25. _____
11. _____   26. _____
12. _____   27. _____
13. _____   28. _____
14. _____   29. _____
15. _____

Disease and Disorder Terms

Not Built from Word Parts

In some of the following terms, you may recognize word parts you have already learned; however, the full meaning of the terms cannot be discerned by the definition of their word parts.

ACUTE CORONARY SYNDROME (ACS)

is an umbrella term used when a patient seeks care at an emergency care facility for symptoms of **acute angina** or **myocardial infarction not yet diagnosed.** Treatment includes rapid assessment to determine the diagnosis and treatment of symptoms to possibly minimize heart damage.

🏛 **ANGINA PECTORIS**

was believed by the ancients to be a disorder of the breast. The Latin angere, meaning to throttle, was used to represent the sudden pain and was added to pectus, meaning breast.

TERM	DEFINITION
CARDIOVASCULAR SYSTEM	
acute coronary syndrome (ACS) (a-KŪT) (KOR-o-nar-ē) (SIN-drōm)	sudden symptoms of insufficient blood supply to the heart indicating **unstable angina** or **acute myocardial infarction**
aneurysm (AN-ū-rizm)	ballooning of a weakened portion of an arterial wall (Figure 10-9)
angina pectoris (an-JĪ-na) (PEK-to-ris)	chest pain, which may radiate to the left arm and jaw, that occurs when there is an insufficient supply of blood to the heart muscle
arrhythmia (ā-RITH-mē-a)	any disturbance or abnormality in the heart's normal rhythmic pattern

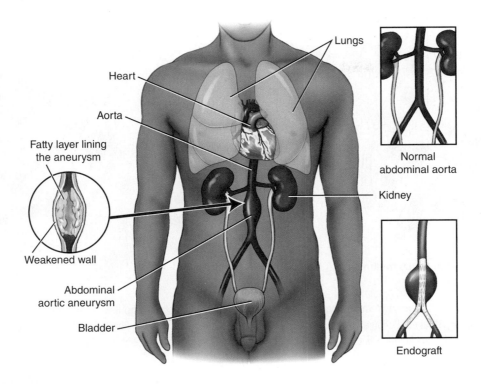

FIGURE 10-9

Abdominal aortic aneurysm (AAA). An AAA is located in the abdominal area of the aorta, the main blood vessel that transports blood away from the heart. Because the success rate of surgery is much lower once an aneurysm has ruptured, more emphasis is being placed on diagnosis. AAAs can be detected by physical examination but are more frequently detected by abdominal sonography. The preferred surgical intervention, called **endovascular stenting,** is performed through a puncture in the femoral artery, using a radiographic device called fluoroscopy. With this technique, a rigid **endograft** can be placed within an aneurysm.

TERM	DEFINITION
atrial fibrillation (AFib) (Ā-trē-al) (fi-bri-LĀ-shun)	cardiac arrhythmia characterized by chaotic, rapid electrical impulses in the atria. The atria quiver instead of contracting, causing irregular ventricular response and the ejection of a reduced amount of blood from both the atria and ventricles. The blood that remains in the atria becomes static, increasing the risk of clot formation, which may lead to a stroke. Two types of AFib are **paroxysmal atrial fibrillation (PAF),** which is intermittent, and **chronic atrial fibrillation,** which is sustained (Figure 10-10).
cardiac arrest (KAR-dē-ak) (a-REST)	sudden cessation of cardiac output and effective circulation, which requires cardiopulmonary resuscitation (CPR)
cardiac tamponade (KAR-dē-ak) (tam-po-NĀD)	acute compression of the heart caused by fluid accumulation in the pericardial cavity
coarctation of the aorta (kō-ark-TĀ-shun) (ā-OR-ta)	congenital cardiac condition characterized by a narrowing of the aorta (Figure 10-11)

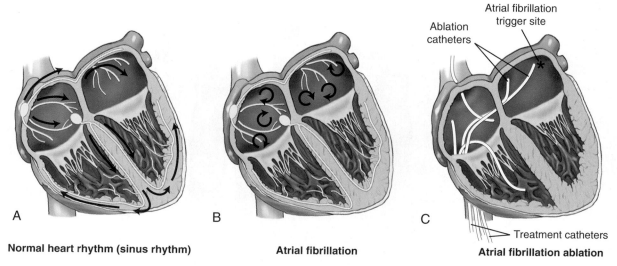

Normal heart rhythm (sinus rhythm)   **Atrial fibrillation**   **Atrial fibrillation ablation**

FIGURE 10-10

Atrial fibrillation (AF). **A,** Normal heart rhythm. Arrows indicate the normal travel of electrical impulses though the heart, stimulating coordinated contraction of chambers. **B,** Atrial fibrillation showing chaotic, rapid electrical impulses. **C,** Atrial fibrillation ablation, which destroys the abnormal cells that trigger atrial fibrillation. Ablation is used to treat atrial fibrillation if drug therapy is not effective.

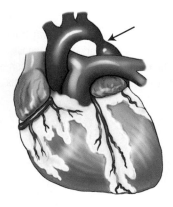

FIGURE 10-11
Coarctation of the aorta.

🏛 **CORONARY**
is derived from the Latin coronalis, meaning crown or wreath. It describes the arteries encircling the heart.

🏛 **RAYNAUD (RĀ-NŌ) PHENOMENON**
is classified as a **peripheral arterial disease (PAD)**. The condition was first described by Maurice Raynaud, a French physician, in 1862. Symptoms include intermittent, symmetric attacks of cyanosis and pallor of the distal ends of the fingers and toes often caused by exposure to cold temperature.

Disease and Disorder Terms—cont'd

Not Built from Word Parts

TERM	DEFINITION
congenital heart disease (kon-JEN-i-tal) (hart) (di-ZĒZ)	heart abnormality present at birth
coronary artery disease (CAD) (KOR-o-*nar*-ē) (AR-te-rē) (di-ZĒZ)	condition that reduces the flow of blood through the coronary arteries to the myocardium that may progress to denying the heart tissue sufficient oxygen and nutrients to function normally; most often caused by coronary atherosclerosis. CAD is a common cause of **heart failure** or **myocardial infarction**.
deep vein thrombosis (DVT) (dēp) (vān) (throm-BŌ-sis)	condition of thrombus in a deep vein of the body. Most often occurs in the lower extremities. A clot, or part of a clot, can break off and travel to the lungs, causing a pulmonary embolism.
heart failure (HF) (hart) (fāl-ŪR)	condition in which there is an inability of the heart to pump enough blood through the body to supply the tissues and organs with nutrients and oxygen (also called **congestive heart failure [CHF]**).
hypertensive heart disease (HHD) (*hī*-per-TEN-siv) (hart) (di-ZĒZ)	disorder of the heart caused by persistent high blood pressure
intermittent claudication (*in*-ter-MIT-nt) (*klaw*-di-KĀ-shun)	pain and discomfort in calf muscles while walking; a condition seen in peripheral arterial disease.

TERM	DEFINITION
ischemia (is-KĒ-mē-a)	condition of deficient blood flow due to constriction or obstruction of a blood vessel. Myocardial ischemia, or deficient blood to the heart muscle through coronary arteries, is most commonly caused by vessel constriction due to atherosclerosis and can lead to myocardial infarction.
mitral valve stenosis (MĪ-tral) (ste-NŌ-sis)	narrowing of the mitral valve from scarring, usually caused by episodes of **rheumatic fever**
myocardial infarction (MI) (mī-ō-KAR-dē-al) (in-FARK-shun)	death (necrosis) of a portion of the myocardium caused by lack of oxygen resulting from an interrupted blood supply (also called **heart attack**)
peripheral arterial disease (PAD) (pe-RIF-er-al) (ar-TER-ē-al) (di-ZĒZ)	disease of the arteries in the arms and legs, resulting in narrowing or complete obstruction of the artery. This is caused most commonly by atherosclerosis, but occasionally by inflammatory diseases, emboli, or thrombus formation. The most common symptom of peripheral arterial disease is intermittent claudication. (also called **peripheral vascular disease [PVD]**).
rheumatic heart disease (rū-MAT-ik) (hart) (di-ZĒZ)	damage to the heart muscle or heart valves caused by one or more episodes of **rheumatic fever**
varicose veins (VAR-i-kōs) (vānz)	distended or tortuous veins usually found in the lower extremities (Figure 10-12)

VARICOSE VEINS AND CURRENT TREATMENT

Varicose veins usually occur in the superficial veins of the legs, which return approximately 15% of the blood back to the heart. One-way valves in the veins help move the blood upward. When these valves fail, or the veins lose their elasticity, the blood flows backward, pools, and forms varicose veins. Approximately 80 million Americans, mostly women, have varicose veins or small, shallow spider veins. Causes are heredity, obesity, pregnancy, illness, or injury. Ligation and stripping was previously considered the primary surgical procedure for treatment.

Current Treatment

Endovenous laser ablation—Closure of varicose veins by application of heat within the vein.

Ambulatory phlebectomy—Tiny punctures are made in the skin through which the varicose veins are pulled out. Local anesthetic is used, and the procedure is minimally invasive.

Sclerotherapy—Injection of a liquid or foam sclerosant solution into a varicose vein causing it to thrombose and close over a month or two. Sclerosants have been used in large and small veins. This therapy usually takes less than an hour and requires no anesthesia.

Laser or intense pulsed light—Noninvasive technique used to remove spider veins. The light causes the veins to shrink and collapse.

RHEUMATIC FEVER

is an inflammatory disease, usually occurring in children and young adults after an upper respiratory tract streptococcal infection.

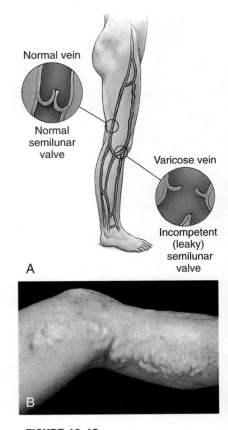

FIGURE 10-12
A, Normal and varicose veins.
B, Appearance of varicose veins.

COMMON TYPES OF ANEMIA

- **Acute blood loss anemia:** reduction in red blood cells as a result of hemorrhage
- **Iron-deficiency anemia:** insufficient amount of iron in the body to produce hemoglobin; frequently caused by chronic blood loss
- **Pernicious anemia:** ineffective production of red blood cells from vitamin B$_{12}$ deficiency
- **Hemolytic anemia:** reduced life of red blood cells (e.g., sickle cell anemia)
- **Anemia of chronic inflammation:** ineffective red blood cell production from chronic disease
- **Aplastic anemia:** resulting from bone marrow failure

SEPSIS OR SEPTICEMIA

can result when a severe bacterial infection, such as **pneumonia** or **pyelonephritis**, is untreated or treated with incomplete antibiotic therapy; the microorganism can enter the bloodstream, causing sepsis. **Sepsis** is the tenth most common cause of death in the United States. Patients in intensive care units or patients with impaired immune function are vulnerable to developing septicemia.

🏛 HODGKIN DISEASE

was first described in 1832 by Thomas Hodgkin, a pathologist at Guy's Hospital in London. In 1865 the name Hodgkin's disease was given to the condition by another English physician, Sir Samuel Wilks.

Disease and Disorder Terms—cont'd

Not Built from Word Parts

TERM	DEFINITION
BLOOD	
anemia (a-NĒ-mē-a)	condition in which there is a reduction in the number of erythrocytes. Anemia may be caused by blood loss or decrease in the production or increase in the destruction of red blood cells.
embolus (*pl.* emboli) (EM-bō-lus) (EM-bo-lī)	blood clot or foreign material, such as air or fat, that enters the bloodstream and moves until it lodges at another point in the circulation
hemophilia (hē-mō-FIL-ē-a)	inherited bleeding disease most commonly caused by a deficiency of the coagulation factor VIII
leukemia (lū-KĒ-mē-a)	malignant disease characterized by excessive increase in abnormal leukocytes formed in the bone marrow
sepsis (SEP-sis)	condition in which pathogenic microorganisms, usually bacteria, enter the bloodstream, causing a systemic inflammatory response to the infection (also called **septicemia**)
LYMPHATIC SYSTEM	
Hodgkin disease (HOJ-kin) (di-ZĒZ)	malignant disorder of the lymphatic tissue characterized by progressive enlargement of the lymph nodes, usually beginning in the cervical nodes
infectious mononucleosis (in-FEK-shus) (*mon*-ō-*nū*-klē-Ō-sis)	acute infection caused by the Epstein-Barr virus characterized by swollen lymph nodes, sore throat, fatigue, and fever. The disease affects mostly young people and is usually transmitted by saliva.

To watch animations go to evolve.elsevier.com. Select:
Chapter 10, **Animations,** Cardiac Ischemia
Arrhythmia
Hemophilia
Sepsis

Refer to p. 10 for your Evolve Access Information.

Table 10-1

Leukemia

Leukemia is differentiated by the type of leukocyte that is affected and how quickly the disease develops and progresses.

Acute Leukemia develops quickly with rapid progression of the disease. Both adults and children may develop acute leukemia. Acute leukemia is the most common form of cancer in children and adolescents.

Chronic Leukemia develops slowly with gradual disease progression and is only present in adults.

TYPES OF LEUKEMIA

- Acute lymphoblastic leukemia (ALL)
- Chronic lymphocytic leukemia (CLL)
- Acute myeloid leukemia (AML)
- Chronic myeloid leukemia (CML)
- Hairy cell leukemia (HCL)

EXERCISE 15

Practice saying aloud each of the disease and disorder terms not built from word parts on pp. 402–406.

To hear the terms, go to evolve.elsevier.com. Select: Chapter 10, **Exercises**, Pronunciation.

Refer to p. 10 for your Evolve Access Information.

☐ Place a check mark in the box when you have completed this exercise.

EXERCISE 16

Fill in the blanks with the correct terms.

1. A congenital cardiac condition characterized by a narrowing of the aorta is called _____ of the aorta.

2. A blood clot or foreign material that enters the bloodstream and moves until it lodges at another point in the circulation is called a(n) _____.

3. Sudden cessation of cardiac output and effective circulation is referred to as a(n) _____ _____.

4. _____ heart disease is the name given to a heart abnormality present at birth.

5. Veins that are distended or tortuous are called _____ _____.

6. Obstruction or constriction of a vessel causing deficient blood flow is called _____.

7. _____ is the name given to the ballooning of a weakened portion of an artery wall.

8. _____ _____ is the name given to a malignant disorder of lymphatic tissue characterized by enlarged lymph nodes.

9. _____ _____ _____ is a condition most often caused by coronary atherosclerosis.

10. _____ _____ is a cardiac condition characterized by chest pain caused by an insufficient blood supply to the cardiac muscle.

11. Death of a portion of myocardial muscle caused by lack of oxygen resulting from an interrupted blood supply is called a(n) _____ _____.

12. _____ _____ is a cardiac arrhythmia.

13. Any disturbance or abnormality in the heart's normal rhythmic pattern is called a(n) _____.

14. A disorder of the heart caused by a persistently high blood pressure is called _____ heart disease.

15. _____ _____ is the inability of the heart to pump enough blood through the body to supply tissues and organs.

16. _____ _____ _____ is a disease of the arteries in the arms and legs resulting in narrowing or complete obstruction of an artery.

17. _____ is an inherited bleeding disease most commonly caused by a deficiency of the coagulation factor VIII.

18. _____ is a malignant disease in which the number of abnormal white blood cells formed in the bone marrow is excessively increased.

19. A reduction in the number of erythrocytes results in a condition known as

_____.

20. _____ _____ is an infection caused by the Epstein-Barr virus.

21. _____ _____ is a condition in which a patient has pain and discomfort in calf muscles while walking.

22. Acute compression of the heart caused by fluid accumulation in the pericardial cavity is known as _____ _____.

23. Episodes of rheumatic fever can cause _____

_____ _____ and _____

_____ _____.

24. _____ _____ _____ is the condition of a thrombus, most often occurring in the lower extremities.

25. _____ _____ _____ is insufficient blood supply to the heart, indicating unstable angina or myocardial infarction.

26. _____ is a systemic inflammatory response to an infection.

EXERCISE 17

Match the terms in the first column with the correct definitions in the second column.

_____ 1. anemia
_____ 2. aneurysm
_____ 3. angina pectoris
_____ 4. arrhythmia
_____ 5. cardiac arrest
_____ 6. cardiac tamponade
_____ 7. coarctation of the aorta
_____ 8. congenital heart disease
_____ 9. heart failure
_____ 10. ischemia
_____ 11. intermittent claudication
_____ 12. deep vein thrombosis
_____ 13. coronary artery disease
_____ 14. peripheral arterial disease

a. sudden cessation of cardiac output and effective circulation
b. deficient blood flow due to constriction or obstruction of a blood vessel
c. ballooning of a weak portion of an arterial wall
d. reduction in the number of erythrocytes in the blood
e. any disturbance or abnormality in the heart's normal rhythmic pattern
f. chest pain occurring because of insufficient blood supply to the heart muscle
g. inability of the heart to pump enough blood through the body to supply tissues or organs
h. pain in calf muscles while walking
i. congenital cardiac condition with narrowing of the aorta
j. acute compression of the heart caused by fluid in the pericardial cavity
k. heart abnormality present at birth
l. clot in a deep vein
m. disease of the arteries in the arms and legs resulting in narrowing or complete obstruction of the artery
n. condition that reduces the flow of blood through the coronary arteries

EXERCISE 18

Match the terms in the first column with the correct definitions in the second column.

_____ 1. embolus

_____ 2. atrial fibrillation

_____ 3. hemophilia

_____ 4. infectious mononucleosis

_____ 5. Hodgkin disease

_____ 6. hypertensive heart disease

_____ 7. leukemia

_____ 8. myocardial infarction

_____ 9. mitral valve stenosis

_____ 10. acute coronary syndrome

_____ 11. varicose veins

_____ 12. rheumatic heart disease

_____ 13. sepsis

a. inherited bleeding disease most commonly caused by a deficiency of the coagulation factor VIII

b. heart disorder brought on by persistent high blood pressure

c. distended or tortuous veins

d. malignant disease, characterized by excessive increase of abnormal white blood cells formed in the bone marrow

e. characterized by chaotic, rapid electrical impulses of the atria

f. systemic inflammatory response to an infection

g. symptoms indicating unstable angina or myocardial infarction

h. infectious disease that affects mostly young people; characterized by swollen lymph glands

i. blood clot or foreign material that enters the bloodstream and moves until it lodges at another point

j. malignant disorder of lymphatic tissue with enlargement of lymph nodes

k. death of a portion of myocardium caused by lack of oxygen resulting from an interrupted blood supply

l. narrowing of the valve between the left atrium and left ventricle

m. damage to the heart caused by episodes of rheumatic fever

EXERCISE 19

Spell each of the disease and disorder terms not built from word parts on pp. 402–406 by having someone dictate them to you.

> To hear and spell the terms, go to evolve.elsevier.com. Select: Chapter 10, **Exercises**, Spelling.
>
> (e) Refer to p. 10 for your Evolve Access Information.
>
> ☐ Place a check mark in the box if you have completed this exercise online.

1. _____
2. _____
3. _____
4. _____
5. _____
6. _____
7. _____
8. _____
9. _____
10. _____
11. _____
12. _____
13. _____
14. _____

15. _____
16. _____
17. _____
18. _____
19. _____
20. _____
21. _____
22. _____
23. _____
24. _____
25. _____
26. _____
27. _____

Surgical Terms

Built from Word Parts

The following terms are built from word parts you have already learned and can be translated literally to find their meanings. Further explanation of terms beyond the definition of their word parts, if needed, is included in parentheses.

TERM	DEFINITION
CARDIOVASCULAR SYSTEM	
angioplasty (AN-jē-ō-*plas*-tē)	surgical repair of a blood vessel
atherectomy (ath-er-EK-to-mē)	excision of fatty plaque (from a blocked artery using a specialized catheter and a rotary cutter)
endarterectomy (*end*-ar-ter-EK-to-mē) *(NOTE: the o from endo- is dropped for easier pronunciation)*	excision within the artery (excision of plaque from the arterial wall). This procedure is usually named for the artery to be cleaned out, such as carotid endarterectomy, which means removal of plaque from the wall of the carotid artery (Exercise Figure D).
pericardiocentesis (*per*-i-kar-dē-ō-sen-TĒ-sis)	surgical puncture to aspirate fluid from the sac surrounding the heart (pericardium) (used to remove fluid or air, usually to relieve cardiac tamponade) (see Figure 10-13)
phlebectomy (fle-BEK-to-mē)	excision of a vein
phlebotomy (fle-BOT-o-mē)	incision into a vein (with a needle to remove blood or to give blood or intravenous fluids) (also called **venipuncture**)
valvuloplasty (VAL-vū-lō-*plas*-tē)	surgical repair of a valve (cardiac or venous)
LYMPHATIC SYSTEM	
splenectomy (splē-NEK-to-mē)	excision of the spleen
splenopexy (SPLĒ-nō-*peks*-ē)	surgical fixation of the spleen
thymectomy (thī-MEK-to-mē)	excision of the thymus gland

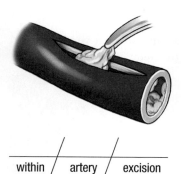

EXERCISE FIGURE **D**

Fill in the blanks to label the diagram.

within / artery / excision

To watch animations, go to evolve.elsevier.com. Select:
Chapter 10, **Animations**, Pericardiocentesis
Angioplasty

Refer to p. 10 for your Evolve Access Information.

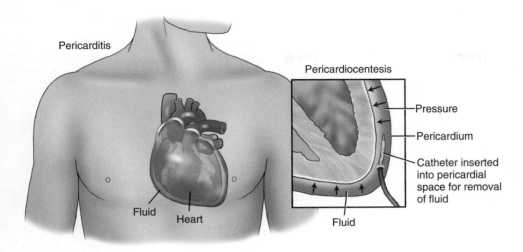

FIGURE 10-13
Pericarditis may produce excess fluid in the pericardium. If the fluid seriously affects the heart's ability to pump blood, pericardiocentesis may be performed to remove the fluid.

EXERCISE 20

Practice saying aloud each of the surgical terms built from word parts.

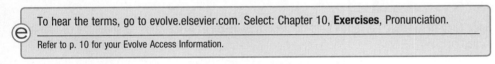

To hear the terms, go to evolve.elsevier.com. Select: Chapter 10, **Exercises**, Pronunciation.

Refer to p. 10 for your Evolve Access Information.

☐ Place a check mark in the box when you have completed this exercise.

EXERCISE 21

Analyze and define the following surgical terms.

1. pericardiocentesis _____
2. thymectomy _____
3. angioplasty _____
4. splenopexy _____
5. valvuloplasty _____
6. endarterectomy _____
7. phlebotomy _____
8. splenectomy _____
9. phlebectomy _____
10. atherectomy _____

EXERCISE 22

Build surgical terms for the following definitions by using the word parts you have learned.

1. excision within the artery   _____ / _____ / _____
                                     P   WR   S

2. surgical fixation of the spleen _____ / _____ / _____
                                       WR   CV   S

3. surgical repair of a valve

_____
WR   /CV/   S

4. incision into a vein

_____
WR   /CV/   S

5. excision of the thymus gland

_____
WR   /   S

6. surgical puncture to aspirate fluid from the sac surrounding the heart

_____
P   /   WR   /CV/   S

7. surgical repair of a blood vessel

_____
WR   /CV/   S

8. excision of the spleen

_____
WR   /   S

9. excision of a vein

_____
WR   /   S

10. excision of fatty plaque

_____
WR   /   S

EXERCISE 23

Spell each of the surgical terms built from word parts on p. 410 by having someone dictate them to you.

> To hear and spell the terms, go to evolve.elsevier.com. Select: Chapter 10, **Exercises**, Spelling.
>
> (e) Refer to p. 10 for your Evolve Access Information.
>
> ☐ Place a check mark in the box if you have completed this exercise online.

1. _____   6. _____

2. _____   7. _____

3. _____   8. _____

4. _____   9. _____

5. _____   10. _____

Surgical Terms

Not Built from Word Parts

In some of the following terms, you may recognize word parts you have already learned; however, the full meaning of the terms cannot be discerned by the definition of their word parts.

TERM	DEFINITION
CARDIOVASCULAR SYSTEM	
aneurysmectomy (*an*-ū-riz-MEK-to-mē)	surgical excision of an aneurysm
atrial fibrillation ablation (Ā-tre-al) (fi-bri-LĀ-shun) (ab-LĀ-shun)	procedure in which abnormal cells that trigger atrial fibrillation are destroyed by using a device that heats or freezes the cells (see Figure 10-10)
cardiac pacemaker (KAR-dē-ak) (PĀS-mā-kr)	battery-powered apparatus implanted under the skin with leads placed on the heart (Figure 10-15, *A*) or in the chamber of the heart (Figure 10-15, *B*); used to treat an abnormal heart rhythm, usually one that is too slow, secondary to an abnormal sinus node
coronary artery bypass graft (CABG) (KOR-o-*nar*-ē) (AR-te-rē) (BĪ-pas) (graft)	surgical technique to bring a new blood supply to heart muscle by detouring around blocked arteries (Figure 10-14)
coronary stent (KOR-o-*nar*-ē) (stent)	supportive scaffold device placed in the coronary artery; used to prevent closure of the artery after angioplasty or atherectomy (Figure 10-16); used to treat an artery occluded by plaque

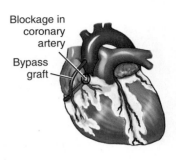

FIGURE 10-14
Coronary artery bypass graft (CABG). The abbreviation is pronounced "cabbage" like the vegetable.

STENT

is the name of a **supporting device**, such as a stiff cylinder or a mold, fashioned to anchor a graft. It is used to preserve dilation during healing or to provide support to keep a skin graft in place. Stent is not related to the term **stenosis**.

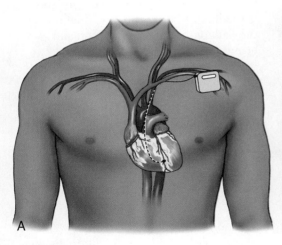

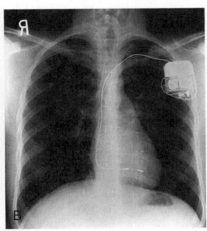

FIGURE 10-15
A, Cardiac pacemaker. The leads are implanted surgically on the epicardium through a thoracotomy. **B,** Chest radiograph of a patient with a cardiac pacemaker in which leads are implanted transvenously under fluoroscopic guidance. A pacemaker is primarily used to treat bradycardia, which is caused by an abnormality of the sinus node or conduction mechanism.

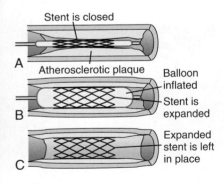

FIGURE 10-16
Coronary stent. **A,** Stent at the site of plaque formation. **B,** Inflated balloon and expanded stent. **C,** Inflated stent with balloon removed.

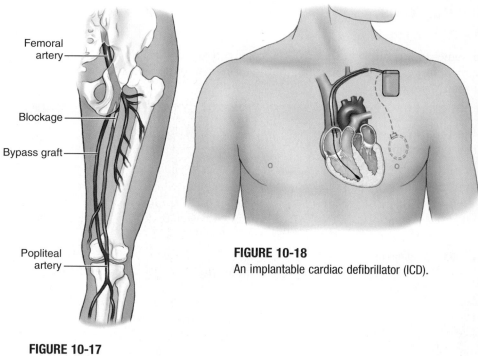

Femoral artery

Blockage

Bypass graft

Popliteal artery

FIGURE 10-17
Femoropopliteal bypass.

FIGURE 10-18
An implantable cardiac defibrillator (ICD).

CARDIAC RESYNCHRONIZATION THERAPY (CRT)

also called **biventricular pacing**, is the use of an **implantable device**, alone or in combination with an **ICD**, that provides simultaneous pacing of both ventricles of the heart. **CRT** is used in the treatment of severe heart failure (see Figure 10-18)

Surgical Terms—cont'd

Not Built from Word Parts

TERM	DEFINITION
embolectomy (*em*-bo-LEK-to-mē)	surgical removal of an embolus or clot, usually with a balloon catheter, inflating the balloon beyond the clot, then pulling the balloon back to the incision and bringing the clot with it
femoropopliteal bypass (*fem*-o-rō-pop-LIT-ē-al) (BĪ-pass)	surgery to establish an alternate route from femoral artery to popliteal artery to bypass an obstruction (Figure 10-17)
implantable cardiac defibrillator (ICD) (im-PLANT-a-bl) (KAR-dē-ak) (dē-FIB-ri-lā-tor)	device implanted in the body that continuously monitors the heart rhythm. If life-threatening arrhythmias occur, the device delivers an electric shock to convert the arrhythmia back to a normal rhythm (Figure 10-18).
intracoronary thrombolytic therapy (in-tra-KOR-o-nar-ē) (*throm*-bō-LIT-ik) (THER-a-pē)	injection of a medication either intravenously or intraarterially to dissolve blood clots in the coronary arteries before they become hardened. It is often used in emergency departments for acute myocardial infarction.

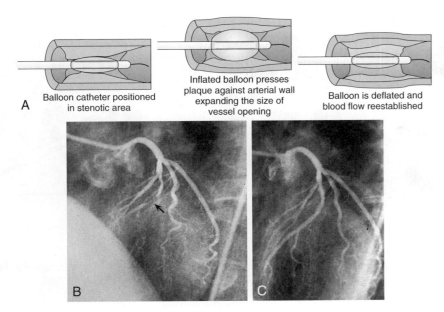

A, Balloon catheter positioned in stenotic area

Inflated balloon presses plaque against arterial wall expanding the size of vessel opening

Balloon is deflated and blood flow reestablished

B

C

FIGURE 10-19
Percutaneous transluminal coronary angioplasty (PTCA). **A,** Balloon dilation. **B,** Coronary arteriogram before PTCA. The *arrow* indicates the stenotic area with blockage, estimated at 95% minimum blood flow distal to the lesion. **C,** Coronary arteriogram after PTCA in the same patient. Blood flow is estimated to be 100%.

TERM	DEFINITION
percutaneous transluminal coronary angioplasty (PTCA) (*per*-kū-TĀ-nē-us) (trans-LŪ-min-al) (KOR-o-*nar*-ē) (AN-jē-ō-*plas*-tē)	procedure in which a balloon is passed through a blood vessel into a coronary artery to the area where plaque is formed. Inflation of the balloon compresses the plaque against the vessel wall, expanding the inner diameter of the blood vessel, which allows the blood to circulate more freely (also called **balloon angioplasty**) (Figure 10-19).
BLOOD	
bone marrow aspiration (bōn) (MAR-ō) (*as*-pi-RĀ-shun)	procedure to aspirate a sample of the liquid portion of the bone marrow, usually from the ilium, for study; used to diagnose, stage, and monitor disease and condition of blood cells (Figure 10-20)
bone marrow biopsy (bōn) (MAR-ō) (BĪ-op-sē)	procedure to obtain a sample of bone marrow, usually from the ilium, for study; used to diagnose, stage, and monitor disease and condition of blood cells
bone marrow transplant (bōn) (MAR-ō) (TRANS-plant)	infusion of healthy bone marrow cells to a recipient with matching cells from a donor

PERCUTANEOUS CORONARY INTERVENTION (PCI)

is an umbrella term that encompasses a variety of minimally invasive cardiovascular procedures. Specialized endovascular devices such as **stents** and **balloons** are inserted through a puncture in the skin, guided to heart vessels, and utilized to open narrowed or blocked coronary arteries. PCI results in significantly less recovery time and fewer complications than open cardiac surgery. PCI procedures are usually performed by an interventional cardiologist.

To watch animations, go to evolve.elsevier.com. Select:
Chapter 10, **Animations**, Coronary Artery Bypass Graft
                      PTCA

Refer to p. 10 for your Evolve Access Information.

● PERIPHERAL BLOOD STEM CELL TRANSPLANT (PBSCT)

is similar to **bone marrow transplant**. Stem cells are collected by apheresis, a process in which blood is removed from the patient or a matched donor and spun through a machine to harvest stem cells. The concentrated stem cells are given to the recipient by infusion. Both types of transplant are used to treat certain blood-related cancers and disorders, such as **leukemia** or **anemia**.

BONE MARROW

is a spongy tissue found in the hollow part of the larger bones of the body. It is made up of both a solid and liquid portion. Stem cells within the bone marrow turn into platelets, red blood cells, and white blood cells. **Bone marrow aspiration** and **bone marrow biopsy** are both used to obtain specimens for study. Each provides complementary information about the condition of blood cells. Bone marrow aspiration is performed first if both are being performed on the patient. Information from both procedures is used for **staging, monitoring,** and **diagnosing diseases** and conditions of the blood such as **anemia, leukemia, lymphoma,** and **multiple myeloma**.

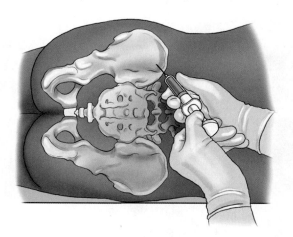

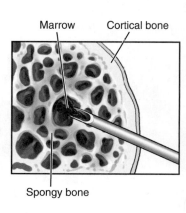

Marrow   Cortical bone

Spongy bone

FIGURE 10-20
Bone marrow aspiration. Study of the bone marrow can be used to identify the presence of leukemia or other malignancies or to determine the cause of anemia.

EXERCISE 24

Practice saying aloud each of the surgical terms not built from word parts on pp. 413–415.

> ⒠ To hear the terms, go to evolve.elsevier.com. Select: Chapter 10, **Exercises**, Pronunciation.
>
> Refer to p. 10 for your Evolve Access Information.

☐ Place a check mark in the box when you have completed this exercise.

EXERCISE 25

1. The procedure used to treat atrial fibrillation using a device that heats or freezes the cells is called atrial fibrillation _____.
2. The procedure in which a balloon is passed through a blood vessel into a coronary artery to compress plaque against the vessel wall when the balloon is inflated is called _____ _____

   _____ _____.

3. To regulate the heart rate, the physician may insert a(n) _____

   _____ with leads on or in the patient's heart.
4. Bone marrow aspiration and biopsy are used to diagnose, stage, and monitor disease and conditions of _____ _____.

5. The surgery performed to detour blood around a blocked artery so that a new

   blood supply can be given to heart muscles is called _____

   _____ _____ _____.

6. The surgical excision of an aneurysm is called a(n) _____.

7. A(n) _____ _____ is the name of the surgery
   performed to establish an alternate route from femoral artery to popliteal
   artery to bypass an obstruction.

8. An injection of a medication in a blocked coronary vessel to dissolve blood

   clots is called _____ _____ therapy.

9. _____ _____ _____ is a
   procedure to infuse healthy bone marrow cells to a recipient from a donor with
   matching tissue.

10. _____ is the surgical removal of an embolus, or clot.

11. A supportive scaffold device used to prevent closure of a coronary artery is

    called a(n) _____ _____.

12. _____ _____ _____ is
    used to treat life-threatening arrhythmias.

EXERCISE 26

Match the terms in the first column with their correct definitions in the second column.

_____ 1. aneurysmectomy

_____ 2. coronary artery bypass graft

_____ 3. femoropopliteal bypass

_____ 4. bone marrow aspiration

_____ 5. cardiac pacemaker

_____ 6. atrial fibrillation ablation

_____ 7. percutaneous transluminal coronary angioplasty

_____ 8. bone marrow biopsy

_____ 9. bone marrow transplant

_____ 10. intracoronary thrombolytic therapy

_____ 11. embolectomy

_____ 12. coronary stent

_____ 13. implantable cardiac defibrillator

a. compressing plaque against a blood vessel wall by inflating a balloon passed through the blood vessel

b. use of medication to dissolve blood clots in a blocked coronary vessel

c. used to obtain a sample of bone marrow

d. apparatus implanted under the skin to regulate the heartbeat

e. procedure using radiofrequency energy

f. monitors and corrects heart rhythms

g. supportive scaffold device placed in an artery

h. excision of a weakened, ballooning blood vessel wall

i. healthy bone marrow cells infused to a recipient with matching cells from a donor

j. surgical removal of an embolus

k. surgical procedure to establish an alternate route from the femoral artery to the popliteal artery to bypass an obstruction

l. aspiration of a sample of the liquid portion of bone marrow

m. diverts blood flow past a blocked artery in the heart

EXERCISE 27

Spell each of the surgical terms not built from word parts on pp. 413–415 by having someone dictate them to you.

> To hear and spell the terms, go to evolve.elsevier.com. Select: Chapter 10, **Exercises**, Spelling.
>
> Refer to p. 10 for your Evolve Access Information.
>
> ☐ Place a check mark in the box if you have completed this exercise online.

1. _____
2. _____
3. _____
4. _____
5. _____
6. _____
7. _____

8. _____
9. _____
10. _____
11. _____
12. _____
13. _____

Diagnostic Terms

Built from Word Parts

The following terms are built from word parts you have already learned and can be translated literally to find their meanings. Further explanation of terms beyond the definition of their word parts, if needed, is included in parentheses.

TERM	DEFINITION
CARDIOVASCULAR SYSTEM	
DIAGNOSTIC IMAGING	
angiography (*an*-jē-OG-ra-fē)	radiographic imaging of blood vessels (the procedure is named for the vessel to be studied, e.g., **femoral angiography** or **coronary angiography**) (Table 10-1)
angioscope (AN-jē-ō-skōp)	instrument used for visual examination (of the lumen) of a blood vessel
angioscopy (*an*-jē-OS-ko-pē)	visual examination (of the lumen) of a blood vessel
aortogram (ā-ŌR-to-gram)	radiographic image of the aorta (after an injection of contrast media)
arteriogram (ar-TĔR-ē-ō-gram)	radiographic image of an artery (after an injection of contrast media) (Figure 10-21)
venogram (VĒ-nō-gram)	radiographic image of a vein (after an injection of contrast media) (Figure 10-22)

TERM	DEFINITION
CARDIOVASCULAR PROCEDURES	
echocardiogram (ECHO) (*ek*-ō-KAR-dē-ō-gram)	record of the heart (structure and motion) using sound (used to detect valvular disease and evaluate heart function)
electrocardiogram (ECG, EKG) (ē-*lek*-trō-KAR-dē-ō-gram)	record of the electrical activity of the heart (Exercise Figure E)
electrocardiograph (ē-*lek*-trō-KAR-dē-ō-graf)	instrument used to record the electrical activity of the heart
electrocardiography (ē-*lek*-trō-*kar*-dē-OG-ra-fē)	process of recording the electrical activity of the heart

To watch animations, go to evolve.elsevier.com. Select:
Chapter 10, **Animations,** Subaortic Stenosis and Echocardiography
Pericardial Effusion and Echocardiography

Refer to p. 10 for your Evolve Access Information.

Table 10-2

Types of Angiography

CORONARY ARTERY VISUALIZATION

Coronary angiography, commonly called cardiac catheterization, is an **invasive procedure** in which a catheter is inserted into the coronary vessels, contrast media are injected, and images are recorded. It is considered the best technique for determining the percentage of blockage in the coronary arteries.

OTHER VASCULAR VISUALIZATION

Magnetic resonance angiography (MRA) is a **noninvasive procedure** that does not require catheterization or the injection of dye and uses specialized MR imaging to study vascular structures of the body. MRA may be chosen over computed tomography angiography because there is no exposure to ionizing radiation and contrast media.

Computed tomography angiography (CTA) is a **noninvasive procedure** that uses a high-resolution CT system to study vascular structures of the body after the injection of intravenous contrast media.

Digital subtraction angiography (DSA) is a procedure in which an image is taken and stored in the computer, then contrast medium is injected. A second image is taken and stored in the computer. The computer compares the two images and subtracts the first image from the second, removing structures not being studied. DSA enables better visualization of the arteries than regular angiography (Figure 10-23).

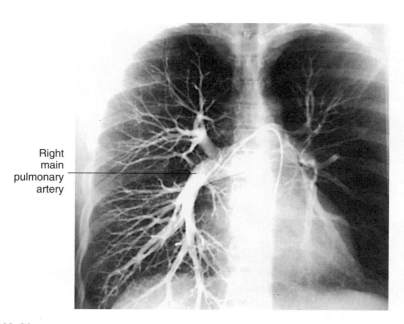

FIGURE 10-21

Arteriogram showing the right main pulmonary artery. This procedure (arteriography) is performed after injection of contrast material.

Right main pulmonary artery

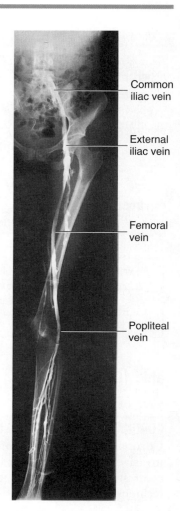

Common iliac vein

External iliac vein

Femoral vein

Popliteal vein

FIGURE 10-22

Normal venogram, lower left limb.

EXERCISE FIGURE **E**

Fill in the blanks to complete labeling of the diagram.

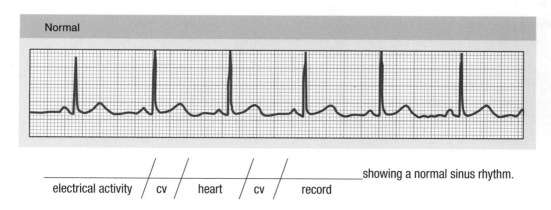

Normal

_____ / cv / _____ / cv / _____ showing a normal sinus rhythm.

electrical activity / cv / heart / cv / record

EXERCISE 28

Practice saying aloud each of the diagnostic terms built from word parts on pp. 418–419.

> To hear the terms, go to evolve.elsevier.com.
> ⓔ Select: Chapter 10, **Exercises**, Pronunciation.
> _____
> Refer to p. 10 for your Evolve Access Information.

☐ Place a check mark in the box when you have completed this exercise.

EXERCISE 29

Analyze and define the following diagnostic terms.

1. electrocardiograph _____

2. venogram_____

3. angiography _____

4. echocardiogram _____

5. aortogram _____

6. electrocardiogram_____

7. arteriogram _____

8. electrocardiography _____

9. angioscopy_____

10. angioscope_____

EXERCISE 30

Build diagnostic terms that correspond to the following definitions by using the word parts you have learned.

1. instrument used to record the electrical activity of the heart

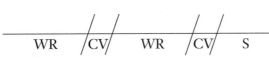

2. radiographic image of an artery (after an injection of contrast media)

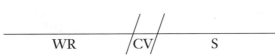

3. radiographic image of a vein (after an injection of contrast media)

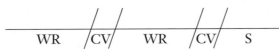

4. radiographic imaging of a blood vessel

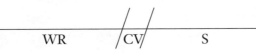

5. record of the electrical activity of the heart

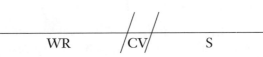

6. record of the heart (structure and motion) by using sound

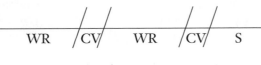

7. radiographic image of the aorta (after an injection of contrast media)

$$\underline{\hspace{2cm}} \quad \underline{/CV/} \quad \underline{\hspace{1cm}}$$
WR   CV   S

8. process of recording the electrical activity of the heart

$$\underline{\hspace{2cm}} \quad \underline{/CV/} \quad \underline{\hspace{1cm}} \quad \underline{/CV/} \quad \underline{\hspace{1cm}}$$
WR   CV   WR   CV   S

9. visual examination (of the lumen) of a blood vessel

$$\underline{\hspace{2cm}} \quad \underline{/CV/} \quad \underline{\hspace{1cm}}$$
WR   CV   S

10. instrument used for visual examination (of the lumen) of a blood vessel

$$\underline{\hspace{2cm}} \quad \underline{/CV/} \quad \underline{\hspace{1cm}}$$
WR   CV   S

EXERCISE 31

Spell each of the diagnostic terms built from word parts on pp. 418–419 by having someone dictate them to you.

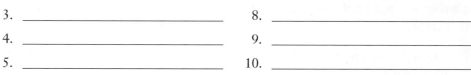

To hear and spell the terms, go to evolve.elsevier.com. Select: Chapter 10, **Exercises**, Spelling.

Refer to p. 10 for your Evolve Access Information.

☐ Place a check mark in the box if you have completed this exercise online.

1. _____   6. _____

2. _____   7. _____

3. _____   8. _____

4. _____   9. _____

5. _____   10. _____

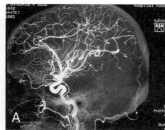

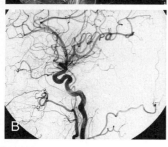

FIGURE 10-23
Digital subtraction angiography (DSA). **A,** Lateral digital **nonsubtracted** carotid artery. **B,** Lateral digital **subtracted** carotid artery. By removing unwanted anatomy, the image of the carotid artery is of high quality.

Diagnostic Terms

Not Built from Word Parts

In some of the following terms, you may recognize word parts you have already learned; however, the full meaning of the terms cannot be discerned by the definition of their word parts.

TERM	DEFINITION
CARDIOVASCULAR SYSTEM	
DIAGNOSTIC IMAGING	
digital subtraction angiography (DSA) (DIJ-i-tal) (sub-TRAK-shun) (*an*-jē-OG-ra-fē)	process of digital radiographic imaging of the blood vessels that "subtracts" or removes structures not being studied (Figure 10-23 and Table 10-1)

TERM	DEFINITION
Doppler ultrasound (DOP-ler) (UL-tra-sound)	study that uses high-frequency sound waves for detection of blood flow within the vessels; used to assess intermittent claudication, deep vein thrombosis, and other blood flow abnormalities (Figure 10-24)
exercise stress test (EK-ser-sīz) (stres) (test)	study that evaluates cardiac function during physical stress by riding a bike or walking on a treadmill. **Electrocardiography, echocardiography,** and **nuclear medicine scanning** are three types of stress tests performed to measure cardiac function while exercising.
single-photon emission computed tomography (SPECT) (SING-el-fō-ton) (ē-MISH-on) (com-PŪ-td) (tō-MOG-ra-fē)	nuclear medicine scan that visualizes the heart from several different angles, producing three-dimensional images; used to assess damage to cardiac tissue (Figure 10-25).

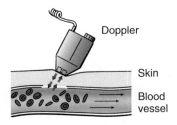

FIGURE 10-24
Doppler ultrasound showing the red blood cells reflecting sound.

CHEMICAL STRESS TESTING

is the **use of drugs to simulate the stress of physical exercise** on the body. It is used to study patients who are unable to exercise.

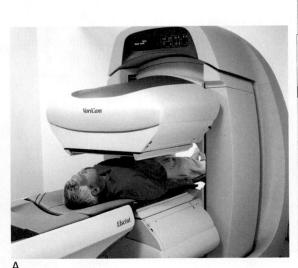

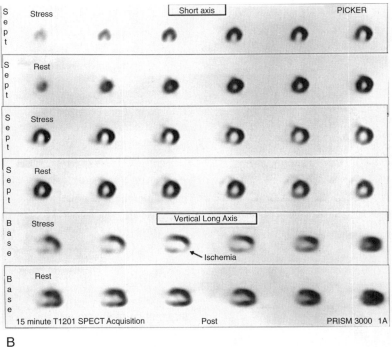

A   B

FIGURE 10-25
A, Single-photon emission computed tomography (SPECT) camera system. **B,** Thallium-201 myocardial perfusion scan comparing stress and redistribution (resting) images in various planes of the heart (short axis and long axis). A perfusion defect is identified in the stress images but not seen in the redistribution (rest) images. This finding is indicative of ischemia.

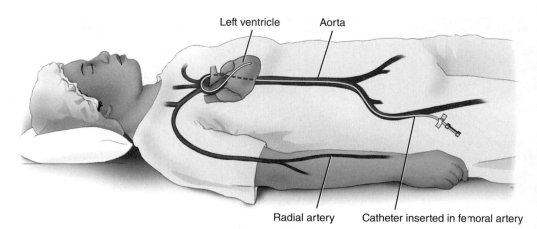

Left ventricle   Aorta

Radial artery   Catheter inserted in femoral artery

FIGURE 10-26
Cardiac catheterization

Diagnostic Terms—cont'd

Not Built from Word Parts

TERM	DEFINITION
thallium test (THĀL-ē-um) (test)	nuclear medicine test used to diagnose coronary artery disease and assess revascularization after coronary artery bypass surgery. Thallium, a radioactive isotope, is taken up by normal myocardial cells, but not in ischemia or infarction. These areas are identified as "cold" spots on the images produced. Thallium testing can be performed when the patient is at rest or it can be part of a stress test.
transesophageal echocardiogram (TEE) (*trans*-e-*sof*-a-JĒ-al) (*ek*-ō-KAR-dē-ō-gram)	ultrasound test that examines cardiac function and structure by using an ultrasound probe placed in the esophagus, which provides views of the heart structures
CARDIOVASCULAR STUDIES **cardiac catheterization** (KAR-dē-ak) (*kath*-e-ter-i-ZĀ-shun)	diagnostic procedure performed by passing a catheter into the heart through a blood vessel to examine the condition of the heart and surrounding blood vessels; used to diagnose and treat cardiovascular conditions such as coronary artery disease (also called **coronary angiography**) (Figure 10-26).
impedance plethysmography (IPG) (im-PĒD-ans) (*ple*-thiz-MOG-ra-fē)	measures venous flow of the extremities with a plethysmograph to detect clots by measuring changes in blood volume and resistance (impedance) in the vein; used to detect deep vein thrombosis
OTHER **blood pressure (BP)**	pressure exerted by the blood against the blood vessel walls. A blood pressure measurement written as **systolic** pressure (120) and **diastolic** pressure (80) is commonly recorded as 120/80 (Figure 10-27).

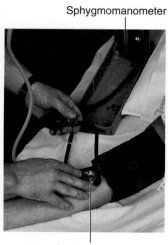

Sphygmomanometer

Stethoscope

FIGURE 10-27
Measurement of blood pressure.

TERM	DEFINITION
pulse (puls)	rhythmic expansion of an artery, created by the contraction of the heart, that can be felt with a fingertip. The pulse is most commonly felt over the radial artery (in the wrist); however, the pulsations can be felt over a number of sites, including the femoral (groin) and carotid (neck) arteries.
sphygmomanometer (*sfig*-mō-ma-NOM-e-ter)	device used for measuring blood pressure (see Figure 10-27)
LABORATORY **C-reactive protein (CRP)** (rē-AK-tiv) (PRŌ-tēn)	blood test to measure the amount of C-reactive protein in the blood, which, when elevated, indicates inflammation in the body. It is sometimes used in assessing the risk of cardiovascular disease.
creatine phosphokinase (CPK) (KRĒ-a-tin) (*fos*-fō-KĪ-nās)	blood test used to measure the level of creatine phosphokinase, an enzyme of heart and skeletal muscle released into the blood after muscle injury or necrosis. The test is useful in evaluating patients with acute myocardial infarction.
homocysteine (*hō*-mō-SIS-tēn)	blood test used to measure the amount of homocysteine in the blood. Homocysteine is an amino acid that, if elevated, may indicate an increased risk of cardiovascular disease.
lipid profile (LIP-id) (PRŌ-fil)	blood test used to measure the amount and type of lipids in a sample of blood. This test is used to evaluate the risk of developing cardiovascular disease and to monitor therapy of existing disease. Results provide levels of total cholesterol, high-density lipoprotein (HDL), low-density lipoprotein (LDL), very-low-density lipoprotein (VLDL), and triglycerides (Table 10-2).
troponin (TRŌ-pō-nin)	blood test that measures troponin, a heart muscle enzyme. Troponins are released into the blood approximately 3 hours after necrosis of the heart muscle and may remain elevated from 7 to 10 days. The test is useful in the diagnosis of a myocardial infarction.

BLOOD

LABORATORY

coagulation time (kō-*ag*-ū-LĀ-shun)	blood test to determine the time it takes for blood to form a clot
complete blood count (CBC) and differential count (Diff)	laboratory test for basic blood screening that measures various aspects of erythrocytes, leukocytes, and platelets; this automated test quickly provides a tremendous amount of information about the blood. (Figure 10-28)

A BIOMARKER

is a naturally occurring substance of certain body cells that can be measured in the blood and used to aid in the diagnosis of various disorders. **Troponin, creatinine phosphokinase, homocysteine,** and **C-reactive protein** are biomarkers, and elevated levels are used in diagnosing various disorders occurring in the body.

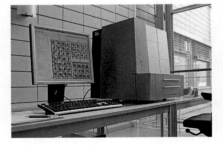

FIGURE 10-28
Complete blood count (CBC) results are obtained from a blood sample processed by an automated hematology analyzer.

Diagnostic Terms—cont'd

Not Built from Word Parts

TERM	DEFINITION
hematocrit (HCT) (hē-MAT-o-crit)	blood test to measure the volume of erythrocytes. It is used in the diagnosis and evaluation of anemic patients.
hemoglobin (Hgb) (HĒ-mō-*glō*-bin)	blood test used to determine the concentration of oxygen-carrying components (hemoglobin) in erythrocytes
prothrombin time (PT) (prō-THROM-bin)	blood test used to determine certain coagulation activity defects and to monitor anticoagulation therapy for patients taking Coumadin, an oral anticoagulant medication. (Activated partial thromboplastin time [APTT] is used to monitor anticoagulation therapy for patients taking heparin, an intravenous anticoagulant medication.)

PT/INR

stands for **prothrombin time/ international normalized ratio.** Most institutions now, on the recommendation of the World Health Organization, report both absolute numbers and INR numbers, which provide uniform PT results to physicians worldwide.

Table 10-3

Understanding a Lipid Profile

TERMS

Cholesterol—a compound important in the production of sex hormones, steroids, cell membranes, and bile acids. Cholesterol is produced by the body and contained in foods such as animal fats. Cholesterol is transported by lipoproteins.

High-density lipoprotein (HDL)—a type of lipoprotein that removes cholesterol from the tissues and transports it to the liver to be excreted in the bile. Elevated levels of HDL are considered protective against development of atherosclerosis, which may lead to coronary artery disease. HDL is often referred to as the "good" cholesterol.

Low-density lipoprotein (LDL)—a type of lipoprotein that transports cholesterol to the tissue and deposits it on the walls of the arteries. High levels of LDL are associated with the presence of atherosclerosis, which may lead to coronary artery disease. LDL is often referred to as the "bad" cholesterol.

Total cholesterol—the total amount of cholesterol contained in the HDL and LDL.

Triglycerides (TGs)—a form of fat in the blood. Triglycerides are synthesized in the liver and used to store energy. Test results are used to assess the risk of coronary artery disease.

Very-low-density lipoprotein (VLDL)—a type of lipoprotein that transports most of the triglycerides in the blood. Elevated levels of VLDL, to a lesser degree than LDL, indicate a risk for developing coronary artery disease.

EXAMPLE OF LIPID PROFILE LAB REPORT

TESTS	RESULTS	FLAG	NORMAL RANGE
Cholesterol, total	188 mg/dL		100-199 mg/dL
Triglycerides	287 mg/dL	High	0-149 mg/dL
HDL cholesterol	50 mg/dL		40-59 mg/dL
VLDL cholesterol calc	57 mg/dL	High	5-40 mg/dL
LDL cholesterol calc	81 mg/dL		0-99 mg/dL

EXERCISE 32

Practice saying aloud each of the diagnostic terms not built from word parts on pp. 422–426.

> (e) To hear the terms, go to evolve.elsevier.com. Select: Chapter 10, **Exercises**, Pronunciation.
>
> Refer to p. 10 for your Evolve Access Information.

☐ Place a check mark in the box when you have completed this exercise.

EXERCISE 33

Fill in the blanks with the correct terms.

1. A device for measuring blood pressure is called a(n) _____.
2. _____ _____ is a blood test that determines the time it takes for blood to form a clot.
3. _____ _____ and _____ _____ are the names of basic blood-screening tests.
4. A study that uses high-frequency sound waves for detection of blood flow within blood vessels is called_____ _____.
5. Pressure exerted by blood against the blood vessel walls is called_____ _____.
6. A blood test used to determine certain coagulation activity defects and to monitor oral anticoagulation therapy is called _____ _____.
7. _____ _____ is a procedure in which a catheter is introduced into the heart to record pressures and enable the visualization of the heart chambers.
8. A blood test used to determine the oxygen-carrying component in erythrocytes is called_____.
9. _____ _____ measures venous flow of the extremities and is used to detect deep vein thrombosis.
10. A nuclear medicine test used to diagnose coronary artery disease is _____ _____.
11. _____ _____ is a test in which an ultrasound probe provides views of the heart structures from the esophagus.
12. A nuclear medicine test that visualizes the heart from different angles is called a(n) _____ _____ _____ _____.

13. _____ _____ _____ evaluates cardiac function during physical stress.

14. A process of radiographic imaging of blood vessels that removes structures not being studied is called _____ _____

_____.

15. A blood test to measure an enzyme of the heart released into the bloodstream after muscle injury is called_____ _____.

16. An elevated_____ _____ indicates inflammation in the body.

17. _____ is the rhythmic expansion of an artery created by contraction of the heart that can be felt with a fingertip.

18. _____ is an amino acid that if elevated, indicates an increased risk of cardiovascular disease.

19. _____ is a heart muscle enzyme released into the bloodstream approximately 3 hours after heart muscle necrosis.

20. _____ _____ is the name of the blood test that measures the amount and type of lipids in the blood.

21. A test to measure the volume of erythrocytes and used in the diagnosis and evaluation of anemic patients is called _____.

EXERCISE 34

Match the terms in the first column with their correct definition in the second column.

_____ 1. cardiac catheterization

_____ 2. complete blood count and differential count

_____ 3. coagulation time

_____ 4. hemoglobin

_____ 5. Doppler ultrasound

_____ 6. prothrombin time

_____ 7. sphygmomanometer

_____ 8. single-photon emission computed tomography

_____ 9. digital subtraction angiography

_____ 10. thallium test

_____ 11. transesophageal echocardiogram

a. device used for measuring blood pressure

b. digital radiographic imaging of blood vessels

c. test to determine certain coagulation activity defects

d. passage of a catheter into the heart to evaluate coronary artery disease

e. visualizes the heart from several different angles

f. used to assess revascularization after CABG

g. oxygen-carrying component of erythrocytes

h. basic blood-screening test

i. an ultrasound test that provides views of the heart from the esophagus

j. study in which high-frequency sound waves are used to determine the flow of blood within the vessels

k. determines the time it takes for blood to form a clot

EXERCISE 35

Match the terms in the first column with the correct definitions in the second column.

_____ 1. exercise stress test

_____ 2. impedance plethysmography

_____ 3. C-reactive protein

_____ 4. blood pressure

_____ 5. creatine phosphokinase

_____ 6. hematocrit

_____ 7. homocysteine

_____ 8. pulse

_____ 9. lipid profile

_____ 10. troponin

a. measures the volume and number of erythrocytes

b. blood test to determine inflammation or risk of cardiovascular disease

c. measures cardiac function during physical stress

d. measures the level of an enzyme released into the blood after muscle injury

e. measures blood flow of the extremities

f. pressure exerted by blood against the blood vessel walls

g. measures the amount of an amino acid in the blood

h. measured most often over the radial artery

i. results provide levels of cholesterol, HDL, LDL, VLDL, and triglycerides

j. measures an enzyme released within hours after damage to the heart muscle

EXERCISE 36

Spell each of the diagnostic terms not built from word parts on pp. 422–426 by having someone dictate them to you.

To hear and spell the terms, go to evolve.elsevier.com. Select: Chapter 10, **Exercises**, Spelling.

Refer to p. 10 for your Evolve Access Information.

☐ Place a check mark in the box if you have completed this exercise online.

1. _____

2. _____

3. _____

4. _____

5. _____

6. _____

7. _____

8. _____

9. _____

10. _____

11. _____

12. _____

13. _____

14. _____

15. _____

16. _____

17. _____

18. _____

19. _____

20. _____

21. _____

Complementary Terms

Built from Word Parts

The following terms are built from word parts you have already learned and can be translated literally to find their meanings. Further explanation of terms beyond the definition of their word parts, if needed, is included in parentheses.

TERM	DEFINITION
CARDIOVASCULAR SYSTEM	
atrioventricular (AV) (ā-trē-ō-ven-TRIK-ū-ler)	pertaining to the atrium and ventricle
cardiac (KAR-dē-ak)	pertaining to the heart
cardiogenic (kar-dē-ō-JEN-ik)	originating in the heart
cardiologist (kar-dē-OL-o-jist)	physician who studies and treats diseases of the heart
cardiology (kar-dē-OL-o-jē)	study of the heart (a branch of medicine that deals with diseases of the heart)
hypothermia (hī-pō-THER-mē-a)	condition of (body) temperature that is below (normal) (sometimes induced for various surgical procedures, such as bypass surgery)
intravenous (IV) (in-tra-VĒ-nus)	pertaining to within the vein (Exercise Figure F)
phlebologist (fle-BOL-o-jist)	physician who studies and treats diseases of the veins
phlebology (fle-BOL-o-jē)	study of veins (a branch of medicine that deals with diseases of the veins)
BLOOD	
hematologist (hē-ma-TOL-o-jist)	physician who studies and treats diseases of the blood
hematology (hē-ma-TOL-o-jē)	study of the blood (a branch of medicine that deals with diseases of the blood)
hematopoiesis (hē-ma-tō-poy-Ē-sis)	formation of blood (cells)
hemolysis (hē-MOL-i-sis)	dissolution of (red) blood (cells)
hemostasis (hē-mō-STĀ-sis)	stoppage of bleeding
myelopoiesis (mī-e-lō-poy-Ē-sis)	formation of bone marrow
plasmapheresis (plaz-ma-fe-RĒ-sis)	removal of plasma (from withdrawn blood)
thrombolysis (throm-BOL-i-sis)	dissolution of a clot

ELECTRO-PHYSIOLOGIST

is a **cardiologist** who specializes in the diagnosis and treatment of patients with arrhythmias.

INTRAVENOUS (IV) THERAPY

is **the infusion of a substance directly into a vein** for therapeutic purposes. **IV therapy** is a very common and essential component of medical care, serving as a direct, efficient route for the administration of fluids, medications, and blood products.

EXERCISE FIGURE

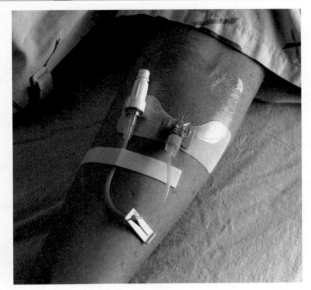

Patient's arm with an ————/————/———————— (IV) catheter.
                        within / vein / pertaining to

EXERCISE 37

Practice saying aloud each of the complementary terms built from word parts.

 To hear the terms, go to evolve.elsevier.com. Select: Chapter 10, **Exercises**, Pronunciation.

Refer to p. 10 for your Evolve Access Information.

☐ Place a check mark in the box when you have completed this exercise.

EXERCISE 38

Analyze and define the following complementary terms.

1. hypothermia _____
2. hematopoiesis _____
3. cardiology _____
4. cardiologist _____
5. hemolysis _____
6. hematologist _____
7. cardiac _____
8. hematology _____
9. plasmapheresis _____
10. hemostasis _____
11. cardiogenic _____
12. myelopoiesis _____
13. thrombolysis _____
14. atrioventricular _____
15. intravenous _____
16. phlebologist_____
17. phlebology_____

EXERCISE 39

Build the complementary terms for the following definitions by using the word parts you have learned.

1. study of the heart

   _____ / CV / _____
   WR   CV   S

2. formation of blood (cells)

   _____ / CV / _____
   WR   CV   S

3. condition of (body) temperature that is below (normal)

   _____ / _____ / _____
   P   WR   S

4. dissolution of (red) blood (cells)

   _____ / CV / _____
   WR   CV   S

5. removal of plasma (from withdrawn blood)

   _____ / _____
   WR   S

6. physician who studies and treats diseases of the blood

   _____ / CV / _____
   WR   CV   S

7. pertaining to the heart

   _____ / _____
   WR   S

8. physician who studies and treats diseases of the heart

   _____ / CV / _____
   WR   CV   S

9. study of the blood

   _____ / CV / _____
   WR   CV   S

10. stoppage of bleeding

    _____ / CV / _____
    WR   CV   S

11. formation of bone marrow

    _____ / CV / _____
    WR   CV   S

12. originating in the heart

    _____ / CV / _____
    WR   CV   S

13. dissolution of a clot

    _____ / CV / _____
    WR   CV   S

14. pertaining to the atrium and ventricle

    _____ / CV / _____ / _____
    WR   CV   WR   S

15. pertaining to within the vein

    _____ / _____ / _____
    P   WR   S

16. study of veins

    _____ / CV / _____
    WR   CV   S

17. physician who studies and treats diseases of the vein

    _____ / CV / _____
    WR   CV   S

EXERCISE 40

Spell each of the complementary terms built from word parts on p. 430 by having someone dictate them to you.

To hear and spell the terms, go to evolve.elsevier.com. Select: Chapter 10, **Exercises**, Spelling.

Refer to p. 10 for your Evolve Access Information.

☐ Place a check mark in the box if you have completed this exercise online.

1. _____   10. _____

2. _____   11. _____

3. _____   12. _____

4. _____   13. _____

5. _____   14. _____

6. _____   15. _____

7. _____   16. _____

8. _____   17. _____

9. _____

For review and/or assessment, go to evolve.elsevier.com. Select:
Chapter 10, **Activities**, Terms Built from Word Parts
Chapter 10, **Games**,   Term Storm

Refer to p. 10 for your Evolve Access Information.

Complementary Terms

Not Built from Word Parts

In some of the following terms, you may recognize word parts you have already learned; however, the full meaning of the terms cannot be discerned by the definition of their word parts.

TERM	DEFINITION
CARDIOVASCULAR SYSTEM	
bruit (broo-Ē)	abnormal vascular sound heard through auscultation, caused by turbulent blood flow through arteries or veins. Cardiovascular system abnormalities, such as **aneurysm**, create a distinctive bruit. Bruits may occur in numerous sites throughout the body where blood flow or body system functioning is abnormal.
cardiopulmonary resuscitation (CPR) (*kar*-dē-ō-PUL-mo-nar-ē) (rē-*sus*-i-TĀ-shun)	emergency procedure consisting of external cardiac compressions and artificial ventilation
defibrillation (dē-*fib*-ri-LĀ-shun)	application of an electric shock to the myocardium through the chest wall to restore normal cardiac rhythm (Figure 10-29)

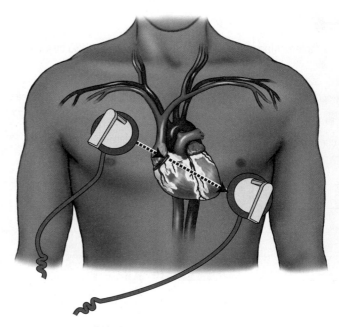

FIGURE 10-29
Placement of defibrillator paddles on the chest.

TERM	DEFINITION
diastole (dī-AS-tō-lē)	phase in the cardiac cycle in which the ventricles relax and fill with blood between contractions (diastolic is the lower number of a blood pressure reading)
extracorporeal (*ek*-stra-kōr-POR-ē-al)	occurring outside the body. During open-heart surgery extracorporeal circulation occurs when blood is diverted outside the body to a heart-lung machine.
extravasation (ek-*strav*-a-SĀ-shun)	escape of blood from the blood vessel into the tissue
fibrillation (fi-bri-LĀ-shun)	rapid, quivering, noncoordinated contractions of the atria or ventricles
hypercholesterolemia (*hī*-per-k-*les*-ter-ol-Ē-mē-a)	excessive amount of cholesterol in the blood; associated with heightened risk of cardiovascular disease
hyperlipidemia (*hī*-per-*lip*-i-DĒ-mē-a)	excessive amount of fats (lipids, triglycerides, and cholesterol) in the blood
hypertension (*hī*-per-TEN-shun)	blood pressure that is above normal (greater than 140/90)
hypertriglyceridemia (*hī*-per-trī-*glis*-er-rī-DĒ-mē-a)	excessive amount of triglycerides in the blood; associated with an increased risk of cardiovascular disease
hypotension (*hī*-pō-TEN-shun)	blood pressure that is below normal (less than 90/60)
lipids (LIP-ids)	fats and fatlike substances that serve as a source of fuel in the body and are an important constituent of cell structure

TERM	DEFINITION
lumen (LŪ-men)	space within a tubular part or organ, such as the space within a blood vessel
murmur (MER-mer)	abnormal cardiac sound heard through auscultation, caused by turbulent blood flow through the heart. Murmurs are short-duration sounds heard in the cardiac region that are distinct from normal heart sounds. Heart valve defects, such as **mitral valve stenosis**, create a distinctive murmur.
occlude (o-KLŪD)	to close tightly, to block
systole (SIS-tō-lē)	phase in the cardiac cycle in which the ventricles contract and eject blood (systolic is the upper number of a blood pressure reading)
vasoconstrictor (*vās*-ō-kon-STRIK-tor)	agent or nerve that narrows the blood vessels
vasodilator (*vās*-ō-DĪ-lā-tor)	agent or nerve that enlarges the blood vessels
venipuncture (VEN-i-*punk*-chur)	procedure used to puncture a vein with a needle to remove blood, instill a medication, or start an intravenous infusion
BLOOD **anticoagulant** (*an*-tī-kō-AG-ū-lant)	agent that slows the blood clotting process
blood dyscrasia (blud) (dis-KRĀ-zha)	abnormal or pathologic condition of the blood
hemorrhage (HEM-o-rij)	rapid loss of blood, as in bleeding

EXERCISE 41

Practice saying aloud each of the complementary terms not built from word parts on pp. 433–435.

> ⓔ To hear the terms, go to evolve.elsevier.com. Select: Chapter 10, **Exercises**, Pronunciation.
>
> Refer to p. 10 for your Evolve Access Information.

☐ Place a check mark in the box when you have completed this exercise.

EXERCISE 42

Write the term for each of the following definitions.

1. agent that narrows the blood vessels _____

2. space within a tubelike structure _____

3. emergency procedure consisting of external cardiac compressions and artificial ventilation _____ _____

4. phase in the cardiac cycle in which the ventricles relax

_____

5. noncoordinated contractions of the atria or ventricles

_____

6. blood pressure that is below normal

_____

7. escape of blood from the blood vessel into the tissue

_____

8. puncture of a vein to remove blood

_____

9. phase in the cardiac cycle in which the ventricles contract

_____

10. agent that enlarges the blood vessels

_____

11. blood pressure that is above normal

_____

12. to close tightly

_____

13. excessive amount of triglycerides in the blood

_____

14. excessive amount of fats in the blood

_____

15. rapid loss of blood

_____

16. excessive amount of cholesterol in the blood

_____

17. pathologic condition of the blood

_____ _____

18. abnormal cardiac sound heard through auscultation

_____

19. occurring outside the body

_____

20. fats and fatlike substances

_____

21. used to restore normal cardiac rhythm

_____

22. agent that slows the clotting process

_____

23. abnormal vascular sound heard through auscultation

_____

EXERCISE 43

Write the definitions of the following terms.

1. lumen_____

2. extravasation _____

3. hypercholesterolemia_____

4. venipuncture_____

5. vasodilator _____

6. hypertension _____

7. cardiopulmonary resuscitation _____

8. systole _____

9. hypotension_____

10. vasoconstrictor _____

11. diastole _____

12. fibrillation _____

13. occlude _____

14. hyperlipidemia _____

15. hypertriglyceridemia _____

16. blood dyscrasia _____

17. hemorrhage_____

18. anticoagulant_____

19. extracorporeal_____

20. murmur _____

21. lipid _____

22. defibrillation _____

23. bruit_____

EXERCISE 44

Spell each of the complementary terms not built from word parts on pp. 433–435 by having someone dictate them to you.

To hear and spell the terms, go to evolve.elsevier.com. Select: Chapter 10, **Exercises**, Spelling.

Refer to p. 10 for your Evolve Access Information.

☐ Place a check mark in the box if you have completed this exercise online.

1. _____   13. _____

2. _____   14. _____

3. _____   15. _____

4. _____   16. _____

5. _____   17. _____

6. _____   18. _____

7. _____   19. _____

8. _____   20. _____

9. _____   21. _____

10. _____   22. _____

11. _____   23. _____

12. _____

Complementary Terms

Not Built From Word Parts

TERM	DEFINITION
IMMUNE SYSTEM	
allergen (AL-er-jen)	environmental substance capable of producing an immediate hypersensitivity in the body (allergy). Common allergens are house dust, pollen, animal dander, and various foods.
allergist (AL-er-jist)	physician who studies and treats allergic conditions
allergy (AL-er-jē)	hypersensitivity to a substance, resulting in an inflammatory immune response
anaphylaxis (*an*-a-fe-LAK-sis)	exaggerated, life-threatening reaction to a previously encountered antigen such as bee venom, peanuts, or latex. Symptoms range from mild, with patients experiencing hives or sneezing, to severe symptoms such as drop in blood pressure and blockage of the airway, which can lead to death within minutes (also called **anaphylactic shock**).
antibody (AN-ti-*bod*-ē)	substance produced by lymphocytes that inactivates or destroys antigens (also called **immunoglobulins**)
antigen (AN-ti-jen)	substance that triggers an immune response when introduced into the body. Examples of antigens are transplant tissue, toxins, and infectious organisms.
autoimmune disease (*aw*-tō-i-MŪN) (di-ZĒZ)	disease caused by the body's inability to distinguish its own cells from foreign bodies, thus producing antibodies that attack its own tissue. **Rheumatoid arthritis** and **systemic lupus erythematosus** are examples of autoimmune diseases.
immune (i-MŪN)	being resistant to specific invading pathogens
immunodeficiency (*im*-ū-nō-de-FISH-en-sē)	deficient immune response caused by the immune system dysfunction brought on by disease (HIV infection) or immunosuppressive drugs (prednisone)
immunologist (*im*-ū-NOL-o-jist)	physician who studies and treats immune system disorders
immunology (*im*-ū-NOL-o-jē)	the branch of medicine dealing with immune system disorders
phagocytosis (*fā*-gō-sī-TŌ-sis)	process in which some of the white blood cells destroy the invading microorganism and old cells
vaccine (vak-SĒN)	suspension of inactivated microorganisms administered by injection, mouth, or nasal spray to prevent infectious diseases by inducing immunity

IMMUNITY

occurs in three ways:

- **natural immunity** between mother and child before birth and after birth through breast milk
- **active immunity** by the body producing antibodies in response to an infectious disease such as tuberculosis
- **artificial immunity** by receiving vaccinations to produce antibodies. Artificial immunity is used to prevent previously common diseases such as measles and mumps.

To watch animations, go to evolve.elsevier.com. Select:
Chapter 10, **Animations,** Allergy
                                Phagocytosis
                                Antibiotics

Refer to p. 10 for your Evolve Access Information.

Refer to **Appendix D** for pharmacology terms related to the cardiovascular system and blood.

EXERCISE 45

Practice saying aloud each of the complementary terms not built from word parts on p. 438.

To hear the terms, go to evolve.elsevier.com. Select: Chapter 10, **Exercises,** Pronunciation.

Refer to p. 10 for your Evolve Access Information.

☐ Place a check mark in the box when you have completed this exercise.

EXERCISE 46

Match the immune system terms in the first column with the phrases in the second column.

_____ 1. allergen
_____ 2. autoimmune disease
_____ 3. immunologist
_____ 4. antigen
_____ 5. immune
_____ 6. allergist
_____ 7. antibodies
_____ 8. immunodeficiency
_____ 9. phagocytosis
_____ 10. vaccine
_____ 11. allergy
_____ 12. immunology
_____ 13. anaphylaxis

a. deficient immune response
b. branch of medicine dealing with immune system disorders
c. administered by injection, nasal spray, or orally to prevent infectious diseases
d. inactivates or destroys antigens
e. house dust, pollen, animal dander
f. transplant tissue, toxin, infectious organisms
g. treats allergic conditions
h. white blood cells destroy invading microorganisms
i. hypersensitivity to a substance
j. rheumatoid arthritis
k. life-threatening reaction
l. resistant to invading pathogens
m. treats immune system disorders

EXERCISE 47

Spell each of the complementary terms not built from word parts on p. 438 by having someone dictate them to you.

To hear and spell the terms, go to evolve.elsevier.com. Select: Chapter 10, **Exercises,** Spelling.

Refer to p. 10 for your Evolve Access Information.

☐ Place a check mark in the box if you have completed this exercise online.

1. _____   8. _____

2. _____   9. _____

3. _____   10. _____

4. _____   11. _____

5. _____   12. _____

6. _____   13. _____

7. _____

For review and/or assessment, go to evolve.elsevier.com. Select:

Chapter 10, **Activities**, Terms Not Built from Word Parts

Hear It and Type It: Clinical Vignettes

Chapter 10, **Games**,   Term Explorer

Termbusters

Medical Millionaire

Refer to p. 10 for your Evolve Access Information.

Abbreviations

ABBREVIATION	MEANING
ACS	acute coronary syndrome
AFib	atrial fibrillation
AV	atrioventricular
BP	blood pressure
CABG	coronary artery bypass graft
CAD	coronary artery disease
CBC and Diff	complete blood count and differential
CCU	coronary care unit
CPK	creatine phosphokinase
CPR	cardiopulmonary resuscitation
CRP	C-reactive protein
DSA	digital subtraction angiography
DVT	deep vein thrombosis
ECG, EKG	electrocardiogram
ECHO	echocardiogram
Hct	hematocrit
HF	heart failure
Hgb	hemoglobin
HHD	hypertensive heart disease
ICD	implantable cardiac defibrillator
IPG	impedance plethysmography
IV	intravenous
MI	myocardial infarction
PAD	peripheral arterial disease

ABBREVIATION	MEANING
PT	prothrombin time
PTCA	percutaneous transluminal coronary angioplasty
RBC	red blood cell (erythrocyte)
SPECT	single-photon emission computed tomography
TEE	transesophageal echocardiogram
WBC	white blood cell (leukocyte)

🔍 Refer to **Appendix C** for a complete list of abbreviations.

EXERCISE 48

Write the meaning of the abbreviation in the blanks.

1. **CAD** _____ _____ _____ has
   received growing interest over the past 20 years. Diagnostic procedures for
   new patients

   usually begin with an exercise **ECG** _____. Patients whose stress
   tests are borderline usually proceed to noninvasive imaging such as **SPECT**

   _____ _____ _____

   _____ and stress **ECHO**_____.

2. **DVT** _____ _____ _____ is
   common in hospitalized patients. Early detection is important because DVT
   can result in death from a pulmonary embolism. Doppler ultrasound and **IPG**

   _____ _____ are two noninvasive diagnostic
   procedures used to diagnose DVT. MRI and venography may be used as well.

3. The **CBC** _____ _____ _____ and

   _____ count are a series of automated laboratory tests of the
   peripheral blood that provide a great deal of information about the blood and
   other body

   organs. Tests performed as part of the CBC are **RBC** _____

   _____ _____ count, **WBC** _____

   _____ _____ count and differential count, **Hgb**

   _____, and **Hct** _____.

4. Standard surgical treatment for CAD includes **CABG** _____

   _____ _____ _____. There is a
   growth in the use of minimally invasive techniques to treat CAD, which
   include

   transmyocardial laser revascularization and **PTCA** _____

   _____ _____ _____, atherectomy,
   and stent placement.

5. Hospitalized patients diagnosed with **MI** _____ _____
   are cared for in the **CCU** _____ _____

   _____.

6. A sphygmomanometer is used to measure **BP** _____ _____.

7. Diagnosis used to indicate that a patient's heart is unable to pump enough blood through the body to supply tissues is **HF** _____ _____.

8. If the patient's heart and/or lungs have ceased to function, the medical team must begin **CPR** _____ _____.

9. A patient with persistently elevated blood pressure is likely to be diagnosed with **HHD** _____ _____ _____.

10. When scheduling blood tests for a patient on oral anticoagulant medication, the doctor is likely to include a **PT** _____ _____.

11. Any interruption of the conduction of electrical impulses from the atria to the ventricles is called **AV** _____ block.

12. The treatment of **ACS** _____ _____ _____ is aimed at preventing thrombus formation and restoring blood flow to the occluded coronary artery.

13. Stopping smoking, exercising, and proper diet are important in the medical management of **PAD** _____ _____ _____.

14. **DSA** _____ _____ _____ is especially valuable in cardiac diagnostic applications.

15. The physician ordered a **TEE** _____ _____ to examine the patient's heart structure and function.

16. Two blood tests used in assessing and evaluating cardiovascular diseases are **CRP** _____ _____ and **CPK** _____ _____.

17. A patient experiencing **AFib** _____ _____ may be referred to an electrophysiologist, a cardiology subspecialist.

18. An **ICD** _____ _____ _____ delivers an electric shock to convert an arrhythmia back to normal rhythm.

19. The patient with dehydration was ordered **IV** _____ fluids by her physician.

For more practice with abbreviations, go to evolve.elsevier.com. Select:
Chapter 10, **Flashcards**
ⓔ Chapter 10, **Games,** Crossword Puzzle

Refer to p. 10 for your Evolve Access Information.

PRACTICAL APPLICATION

EXERCISE 49 *Interact with Medical Documents and Electronic Health Records*

A. Complete the inpatient progress note by writing the medical terms in the blanks. Use the list of definitions with the corresponding numbers on the next page.

20922-CVR WILLAMETT, Josephine   _ □ X

File   Patient   Navigate   Custom Fields   Help

Chart Review | Encounters | Notes | Labs | Imaging | Procedures | Rx | Documents | Referrals | Scheduling | Billing

| Name: **WILLAMETT, Josephine** | MR#: **20922-CVR** | Gender: F | **Allergies:** ASA |
| | DOB: **03/12/19XX** | Age: 76 | **PCP:** Julian Giverne, MD |

Inpatient progress note:

Chief complaint: Josephine Willamett is a 76-year-old woman who was admitted to the hospital for recurrent chest pain.

History of present illness: The patient has a long history of stable 1._____. She had a positive treadmill stress test in 1998. A 2._____ in 2008 showed reversible 3._____. In May 2011 she underwent cataract surgery, and during her postoperative care she developed severe chest pain. An ECG at that time showed ischemic ST changes in the anterior leads. Subsequent coronary 4._____ revealed a 90% focal 5._____ left anterior descending coronary artery. The patient then underwent 6._____ of this lesion. The 90% stenosis was dilated to a 20% stenosis. The patient had an uncomplicated course.

Over the last 10 days the patient has had at least five episodes of chest pain, all relieved by rest or a single nitroglycerin tablet. She had an episode yesterday while gardening, which lasted almost 5 minutes before subsiding after a second nitroglycerin tablet. She went to her 7._____ office yesterday. 8._____ was performed, which showed marked T-wave inversion in the anterior leads, and she was immediately sent to this hospital for further evaluation. Atherogenic risk factors for her age include hypercholesterolemia and hypertension; she also smokes one pack of cigarettes per day. She is not a diabetic. Her family history reveals a brother who has had a coronary artery bypass graft.

Physical exam: On exam today, blood pressure is 138/86. She has tachycardia with a pulse of 120. She is in no acute distress. Her lungs are clear and she has regular rhythm without a murmur. There is no edema or distention of neck veins.

Current medications:
1. Lovastatin 20 mg with evening meal.
2. Enalapril 20 mg bid.
3. Nifedipine 10 mg tid.
4. Nitroglycerin 0.4 mg sublingual prn.

Plan: 9._____ with possible coronary stent if necessary. Serial ECGs, 10._____ _____ and 11._____ will be obtained to rule out 12._____.

Electronically signed: Marguerite DeRouge, DO 04/07/20XX 07:32

Start | Log On/Off | Print | Edit

---

1. chest pain, occurs when there is an insufficient supply of blood to the heart muscle
2. nuclear medicine test used to determine blood flow to the myocardium
3. deficient supply of blood to the heart's blood vessels
4. radiographic imaging a blood vessel
5. narrowing
6. surgical repair of a blood vessel
7. physician who studies and treats diseases of the heart
8. process of recording electrical activity of the heart
9. introduction of a catheter into the heart by way of a blood vessel to determine coronary artery disease
10. enzyme of heart and skeletal muscles
11. blood test that measures the amount of a certain enzyme approximately 3 hours after necrosis of the heart muscle
12. death of a portion of the myocardial muscle caused by lack of oxygen resulting from an interrupted blood supply

B. Read the progress note and answer the questions following it.

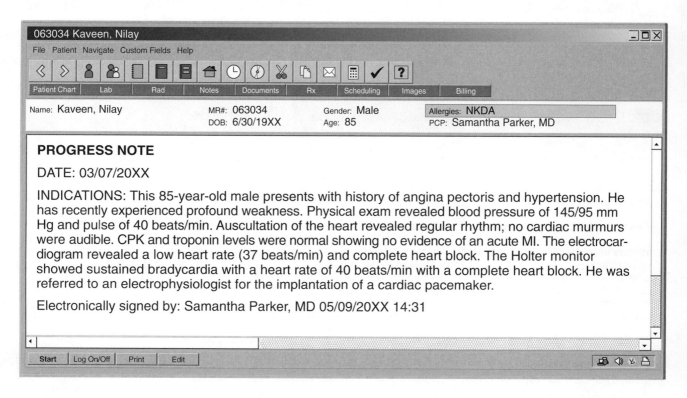

1. The patient had a history of (high or low) BP?
2. Cardiac murmur was ruled out by:
   a. diagnostic imaging test
   b. laboratory test
   c. stethoscope
3. An acute myocardial infarction was ruled out by:
   a. an EKG
   b. an ultrasound test
   c. a laboratory test

4. A cardiac pacemaker is used to:
   a. lower blood pressure
   b. regulate heart rate
   c. treat atrial fibrillation

C. Complete the **three medical documents** within the electronic health record (EHR) on Evolve.

> Many healthcare records today are stored and used in an electronic system called **Electronic Health Records (EHRs).** Electronic health records contain a collection of health information of an individual patient; the digitally formatted record can be shared through computer networks with patients, physicians, and other health care providers.

> For practice with medical terms using electronic health records, go to http:evolve.elsevier.com. Select: Chapter 10, **Electronic Health Records.**
>
> Refer to p. 10 for your Evolve Access Information.

EXERCISE 50   *Interpret Medical Terms*

To test your understanding of the terms introduced in this chapter, circle the words that correctly complete the sentences. The italicized words refer to the correct answer.

1. *Yellowish, fatty plaque within the arteries* is (**arteriosclerosis, atherosclerosis, aortosclerosis**).
2. *Inflammation of a vein associated with a clot* is called a (**thrombosis, phlebitis, thrombophlebitis**).
3. *Inflammation of the middle muscular layer of the heart* is (**endocarditis, myocarditis, pericarditis**).
4. Another name for a *heart attack* is (**myocardial infarction, coronary fibrillation, angina pectoris**).
5. The *surgical excision of a thickened artery interior* is an (**atherectomy, angioplasty, endarterectomy**).
6. An *acute infection caused by the Epstein-Barr virus* is (**anemia, infectious mononucleosis, rheumatic heart disease**).
7. *Reduction of body temperature to a level below normal* results in a condition called (**hypothermia, hypertension, hyperthermia**).
8. (**Impedance plethysmography, cardiac scan, aortogram**) is used to *determine if a patient has a blood clot in the femoral vein.*
9. *An abnormal cardiac sound heard through auscultation* or (**hemorrhage, murmur, pulse**) is sometimes the result of many episodes of rheumatic fever, an inflammatory disease occurring in children.
10. The doctor uses an (**echocardiograph, electrocardiogram, angioscope**) to *visualize the blood vessel* and guide the laser beam to open blocked arteries; this procedure is called (**echocardiography, angioscopy**).
11. The following is *a nuclear medicine test used to diagnose coronary artery disease* (**coronary stent, thallium test, transesophageal echocardiogram**).
12. Each time *the patient came in contact with house dust she immediately began to sneeze and experienced rhinorrhea.* She visited a(n) (**allergist, immunologist, hematologist**) to seek relief from her symptoms.
13. Peanuts are an antigen that can trigger an *exaggerated life-threatening reaction* or (**allergen, anaphylaxis, allergies**).

 WEB LINK

For additional information on the cardiovascular system, visit the **American Heart Association** at *www.heart.org.*

WEB LINK

For additional information on the lymphatic system and blood, visit the **Leukemia and Lymphoma Society** at *www.lls.org.*

EXERCISE 51 *Read Medical Terms in Use*

Practice pronunciation of terms by reading the following medical document. Use the pronunciation key following the medical terms to assist you in saying the word.

> To hear these terms, go to evolve.elsevier.com.
> Select: Chapter 10, **Exercises**, Read Medical Terms in Use.
>
> Refer to p. 10 for your Evolve Access Information.

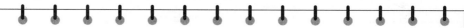

A 55-year-old man presented to his doctor with pain in the calf and swelling in the left foot and ankle. Three days prior, the patient had completed trans-Pacific airline travel, spending several hours in a sitting position. He has a history of **varicose** (VAR-i-kōs) **veins** (vānz). No previous history of **hypertension** (hī-per-TEN-shun) or **thrombophlebitis** (*throm*-bō-fle-BĪ-tis) existed. Physical examination revealed an edematous left lower extremity and a tender calf. The pedal **pulse** (puls) was intact. A **Doppler ultrasound** (DOP-ler) (UL-tra-sound) was obtained, which revealed **deep vein thrombosis** (throm-BŌ-sis). The patient was hospitalized and subcutaneous low molecular weight heparin was begun. Concurrently, Coumadin was started and will continue for 6 months. The oral **anticoagulant** (*an*-tī-cō-AG-ū-lant) therapy will be monitored monthly by **prothrombin** (prō-THROM-bin) **time.**

EXERCISE 52 *Comprehend Medical Terms in Use*

Test your comprehension of the terms in the previous medical document by circling the correct answer.

1. T F A radiographic image was used to diagnose deep vein thrombosis.
2. The patient was diagnosed with:
   a. inflammation of the vein
   b. vascular inflammatory disorder
   c. a clot in a vein in the lower extremity
   d. a clot in the blood vessels of the heart
3. A blood test will be used to determine:
   a. bleeding time
   b. the time it takes for blood to form a clot
   c. the oxygen-carrying capacity of the red blood cell
   d. certain coagulation activity defects

> For a snapshot assessment of your knowledge of cardiovascular, immune, lymphatic systems, and blood terms, go to http:evolve.elsevier.com.
> Select: Chapter 10, **Quick Quizzes.**
>
> Refer to p. 10 for your Evolve Access Information.

CHAPTER REVIEW

 Review of Evolve

Keep a record of the online activities you have completed by placing a check mark in the box. You may also record your scores. All activities have been referenced throughout the chapter.

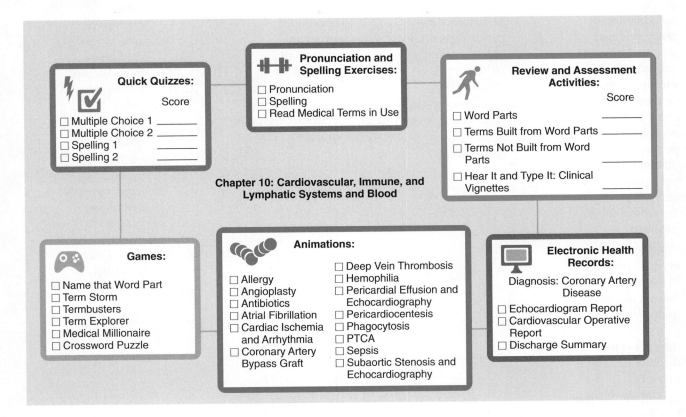

Quick Quizzes:

Score

☐ Multiple Choice 1 _____
☐ Multiple Choice 2 _____
☐ Spelling 1 _____
☐ Spelling 2 _____

Pronunciation and Spelling Exercises:

☐ Pronunciation
☐ Spelling
☐ Read Medical Terms in Use

Review and Assessment Activities:

Score

☐ Word Parts _____
☐ Terms Built from Word Parts _____
☐ Terms Not Built from Word Parts _____
☐ Hear It and Type It: Clinical Vignettes

Chapter 10: Cardiovascular, Immune, and Lymphatic Systems and Blood

Games:

☐ Name that Word Part
☐ Term Storm
☐ Termbusters
☐ Term Explorer
☐ Medical Millionaire
☐ Crossword Puzzle

Animations:

☐ Allergy
☐ Angioplasty
☐ Antibiotics
☐ Atrial Fibrillation
☐ Cardiac Ischemia and Arrhythmia
☐ Coronary Artery Bypass Graft
☐ Deep Vein Thrombosis
☐ Hemophilia
☐ Pericardial Effusion and Echocardiography
☐ Pericardiocentesis
☐ Phagocytosis
☐ PTCA
☐ Sepsis
☐ Subaortic Stenosis and Echocardiography

Electronic Health Records:

Diagnosis: Coronary Artery Disease

☐ Echocardiogram Report
☐ Cardiovascular Operative Report
☐ Discharge Summary

Review of Word Parts

Can you define and spell the following word parts?

COMBINING FORMS		PREFIXES	SUFFIXES
angi/o	myel/o	brady-	-ac
aort/o	phleb/o	pan-	-apheresis
arteri/o	plasm/o		-penia
ather/o	splen/o		-poiesis
atri/o	therm/o		-sclerosis
cardi/o	thromb/o		
ech/o	thym/o		
electr/o	valv/o		
isch/o	valvul/o		
lymph/o	ven/o		
lymphaden/o	ventricul/o		

Review of Terms

Can you define, pronounce, and spell the following terms *built from word parts?*

DISEASES AND DISORDERS	SURGICAL	DIAGNOSTIC	COMPLEMENTARY
Cardiovascular System	***Cardiovascular System***	***Cardiovascular System***	***Cardiovascular System***
angioma	angioplasty	angiography	atrioventricular (AV)
angiostenosis	atherectomy	angioscope	cardiac
aortic stenosis	endarterectomy	angioscopy	cardiogenic
arteriosclerosis	pericardiocentesis	aortogram	cardiologist
atherosclerosis	phlebectomy	arteriogram	cardiology
bradycardia	phlebotomy	echocardiogram (ECHO)	hypothermia
cardiomegaly	valvuloplasty	electrocardiogram (ECG, EKG)	intravenous (IV)
cardiomyopathy		electrocardiograph	phlebologist
endocarditis	***Lymphatic System***	electrocardiography	phlebology
myocarditis	splenectomy	venogram	
pericarditis	splenopexy		***Blood***
phlebitis	thymectomy		hematologist
polyarteritis			hematology
tachycardia			hematopoiesis
thrombophlebitis			hemolysis
valvulitis			hemostasis
			myelopoiesis
Blood			plasmapheresis
erythrocytopenia			thrombolysis
hematoma			
leukocytopenia			
multiple myeloma			
pancytopenia			
thrombocytopenia			
thrombosis			
thrombus			
Lymphatic System			
lymphadenitis			
lymphadenopathy			
lymphoma			
splenomegaly			
thymoma			

Can you define, pronounce, and spell the following terms *not built from word parts?*

DISEASES AND DISORDERS	SURGICAL	DIAGNOSTIC	COMPLEMENTARY
Cardiovascular System	***Cardiovascular System***	***Cardiovascular System***	***Cardiovascular System***
acute coronary syndrome (ACS)	aneurysmectomy	blood pressure (BP)	bruit
aneurysm	atrial fibrillation ablation	cardiac catheterization	cardiopulmonary resuscitation (CPR)
angina pectoris	cardiac pacemaker	C-reactive protein (CRP)	defibrillation
arrhythmia	coronary artery bypass graft (CABG)	creatine phosphokinase (CPK)	diastole
atrial fibrillation (AFib)	coronary stent	digital subtraction angiography (DSA)	extracorporeal
cardiac arrest	embolectomy	Doppler ultrasound	extravasation
cardiac tamponade	femoropopliteal bypass	exercise stress test	fibrillation
coarctation of the aorta	implantable cardiac defibrillator (ICD)	homocysteine	heart murmur
congenital heart disease	intracoronary thrombolytic therapy	impedance plethysmography (IPG)	hypercholesterolemia
coronary artery disease (CAD)	percutaneous transluminal coronary angioplasty (PTCA)	lipid profile	hyperlipidemia
deep vein thrombosis (DVT)		pulse	hypertension
heart failure (HF)	***Blood***	single-photon emission computed tomography (SPECT)	hypertriglyceridemia
hypertensive heart disease (HHD)	bone marrow aspiration	sphygmomanometer	hypotension
intermittent claudication	bone marrow biopsy	thallium test	lipids
ischemia	bone marrow transplant	transesophageal echocardiogram (TEE)	lumen
mitral valve stenosis		troponin	murmur
myocardial infarction (MI)			occlude
peripheral arterial disease (PAD)		***Blood***	systole
rheumatic heart disease		coagulation time	vasoconstrictor
varicose veins		complete blood count and differential (CBC and Diff)	vasodilator
		hematocrit (Hct)	venipuncture
Blood		hemoglobin (Hgb)	
anemia		prothrombin time (PT)	***Blood***
embolus, *pl.* emboli			anticoagulant
hemophilia			blood dyscrasia
leukemia			hemorrhage
sepsis			
			Immune System
Lymphatic System			allergen
Hodgkin disease			allergist
infectious mononucleosis			allergy
			anaphylaxis
			antibody
			antigen
			autoimmune disease
			immune
			immunodeficiency
			immunologist
			immunology
			phagocytosis
			vaccine

ANSWERS

ANSWERS TO CHAPTER 10 EXERCISES
Exercise Figures

Exercise Figure

A.
1. blood vessel: angi/o
2. valve: valv/o, valvul/o
3. heart: cardi/o
4. aorta: aort/o
5. artery: arteri/o
6. atrium: atri/o
7. ventricle: ventricul/o

Exercise Figure

B. thromb/osis, ather/o/sclerosis

Exercise Figure

C. hemat/oma

Exercise Figure

D. end/arter/ectomy

Exercise Figure

E. electr/o/cardi/o/gram

Exercise Figure

F. intra/ven/ous

Exercise 1
1. e	6. f
2. g	7. d
3. c	8. b
4. h	9. i
5. a	

Exercise 2
1. j	6. a
2. b	7. e
3. g	8. c
4. d	9. f
5. i	

Exercise 3
1. plasma
2. erythrocytes
3. leukocytes
4. platelets
5. platelets
6. serum
7. lymph
8. lymph nodes
9. spleen
10. thymus

Exercise 4
1. protect the body against pathogens, foreign agents, and abnormal body cells

2. a. spleen
   b. liver
   c. intestinal tract
   d. lymph nodes
   e. bone marrow
3. a. prevention of foreign bodies from entering the body
   b. phagocytosis, inflammation, fever, and activation of protective proteins and natural killer cells
   c. forms specific antibodies to fight infectious agents

Exercise 5
1. heart
2. atrium
3. plasma
4. vessel
5. vein
6. aorta
7. valve
8. spleen
9. thymus gland
10. vein
11. ventricle
12. artery
13. valve
14. lymph, lymph tissue
15. lymph node
16. bone marrow

Exercise 6
1. arteri/o
2. a. phleb/o
   b. ven/o
3. cardi/o
4. atri/o
5. ventricul/o
6. lymph/o
7. aort/o
8. angi/o
9. a. valv/o
   b. valvul/o
10. splen/o
11. plasm/o
12. thym/o
13. lymphaden/o
14. myel/o

Exercise 7
1. sound
2. clot
3. deficiency, blockage
4. heat

5. yellowish, fatty plaque
6. electricity, electrical activity

Exercise 8
1. thromb/o
2. ech/o
3. isch/o
4. ather/o
5. therm/o
6. electr/o

Exercise 9
1. slow
2. all, total
3. abnormal reduction in number
4. hardening
5. removal
6. formation
7. pertaining to

Exercise 10
1. -poiesis
2. -ac
3. -sclerosis
4. pan-
5. -penia
6. brady-
7. -apheresis

Exercise 11
Pronunciation Exercise

Exercise 12
Note: The combining form is identified by italic and bold print.

1.   P   WR S
   endo/card/itis
   inflammation of the inner (lining) of the heart

2.   P   WR S
   brady/card/ia
   condition of slow heart (rate)

3.   WR CV S
   cardi/o/megaly
       CF
   enlargement of the heart

4.   WR CV   S
   arteri/o/sclerosis
       CF
   hardening of the arteries

5.   WR   S
   valvul/itis
   inflammation of a valve (of the heart)

6.   WR   S
(multiple) myel/oma
tumors of the bone marrow

7.   P   WR S
tachy/card/ia
condition of a rapid heart (rate)

8. WR CV   S
angi/o/stenosis
   CF
narrowing of a blood vessel

9.   WR   S
thromb/us
(blood) clot

10.   P WR S
peri/card/itis
inflammation of the sac surrounding
the heart

11. WR S
aort/ic stenosis
narrowing, pertaining to the aorta
(narrowing of the aortic valve)

12.   WR   S
thromb/osis
abnormal condition of a (blood) clot

13.   WR CV S
ather/o/sclerosis
   CF
hardening of fatty plaque (deposited
on the arterial wall)

14. WR CV WR S
my/o/card/itis
  CF
inflammation of the muscle of the
heart

15.   WR   S
angi/oma
tumor composed of blood vessels

16.   WR   S
thym/oma
tumor of the thymus gland

17.   WR   S
lymph/oma
tumor of lymphatic tissue

18.   WR   S
lymphaden/itis
inflammation of lymph nodes

19. WR CV   S
splen/o/megaly
   CF
enlargement of the spleen

20.   WR   S
hemat/oma
tumor of blood

21.   P   WR S
poly/arter/itis
inflammation of many (sites in the)
arteries

22.   WR CV WR CV S
cardi/o/my/o/pathy
   CF   CF
disease of the heart muscle

23.   WR   CV S
lymphaden/o/pathy
      CF
disease of lymph nodes

24.   WR CV WR S
thromb/o/phleb/itis
    CF
inflammation of a vein associated
with a clot

25.   WR   S
phleb/itis
inflammation of a vein

26.   P WR CV S
pan/*cyt/o*/penia
     CF
abnormal reduction of all (blood)
cells

27. WR CV WR CV S
erythr/o/cyt/o/penia
   CF   CF
abnormal reduction of red (blood)
cells

28. WR CV WR CV S
leuk/o/cyt/o/penia
   CF   CF
abnormal reduction of white (blood)
cells

29.   WR   CV WR CV S
thromb/o/cyt/o/penia
     CF   CF
abnormal reduction of (blood)
clotting cells

Exercise 13
1. myel/oma
2. cardi/o/megaly
3. endo/card/itis
4. brady/card/ia
5. arteri/o/sclerosis
6. thromb/osis
7. my/o/card/itis
8. angi/o/stenosis
9. tachy/card/ia
10. ather/o/sclerosis
11. angi/oma
12. valvul/itis
13. aort/ic (stenosis)
14. peri/card/itis
15. lymph/oma
16. thym/oma
17. splen/o/megaly
18. hemat/oma
19. lymphaden/itis
20. cardi/o/my/o/pathy
21. poly/arter/itis

22. lymphaden/o/pathy
23. thromb/o/phleb/itis
24. phleb/itis
25. thromb/us
26. pan/cyt/o/penia
27. erythr/o/cyt/o/penia
28. leuk/o/cyt/o/penia
29. thromb/o/cyt/o/penia

Exercise 14
Spelling Exercise; see text p. 402.

Exercise 15
Pronunciation Exercise

Exercise 16
1. coarctation
2. embolus
3. cardiac arrest
4. congenital
5. varicose veins
6. ischemia
7. aneurysm
8. Hodgkin disease
9. coronary artery disease
10. angina pectoris
11. myocardial infarction
12. atrial fibrillation
13. arrhythmia
14. hypertensive
15. heart failure
16. peripheral arterial disease
17. hemophilia
18. leukemia
19. anemia
20. infectious mononucleosis
21. intermittent claudication
22. cardiac tamponade
23. mitral valve stenosis and rheumatic
heart disease
24. deep vein thrombosis
25. acute coronary syndrome
26. sepsis

Exercise 17
1. d	8. k
2. c	9. g
3. f	10. b
4. e	11. h
5. a	12. l
6. j	13. n
7. i	14. m

Exercise 18
1. i	8. k
2. e	9. l
3. a	10. g
4. h	11. c
5. j	12. m
6. b	13. f
7. d	

Exercise 19
Spelling Exercise; see text p. 409.

Exercise 20
Pronunciation Exercise

Exercise 21
Note: The combining form is identified by italic and bold print.

1. P   WR CV   S
    peri/***cardi/o***/centesis
    　　　　CF
    surgical puncture to aspirate fluid from the sac surrounding the heart (pericardium)

2. WR　　　S
    thym/ectomy
    excision of the thymus gland

3. WR CV   S
    angi/o/plasty
    　　CF
    surgical repair of a blood vessel

4. WR CV   S
    splen/o/pexy
    　　CF
    surgical fixation of the spleen

5. WR CV   S
    valvul/o/plasty
    　　CF
    surgical repair of a valve

6. P   WR　　S
    end/arter/ectomy
    excision within an artery

7. WR CV   S
    phleb/o/tomy
    　　CF
    incision into a vein

8. WR　　S
    splen/ectomy
    excision of the spleen

9. WR　　S
    phleb/ectomy
    excision of a vein

10. WR　　S
    ather/ectomy
    excision of fatty plaque

Exercise 22
1. end/arter/ectomy
2. splen/o/pexy
3. valvul/o/plasty
4. phleb/o/tomy
5. thym/ectomy
6. peri/cardi/o/centesis
7. angi/o/plasty
8. splen/ectomy
9. phleb/ectomy
10. ather/ectomy

Exercise 23
Spelling Exercise; see text p. 412.

Exercise 24
Pronunciation Exercise

Exercise 25
1. ablation
2. percutaneous transluminal coronary angioplasty
3. cardiac pacemaker
4. blood cells
5. coronary artery bypass graft
6. aneurysmectomy
7. femoropopliteal bypass
8. intracoronary thrombolytic
9. bone marrow transplant
10. embolectomy
11. coronary stent
12. implantable cardiac defibrillator

Exercise 26
1. h	8. c
2. m	9. i
3. k	10. b
4. l	11. j
5. d	12. g
6. e	13. f
7. a	

Exercise 27
Spelling Exercise; see text p. 418.

Exercise 28
Pronunciation Exercise

Exercise 29
Note: The combining form is identified by italic and bold print.

1. WR CV WR CV   S
    electr/o/***cardi/o***/graph
    　　CF　　CF
    instrument used to record the electrical activity of the heart

2. WR CV   S
    ven/o/gram
    　　CF
    radiographic image of the veins (after an injection of contrast medium)

3. WR CV　　S
    angi/o/graphy
    　　CF
    radiographic imaging of a blood vessel

4. WR CV   WR CV S
    ech/o/***cardi/o***/gram
    　　CF　　CF
    record of the heart by using sound

5. WR CV   S
    aort/o/gram
    　　CF
    radiographic image of the aorta (after an injection of contrast media)

6. WR CV WR CV   S
    electr/o/***cardi/o***/gram
    　　CF　　CF
    record of the electrical activity of the heart

7. WR CV   S
    arteri/o/gram
    　　CF
    radiographic image of an artery (after an injection of contrast media)

8. WR CV WR CV   S
    electr/o/***cardi/o***/graphy
    　　CF　　CF
    process of recording the electrical activity of the heart

9. WR CV   S
    angi/o/scopy
    　　CF
    visual examination of a blood vessel

10. WR CV   S
    angi/o/scope
    　　CF
    instrument used for visual examination of a blood vessel

Exercise 30
1. electr/o/cardi/o/graph
2. arteri/o/gram
3. ven/o/gram
4. angi/o/graphy
5. electr/o/cardi/o/gram
6. ech/o/cardi/o/gram
7. aort/o/gram
8. electr/o/cardi/o/graphy
9. angi/o/scopy
10. angi/o/scope

Exercise 31
Spelling Exercise; see text p. 422.

Exercise 32
Pronunciation Exercise

Exercise 33
1. sphygmomanometer
2. coagulation time
3. complete blood count and differential count
4. Doppler ultrasound
5. blood pressure
6. prothrombin time
7. cardiac catheterization
8. hemoglobin
9. impedance plethysmography

10. thallium test
11. transesophageal echocardiogram
12. single-photon emission computed tomography
13. exercise stress test
14. digital subtraction angiography
15. creatine phosphokinase
16. C-reactive protein
17. pulse
18. homocysteine
19. troponin
20. lipid profile
21. hematocrit

Exercise 34

1. d		7. a
2. h		8. e
3. k		9. b
4. g		10. f
5. j		11. i
6. c		

Exercise 35

1. c		6. a
2. e		7. g
3. b		8. h
4. f		9. i
5. d		10. j

Exercise 36

Spelling Exercise; see text p. 429.

Exercise 37

Pronunciation Exercise

Exercise 38

Note: The combining form is identified by italic and bold print.

1.   P   WR   S
    hypo/therm/ia
    condition of (body) temperature that is below (normal)

2.   WR CV   S
    hemat/o/poiesis
           CF
    formation of blood (cells)

3.   WR CV   S
    cardi/o/logy
           CF
    study of the heart

4.   WR CV   S
    cardi/o/logist
           CF
    physician who studies and treats diseases of the heart

5.   WR CV   S
    hem/o/lysis
           CF
    dissolution of blood (cells)

6.   WR CV   S
    hemat/o/logist
           CF
    physician who studies and treats diseases of the blood

7.   WR   S
    cardi/ac
    pertaining to the heart

8.   WR CV   S
    hemat/o/logy
           CF
    study of the blood

9.   WR   S
    plasm/apheresis
    removal of plasma (from withdrawn blood)

10. WR CV   S
    hem/o/stasis
           CF
    stoppage of bleeding

11. WR CV   S
    cardi/o/genic
           CF
    originating in the heart

12. WR CV   S
    myel/o/poiesis
           CF
    formation of bone marrow

13. WR   CV   S
    thromb/o/lysis
           CF
    dissolution of a clot

14. WR CV WR   S
    atri/o/ventricul/ar
           CF
    pertaining to the atrium and ventricle

15.   P   WR   S
    intra/ven/ous
    pertaining to within the vein

16. WR CV   S
    phleb/o/logist
           CF
    physician who studies and treats disease of the veins

17. WR CV   S
    phleb/o/logy
           CF
    study of veins

Exercise 39

1. cardi/o/logy
2. hemat/o/poiesis
3. hypo/therm/ia
4. hem/o/lysis
5. plasm/apheresis
6. hemat/o/logist

7. cardi/ac
8. cardi/o/logist
9. hemat/o/logy
10. hem/o/stasis
11. myel/o/poiesis
12. cardi/o/genic
13. thromb/o/lysis
14. atri/o/ventricul/ar
15. intra/ven/ous
16. phleb/o/logy
17. phleb/o/logist

Exercise 40

Spelling Exercise; see text p. 433.

Exercise 41

Pronunciation Exercise

Exercise 42

1. vasoconstrictor
2. lumen
3. cardiopulmonary resuscitation
4. diastole
5. fibrillation
6. hypotension
7. extravasation
8. venipuncture
9. systole
10. vasodilator
11. hypertension
12. occlude
13. hypertriglyceridemia
14. hyperlipidemia
15. hemorrhage
16. hypercholesterolemia
17. blood dyscrasia
18. murmur
19. extracorporeal
20. lipids
21. defibrillation
22. anticoagulant
23. bruit

Exercise 43

1. space within a tubelike structure
2. escape of blood from the blood vessel into the tissues
3. excessive amount of cholesterol in the blood
4. puncture of a vein with a needle to remove blood, start an intravenous infusion, or instill medication
5. agent or nerve that enlarges the blood vessels
6. blood pressure that is above normal
7. emergency procedure consisting of external cardiac compressions and artificial ventilation
8. phase in the cardiac cycle in which ventricles contract

9. blood pressure that is below normal
10. agent or nerve that narrows blood vessels
11. cardiac cycle phase in which ventricles relax
12. rapid, quivering, noncoordinated contractions of the atria or ventricles
13. to close tightly
14. excessive amount of fats in the blood
15. excessive amount of triglycerides in the blood
16. abnormal or pathologic condition of the blood
17. rapid loss of blood
18. agent that slows down the clotting process
19. occurring outside the body
20. abnormal cardiac sound heard through auscultation
21. fats and fatlike substances that serve as a source of fuel in the body
22. application of electric shock to the myocardium to restore normal heart rhythm
23. abnormal vascular sound heard through auscultation

Exercise 44

Spelling Exercise; see text p. 437.

Exercise 45

Pronunciation Exercise

Exercise 46

1. e		8. a	
2. j		9. h	
3. m		10. c	
4. f		11. i	
5. l		12. b	
6. g		13. k	
7. d			

Exercise 47

Spelling Exercise; see text pp. 439–440.

Exercise 48

1. coronary artery disease; electrocardiogram; single-photon emission computed tomography; echocardiogram
2. deep vein thrombosis; impedance plethysmography
3. complete blood count, diff; red blood cell, white blood cell, hemoglobin, hematocrit
4. coronary artery bypass graft; percutaneous transluminal coronary angioplasty
5. myocardial infarction; coronary care unit
6. blood pressure
7. heart failure
8. cardiopulmonary resuscitation
9. hypertensive heart disease
10. prothrombin time
11. atrioventricular
12. acute coronary syndrome
13. peripheral arterial disease
14. digital subtraction angiography
15. transesophageal echocardiogram
16. C-reactive protein, creatine phosphokinase
17. atrial fibrillation
18. implantable cardiac defibrillator
19. intravenous

Exercise 49

A. 1. angina pectoris
2. thallium test
3. ischemia
4. angiography
5. stenosis
6. angioplasty
7. cardiologist

8. electrocardiography
9. cardiac catheterization
10. creatine phosphokinase
11. troponin
12. myocardial infarction
B. 1. high
2. c
3. c
4. b
C. Online Exercise.

Exercise 50

1. atherosclerosis
2. thrombophlebitis
3. myocarditis
4. myocardial infarction
5. endarterectomy
6. infectious mononucleosis
7. hypothermia
8. impedance plethysmography
9. murmur
10. angioscope, angioscopy
11. thallium test
12. allergist
13. anaphylaxis

Exercise 51

Reading Exercise

Exercise 52

1. *F*, the diagnosis was made with an ultrasound procedure.
2. c
3. d

Digestive System

Outline

Objectives

Upon completion of this chapter you will be able to:

1 Identify organs and structures of the digestive system.

2 Define and spell word parts related to the digestive system.

3 Define, pronounce, and spell disease and disorder terms related to the digestive system.

4 Define, pronounce, and spell surgical terms related to the digestive system.

5 Define, pronounce, and spell diagnostic terms related to the digestive system.

6 Define, pronounce, and spell complementary terms related to the digestive system.

7 Interpret the meaning of abbreviations related to the digestive system.

8 Interpret, read, and comprehend medical language in simulated medical statements, documents, and electronic health records.

🔍 ANATOMY

The digestive tract, also known as the alimentary canal or the gastrointestinal tract and abbreviated as GI tract, is a long continuous tube comprising the mouth, pharynx, esophagus, stomach, small intestine, large intestine, rectum, and anus. Accessory organs of the digestive tract are the salivary glands, liver, bile ducts, gallbladder, and pancreas (Figures 11-1 through 11-5).

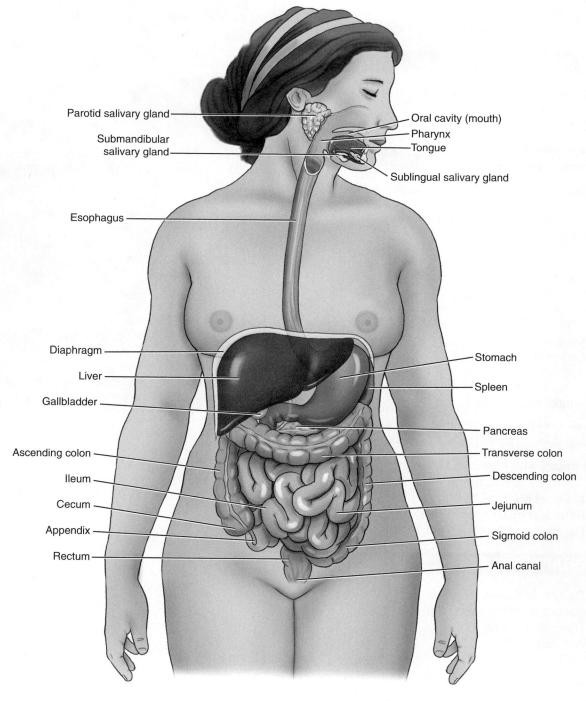

FIGURE 11-1
Organs of the digestive system.

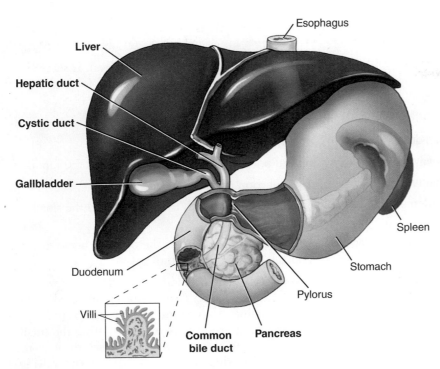

FIGURE 11-2
Accessory organs: liver, hepatic duct, cystic duct, gallbladder, common bile duct, and pancreas.

Function

Functions of the digestive tract are **ingestion**, the taking in of nutrients through the mouth; **digestion**, the mechanical and chemical breakdown of food for use by body cells; **absorption**, the transfer of digested food from the small intestine to the blood stream; and **elimination**, the removal of solid waste from the body.

Organs of the Digestive Tract

TERM	DEFINITION
mouth	opening through which food passes into the body; breaks food into small particles by mastication (chewing) and mixing with saliva (Figure 11-3)
tongue	consists mostly of skeletal muscle; attached in the posterior region of the mouth. It provides movement of food for mastication, directs food to the pharynx for swallowing, and is a major organ for taste and speech.
palate	separates the nasal cavity from the oral cavity
soft palate	posterior portion, not supported by bone
hard palate	anterior portion, supported by bone
uvula	soft V-shaped structure that extends from the soft palate; directs food into the throat
pharynx, throat	performs the swallowing action that passes food from the mouth into the esophagus
esophagus	10-inch (25 cm) tube that is a passageway for food extending from the pharynx to the stomach. **Peristalsis**, involuntary wavelike movements that propel food along the digestive tract, begins in the esophagus.

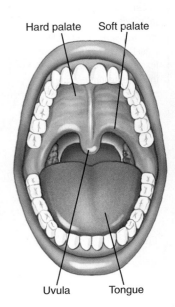

FIGURE 11-3
The oral cavity.

Organs of the Digestive Tract—cont'd

TERM	DEFINITION
stomach	J-shaped sac that mixes and stores food. It secretes chemicals for digestion and hormones for local communication control.
cardia	area around the opening of the esophagus
fundus	proximal domed portion of the stomach
body	central portion of the stomach, distal to the fundus
antrum	distal portion of the stomach
pylorus	portion of the stomach that connects to the small intestine
pyloric sphincter	ring of muscle that guards the opening between the stomach and the duodenum
small intestine	20-foot (6 m) tube extending from the pyloric sphincter to the large intestine. **Digestion** is completed in the small intestine. **Absorption**, the passage of the nutrients (end products of digestion) from the small intestine to the bloodstream, takes place through the **villi**, tiny fingerlike projections that line the walls of the small intestine.
duodenum	first 10 to 12 inches (25 cm) of the small intestine
jejunum	second portion of the small intestine, approximately 8 feet (2.4 m) long
ileum	third portion of the small intestine, approximately 11 feet (3.3 m) long, which connects with the large intestine
large intestine	approximately 5 feet (1.5 m) long tube that extends from the ileum to the anus (Figure 11-4). **Absorption** of water and transit of the solid waste products of digestion take place in the large intestine.
cecum	blind U-shaped pouch that is the first portion of the large intestine
colon	next portion of the large intestine. The colon is divided into four parts: ascending colon, transverse colon, descending colon, and sigmoid colon
rectum	distal portion of the large intestine, approximately 8 to 10 inches (20 cm) long, extending from the sigmoid colon to the anus
anus	sphincter muscle (ringlike band of muscle fiber that keeps an opening tight) at the end of the digestive tract. Provides for elimination of solid waste products of digestion.

ACCESSORY ORGANS (see Figure 11-2)

salivary glands	produce saliva, which flows into the mouth
liver	produces bile, which is necessary for the digestion of fats. The liver performs many other functions concerned with digestion and metabolism.

🏛 **DUODENUM** is derived from the Latin **duodeni**, meaning **12 each**, a reference to its length. It was named in 240 BC by a Greek physician.

Jejunum is derived from the Latin **jejunus**, meaning **empty**; it was so named because the early anatomists always found it empty.

Ileum is derived from the Greek **eilein**, meaning **to roll**, a reference to the peristaltic waves that move food along the digestive tract. This term was first used in the early part of the seventeenth century.

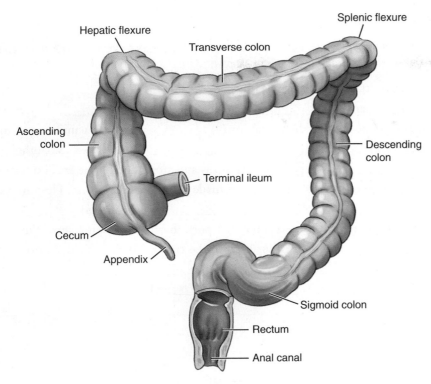

FIGURE 11-4
Anatomy of the large intestine.

TERM	DEFINITION
bile ducts	passageways that carry bile: the **hepatic duct** is a passageway for bile from the liver, and the **cystic duct** carries bile to and from the gallbladder. They join to form the **common bile duct**, which conveys bile to the duodenum. Collectively, these passageways are referred to as the **biliary tract**.
gallbladder	small, saclike structure that stores bile produced by the liver
pancreas	produces pancreatic juice, which helps digest all types of food and secretes insulin for carbohydrate metabolism
OTHER STRUCTURES	
peritoneum	serous saclike lining of the abdominal and pelvic cavities
appendix	small pouch, which has no known function in digestion, attached to the cecum (also called **vermiform appendix**)
abdomen	portion of the body between the thorax and the pelvis

BILIARY SYSTEM

The liver, bile ducts, and gallbladder comprise the biliary system, which creates, transports, stores, and releases bile into the small intestine to facilitate the absorption of fat.

🏛 PANCREAS
is derived from the Greek **pan**, meaning **all**, and **krea**, meaning **flesh.** The pancreas was first described in 300 BC. It was so named because of its fleshy appearance.

A&P Booster
For more anatomy and physiology, go to evolve.elsever.com.
Select: **Extra Content**, A & P Booster, Chapter 11.

Refer to p. 10 for your Evolve Access Information.

EXERCISE 1

Fill in the blanks with the correct terms. *To check your answers to the exercises in this chapter, go to Answers, p. 510, at the end of the chapter.*

The digestive tract, also known as the (1) _____
_____ and (2) _____ _____, begins with
the mouth, connects with the throat, or (3) _____, and continues on to a
10-inch tube called the (4) _____; this connects with the
(5) _____, a J-shaped sac that mixes and stores food. The small intestine,
the next portion of the digestive tract, is made up of three portions. They are called
the (6) _____, (7) _____, and (8) _____.
The small intestine connects with the first portion of the large intestine, the
(9) _____, and then connects with the colon, which is divided into
four parts called (10) _____ _____,
(11) _____ _____, (12) _____
_____, and (13) _____ _____. The (14) _____
extends from the sigmoid colon to the (15) _____.

EXERCISE 2

Match the definitions in the first column with the correct terms in the second column.

_____ 1. distal portion of the stomach

_____ 2. hangs from the roof of the mouth

_____ 3. produce saliva

_____ 4. produces bile

_____ 5. separates the nasal cavity from the oral cavity

_____ 6. guards the opening between the stomach and the duodenum

_____ 7. secretes insulin for carbohydrate metabolism

_____ 8. small pouch that has no function in digestion

_____ 9. lining of the abdominal and pelvic cavities

_____ 10. portion of the body between the pelvis and thorax

_____ 11. stores bile produced by the liver

_____ 12. proximal domed portion of the stomach

_____ 13. directs food to the pharynx for swallowing

a. salivary glands
b. pancreas
c. peritoneum
d. uvula
e. gallbladder
f. tongue
g. abdomen
h. liver
i. appendix
j. pyloric sphincter
k. fundus
l. antrum
m. palate

WORD PARTS

Word parts you need to learn to complete this chapter are listed on the following pages. The exercises at the end of each list will help you learn their definitions and spellings.

Use the flashcards accompanying this text or electronic flashcards to assist you in memorizing the word parts for this chapter.

To use electronic flashcards, go to evolve.elsevier.com. Select: Chapter 11, **Flashcards**.

Refer to p. 10 for your Evolve Access Information.

Combining Forms of the Digestive Tract

COMBINING FORM	DEFINITION
an/o	anus
antr/o	antrum
cec/o	cecum
col/o, colon/o	colon (large intestine)
duoden/o	duodenum
enter/o	intestine (small intestine)
esophag/o (NOTE: esophag/o *was covered in* Chapter 9)	esophagus
gastr/o	stomach
ile/o	ileum
jejun/o	jejunum
or/o, stomat/o	mouth
proct/o, rect/o	rectum
sigmoid/o	sigmoid colon

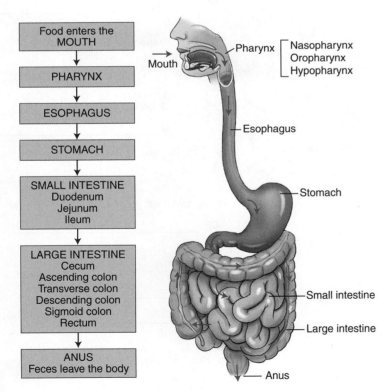

FIGURE 11-5
Pathway of food.

EXERCISE FIGURE **A**

Fill in the blanks with combining forms in this diagram of the digestive system. *To check your answers, go to p. 510.*

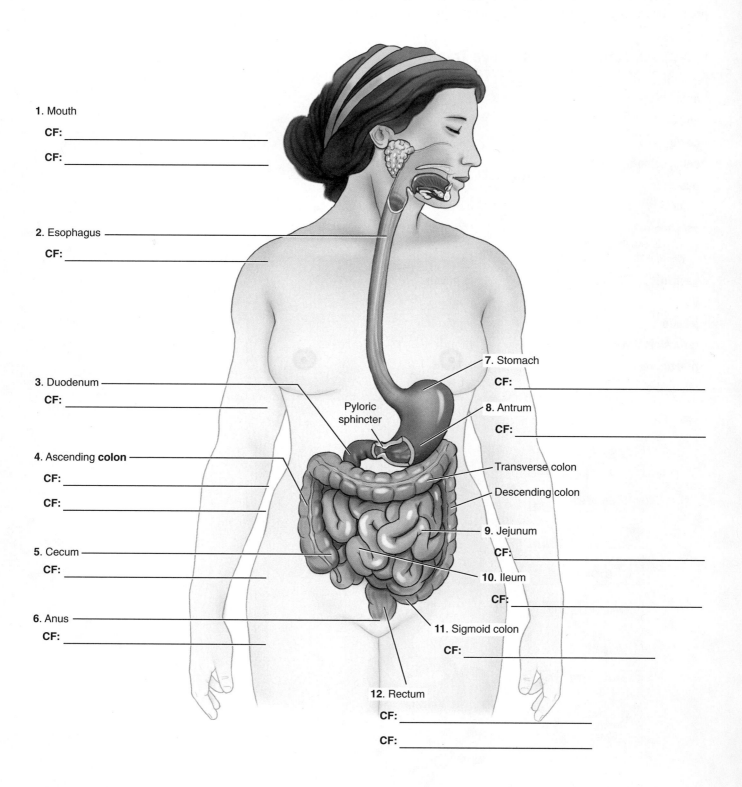

1. Mouth

CF:_____

CF:_____

2. Esophagus

CF:_____

3. Duodenum

CF:_____

4. Ascending **colon**

CF:_____

CF:_____

5. Cecum

CF:_____

6. Anus

CF:_____

Pyloric
sphincter

7. Stomach

CF:_____

8. Antrum

CF:_____

Transverse colon

Descending colon

9. Jejunum

CF:_____

10. Ileum

CF:_____

11. Sigmoid colon

CF:_____

12. Rectum

CF:_____

CF:_____

EXERCISE 3

Write the definitions of the following combining forms.

1. proct/o _____
2. gastr/o _____
3. an/o _____
4. cec/o _____
5. ile/o _____
6. stomat/o _____
7. duoden/o _____
8. col/o _____

9. or/o _____
10. enter/o _____
11. rect/o _____
12. antr/o _____
13. esophag/o _____
14. jejun/o _____
15. sigmoid/o _____
16. colon/o _____

EXERCISE 4

Write the combining form for each of the following terms.

1. cecum _____
2. stomach _____
3. ileum _____
4. jejunum _____
5. sigmoid colon _____
6. esophagus _____
7. rectum a. _____
         b. _____

8. intestine _____
9. duodenum _____
10. colon a. _____
         b. _____
11. mouth a. _____
         b. _____
12. anus _____
13. antrum _____

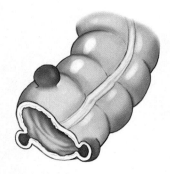

FIGURE 11-6
Diverticula of the large intestine.

HERNIA

The layman's term for hernia is **rupture**. Types in the digestive system include abdominal, hiatal or diaphragmatic, inguinal, and umbilical hernia.

Combining Forms of the Accessory Organs/Combining Forms Commonly Used with Digestive System Terms

COMBINING FORM	DEFINITION
abdomin/o, celi/o, lapar/o	abdomen, abdominal cavity
append/o, appendic/o	appendix
cheil/o	lip
cholangi/o	bile duct
chol/e (NOTE: the combining vowel is e)	gall, bile
choledoch/o	common bile duct
diverticul/o	diverticulum, or blind pouch, extending from a hollow organ (pl. diverticula) (Figure 11-6)
gingiv/o	gum
gloss/o, lingu/o	tongue
hepat/o	liver
herni/o	hernia, or protrusion of an organ through a membrane or cavity wall (Figure 11-7)
palat/o	palate
pancreat/o	pancreas
peritone/o	peritoneum
polyp/o	polyp, small growth
pylor/o (NOTE: pylor/o *was covered in Chapter 9*)	pylorus, pyloric sphincter
sial/o	saliva, salivary gland
steat/o	fat
uvul/o	uvula

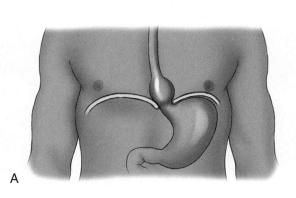
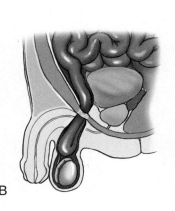
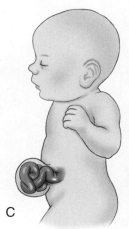

FIGURE 11-7
Types of hernias. **A**, Hiatal. **B**, Inguinal. **C**, Umbilical.

EXERCISE FIGURE B

Fill in the blanks with combining forms in this diagram of the digestive system and associated structures.

1. Palate

   CF: _____

2. Uvula

   CF: _____

3. Tongue

   CF: _____

   CF: _____

4. Gallbladder

   CF: _____ (gall)

   CF: _____ (bladder)

5. Pyloric sphincter

   CF: _____

6. Appendix

   CF: _____

   CF: _____

7. Gums

   CF: _____

8. Lips

   CF: _____

9. Salivary glands

   CF: _____

10. Liver

    CF: _____

11. Bile ducts

    CF: _____

12. Common bile duct

    CF: _____

13. Pancreas

    CF: _____

14. Abdomen, abdominal cavity

    CF: _____

    CF: _____

    CF: _____

EXERCISE 5

Write the definitions of the following combining forms.

1. herni/o _____
2. abdomin/o _____
3. sial/o _____
4. chol/e _____
5. diverticul/o _____
6. gingiv/o _____
7. appendic/o _____
8. gloss/o _____
9. hepat/o _____
10. cheil/o _____
11. peritone/o _____
12. palat/o _____

13. pancreat/o _____
14. lapar/o _____
15. lingu/o _____
16. choledoch/o _____
17. pylor/o _____
18. uvul/o _____
19. cholangi/o _____
20. polyp/o _____
21. celi/o _____
22. steat/o _____
23. append/o _____

EXERCISE 6

Write the combining form for each of the following.

1. palate _____
2. saliva, salivary gland _____
3. pancreas _____
4. peritoneum _____
5. tongue   a. _____
            b. _____
6. gum _____
7. pylorus, pyloric
   sphincter _____
8. liver _____
9. gall, bile _____
10. abdomen, abdominal
    cavity   a. _____
             b. _____
             c. _____

11. hernia _____
12. diverticulum _____
13. lip _____
14. appendix   a. _____
               b. _____
15. uvula _____
16. bile duct _____
17. common bile duct _____
18. small growth _____
19. fat _____

Prefix

Prefix	Definition
hemi-	half

Suffix

Suffix	Definition
-pepsia	digestion

 Refer to Appendix A and Appendix B for a complete listing of word parts.

EXERCISE 7

Write the definition of the following prefix and suffix.

1. -pepsia _____

2. hemi- _____

EXERCISE 8

Write the prefix and suffix for the following definition.

1. digestion _____

2. half _____

For review and/or assessment, go to evolve.elsevier.com. Select:
Chapter 11, **Activities**, Word Parts
Chapter 11, **Games**, Name that Word Part
Refer to p. 10 for your Evolve Access Information.

MEDICAL TERMS

The terms you need to learn to complete this chapter are presented on the following pages. The exercises following each list will help you learn the definition and the spelling of each word.

Disease and Disorder Terms

Built from Word Parts

The following terms are built from word parts you have already learned and can be translated literally to find their meanings. Further explanation of terms beyond the definition of their word parts, if needed, is included in parentheses.

TERM	DEFINITION
appendicitis (a-*pen*-di-SĪ-tis)	inflammation of the appendix (Exercise Figure C)
cholangioma (kō-*lan*-jē-Ō-ma)	tumor of the bile duct

EXERCISE FIGURE C

Fill in the blanks to complete labeling of the diagram.

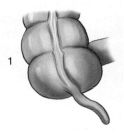

1. Normal appendix.

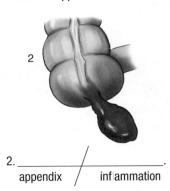

2. _____ / _____ .
       appendix   inflammation

Disease and Disorder Terms—cont'd

Built from Word Parts

TERM	DEFINITION
cholecystitis (kō-lē-sis-TĪ-tis)	inflammation of the gallbladder
choledocholithiasis (kō-*led*-o-kō-li-THĪ-a-sis)	condition of stones in the common bile duct (Exercise Figure D)
cholelithiasis (kō-le-li-THĪ-a-sis)	condition of gallstones (Exercise Figure D)
colitis (ko-LĪ-tis)	inflammation of the colon
diverticulitis (dī-ver-*tik*-ū-LĪ-tis)	inflammation of a diverticulum (Figure 11-6)
diverticulosis (dī-ver-*tik*-ū-LŌ-sis)	abnormal condition of having diverticula (see Figures 11-6 and 11-15, *B*)
esophagitis (e-*sof*-a-JĪ-tis)	inflammation of the esophagus
gastritis (gas-TRĪ-tis)	inflammation of the stomach
gastroenteritis (*gas*-trō-*en*-te-RĪ-tis)	inflammation of the stomach and intestines

ANTIBIOTIC-ASSOCIATED COLITIS

is caused by *Clostridium difficile* (*C. difficile* or *C. diff*) and mostly occurs in older, hospitalized patients who have been treated with antibiotics. Symptoms range from diarrhea to severe inflammation of the colon. Treatment includes using a different antibiotic or **fecal microbiota transplantation** (FMT), a fecal transplant, which is the infusion of fecal bacteria by enema or nasoenteric tube.

EXERCISE FIGURE D

Fill in the blanks to complete labeling of the diagram.

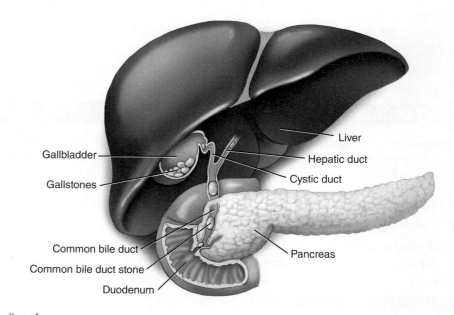

Liver
Hepatic duct
Gallbladder
Cystic duct
Gallstones
Common bile duct
Common bile duct stone
Pancreas
Duodenum

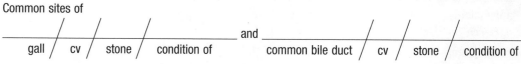

Common sites of

_____ / _____ / _____ / _____ and _____ / _____ / _____ / _____
gall / cv / stone / condition of   common bile duct / cv / stone / condition of

TERM	DEFINITION
gastroenterocolitis (*gas*-trō-*en*-ter-ō-kōl-Ĭ-tis)	inflammation of the stomach, intestines, and colon
gingivitis (*jin*-ji-VĬ-tis)	inflammation of the gums
glossitis (glos-Ĭ-tis)	inflammation of the tongue
hepatitis (*hep*-a-TĬ-tis)	inflammation of the liver
hepatoma (*hep*-a-TŌ-ma)	tumor of the liver
palatitis (*pal*-a-TĬ-tis)	inflammation of the palate
pancreatitis (*pan*-krē-a-TĬ-tis)	inflammation of the pancreas
peritonitis (*per*-i-tō-NĬ-tis) *(NOTE: the e is dropped from the combining form peritone/o)*	inflammation of the peritoneum
polyposis (*pol*-i-PŌ-sis)	abnormal condition of (multiple) polyps (in the mucous membrane of the intestine, especially the colon; high potential for malignancy if not removed when small) (Figure 11-8)
proctoptosis (*prok*-top-TŌ-sis)	prolapse of the rectum
rectocele (REK-tō-sēl)	protrusion of the rectum
sialolith (sī-AL-ō-lith)	stone in the salivary gland
steatohepatitis (*stē*-a-tō-*hep*-a-TĬ-tis)	inflammation of the liver associated with (excess) fat; (often caused by alcohol abuse and obesity; over time may cause cirrhosis)
uvulitis (*ū*-vū-LĬ-tis)	inflammation of the uvula

NASH SYNDROME

or **nonalcoholic steatohepatitis** may occur in nonalcoholic patients who are obese and/or suffer from type 2 diabetes mellitus.

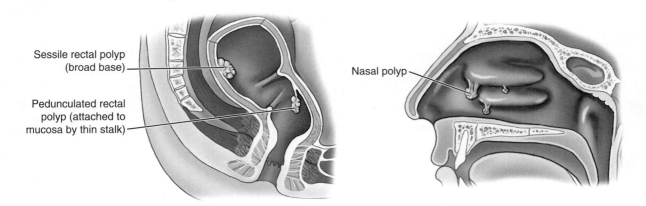

FIGURE 11-8

Polyp is a general term used to describe a protruding growth from a mucous membrane. Polyps are commonly found in the nose, throat, intestines, uterus, and urinary bladder.

> ⓔ To watch animations, go to evolve.elsevier.com. Select:
> Chapter 11, **Animations**, Appendicitis
> Cholecystitis
> Diverticulitis
> Peritonitis
>
> Refer to p. 10 for your Evolve Access Information.

> ⓔ For nutritional terms and dental terms, go to evolve.elsevier.com. Select:
> **Extra Content,** Appendices, Appendix J, Nutritional Term
> Appendix K, Dental Terms
>
> Refer to p. 10 for your Evolve Access Information.

EXERCISE 9

Practice saying aloud each of the disease and disorder terms built from word parts on pp. 467–469.

> ⓔ To hear the terms, go to evolve.elsevier.com. Select: Chapter 11, **Exercises**, Pronunciation.
>
> Refer to p. 10 for your Evolve Access Information.

☐ Place a check mark in the box when you have completed this exercise.

EXERCISE 10

Analyze and define the following terms.

1. cholelithiasis _____
2. diverticulosis _____
3. sialolith _____
4. hepatoma_____
5. uvulitis_____
6. pancreatitis _____
7. proctoptosis_____
8. gingivitis _____
9. gastritis _____
10. rectocele _____
11. palatitis _____
12. hepatitis_____
13. appendicitis_____
14. cholecystitis_____
15. diverticulitis _____
16. gastroenteritis_____
17. gastroenterocolitis _____
18. choledocholithiasis_____
19. cholangioma _____

20. polyposis _____

21. esophagitis _____

22. peritonitis _____

23. steatohepatitis _____

24. glossitis _____

25. colitis _____

EXERCISE 11

Build disease and disorder terms for the following definitions by using the word parts you have learned.

1. tumor of the liver

    _____
    WR   /   S

2. inflammation of the stomach

    _____
    WR   /   S

3. stone in the salivary gland

    _____
    WR   /CV/   WR

4. inflammation of the appendix

    _____
    WR   /   S

5. inflammation of a diverticulum

    _____
    WR   /   S

6. inflammation of the gallbladder

    _____
    WR   /CV/   WR   /   S

7. abnormal condition of having diverticula

    _____
    WR   /   S

8. inflammation of the stomach and intestines

    _____
    WR   /CV/   WR   /   S

9. prolapse of the rectum

    _____
    WR   /CV/   S

10. protrusion of the rectum

    _____
    WR   /CV/   S

11. inflammation of the uvula

    _____
    WR   /   S

12. inflammation of the gums

    _____
    WR   /   S

13. inflammation of the liver

    _____
    WR   /   S

14. inflammation of the palate

    _____
    WR   /   S

15. condition of gallstones

    _____
    WR   /CV/   WR   /   S

16. inflammation of the liver associated with (excess) fat

_____/_/_____/____
WR /CV/ WR / S

17. inflammation of the stomach, intestines, and colon

___/_/____/_/___/__
WR /CV/ WR /CV/ WR / S

18. inflammation of the pancreas

_____/_____
WR / S

19. tumor of the bile duct

_____/_____
WR / S

20. inflammation of the esophagus

_____/_____
WR / S

21. condition of stones in the common bile duct

_____/_/_____/____
WR /CV/ WR / S

22. abnormal condition of (multiple) polyps

_____/_____
WR / S

23. inflammation of the peritoneum

_____/_____
WR / S

24. inflammation of the tongue

_____/_____
WR / S

25. inflammation of the colon

_____/_____
WR / S

EXERCISE 12

Spell each of the disease and disorder terms built from word parts on pp. 467–469 by having someone dictate them to you.

> To hear and spell the terms, go to evolve.elsevier.com. Select: Chapter 11, **Exercises**, Spelling.
>
> (e) Refer to p. 10 for your Evolve Access Information.
>
> ☐ Place a check mark in the box if you have completed this exercise online.

1. _____   14. _____
2. _____   15. _____
3. _____   16. _____
4. _____   17. _____
5. _____   18. _____
6. _____   19. _____
7. _____   20. _____
8. _____   21. _____
9. _____   22. _____
10. _____   23. _____
11. _____   24. _____
12. _____   25. _____
13. _____

Disease and Disorder Terms

Not Built from Word Parts

In some of the following terms, you may recognize word parts you have already learned; however, the full meaning of the terms cannot be discerned by the definition of their word parts.

TERM	DEFINITION
adhesion (ad-HĒ-zhun)	abnormal growing together of two peritoneal surfaces that normally are separated. This may occur after abdominal surgery. Surgical treatment is called **adhesiolysis** or **adhesiotomy** (Figure 11-9, *A*).
celiac disease (SĒ-lē-ak) (di-ZĒZ)	malabsorption syndrome caused by an immune reaction to gluten (a protein in wheat, rye, and barley), which may damage the lining of the small intestine that is responsible for absorption of food into the bloodstream. Celiac disease is considered a multisystem disorder with varying signs and symptoms, including abdominal bloating and pain, chronic diarrhea or constipation, steatorrhea, vomiting, weight loss, fatigue, and iron deficiency anemia. A pruritic skin rash known as dermatitis herpetiformis may be associated with celiac disease (also called **gluten enteropathy**).

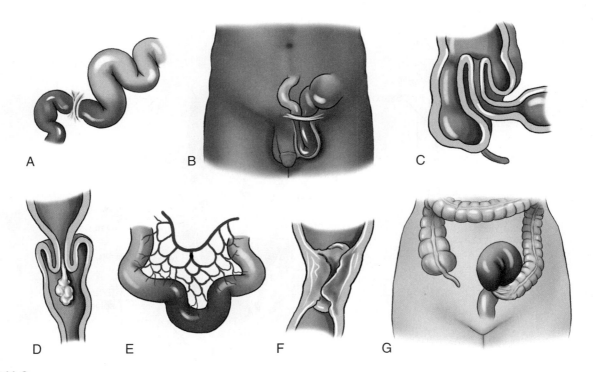

FIGURE 11-9
Causes of intestinal obstruction. **A**, Adhesions. **B**, Strangulated inguinal hernia. **C**, Ileocecal intussusception. **D**, Intussusception caused by polyps. **E**, Mesenteric vascular occlusion. **F**, Neoplasm. **G**, Volvulus of the sigmoid colon.

Disease and Disorder Terms—cont'd

Not Built from Word Parts

TERM	DEFINITION
cirrhosis (sir-RŌ-sis)	chronic disease of the liver with gradual destruction of cells and formation of scar tissue; commonly caused by alcoholism and certain types of viral hepatitis
Crohn disease (krōn) (di-ZĒZ)	chronic inflammation of the intestinal tract usually affecting the ileum and colon; characterized by cobblestone ulcerations and the formation of scar tissue that may lead to intestinal obstruction (also called **regional ileitis** or **regional enteritis.**)
gastroesophageal reflux disease (GERD) (gas-trō-e-sof-a-JĒ-al) (RĒ-fluks) (di-ZĒZ)	abnormal backward flow of the gastrointestinal contents into the esophagus, causing heartburn and the gradual breakdown of the mucous barrier of the esophagus
hemochromatosis (hē-mō-krō-ma-TŌ-sis)	iron metabolism disorder that occurs when too much iron is absorbed from food, resulting in excessive deposits of iron in the tissue; can cause heart failure, diabetes, cirrhosis, or cancer of the liver
hemorrhoids (HEM-o-roydz)	swollen or distended veins in the rectal area, which may be internal or external, and can be a source of rectal bleeding and pain (Figure 11-10)
ileus (IL-ē-us)	non-mechanical obstruction of the intestine, often caused by failure of peristalsis

GASTROESOPHAGEAL REFLUX DISEASE (GERD)

is a common gastrointestinal disorder. The acidity of the regurgitated stomach contents causes irritation and inflammation of the esophagus (reflux esophagitis). **Chronic GERD** may cause cellular changes in the lower esophagus called **Barrett esophagus** which increases the risk of cancer.

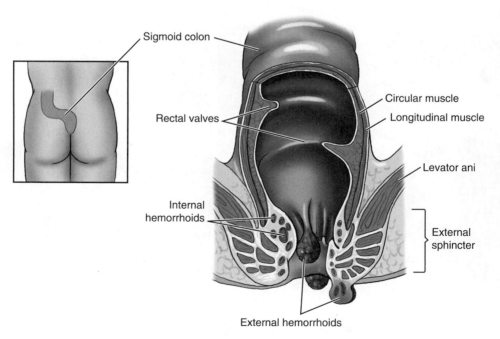

FIGURE 11-10
Hemorrhoids.

TERM	DEFINITION
intussusception (*in*-tu-sus-SEP-shun)	telescoping of a segment of the intestine (see Figure 11-9, *C* and *D*)
irritable bowel syndrome (IBS) (IR-i-ta-bl) (BOW-el) (SIN-drōm)	periodic disturbances of bowel function, such as diarrhea and/or constipation, usually associated with abdominal pain
obesity (ō-BĒS-i-tē)	excess of body fat (not body weight)
peptic ulcer (PEP-tik) (UL-ser)	erosion of the mucous membrane of the stomach or duodenum associated with increased secretion of acid from the stomach, bacterial infection (*H. pylori*), or nonsteroidal anti-inflammatory drugs (often referred to as **gastric** or **duodenal ulcer**, depending on its location) (Figure 11-11)
polyp (POL-ip)	tumorlike growth extending outward from a mucous membrane; usually benign; common sites are in the nose, throat, and intestines (see Figures 11-8 and 11-13)
ulcerative colitis (UL-ser-a-tiv) (kō-LĪ-tis)	inflammation of the colon with the formation of ulcers that produces bloody diarrhea. A proctocolectomy with a permanent ileostomy is a standard treatment.
volvulus (VOL-vū-lus)	twisting or kinking of the intestine, causing intestinal obstruction (see Figure 11-9, *G*)

🍃 **CAM TERM**

Hypnotherapy is the use of the power of suggestion and a state of altered consciousness involving focused attention to promote wellness. Studies have demonstrated that hypnosis has provided relief of symptoms and improvement in quality of life for patients with **irritable bowel syndrome**.

OBESITY

is a condition in which the BMI (body mass index) is greater than 30 kg/m². **Overweight** is defined as BMI between 25 and 29.9 kg/m². **Morbid obesity** is defined as BMI over 40 kg/m². BMI is calculated by dividing weight in kilograms by the square of height in meters (or by dividing weight in pounds by height in inches squared and then multiplying by 703).

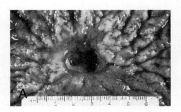

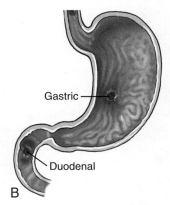

FIGURE 11-11
A, Peptic ulcer as viewed by endoscopy. **B**, Sites of peptic ulcers.

To watch animations, go to evolve.elsevier.com. Select:
Chapter 11, **Animations**, Adhesion-Bowel Obstruction
                Cirrhosis
                Duodenal Ulcer
                Ileus
                Irritable Bowel Syndrome
                Volvulus

Refer to p. 10 for your Evolve Access Information.

EXERCISE 13

Practice saying aloud each of the disease and disorder terms not built from word parts on pp. 473–475.

To hear the terms, go to evolve.elsevier.com. Select: Chapter 11, **Exercises**, Pronunciation.

Refer to p. 10 for your Evolve Access Information.

☐ Place a check mark in the box when you have completed this exercise.

EXERCISE 14

Match the definitions in the first column with the correct terms in the second column.

_____ 1. chronic disease of the liver

_____ 2. chronic inflammation of the intestinal tract usually affecting the ileum and colon

_____ 3. abnormal growing together of two peritoneal surfaces

_____ 4. twisted intestine

_____ 5. eroded area of the mucous membrane of the stomach or duodenum

_____ 6. telescoping of a segment of the intestine

_____ 7. tumorlike growth

_____ 8. formation of ulcers in the colon

_____ 9. non-mechanical obstruction of the intestine

_____ 10. periodic disturbance of bowel function

_____ 11. abnormal backward flow of the gastrointestinal contents into the esophagus

_____ 12. excess of body fat

_____ 13. malabsorption syndrome caused by an immune reaction to gluten

_____ 14. swollen or distended veins in the rectal area

_____ 15. iron metabolism disorder

a. intussusception
b. cirrhosis
c. gastroesophageal reflux disease
d. volvulus
e. Crohn disease
f. peptic ulcer
g. ulcerative colitis
h. irritable bowel syndrome
i. polyp
j. obesity
k. ileus
l. adhesion
m. celiac disease
n. hemorrhoids
o. hemochromatosis

EXERCISE 15

Write the definitions of the following terms.

1. peptic ulcer _____

2. Crohn disease _____

3. volvulus _____

4. adhesion _____

5. cirrhosis _____

6. intussusception _____

7. celiac disease _____

8. ulcerative colitis _____

9. hemorrhoids _____

10. polyp _____

11. irritable bowel syndrome _____

12. ileus _____

13. gastroesophageal reflux disease _____

14. obesity _____

15. hemochromatosis _____

EXERCISE 16

Spell each of the disease and disorder terms not built from word parts on pp. 473–475 by having someone dictate them to you.

> To hear and spell the terms, go to evolve.elsevier.com. Select: Chapter 11, **Exercises**, Spelling.
>
> Refer to p. 10 for your Evolve Access Information.
>
> ☐ Place a check mark in the box if you have completed this exercise online.

1. _____   9. _____
2. _____   10. _____
3. _____   11. _____
4. _____   12. _____
5. _____   13. _____
6. _____   14. _____
7. _____   15. _____
8. _____

Surgical Terms

Built from Word Parts

The following terms are built from word parts you have already learned and can be translated literally to find their meanings. Further explanation of terms beyond the definition of their word parts, if needed, is included in parentheses.

TERM	DEFINITION
abdominocentesis (ab-*dom*-i-nō-sen-TĒ-sis)	surgical puncture to aspirate fluid from the abdominal cavity (also called **paracentesis**)
abdominoplasty (ab-DOM-i-nō-*plas*-tē)	surgical repair of the abdomen
anoplasty (Ā-nō-*plas*-tē)	surgical repair of the anus
antrectomy (an-TREK-to-mē)	excision of the antrum (of the stomach)
appendectomy (*ap*-en-DEK-to-mē)	excision of the appendix
celiotomy (sē-lē-OT-o-mē)	incision into the abdominal cavity
cheilorrhaphy (kī-LOR-a-fē)	suturing of the lip
cholecystectomy (kō-le-sis-TEK-to-mē)	excision of the gallbladder (Figure 11-12)
choledocholithotomy (kō-*led*-o-kō-li-THOT-o-mē)	incision into the common bile duct to remove a stone
colectomy (kō-LEK-to-mē)	excision of the colon

🏛 **CHOLECYSTECTOMY** was first performed in 1882 by a German surgeon. **Laparoscopic cholecystectomy** was first performed in 1987 in France.

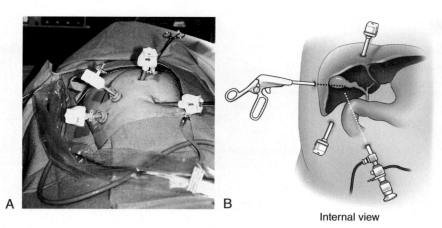

A   B

Internal view

FIGURE 11-12
In **laparoscopic cholecystectomy**, a type of endoscopic surgery, CO_2 is used to insufflate the surgical area for better visualization. A tiny camera and surgical instruments, including a laparoscope, are passed through small incisions. External view (**A**), Internal view (**B**).

Surgical Terms—cont'd

Built from Word Parts

TERM	DEFINITION
colostomy (ko-LOS-to-mē)	creation of an artificial opening into the colon (through the abdominal wall). (Used for the passage of stool. A colostomy, which creates a mouthlike opening on the abdominal wall called a **stoma**, may be permanent or temporary; performed as treatment for bowel obstruction, cancer, or diverticulitis.) (Exercise Figure E)
diverticulectomy (*dī*-ver-*tik*-ū-LEK-to-mē)	excision of a diverticulum
enterorrhaphy (*en*-ter-OR-a-fē)	suturing of the intestine
esophagogastroplasty (e-*sof*-a-gō-GAS-trō-*plas*-tē)	surgical repair of the esophagus and the stomach
gastrectomy (gas-TREK-to-mē)	excision of the stomach (or part of the stomach) (Exercise Figure F)
gastrojejunostomy (*gas*-trō-je-jū-NOS-to-mē)	creation of an artificial opening between the stomach and jejunum
gastroplasty (GAS-trō-*plas*-tē)	surgical repair of the stomach (Table 11-1)
gastrostomy (gas-TROS-to-mē)	creation of an artificial opening into the stomach (through the abdominal wall). (A tube is inserted through the opening for administration of food when swallowing is impossible.) (Exercise Figure G)
gingivectomy (*jin*-ji-VEK-to-mē)	surgical removal of gum (tissue)

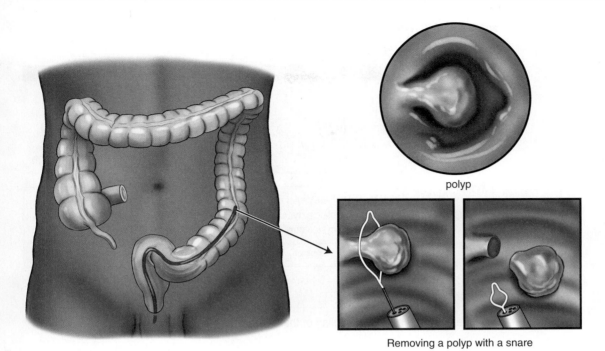

polyp

Removing a polyp with a snare

FIGURE 11-13
Polypectomy performed using a colonoscope.

TERM	DEFINITION
glossorrhaphy (glo-SOR-a-fē)	suturing of the tongue
hemicolectomy (*hem*-ē-kō-LEK-to-mē)	excision of half of the colon
herniorrhaphy (*her*-nē-OR-a-fē)	suturing of a hernia (for repair)
ileostomy (*il*-ē-OS-to-mē)	creation of an artificial opening into the ileum (through the abdominal wall creating a stoma, a mouthlike opening on the abdominal wall). (Used for the passage of stool. It is performed following total proctocolectomy for ulcerative colitis, Crohn disease, or cancer.) (Exercise Figure E)
laparotomy (*lap*-a-ROT-o-mē)	incision into the abdominal cavity
palatoplasty (PAL-a-tō-*plas*-tē)	surgical repair of the palate
polypectomy (*pol*-i-PEK-to-mē)	excision of a polyp (Figure 11-13)
pyloromyotomy (pī-*lor*-ō-mī-OT-o-mē)	incision into the pyloric muscle (performed to correct pyloric stenosis)
pyloroplasty (pī-LOR-ō-*plas*-tē)	surgical repair of the pylorus

Surgical Terms—cont'd

Built from Word Parts

TERM	DEFINITION
uvulectomy (ū-vū-LEK-to-mē)	excision of the uvula
uvulopalatopharyngoplasty (UPPP) (ū-vū-lō-*pal*-a-*tō*-fa-RING-gō-*plas*-tē)	surgical repair of the uvula, palate, and pharynx (performed to correct obstructive sleep apnea) (see Figure 5-7)

To watch animations, go to evolve.elsevier.com. Select:
Chapter 11, **Animations**, Colonoscopy with Polypectomy.
Cholecystectomy

Refer to p. 10 for your Evolve Access Information.

EXERCISE FIGURE E

Fill in the blanks to complete labeling of the diagram.

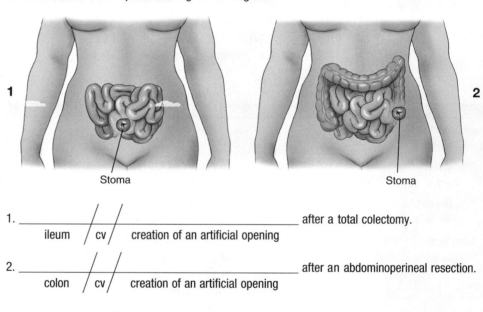

1. _____ / cv / _____ after a total colectomy.
   ileum / cv / creation of an artificial opening

2. _____ / cv / _____ after an abdominoperineal resection.
   colon / cv / creation of an artificial opening

EXERCISE FIGURE F

Fill in the blanks to label the diagram.

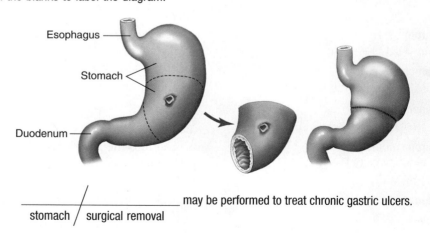

Esophagus

Stomach

Duodenum

_____ / _____ may be performed to treat chronic gastric ulcers.
stomach / surgical removal

EXERCISE FIGURE G

Fill in the blanks to label the diagram.

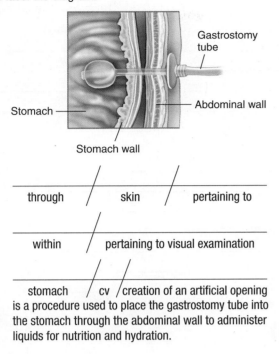

Gastrostomy tube

Stomach

Abdominal wall

Stomach wall

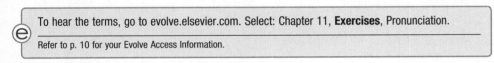

_____ / _____ / _____
through / skin / pertaining to

_____ / _____
within / pertaining to visual examination

_____ / cv / _____
stomach / cv / creation of an artificial opening
is a procedure used to place the gastrostomy tube into
the stomach through the abdominal wall to administer
liquids for nutrition and hydration.

EXERCISE 17

Practice saying aloud each of the surgical terms built from word parts on pp. 477–480.

> (e) To hear the terms, go to evolve.elsevier.com. Select: Chapter 11, **Exercises**, Pronunciation.
>
> Refer to p. 10 for your Evolve Access Information.

☐ Place a check mark in the box when you have completed this exercise.

EXERCISE 18

Analyze and define the following surgical terms.

1. gastrectomy _____
2. esophagogastroplasty _____
3. diverticulectomy _____
4. antrectomy _____
5. palatoplasty _____
6. uvulectomy _____
7. gastrojejunostomy _____
8. cholecystectomy _____
9. colectomy _____
10. colostomy _____
11. pyloroplasty _____
12. anoplasty _____
13. appendectomy _____

14. cheilorrhaphy _____

15. gingivectomy _____

16. laparotomy _____

17. ileostomy _____

18. gastrostomy _____

19. herniorrhaphy _____

20. glossorrhaphy _____

21. choledocholithotomy _____

22. hemicolectomy _____

23. polypectomy _____

24. enterorrhaphy _____

25. abdominoplasty _____

26. pyloromyotomy _____

27. uvulopalatopharyngoplasty _____

28. celiotomy _____

29. gastroplasty _____

30. abdominocentesis _____

EXERCISE 19

Build surgical terms for the following definitions by using the word parts you have learned.

1. excision of the appendix
   _____ / _____
   WR   S

2. suturing of the tongue
   _____ /CV/ _____
   WR   S

3. surgical repair of the esophagus and stomach
   _____ /CV/ _____ /CV/ ____
   WR   WR   S

4. excision of a diverticulum
   _____ / _____
   WR   S

5. creation of artificial opening into the ileum
   _____ /CV/ _____
   WR   S

6. surgical removal of gum tissue
   _____ / _____
   WR   S

7. incision into the abdominal cavity
   a. _____ /CV/ _____
      WR   S
   b. _____ /CV/ _____
      WR   S

8. surgical repair of the anus
   _____ /CV/ _____
   WR   S

9. excision of the antrum
   _____ / _____
   WR   S

10. excision of the gallbladder
    _____ /CV/ _____ / ____
    WR   WR   S

11. excision of the colon

         WR   /   S

12. creation of an artificial opening into the colon

         WR /CV/ S

13. excision of the stomach

         WR   /   S

14. creation of an artificial opening into the stomach

         WR /CV/ S

15. creation of an artificial opening between the stomach and jejunum

     WR /CV/ WR /CV/ S

16. excision of the uvula

         WR   /   S

17. surgical repair of the palate

         WR /CV/ S

18. surgical repair of the pylorus

         WR /CV/ S

19. suturing of a hernia

         WR /CV/ S

20. suturing of the lip

         WR /CV/ S

21. excision of half of the colon

         P   /   WR   /   S

22. incision into the common bile duct to remove a stone

     WR /CV/ WR /CV/ S

23. excision of a polyp

         WR   /   S

24. suturing of the intestine

         WR /CV/ S

25. surgical repair of the abdomen

         WR /CV/ S

26. incision into the pylorus muscle

     WR /CV/ WR /CV/ S

27. surgical repair of the uvula, palate, and pharynx

   WR /CV/ WR /CV/ WR /CV/ S

28. surgical repair of the stomach

         WR /CV/ S

29. surgical puncture to aspirate fluid from the abdominal cavity

         WR /CV/ S

EXERCISE 20

Spell each of the surgical terms built from word parts on pp. 477–480 by having someone dictate them to you.

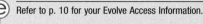

To hear and spell the terms, go to evolve.elsevier.com. Select: Chapter 11, **Exercises**, Spelling.

Refer to p. 10 for your Evolve Access Information.

☐ Place a check mark in the box if you have completed this exercise online.

1. _____	16. _____
2. _____	17. _____
3. _____	18. _____
4. _____	19. _____
5. _____	20. _____
6. _____	21. _____
7. _____	22. _____
8. _____	23. _____
9. _____	24. _____
10. _____	25. _____
11. _____	26. _____
12. _____	27. _____
13. _____	28. _____
14. _____	29. _____
15. _____	30. _____

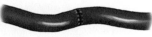

End to end

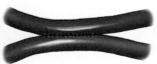

End to side

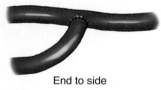

Side to side

FIGURE 11-14
Types of anastomoses.

BARIATRIC

contains the word roots **bar**, meaning **weight**, and **iatr**, meaning **treatment**.

To watch animations, go to evolve.elsevier.com. Select: Chapter 11, **Animations**, Bariatric Surgery.

Refer to p. 10 for your Evolve Access Information.

Surgical Terms

Not Built from Word Parts

In some of the following terms, you may recognize word parts you have already learned; however, the full meaning of the terms cannot be discerned by the definition of their word parts.

TERM	DEFINITION
abdominoperineal resection (A&P resection) (ab-*dom*-i-nō-per-i-NĒ-el) (rē-SEK-shun)	removal of the distal colon and rectum through both abdominal and perineal approaches; performed to treat colorectal cancer and inflammatory diseases of the lower large intestine. The patient will have a colostomy. (see Exercise Figure E, *2*)
anastomosis (pl. anastomoses) (a-*nas*-to-MŌ-sis) (a-*nas*-to-MŌ-sēz)	connection created by surgically joining two structures, such as blood vessels or bowel segments (Figure 11-14)
bariatric surgery (*bar*-ē-AT-rik) (SUR-jer-ē)	surgical reduction of gastric capacity to treat morbid obesity, a condition which can cause serious illness (Table 11-1)
hemorrhoidectomy (*hem*-o-royd-EK-to-mē)	excision of hemorrhoids, the swollen or distended veins in the rectal region
vagotomy (vā-GOT-o-mē)	cutting of certain branches of the vagus nerve, performed with gastric surgery to reduce the amount of gastric acid produced and thus reduce the recurrence of ulcers

Table 11-1

Bariatric Surgery

Bariatric surgery may be used to treat morbid obesity for patients with a BMI greater than 40 or those with a BMI greater than 35 associated with a serious medical condition. During surgery, a small stomach pouch is created for the purpose of restricting the amount of food an individual can eat. The following are three types of surgeries performed.

ROUX-EN-Y GASTRIC BYPASS (RYGB)

Creation of a small gastric pouch with drainage of food to the rest of the gastrointestinal tract through a restricted stoma; the duodenum and part of the jejunum are bypassed. RYGB, the most common form of bariatric surgery performed in the United States, restricts food intake and calorie absorption rate.

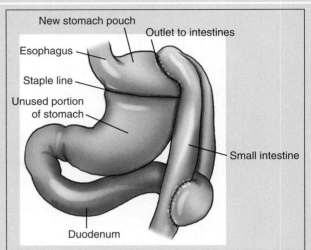

VERTICAL BANDED GASTROPLASTY (VBG)

Creation of a small gastric pouch with a vertical line of staples and the connection of a band for the drainage of food into the small intestine; also called stomach stapling.

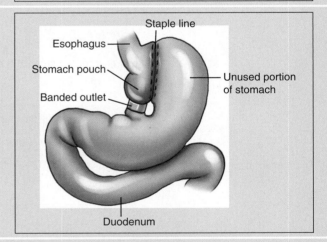

LAPAROSCOPIC ADJUSTABLE GASTRIC BANDING (LAGB)

Creation of a small gastric pouch by the placement of a band around the upper portion of the stomach; the band can be adjusted to change the size of the stomach through a subcutaneous port.

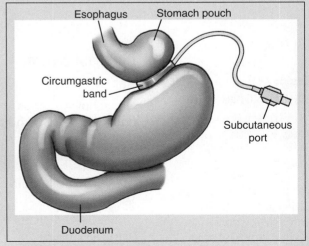

EXERCISE 21

Practice saying aloud each of the surgical terms not built from word parts on p. 484.

 To hear the terms, go to evolve.elsevier.com. Select: Chapter 11, **Exercises**, Pronunciation.

Refer to p. 10 for your Evolve Access Information.

☐ Place a check mark in the box when you have completed this exercise.

EXERCISE 22

Write the term for each of the following definitions.

1. cutting certain branches of the vagus nerve _____
2. connection created by surgically joining two structures _____
3. removal of the distal colon and rectum_____ _____
4. surgical reduction of gastric capacity to treat morbid obesity _____

   _____

5. excision of the swollen or distended veins in the rectal region

   _____

EXERCISE 23

Spell each of the surgical terms not built from word parts on p. 484 by having someone dictate them to you.

 To hear and spell the terms, go to evolve.elsevier.com. Select: Chapter 11, **Exercises**, Spelling.

Refer to p. 10 for your Evolve Access Information.

☐ Place a check mark in the box if you have completed this exercise online.

1. _____   4. _____
2. _____   5. _____
3. _____

Diagnostic Terms

Built from Word Parts

The following terms are built from word parts you have already learned and can be translated literally to find their meanings. Further explanation of terms beyond the definition of their word parts, if needed, is included in parentheses.

TERM	DEFINITION
DIAGNOSTIC IMAGING	
cholangiogram (kō-LAN-jē-ō-gram)	radiographic image of bile ducts
cholangiography (kō-*lan*-jē-OG-ra-fē)	radiographic imaging of the bile ducts (after administration of contrast media to outline the ducts)

OPERATIVE CHOLANGIOGRAPHY

is performed during surgery to check for residual stones after the removal of the gallbladder. Postoperative cholangiography, also called T-tube cholangiography, is performed in the radiology department after a cholecystectomy, also to check for residual stones. Both use the injection of contrast media into the common bile duct.

TERM	DEFINITION
CT colonography (kō-lon-OG-ra-fē)	radiographic imaging of the colon (using a CT scanner and software)
esophagogram (e-SOF-a-gō-gram)	radiographic image of the esophagus (and pharynx). (The contrast medium barium is used to study function and form of swallowing related to the pharynx and esophagus.) (also called **esophagram** and **barium swallow**)

ENDOSCOPY

colonoscope (kō-LON-ō-skōp)	instrument used for visual examination of the colon (see Figure 11-13)
colonoscopy (kō-lon-OS-ko-pē)	visual examination of the colon (Figures 11-15 and 11-16)
endoscope (EN-dō-skōp)	instrument used for visual examination within (a hollow organ)
endoscopy (en-DOS-ko-pē)	visual examination within (a hollow organ) (Figure 11-17)
esophagogastroduodenoscopy (EGD) (e-sof-a-gō-gas-trō-dū-od-e-NOS-ko-pē)	visual examination of the esophagus, stomach, and duodenum
esophagoscopy (e-sof-a-GOS-ko-pē)	visual examination of the esophagus
gastroscope (GAS-trō-skōp)	instrument used for visual examination of the stomach (Exercise Figure H)
gastroscopy (gas-TROS-ko-pē)	visual examination of the stomach (Exercise Figure H)

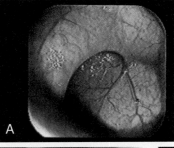
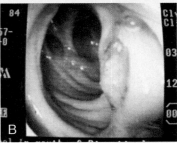
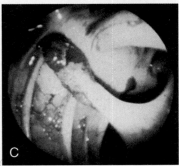
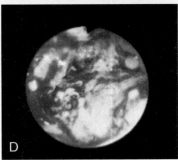

FIGURE 11-15
Images obtained during colonoscopy reveal normal colon (**A**), diverticulosis (**B**), colon polyp (**C**), and colon cancer (**D**).

COMPUTED TOMOGRAPHY (CT) COLONOGRAPHY

also called **virtual colonoscopy**, is a method to screen for colon polyps and colon cancer. It involves using a CT scanner and computer software that allows the physician to see the colon in multiple dimensions. It is less invasive than the conventional method of colonoscopy to screen for colon cancer.

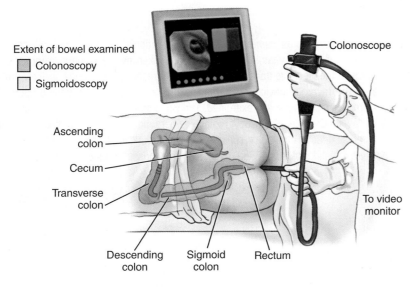

Extent of bowel examined
☐ Colonoscopy
☐ Sigmoidoscopy

Colonoscope

Ascending colon
Cecum
Transverse colon
Descending colon
Sigmoid colon
Rectum
To video monitor

FIGURE 11-16
Sigmoidoscopy, colonoscopy.

Diagnostic Terms—cont'd

Built from Word Parts

TERM	DEFINITION
laparoscope (LAP-a-rō-skōp)	instrument used for visual examination of the abdominal cavity. (Also used to perform laparoscopic surgery, a method that sometimes replaces **laparotomy**, open abdominal incisional surgery.) (See Figure 11-12)
laparoscopy (*lap*-a-ROS-ko-pē)	visual examination of the abdominal cavity
proctoscope (PROK-tō-skōp)	instrument used for visual examination of the rectum
proctoscopy (prok-TOS-ko-pē)	visual examination of the rectum
sigmoidoscopy (*sig*-moy-DOS-ko-pē)	visual examination of the sigmoid colon (see Figure 11-16)

To watch animations, go to evolve.elsevier.com. Select:
Chapter 11, **Animations**, Endoscopy

Refer to p. 10 for your Evolve Access Information.

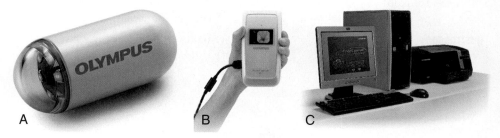

FIGURE 11-17
Capsule endoscopy, also known as *camera endoscopy*. **A**, Patients swallow a capsule containing a camera, about the size of a large vitamin pill. Pictures are taken by the camera every second as it moves naturally through the digestive tract. **B**, The images are recorded on a small device worn around the patient's waist. The recorded device is returned to the physician's office after 8 hours. **C**, The images are transferred to a computer and examined. The video capsule is expelled in the bowel movement and not retrieved. Capsule endoscopy replaces fiberoptic endoscopy of the small intestine because it is much less difficult and yields superior visualization. It is especially helpful in identifying the cause of obscure intestinal bleeding, and diagnosing the causes of abdominal pain.

Fill in the blanks to complete labeling of the diagram.

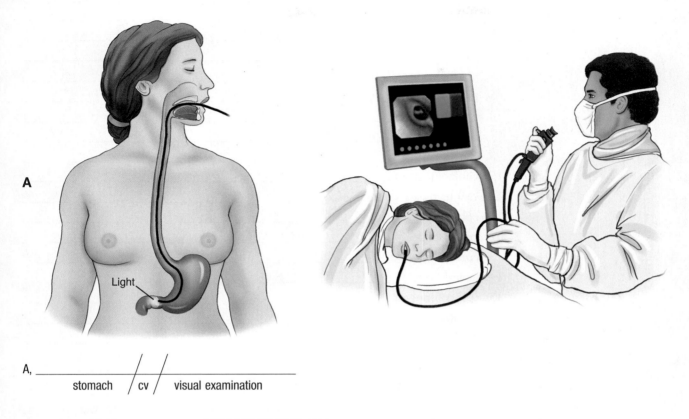

A

Light

A, _____ / _____ / _____
       stomach   cv   visual examination

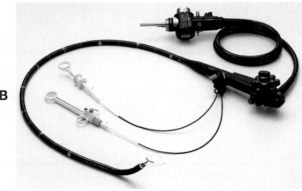

B

B, Fiberscope, a type of _____ / _____ / _____ that
                            stomach   cv   instrument used for visual examination
has glass fibers in a flexible tube, allows for light to be transmitted back to the examiner.

Practice saying aloud each of the diagnostic terms built from word parts on pp. 486–488.

> To hear the terms, go to evolve.elsevier.com. Select: Chapter 11, **Exercises**, Pronunciation.
>
> Refer to p. 10 for your Evolve Access Information.

☐ Place a check mark in the box when you have completed this exercise.

EXERCISE 25

Analyze and define the following diagnostic terms.

1. esophagoscopy _____
2. gastroscope _____
3. gastroscopy _____
4. proctoscope _____
5. proctoscopy _____
6. endoscope _____
7. endoscopy _____
8. sigmoidoscopy _____
9. cholangiogram _____
10. esophagogastroduodenoscopy _____
11. colonoscope _____
12. laparoscope _____
13. colonoscopy _____
14. laparoscopy _____
15. CT colonography _____
16. esophagogram _____
17. cholangiography _____

EXERCISE 26

Build diagnostic terms that correspond to the following definitions by using the word parts you have learned.

1. visual examination within (a hollow organ)

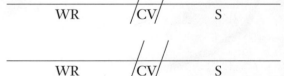

2. instrument used for visual examination of the stomach

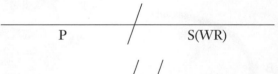

3. instrument used for visual examination of the rectum

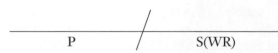

4. instrument used for visual examination within (a hollow organ)

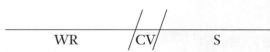

5. visual examination of the rectum

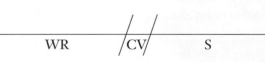

6. visual examination of the esophagus

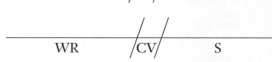

7. visual examination of the sigmoid colon

8. radiographic image of bile ducts

                          WR   /CV/   S

9. visual examination of the stomach

                          WR   /CV/   S

10. instrument used for visual examination of the abdominal cavity

                          WR   /CV/   S

11. visual examination of the esophagus, stomach, and duodenum

     WR /CV/ WR /CV/ WR /CV/ S

12. visual examination of the colon

                          WR   /CV/   S

13. visual examination of the abdominal cavity

                          WR   /CV/   S

14. instrument used for visual examination of the colon

                          WR   /CV/   S

15. radiographic imaging of the colon   CT

                          WR   /CV/   S

16. radiographic imaging of the bile ducts

                          WR   /CV/   S

17. radiographic image of the esophagus

                          WR   /CV/   S

EXERCISE 27

Spell each of the diagnostic terms built from word parts on pp. 486–488 by having someone dictate them to you.

> To hear and spell the terms, go to evolve.elsevier.com. Select: Chapter 11, **Exercises**, Spelling.
>
> Refer to p. 10 for your Evolve Access Information.
>
> ☐ Place a check mark in the box if you have completed this exercise online.

1. _____
2. _____
3. _____
4. _____
5. _____
6. _____
7. _____
8. _____
9. _____
10. _____
11. _____
12. _____
13. _____
14. _____
15. _____
16. _____
17. _____

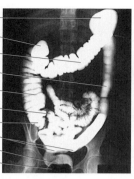

Left (splenic)
colic flexure
Right (hepatic)
colic flexure
Transverse
colon
Descending
colon
Ascending
colon
Terminal
ileum
Cecum
Sigmoid
Rectum
Air-filled
retention tip

FIGURE 11-18
Barium enema (BE); also called
lower GI series.

Endoscope

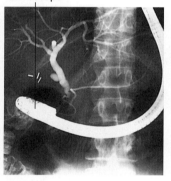

FIGURE 11-19
Endoscopic retrograde cholangiopancreatography (ERCP) is used
to diagnose biliary and pancreatic
pathologic conditions.

**FECAL
IMMUNOCHEMICAL
TEST (FIT) FOR
OCCULT BLOOD**

is becoming the standard test
for screening for colorectal
cancer and large polyps that
may become cancerous. The
FIT test requires only one stool
specimen and is specific for
occult blood in the lower
gastrointestinal tract. The
guaiac-based fecal occult blood
test requires three stool
specimens and is less specific
and sensitive for colorectal
neoplasia.

Diagnostic Terms

Not Built from Word Parts

In some of the following terms, you may recognize word parts you have already learned; however, the full meaning of the terms cannot be discerned by the definition of their word parts.

TERM	DEFINITION
DIAGNOSTIC IMAGING	
abdominal sonography (ab-DOM-i-nal) (so-NOG-ra-fē)	ultrasound test of the abdominal cavity in which the size and structure of organs such as the aorta, liver, gallbladder, bile ducts, and pancreas can be visualized. Liver cysts, abscesses, tumors, cholelithiasis, pancreatitis, and pancreatic tumors may be detected. May also be used to evaluate the kidneys and the portion of the aorta extending through the abdominal cavity (Table 11-2).
barium enema (BE) (BAR-ē-um) (EN-e-ma)	series of radiographic images taken of the large intestine after the contrast agent barium has been administered rectally (also called **lower GI series**) (Figure 11-18)
endoscopic retrograde cholangiopancreatography (ERCP) (en-dō-SKOP-ic) (RET-rō-grād) (kō-lan-jē-ō-pan-krē-a-TOG-rah-fē)	endoscopic procedure involving radiographic imaging of the biliary ducts and pancreatic ducts with contrast media, and fluoroscopy; used to evaluate and diagnose obstructions, strictures, stone diseases, pancreatitis, and pancreatic cancer (Figure 11-19)
upper GI (gastrointestinal) series	series of radiographic images taken of the pharynx, esophagus, stomach, and duodenum after the contrast agent barium has been administered orally
ENDOSCOPY	
endoscopic ultrasound (EUS) (en-dō-SKOP-ic) (UL-tra-sound)	procedure using an endoscope fitted with an ultrasound probe that provides images of layers of the intestinal wall; used to detect tumors and cystic growths and for staging of malignant tumors
LABORATORY	
fecal occult blood test (FOBT) (FĒ-kl) (o-KULT) (blud)	test to detect occult blood in feces. It is used to screen for colon cancer or polyps. Occult blood refers to blood that is present but can only be detected by chemical testing or by microscope. Two types of tests are guaiac-based FOBT and fecal immunochemical test (FIT).
***Helicobacter pylori (H. pylori)* antibodies test** (hel-i-kō-BAK-ter) (pī-LŌ-rē) (AN-ti-bod-ēs)	blood test to determine the presence of *H. pylori* bacteria. The bacteria can be found in the lining of the stomach and can cause peptic ulcers. Tests for *H. pylori* are also performed on biopsy specimens and by breath test.

To watch animations, go to evolve.elsevier.com. Select:
Chapter 11, **Animations**, ERCP.

Refer to p. 10 for your Evolve Access Information.

Table 11-2

Abdominal Sonography

AREAS VISUALIZED AND POSSIBLE FINDINGS

- **Liver**—cysts, abscess, tumors
- **Gallbladder and Bile Ducts**—cholelithiasis, polyps, tumors
- **Pancreas**—inflammation, tumors, abscess, pseudocysts
- **Kidney**—calculi, cysts, tumors, hydronephrosis, malformations, abscess
- **Aorta**—aneurysm

IMAGE

Abdominal ultrasound showing cholelithiasis.
GB = gallbladder
St = stone

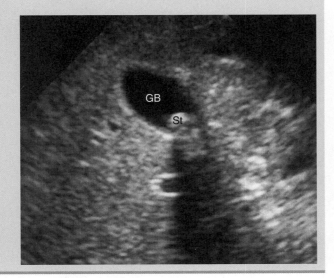

EXERCISE 28

Practice saying aloud each of the diagnostic terms not built from word parts.

 To hear the terms, go to evolve.elsevier.com. Select: Chapter 11, **Exercises**, Pronunciation.

Refer to p. 10 for your Evolve Access Information.

☐ Place a check mark in the box when you have completed this exercise.

EXERCISE 29

Write definitions for the following terms.

1. upper GI series_____ _____

2. barium enema_____ _____

3. endoscopic retrograde cholangiopancreatography _____

_____

4. endoscopic ultrasound_____ _____

5. *Helicobacter pylori* antibodies test_____ _____

6. fecal occult blood test_____ _____

7. abdominal sonography _____ _____

EXERCISE 30

Match the procedures in the first column with their correct definitions in the second column.

_____ 1. fecal occult blood test

_____ 2. barium enema

_____ 3. *Helicobacter pylori* antibodies test

_____ 4. upper GI series

_____ 5. endoscopic retrograde cholangiopancreatography

_____ 6. abdominal sonography

_____ 7. endoscopic ultrasound

a. used to diagnose peptic ulcers
b. radiographic image of the pharynx, esophagus, stomach, and duodenum
c. provides images of layers of the intestinal wall
d. detects blood in feces
e. radiographic image of the esophagus
f. radiographic image of the large intestine
g. ultrasound test of the abdominal cavity
h. radiographic imaging of biliary ducts and pancreatic ducts

EXERCISE 31

Spell each of the diagnostic terms not built from word parts on p. 492 by having someone dictate them to you.

> To hear and spell the terms, go to evolve.elsevier.com. Select: Chapter 11, **Exercises**, Spelling.
> _____
> Refer to p. 10 for your Evolve Access Information.
>
> ☐ Place a check mark in the box if you have completed this exercise online.

1. _____   5. _____

2. _____   6. _____

3. _____   7. _____

4. _____

Complementary Terms

Built from Word Parts

The following terms are built from word parts you have already learned and can be translated literally to find their meanings. Further explanation of terms beyond the definition of their word parts, if needed, is included in parentheses.

TERM	DEFINITION
abdominal (ab-DOM-i-nal)	pertaining to the abdomen
anal (Ā-nal)	pertaining to the anus
aphagia (a-FĀ-ja)	without swallowing (the inability to)
celiac (SĒ-lē-ak)	pertaining to the abdomen
colorectal (kō-lō-REK-tal)	pertaining to the colon and rectum
duodenal (dū-OD-e-nal)	pertaining to the duodenum

TERM	DEFINITION
dyspepsia (dis-PEP-sē-a)	difficult digestion (often used to describe GI symptoms, such as abdominal pain and bloating)
dysphagia (dis-FĀ-ja)	difficult swallowing
enteropathy (*en*-ter-OP-a-thē)	disease of the intestine
esophageal (e-*sof*-a-JĒ-al)	pertaining to the esophagus
gastric (GAS-trik)	pertaining to the stomach
gastroenterologist (*gas*-trō-*en*-ter-OL-o-jist)	physician who studies and treats diseases of the stomach and intestines (GI tract and accessory organs)
gastroenterology (*gas*-trō-*en*-ter-OL-o-jē)	study of the stomach and intestines (branch of medicine that deals with treating diseases of the GI tract and accessory organs)
gastromalacia (*gas*-trō-ma-LĀ-sha)	softening of the stomach
hepatomegaly (*hep*-a-tō-MEG-a-lē)	enlargement of the liver
ileocecal (*il*-ē-ō-SĒ-kal)	pertaining to the ileum and cecum
nasogastric (*nā*-zō-GAS-trik)	pertaining to the nose and stomach
oral (OR-al)	pertaining to the mouth
pancreatic (*pan*-krē-AT-ik)	pertaining to the pancreas
peritoneal (*per*-i-tō-NĒ-al)	pertaining to the peritoneum
proctologist (prok-TOL-o-jist)	physician who studies and treats diseases of the rectum
proctology (prok-TOL-o-jē)	study of the rectum (branch of medicine that deals with disorders of the rectum and anus)
rectal (REK-tal)	pertaining to the rectum
steatorrhea (*stē*-a-tō-RĒ-a)	discharge of fat (excessive amount of fat in the stool, causing frothy, foul-smelling fecal matter usually associated with the malabsorption of fat in conditions such as chronic pancreatitis and celiac disease)
steatosis (*stē*-a-TŌ-sis)	abnormal condition of fat (increased fat at the cellular level often affecting the liver)
stomatitis (*stō*-ma-TĪ-tis)	inflammation of the mouth (mucous membrane)
stomatogastric (*stō*-ma-tō-GAS-trik)	pertaining to the mouth and stomach
sublingual (sub-LING-gwal)	pertaining to under the tongue

To watch animations, go to evolve.elsevier.com. Select:
Chapter 11, **Animations**, Nasogastric Tube Placement.

Refer to p. 10 for your Evolve Access Information.

EXERCISE 32

Practice saying aloud each of the complementary terms built from word parts on pp. 494–495.

 To hear the terms, go to evolve.elsevier.com. Select: Chapter 11, **Exercises**, Pronunciation.

Refer to p. 10 for your Evolve Access Information.

☐ Place a check mark in the box when you have completed this exercise.

EXERCISE 33

Analyze and define the following complementary terms.

1. aphagia_____
2. dyspepsia _____
3. anal_____
4. dysphagia_____
5. hepatomegaly _____
6. ileocecal_____
7. oral_____
8. stomatogastric_____
9. gastromalacia _____
10. pancreatic _____
11. peritoneal _____
12. steatosis _____
13. sublingual _____
14. proctology_____
15. nasogastric_____
16. abdominal _____
17. proctologist_____
18. gastroenterology_____
19. gastroenterologist_____
20. colorectal_____
21. rectal _____
22. steatorrhea_____
23. stomatitis_____
24. enteropathy_____
25. gastric _____
26. duodenal _____
27. esophageal_____
28. celiac _____

EXERCISE 34

Build the complementary terms for the following definitions by using the word parts you have learned.

1. enlargement of the liver

   _____ / ___ / _____
   WR   /CV/   S

2. without swallowing (the inability to)

   _____ / _____
   P   S(WR)

3. pertaining to under the tongue

   ___ / ___ / ___
   P   WR   S

4. pertaining to the nose and the stomach

   ___ / ___ / ___ / ___
   WR /CV/ WR   S

5. pertaining to the mouth and the stomach

   ___ / ___ / ___ / ___
   WR /CV/ WR   S

6. pertaining to the anus

   _____ / ___
   WR   S

7. pertaining to the peritoneum

   _____ / ___
   WR   S

8. pertaining to the abdomen

   a. _____ / ___
      WR   S

   b. _____ / ___
      WR   S

9. difficult swallowing

   _____ / _____
   P   S(WR)

10. pertaining to the ileum and cecum

    ___ / ___ / ___ / ___
    WR /CV/ WR   S

11. softening of the stomach

    ___ / ___ / ___
    WR /CV/   S

12. physician who studies and treats diseases of the rectum

    ___ / ___ / ___
    WR /CV/   S

13. difficult digestion

    _____ / _____
    P   S(WR)

14. pertaining to the pancreas

    _____ / ___
    WR   S

15. study of the rectum

    ___ / ___ / ___
    WR /CV/   S

16. discharge of fat

    ___ / ___ / ___
    WR /CV/   S

17. pertaining to the mouth

    _____ / ___
    WR   S

18. physician who studies and treats diseases of the stomach and intestines

    ___ / ___ / ___ / ___ / ___
    WR /CV/ WR /CV/   S

19. study of the stomach and
    intestines

    _____ / ____ / _____ / ____ / _____
         WR   /CV/   WR   /CV/   S

20. pertaining to the colon and
    rectum

    _____ / ____ / _____ / _____
         WR   /CV/   WR   S

21. pertaining to the rectum

    _____ / _____
         WR   S

22. abnormal condition of fat

    _____ / _____
         WR   S

23. pertaining to the esophagus

    _____ / _____
         WR   S

24. pertaining to the stomach

    _____ / _____
         WR   S

25. pertaining to the duodenum

    _____ / _____
         WR   S

26. disease of the intestine

    _____ / ____ / _____
         WR   /CV/   S

27. inflammation of the mouth
    (mucous membrane)

    _____ / _____
         WR   S

EXERCISE 35

Spell each of the complementary terms built from word parts on pp. 494–495 by having someone
dictate them to you.

> To hear and spell the terms, go to evolve.elsevier.com. Select: Chapter 11, **Exercises**, Spelling.
>
> Refer to p. 10 for your Evolve Access Information.
>
> ☐ Place a check mark in the box if you have completed this exercise online.

1. _____   15. _____
2. _____   16. _____
3. _____   17. _____
4. _____   18. _____
5. _____   19. _____
6. _____   20. _____
7. _____   21. _____
8. _____   22. _____
9. _____   23. _____
10. _____   24. _____
11. _____   25. _____
12. _____   26. _____
13. _____   27. _____
14. _____   28. _____

Complementary Terms

Not Built from Word Parts

In some of the following terms, you may recognize word parts you have already learned; however, the full meaning of the terms cannot be discerned by the definition of their word parts.

TERM	DEFINITION
ascites (a-SĪ-tēz)	abnormal collection of fluid in the peritoneal cavity (Figure 11-20)
diarrhea (dī-a-RĔ-a) *(NOTE: diarrhea is composed* *of* dia-, *meaning through,* *and* -rrhea, *meaning flow)*	frequent discharge of liquid stool
dysentery (DIS-en-*ter*-ē)	disorder that involves inflammation of the intestine (usually the large intestine) associated with diarrhea and abdominal pain
emesis (EM-e-sis)	expelling matter from the stomach through the mouth (also called **vomiting**)
feces (FĔ-sēz)	waste from the digestive tract expelled through the rectum (also called **stool** or **fecal matter**)
flatus (FLĂ-tus)	gas in the digestive tract or expelled through the anus
gastric lavage (GAS-trik) (la-VOZH)	washing out of the stomach
gavage (ga-VOZH)	process of feeding a person through a nasogastric tube
hematemesis (*h*ē-ma-TEM-e-sis)	vomiting of blood
hematochezia (*h*ē-ma-tō-KĔ-zha)	passage of bloody feces
malabsorption (*mal*-ab-SORP-shun)	impaired digestion or intestinal absorption of nutrients
melena (me-LĔ-na)	black, tarry stool that contains digested blood; usually a result of bleeding in the upper GI tract
nausea (NAW-zē-a)	urge to vomit
palpate (PAL-pāt)	to examine by hand; to feel
peristalsis (*per*-i-STAL-sis)	involuntary wavelike contractions that propel food along the digestive tract
reflux (RĔ-fluks)	abnormal backward flow. In esophageal reflux, the stomach contents flow back into the esophagus.

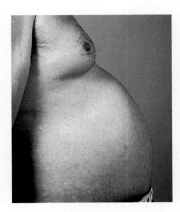

FIGURE 11-20
Ascites.

Complementary Terms—cont'd

Not Built from Word Parts

TERM	DEFINITION
stoma (STŌ-ma)	surgical opening between an organ and the surface of the body, such as the opening established in the abdominal wall by colostomy, ileostomy, or a similar operation. Stoma may also refer to an opening created between body structures or between portions of the intestines. (see Exercise Figure E)
vomiting (VOM-it-ing)	expelling matter from the stomach through the mouth (also called **emesis**)

To watch animations, go to evolve.elsevier.com. Select:
Chapter 11, **Animations**, Nasogastric Lavage
                       Bleeding Ulcers and Hematemesis

Refer to p. 10 for your Evolve Access Information.

Refer to **Appendix D** for pharmacology terms related to the digestive system.

EXERCISE 36

Practice saying aloud each of the complementary terms not built from word parts on pp. 499–500.

To hear the terms, go to evolve.elsevier.com. Select: Chapter 11, **Exercises**, Pronunciation.

Refer to p. 10 for your Evolve Access Information.

☐ Place a check mark in the box when you have completed this exercise.

EXERCISE 37

Match the definitions in the first column with the correct terms in the second column.

_____ 1. abnormal collection of fluid	a. hematemesis
_____ 2. expelling matter from the stomach	b. flatus
_____ 3. feeding a person through a tube	c. gastric lavage
_____ 4. washing out of the stomach	d. reflux
_____ 5. urge to vomit	e. vomiting, emesis
_____ 6. frequent discharge of liquid stool	f. gavage
_____ 7. waste expelled from the rectum	g. melena
_____ 8. vomiting of blood	h. dysentery
_____ 9. abnormal backward flow	i. diarrhea
_____ 10. inflammation of the intestine associated with diarrhea and abdominal pain	j. peristalsis
	k. feces
_____ 11. gas expelled through the anus	l. nausea
_____ 12. involuntary wavelike contractions	m. ascites
_____ 13. black, tarry stools	n. hematochezia
_____ 14. surgical opening between an organ and the surface of the body	o. stoma
	p. malabsorption
_____ 15. to examine by hand	q. palpate
_____ 16. passage of bloody feces	
_____ 17. impaired digestion or intestinal absorption	

EXERCISE 38

Write definitions for each of the following terms.

1. ascites _____
2. gavage _____
3. gastric lavage _____
4. feces _____
5. nausea _____
6. vomiting _____
7. dysentery _____
8. diarrhea _____
9. flatus _____
10. reflux _____
11. hematemesis _____
12. peristalsis _____
13. melena _____
14. stoma _____
15. hematochezia _____
16. emesis _____
17. malabsorption _____
18. palpate _____

EXERCISE 39

Spell each of the complementary terms not built from word parts on pp. 499–500 by having someone dictate them to you.

To hear and spell the terms, go to evolve.elsevier.com. Select: Chapter 11, **Exercises**, Spelling.

Refer to p. 10 for your Evolve Access Information.

☐ Place a check mark in the box if you have completed this exercise online.

1. _____ 10. _____
2. _____ 11. _____
3. _____ 12. _____
4. _____ 13. _____
5. _____ 14. _____
6. _____ 15. _____
7. _____ 16. _____
8. _____ 17. _____
9. _____ 18. _____

For review and/or assessment, go to evolve.elsevier.com. Select:
Chapter 11, **Activities**, Terms Not Built from Word Parts
                   Hear It and Type It: Clinical Vignettes
Chapter 11, **Games**,   Term Explorer
                           Termbusters
                           Medical Millionaire

Refer to p. 10 for your Evolve Access Information.

Abbreviations

ABBREVIATION	MEANING
A&P resection	abdominoperineal resection
BE	barium enema
EGD	esophagogastroduodenoscopy
ERCP	endoscopic retrograde cholangiopancreatography
EUS	endoscopic ultrasound
FOBT	fecal occult blood test
GERD	gastroesophageal reflux disease
GI	gastrointestinal
H. pylori	*Helicobacter pylori*
IBS	irritable bowel syndrome
N&V	nausea and vomiting
PEG	percutaneous endoscopic gastrostomy
UGI	upper gastrointestinal
UPPP	uvulopalatopharyngoplasty

 Refer to **Appendix C** for a complete list of abbreviations.

EXERCISE 40

Write the meaning of the following abbreviations.

1. ERCP _____ _____ _____
2. EUS _____ _____
3. N&V _____ _____ _____
4. IBS _____ _____ _____
5. PEG _____ _____ _____
6. UGI _____ _____
7. UPPP_____
8. GERD _____ _____ _____
9. GI _____
10. *H. pylori* _____ _____
11. BE _____ _____
12. EGD _____
13. A&P resection _____ _____
14. FOBT _____ _____ _____ _____

PRACTICAL APPLICATION

EXERCISE 41 *Interact with Medical Documents and Electronic Health Records*

A. Complete the endoscopy report by writing the medical terms in the blanks. Use the list of definitions with the corresponding numbers.

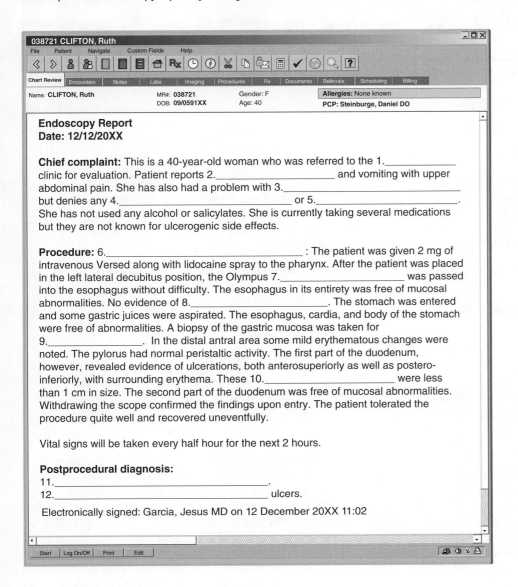

Endoscopy Report
Date: 12/12/20XX

Chief complaint: This is a 40-year-old woman who was referred to the 1._____ clinic for evaluation. Patient reports 2._____ and vomiting with upper abdominal pain. She has also had a problem with 3._____ but denies any 4._____ or 5._____. She has not used any alcohol or salicylates. She is currently taking several medications but they are not known for ulcerogenic side effects.

Procedure: 6._____ : The patient was given 2 mg of intravenous Versed along with lidocaine spray to the pharynx. After the patient was placed in the left lateral decubitus position, the Olympus 7._____ was passed into the esophagus without difficulty. The esophagus in its entirety was free of mucosal abnormalities. No evidence of 8._____. The stomach was entered and some gastric juices were aspirated. The esophagus, cardia, and body of the stomach were free of abnormalities. A biopsy of the gastric mucosa was taken for 9._____. In the distal antral area some mild erythematous changes were noted. The pylorus had normal peristaltic activity. The first part of the duodenum, however, revealed evidence of ulcerations, both anterosuperiorly as well as postero-inferiorly, with surrounding erythema. These 10._____ were less than 1 cm in size. The second part of the duodenum was free of mucosal abnormalities. Withdrawing the scope confirmed the findings upon entry. The patient tolerated the procedure quite well and recovered uneventfully.

Vital signs will be taken every half hour for the next 2 hours.

Postprocedural diagnosis:
11._____.
12._____ ulcers.

Electronically signed: Garcia, Jesus MD on 12 December 20XX 11:02

1. visual examination within a hollow organ
2. urge to vomit
3. difficult digestion
4. vomiting of blood
5. black, tarry stool that contains digested blood
6. visual examination of the esophagus, stomach, and duodenum
7. instrument used for visual examination of the stomach
8. abnormal backward flow
9. abbreviation for *Helicobacter pylori*
10. eroded areas
11. inflammation of the stomach
12. pertaining to the duodenum

B. Read the radiology report and answer the questions following it.

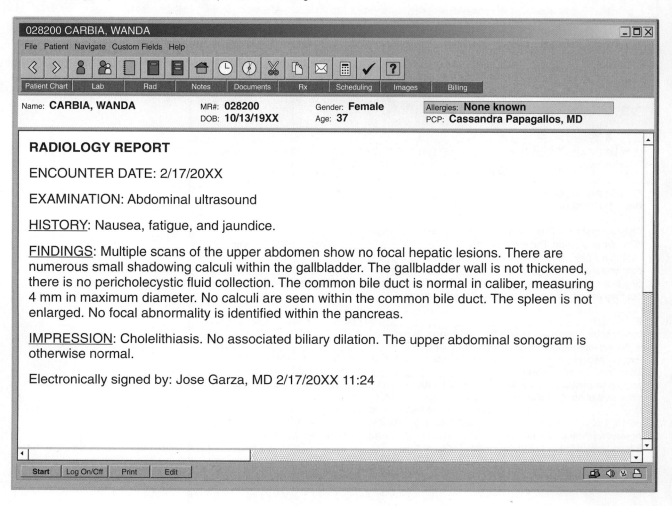

028200 CARBIA, WANDA

File Patient Navigate Custom Fields Help

Patient Chart | Lab | Rad | Notes | Documents | Rx | Scheduling | Images | Billing

Name: **CARBIA, WANDA** MR#: **028200** Gender: **Female** Allergies: **None known**
DOB: **10/13/19XX** Age: **37** PCP: **Cassandra Papagallos, MD**

RADIOLOGY REPORT

ENCOUNTER DATE: 2/17/20XX

EXAMINATION: Abdominal ultrasound

HISTORY: Nausea, fatigue, and jaundice.

FINDINGS: Multiple scans of the upper abdomen show no focal hepatic lesions. There are numerous small shadowing calculi within the gallbladder. The gallbladder wall is not thickened, there is no pericholecystic fluid collection. The common bile duct is normal in caliber, measuring 4 mm in maximum diameter. No calculi are seen within the common bile duct. The spleen is not enlarged. No focal abnormality is identified within the pancreas.

IMPRESSION: Cholelithiasis. No associated biliary dilation. The upper abdominal sonogram is otherwise normal.

Electronically signed by: Jose Garza, MD 2/17/20XX 11:24

Start | Log On/Off | Print | Edit

1. The exam included which diagnostic procedure:
   a. radiographic imaging of the colon with computerized tomography
   b. radiographic imaging of the bile ducts after administration of contrast media
   c. use of an endoscope fitted with an ultrasound probe to obtain images of layers of the intestinal wall
   d. recording images of organs with sound waves produced by a transducer placed directly on the skin
2. The patient's symptoms included:
   a. expelling matter from the stomach through the mouth
   b. condition characterized by a yellow tinge to the skin
   c. bluish discoloration of the skin
   d. erythroderma

3. The examination revealed the presence of:
   a. stones within the gallbladder
   b. stones within the common bile duct
   c. lesions in the liver
   d. inflammation of the pancreas
4. "Biliary dilation" would most likely refer to:
   a. inflammation of the pancreas
   b. the presence of fluid in the upper abdomen
   c. choledocholithiasis
   d. widening of the bile ducts or gallbladder

C. Read the radiology report and answer the questions following it.

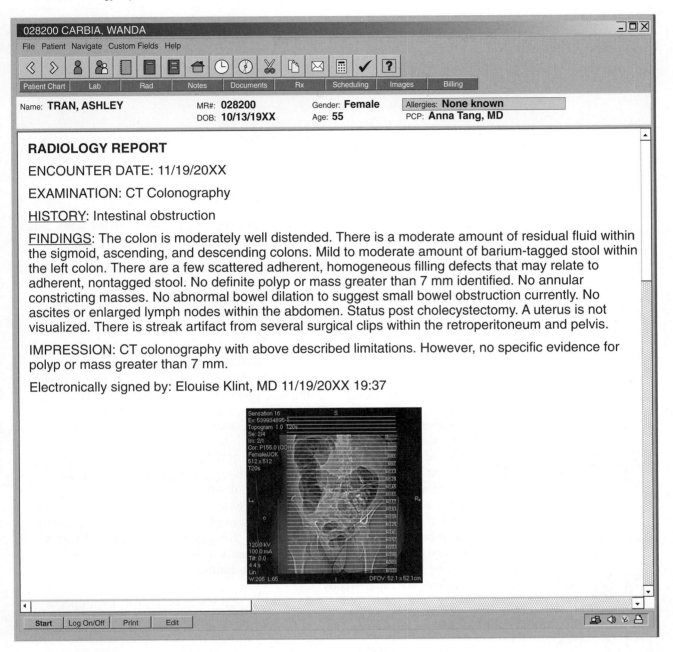

1. No ascites indicates:
   a. no fluid accumulation in the peritoneal cavity
   b. no inflammation of the intestine associated with diarrhea and abdominal pain
   c. no residual fluid within the sigmoid colon
   d. no kinking of the intestine
2. The CT colonography was performed:
   a. before excision of the colon
   b. after excision of the appendix
   c. before creation of an artificial opening into the colon
   d. after excision of the gallbladder
3. The report most clearly suggests that the intestinal obstruction was probably *not* caused by a(n):
   a. adhesion
   b. volvulus
   c. intussusception
   d. polyp or mass

D. Complete the **three medical documents** within the electronic health record (EHR) on Evolve.

> Many healthcare records today are stored and used in an electronic system called **Electronic Health Records (EHR)**. Electronic health records contain a collection of health information of an individual patient documented by various providers at different facilities; the digitally formatted record can be shared through computer networks with patients, physicians, and other health care providers.

> For practice with medical terms using electronic health records, go to evolve.elsevier.com. Select Chapter 11, **Electronic Health Records**.
>
> Refer to p. 10 for your Evolve Access Information.

EXERCISE 42 *Interpret Medical Terms*

To test your understanding of the terms introduced in this chapter, circle the words that correctly complete the sentences. The italicized words refer to the correct answer.

1. Mr. Gomez was tentatively diagnosed with *gallstones,* or (**cholelithiasis, cholecystitis, sialolithiasis**).
2. An abdominal ultrasound confirmed the diagnosis, and Mr. Gomez is now scheduled for a laparoscopic *excision of the gallbladder,* or (**cholecystostomy, cholecystectomy, colectomy**).
3. The plural spelling of the term meaning *connection created by surgically joining two structures* is (**anastomoses, anastomosis, anastomosices**).
4. The patient was diagnosed with a condition of *inflammation of the colon and formation of ulcers,* called (**cirrhosis, ulcerative colitis, peptic ulcer**).
5. A *prolapse of the rectum* is (**rectocele, intussusception, proctoptosis**).
6. An *abnormal growing together of two peritoneal surfaces* is (**anastomosis, adhesion, amniocentesis**).
7. Named for their location, gastric ulcers and duodenal ulcers are forms of *erosions of the mucous membrane of the stomach* and *duodenum* (**irritable bowel syndrome, peptic ulcers, ulcerative colitis**).
8. Tests used to diagnose peptic ulcers include *Helicobacter pylori* antibodies test, *series of radiographic images taken of the stomach and duodenum after the contrast agent barium has been administered orally* (**barium enema, upper GI series, endoscopic ultrasound**), and *visual examination of the pharynx, esophagus, stomach, and duodenum* (**esophagogastroduodenoscopy, endoscopic ultrasound, laparoscopy**).
9. Three surgical procedures that may be performed on a patient with peptic ulcers are (1) *excision of the stomach,* or (**gastrotomy, gastrostomy, gastrectomy**); (2) *surgical repair of the pylorus,* or (**pyloroplasty, cheilorrhaphy, gastrojejunostomy**); and (3) *cutting of certain branches of the vagus nerve,* or (**colostomy, vagotomy, gingivectomy**).
10. *Difficult digestion* is (**dyspepsia, dysphagia, aphagia**).
11. *Feeding* a person *through a gastric tube* is called (**lavage, gavage, gastrostomy**).
12. The *surgical procedures to remove the colon and rectum and create an artificial opening into the colon* are (**colectomy and colostomy, abdominoperineal resection and colostomy, abdominoperineal resection and ileostomy**).
13. To rule out cancer of the colon, the doctor performed a diagnostic procedure to *visually examine the colon* or (**colonoscopy, colonoscope, colostomy**).
14. The doctor diagnosed the patient as having *an obstruction of the intestine* or (**polyp, irritable bowel syndrome, ileus**).
15. The following test is used to screen for colon cancer (**fecal occult blood test, *Helicobacter pylori* antibodies test, upper GI series**).
16. (**Stoma, Stomata, Stomaes**) is the plural spelling of the term meaning *surgical opening between an organ and the surface of the body.*

🛜 WEB LINK

For more information about diseases and disorders of the digestive system and the latest treatments available, please visit the National Digestive Diseases Information Clearing House at **digestive.niddk.nih.gov**.

For a snapshot assessment of your knowledge of digestive system terms, go to evolve.elsevier.com. Select: Chapter 11, **Quick Quizzes**.

Refer to p. 10 for your Evolve Access Information.

EXERCISE **43**   *Read Medical Terms in Use*

Practice pronunciation of terms by reading the following discussion. Use the pronunciation key following the medical term to assist you in saying the word.

To hear these terms, go to evolve.elsevier.com.
Select: Chapter 11, **Exercises**, Read Medical Terms in Use.

Refer to p. 10 for your Evolve Access Information.

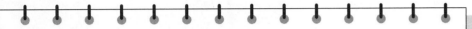

COLORECTAL CANCER

Colorectal (kō-lō-REK-tal) cancer begins in the colon or rectum and is the second leading cause of cancer deaths in the United States. Most are adenocarcinomas that originate as a benign, adenomatous **polyp** (POL-ip).

Many people have no symptoms until the tumor is quite advanced, and symptoms vary depending on the location of the tumor. Warning signs are altered bowel habits, **rectal** (REK-tal) bleeding, **abdominal** (ab-DOM-i-nal) cramps, **flatus** (FLĀ-tus) and bloating, iron deficiency anemia, and weight loss.

Screening and diagnostic tests for colorectal cancer include digital rectal examination, **fecal** (FĒ-kl) **occult** (o-KULT) blood test, **sigmoidoscopy** (*sig*-moy-DOS-ko-pē), **colonoscopy** (kō-lon-OS-ko-pē), and **barium** (BAR-ē-um) **enema** (EN-e-ma). As well as being an important diagnostic tool, colonoscopy may be used for biopsy and for the removal of pedunculated **polyps.** To perform a **polypectomy** (*pol*-i-PEK-to-mē), a braided wire snare is inserted into the **colonoscope** (kō-LON-ō-skōp). A snare loop, like a noose, is placed around the stem of the polyp. With electrosurgical power attached to the snare, the polyp is detached. The polyp is removed from the colon for histologic examination.

For cancer beyond the early stage, conventional surgery is the main treatment. The type of surgery depends on the location and stage of the tumor. Types of surgeries performed are left or right-sided **hemicolectomy** (*hem*-ē-kō-LEK-to-mē) with **anastomosis** (a-*nas*-to-MŌ-sis), sigmoid **colectomy** (kō-LEK-to-mē), and **abdominoperineal** (ab-*dom*-i-nō-*per*-i-NĒ-el) **resection** with **colostomy** (ko-LOS-to-mē).

EXERCISE **44**   *Comprehend Medical Terms in Use*

Test your comprehension of terms in the previous medical discussion by circling the correct answer.

1. Which of the following is used for diagnosing colorectal cancer?
   a. visual exam of the stomach
   b. series of radiographic images of the small intestine
   c. visual exam of the colon
   d. radiographic image of the esophagus
2. T F   A polypectomy may be performed during a colonoscopy.
3. T F   Depending on the location of the tumor, a surgical treatment for colorectal cancer may be performed that creates an opening between the colon and abdominal wall for the passage of stool.
4. T F   Vomiting blood is a warning sign for colorectal cancer.

CHAPTER REVIEW

Review of Evolve

Keep a record of the online activities you have completed by placing a check mark in the box. You may also record your scores. All activities have been referenced throughout the chapter.

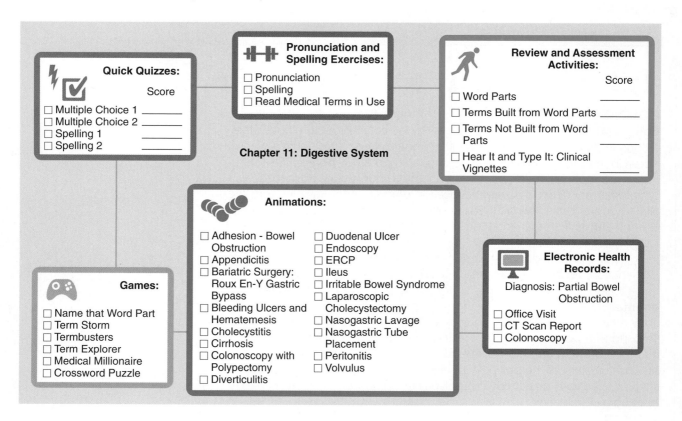

Quick Quizzes:

Score

☐ Multiple Choice 1 _____
☐ Multiple Choice 2 _____
☐ Spelling 1 _____
☐ Spelling 2 _____

Pronunciation and Spelling Exercises:

☐ Pronunciation
☐ Spelling
☐ Read Medical Terms in Use

Chapter 11: Digestive System

Review and Assessment Activities:

Score

☐ Word Parts _____
☐ Terms Built from Word Parts _____
☐ Terms Not Built from Word Parts _____
☐ Hear It and Type It: Clinical Vignettes _____

Animations:

☐ Adhesion - Bowel Obstruction
☐ Appendicitis
☐ Bariatric Surgery: Roux En-Y Gastric Bypass
☐ Bleeding Ulcers and Hematemesis
☐ Cholecystitis
☐ Cirrhosis
☐ Colonoscopy with Polypectomy
☐ Diverticulitis
☐ Duodenal Ulcer
☐ Endoscopy
☐ ERCP
☐ Ileus
☐ Irritable Bowel Syndrome
☐ Laparoscopic Cholecystectomy
☐ Nasogastric Lavage
☐ Nasogastric Tube Placement
☐ Peritonitis
☐ Volvulus

Games:

☐ Name that Word Part
☐ Term Storm
☐ Termbusters
☐ Term Explorer
☐ Medical Millionaire
☐ Crossword Puzzle

Electronic Health Records:

Diagnosis: Partial Bowel Obstruction

☐ Office Visit
☐ CT Scan Report
☐ Colonoscopy

Review of Word Parts

Can you define and spell the following word parts?

COMBINING FORMS			PREFIX	SUFFIX
abdomin/o	duoden/o	palat/o	hemi-	-pepsia
an/o	enter/o	pancreat/o		
antr/o	esophag/o	peritone/o		
append/o	gastr/o	polyp/o		
appendic/o	gingiv/o	proct/o		
cec/o	gloss/o	pylor/o		
celi/o	hepat/o	rect/o		
cheil/o	herni/o	sial/o		
cholangi/o	ile/o	sigmoid/o		
chol/e	jejun/o	steat/o		
choledoch/o	lapar/o	stomat/o		
col/o	lingu/o	uvul/o		
colon/o	or/o			
diverticul/o				

Review of Terms

Can you define, pronounce, and spell the following terms *built from word parts*?

DISEASES AND DISORDERS	SURGICAL	DIAGNOSTIC	COMPLEMENTARY
appendicitis	abdominocentesis	cholangiogram	abdominal
cholangioma	abdominoplasty	cholangiography	anal
cholecystitis	anoplasty	colonoscope	aphagia
choledocholithiasis	antrectomy	colonoscopy	celiac
cholelithiasis	appendectomy	CT colonography	colorectal
colitis	celiotomy	endoscope	duodenal
diverticulitis	cheilorrhaphy	endoscopy	dyspepsia
diverticulosis	cholecystectomy	esophagogastroduodenoscopy (EGD)	dysphagia
esophagitis	choledocholithotomy	esophagogram	enteropathy
gastritis	colectomy	esophagoscopy	esophageal
gastroenteritis	colostomy	gastroscope	gastric
gastroenterocolitis	diverticulectomy	gastroscopy	gastroenterologist
gingivitis	enterorrhaphy	laparoscope	gastroenterology
glossitis	esophagogastroplasty	laparoscopy	gastromalacia
hepatitis	gastrectomy	proctoscope	hepatomegaly
hepatoma	gastrojejunostomy	proctoscopy	ileocecal
palatitis	gastroplasty	sigmoidoscopy	nasogastric
pancreatitis	gastrostomy		oral
peritonitis	gingivectomy		pancreatic
polyposis	glossorrhaphy		peritoneal
proctoptosis	hemicolectomy		proctologist
rectocele	herniorrhaphy		proctology
sialolith	ileostomy		rectal
steatohepatitis	laparotomy		steatorrhea
uvulitis	palatoplasty		steatosis
	polypectomy		stomatitis
	pyloromyotomy		stomatogastric
	pyloroplasty		sublingual
	uvulectomy		
	uvulopalatopharyngoplasty (UPPP)		

Can you build, analyze, define, pronounce, and spell the following terms *not built from word parts*?

DISEASES AND DISORDERS	SURGICAL	DIAGNOSTIC	COMPLEMENTARY
adhesion	abdominoperineal resection (A&P resection)	abdominal sonography	ascites
celiac disease		barium enema (BE)	diarrhea
cirrhosis		endoscopic retrograde cholangiopancreatography (ERCP)	dysentery
Crohn disease	anastomosis (*pl.* anastomoses)		emesis
gastroesophageal reflux disease (GERD)		endoscopic ultrasound (EUS)	feces
	bariatric surgery	fecal occult blood test (FOBT)	flatus
hemochromatosis	hemorrhoidectomy	*Helicobacter pylori* antibodies test	gastric lavage
hemorrhoids	vagotomy	upper GI (gastrointestinal) series	gavage
ileus			hematemesis
intussusception			hematochezia
irritable bowel syndrome (IBS)			malabsorption
obesity			melena
peptic ulcer			nausea
polyp			palpate
ulcerative colitis			peristalsis
volvulus			reflux
			stoma
			vomiting

ANSWERS

ANSWERS TO CHAPTER 11 EXERCISES
Exercise Figures

Exercise Figure

A.
1. mouth: or/o, stomat/o
2. esophagus: esophag/o
3. duodenum: duoden/o
4. colon: col/o, colon/o
5. cecum: cec/o
6. anus: an/o
7. stomach: gastr/o
8. antrum: antr/o
9. jejunum: jejun/o
10. ileum: ile/o
11. sigmoid colon: sigmoid/o
12. rectum: proct/o, rect/o

Exercise Figure

B.
1. palate: palat/o
2. uvula: uvul/o
3. tongue: gloss/o, lingu/o
4. gallbladder: chol/e (gall), cyst/o (bladder)
5. pyloric sphincter: pylor/o
6. appendix: append/o, appendic/o
7. gum: gingiv/o
8. lip: cheil/o
9. salivary glands: sial/o
10. liver: hepat/o
11. bile duct: cholangi/o
12. common bile duct: choledoch/o
13. pancreas: pancreat/o
14. abdomen, abdominal cavity: abdomin/o, celi/o, lapar/o

Exercise Figure

C. 2. appendic/itis

Exercise Figure

D. chol/e/lith/iasis, choledoch/o/lith/iasis

Exercise Figure

E.
1. ile/o/stomy
2. col/o/stomy

Exercise Figure

F. gastr/ectomy

Exercise Figure

G. per/cutane/ous
endo/scopic
gastr/o/stomy

Exercise Figure

H.
A. gastr/o/scopy
B. gastr/o/scope

Exercise 1
1. alimentary canal
2. gastrointestinal tract
3. pharynx
4. esophagus
5. stomach
6. duodenum
7. jejunum
8. ileum
9. cecum
10. ascending colon
11. transverse colon
12. descending colon
13. sigmoid colon
14. rectum
15. anus

Exercise 2
1. l
2. d
3. a
4. h
5. m
6. j
7. b
8. i
9. c
10. g
11. e
12. k
13. f

Exercise 3
1. rectum
2. stomach
3. anus
4. cecum
5. ileum
6. mouth
7. duodenum
8. colon
9. mouth
10. intestine
11. rectum
12. antrum
13. esophagus
14. jejunum
15. sigmoid colon
16. colon

Exercise 4
1. cec/o
2. gastr/o
3. ile/o
4. jejun/o
5. sigmoid/o
6. esophag/o
7. a. rect/o
   b. proct/o
8. enter/o
9. duoden/o
10. a. col/o
    b. colon/o
11. a. or/o
    b. stomat/o
12. an/o
13. antr/o

Exercise 5
1. hernia
2. abdomen, abdominal cavity
3. saliva, salivary gland
4. gall, bile
5. diverticulum
6. gum
7. appendix
8. tongue
9. liver
10. lip
11. peritoneum
12. palate
13. pancreas
14. abdomen, abdominal cavity
15. tongue
16. common bile duct
17. pylorus, pyloric sphincter
18. uvula
19. bile duct
20. polyp, small growth
21. abdomen
22. fat
23. appendix

Exercise 6
1. palat/o
2. sial/o
3. pancreat/o
4. peritone/o
5. a. gloss/o
   b. lingu/o
6. gingiv/o
7. pylor/o
8. hepat/o
9. chol/e
10. a. abdomin/o
    b. celi/o
    c. lapar/o
11. herni/o
12. diverticul/o
13. cheil/o
14. a. append/o
    b. appendic/o
15. uvul/o
16. cholangi/o
17. choledoch/o
18. polyp/o
19. steat/o

Exercise 7
1. digestion
2. half

Exercise 8
1. -pepsia
2. hemi-

Exercise 9
Pronunciation Exercise

Exercise 10
Note: The combining form is identified by italic and bold print.

1.   WR CV WR S
   ***chol/e*/lith/iasis**
       CF
   condition of gallstones

2.   WR   S
diverticul/osis
abnormal condition of having
diverticula

3. WR CV WR
sial/o/lith
    CF
stone in the salivary gland

4. WR   S
hepat/oma
tumor of the liver

5. WR S
uvul/itis
inflammation of the uvula

6.   WR   S
pancreat/itis
inflammation of the pancreas

7. WR CV   S
proct/o/ptosis
    CF
prolapse of the rectum

8.   WR   S
gingiv/itis
inflammation of the gums

9.   WR   S
gastr/itis
inflammation of the stomach

10. WR CV S
rect/o/cele
    CF
protrusion of the rectum

11. WR   S
palat/itis
inflammation of the palate

12.   WR   S
hepat/itis
inflammation of the liver

13.   WR   S
appendic/itis
inflammation of the appendix

14.   WR CV WR S
chol/e/cyst/itis
    CF
inflammation of the gallbladder

15.   WR   S
diverticul/itis
inflammation of a diverticulum

16.   WR CV WR   S
gastr/o/enter/itis
    CF
inflammation of the stomach and
intestines

17.   WR CV WR CV WR S
gastr/o/enter/o/col/itis
      CF   CF
inflammation of the stomach,
intestines, and colon

18.   WR   CV WR S
choledoch/o/lith/iasis
      CF
condition of stones in the common
bile duct

19.   WR   S
cholangi/oma
tumor of the bile duct

20. WR   S
polyp/osis
abnormal condition of (multiple)
polyps

21.   WR   S
esophag/itis
inflammation of the esophagus

22.   WR   S
periton/itis
inflammation of the peritoneum

23.   WR CV WR   S
steat/o/hepat/itis
     CF
inflammation of the liver associated
with (excess) fat

24.   WR   S
gloss/itis
inflammation of the tongue

25. WR   S
col/itis
inflammation of the colon

Exercise 11

1. hepat/oma
2. gastr/itis
3. sial/o/lith
4. appendic/itis
5. diverticul/itis
6. chol/e/cyst/itis
7. diverticul/osis
8. gastr/o/enter/itis
9. proct/o/ptosis
10. rect/o/cele
11. uvul/itis
12. gingiv/itis
13. hepat/itis
14. palat/itis
15. chol/e/lith/iasis
16. steat/o/hepat/itis
17. gastr/o/enter/o/col/itis
18. pancreat/itis
19. cholangi/oma
20. esophag/itis
21. choledoch/o/lith/iasis
22. polyp/osis
23. periton/itis
24. gloss/itis
25. col/itis

Exercise 12
Spelling Exercise; see text p. 472.

Exercise 13
Pronunciation Exercise

Exercise 14

1. b		9. k
2. e		10. h
3. l		11. c
4. d		12. j
5. f		13. m
6. a		14. n
7. i		15. o
8. g		

Exercise 15

1. erosion of the mucous membrane of
the stomach or duodenum
2. chronic inflammation of the
intestinal tract usually affecting the
ileum and colon
3. twisting or kinking of the
intestine
4. abnormal growing together of two
peritoneal surfaces that normally are
separated
5. chronic disease of the liver with
gradual destruction of cells
6. telescoping of segment of the
intestine
7. malabsorption syndrome caused by
an immune reaction to gluten
8. inflammation of the colon with the
formation of ulcers
9. swollen or distended veins in the
rectal area
10. tumorlike growth extending out
from a mucous membrane
11. disturbance of bowel function
12. nonmechanical obstruction of the
intestine, often caused by failure of
peristalsis
13. abnormal backward flow of the
gastrointestinal contents into the
esophagus
14. excess body fat
15. an iron metabolism disorder

Exercise 16
Spelling Exercise; see text p. 477.

Exercise 17
Pronunciation Exercise

Exercise 18
*Note: The combining form is identified by
italic and bold print.*

1.   WR   S
gastr/ectomy
excision of the stomach

2. WR CV WR CV S
esophag/o/gastr/o/plasty
    CF   CF
surgical repair of the esophagus and
the stomach

3. WR   S
diverticul/ectomy
excision of a diverticulum

4. WR   S
antr/ectomy
excision of the antrum

5. WR CV S
palat/o/plasty
    CF
surgical repair of the palate

6. WR   S
uvul/ectomy
excision of the uvula

7. WR CV WR CV S
gastr/o/jejun/o/stomy
   CF   CF
creation of an artificial opening
between the stomach and the
jejunum

8. WR CV WR   S
chol/e/cyst/ectomy
    CF
excision of the gallbladder

9. WR   S
col/ectomy
excision of the colon

10. WR CV S
col/o/stomy
   CF
creation of an artificial opening into
the colon

11. WR CV S
pylor/o/plasty
    CF
surgical repair of the pylorus

12. WR CV S
an/o/plasty
  CF
surgical repair of the anus

13. WR   S
append/ectomy
excision of the appendix

14. WR CV   S
cheil/o/rrhaphy
    CF
suturing of the lip

15. WR   S
gingiv/ectomy
surgical removal of gum (tissue)

16. WR CV S
lapar/o/tomy
    CF
incision into the abdominal cavity

17. WR CV S
ile/o/stomy
   CF
creation of an artificial opening into
the ileum

18. WR CV S
gastr/o/stomy
   CF
creation of an artificial opening into
the stomach

19. WR CV S
herni/o/rrhaphy
   CF
suturing of a hernia

20. WR CV   S
gloss/o/rrhaphy
   CF
suturing of the tongue

21. WR CV WR CV S
choledoch/o/lith/o/tomy
     CF   CF
incision into the common bile duct
to remove a stone

22. P WR   S
hemi/col/ectomy
excision of half of the colon

23. WR   S
polyp/ectomy
excision of a polyp

24. WR CV   S
enter/o/rrhaphy
   CF
suturing of the intestine

25. WR CV S
abdomin/o/plasty
     CF
surgical repair of the abdomen

26. WR CV WR CV S
pylor/o/my/o/tomy
    CF   CF
incision into the pylorus muscle

27. WR CV WR CV WR CV S
uvul/o/palat/o/pharyng/o/plasty
    CF   CF   CF
surgical repair of the uvula, palate,
and pharynx

28. WR CV S
celi/o/tomy
   CF
incision into the abdominal cavity

29. WR CV S
gastr/o/plasty
   CF
surgical repair of the stomach

30. WR CV S
abdomin/o/centesis
     CF
surgical puncture to aspirate fluid
from the abdominal cavity

Exercise 19
1. append/ectomy
2. gloss/o/rrhaphy
3. esophag/o/gastr/o/plasty
4. diverticul/ectomy
5. ile/o/stomy
6. gingiv/ectomy
7. a. lapar/o/tomy
   b. celi/o/tomy
8. an/o/plasty
9. antr/ectomy
10. chol/e/cyst/ectomy
11. col/ectomy
12. col/o/stomy
13. gastr/ectomy
14. gastr/o/stomy
15. gastr/o/jejun/o/stomy
16. uvul/ectomy
17. palat/o/plasty
18. pylor/o/plasty
19. herni/o/rrhaphy
20. cheil/o/rrhaphy
21. hemi/col/ectomy
22. choledoch/o/lith/o/tomy
23. polyp/ectomy
24. enter/o/rrhaphy
25. abdomin/o/plasty
26. pylor/o/my/o/tomy
27. uvul/o/palat/o/pharyng/o/plasty
28. gastr/o/plasty
29. abdomin/o/centesis

Exercise 20
Spelling Exercise; see text p. 484.

Exercise 21
Pronunciation Exercise

Exercise 22
1. vagotomy
2. anastomosis
3. abdominoperineal resection
4. bariatric surgery
5. hemorrhoidectomy

Exercise 23
Spelling Exercise; see text p. 486

Exercise 24
Pronunciation Exercise

Exercise 25
*Note: The combining form is identified by
italic and bold print.*
1. WR CV S
esophag/o/scopy
    CF
visual examination of the esophagus

2. WR CV S
gastr/o/scope
      CF
instrument used for visual
examination of the stomach

3. WR CV S
gastr/o/scopy
      CF
visual examination of the stomach

4. WR CV S
proct/o/scope
      CF
instrument used for visual
examination of the rectum

5. WR CV S
proct/o/scopy
      CF
visual examination of the rectum

6. P   S(WR)
endo/scope
instrument used for visual
examination within (a hollow organ)

7. P   S(WR)
endo/scopy
visual examination within (a hollow
organ)

8. WR CV S
sigmoid/o/scopy
      CF
visual examination of the sigmoid
colon

9. WR CV S
cholangi/o/gram
      CF
radiographic image of bile ducts

10. WR CV WR CV   WR CV S
esophag/o/*gastr/o*/*duoden/o*/scopy
      CF   CF   CF
visual examination of the esophagus,
stomach, and duodenum

11. WR CV S
colon/o/scope
      CF
instrument used for visual
examination of the colon

12. WR CV S
lapar/o/scope
      CF
instrument used for visual
examination of the abdominal cavity

13. WR CV S
colon/o/scopy
      CF
visual examination of the colon

14. WR CV S
lapar/o/scopy
      CF
visual examination of the abdominal
cavity

15. WR CV   S
CT *colon/o*/graphy
      CF
radiographic imaging of the colon

16. WR CV S
esophag/o/gram
      CF
radiographic image of the esophagus

17. WR CV S
cholangi/o/graphy
      CF
radiographic imaging of the bile
ducts

Exercise 26
1. endo/scopy
2. gastr/o/scope
3. proct/o/scope
4. endo/scope
5. proct/o/scopy
6. esophag/o/scopy
7. sigmoid/o/scopy
8. cholangi/o/gram
9. gastr/o/scopy
10. lapar/o/scope
11. esophag/o/gastr/o/duoden/o/scopy
12. colon/o/scopy
13. lapar/o/scopy
14. colon/o/scope
15. CT colon/o/graphy
16. cholangi/o/graphy
17. esophag/o/gram

Exercise 27
Spelling Exercise; see text p. 491.

Exercise 28
Pronunciation Exercise

Exercise 29
1. series of radiographic images taken
of the pharynx, esophagus, stomach,
and duodenum after the contrast
agent barium has been administered
orally
2. series of radiographic images taken
of the large intestine after the
contrast agent barium has been
administered rectally
3. endoscopic procedure involving
radiographic imaging of the biliary
ducts and pancreatic ducts

4. an endoscope fitted with an
ultrasound probe providing images
of layers of the intestinal wall
5. a blood test to determine the
presence of Helicobacter pylori
bacteria, a cause of peptic ulcers
6. a test to detect fecal occult blood
7. ultrasound test of the abdominal
cavity

Exercise 30
1. d
2. f
3. a
4. b
5. h
6. g
7. c

Exercise 31
Spelling Exercise; see text p. 494.

Exercise 32
Pronunciation Exercise

Exercise 33
*Note: The combining form is identified by
italic and bold print.*

1. P   S(WR)
a/phagia
without swallowing (inability to)

2. P   S(WR)
dys/pepsia
difficult digestion

3. WR S
an/al
pertaining to the anus

4. P   S(WR)
dys/phagia
difficult swallowing

5. WR CV   S
hepat/o/megaly
      CF
enlargement of the liver

6. WR CV WR S
ile/o/cec/al
      CF
pertaining to the ileum and cecum

7. WR S
or/al
pertaining to the mouth

8. WR CV WR   S
stomat/o/gastr/ic
      CF
pertaining to the mouth and
stomach

9. WR CV S
gastr/o/malacia
CF
softening of the stomach

10. WR S
pancreat/ic
pertaining to the pancreas

11. WR S
peritone/al
pertaining to the peritoneum

12. WR S
steat/osis
abnormal condition of fat

13. P WR S
sub/lingu/al
pertaining to under the tongue

14. WR CV S
proct/o/logy
CF
study of the rectum

15. WR CV WR S
nas/o/gastr/ic
CF
pertaining to the nose and stomach

16. WR S
abdomin/al
pertaining to the abdomen

17. WR CV S
proct/o/logist
CF
physician who studies and treats
diseases of the rectum

18. WR CV WR CV S
gastr/o/*enter/o*/logy
CF CF
study of the stomach and intestines

19. WR CV WR CV S
gastr/o/*enter/o*/logist
CF CF
physician who studies and treats
diseases of the stomach and
intestines

20. WR CV WR S
col/o/rect/al
CF
pertaining to the colon and rectum

21. WR S
rect/al
pertaining to the rectum

22. WR CV S
steat/o/rrhea
CF
discharge of fat

23. WR S
stomat/itis
inflammation of the mouth (mucous
membrane)

24. WR CV S
enter/o/pathy
CF
disease of the intestine

25. WR S
gastr/ic
pertaining to the stomach

26. WR S
duoden/al
pertaining to the duodenum

27. WR S
esophag/eal
pertaining to the esophagus

28. celi/ac
pertaining to the abdomen

Exercise 34

1. hepat/o/megaly
2. a/phagia
3. sub/lingu/al
4. nas/o/gastr/ic
5. stomat/o/gastr/ic
6. an/al
7. peritone/al
8. abdomin/al, celi/ac
9. dys/phagia
10. ile/o/cec/al
11. gastr/o/malacia
12. proct/o/logist
13. dys/pepsia
14. pancreat/ic
15. proct/o/logy
16. steat/o/rrhea
17. or/al
18. gastr/o/enter/o/logist
19. gastr/o/enter/o/logy
20. col/o/rect/al
21. rect/al
22. steat/osis
23. esophag/eal
24. gastr/ic
25. duoden/al
26. enter/o/pathy
27. stomat/itis

Exercise 35

Spelling Exercise; see text p. 498.

Exercise 36

Pronunciation Exercise

Exercise 37

1. m	10. h
2. e	11. b
3. f	12. j
4. c	13. g
5. l	14. o
6. i	15. q
7. k	16. n
8. a	17. p
9. d	

Exercise 38

1. abnormal collection of fluid in the
peritoneal cavity
2. process of feeding a person through
a nasogastric tube
3. washing out of the stomach
4. waste from the digestive tract
expelled through the rectum
5. urge to vomit
6. expelling matter from the stomach
through the mouth
7. disorder that involves inflammation
of the intestine
8. frequent discharge of liquid stool
9. gas expelled through the anus
10. abnormal backward flow
11. vomiting of blood
12. involuntary wavelike contractions
that propel food along the digestive
tract
13. black, tarry stools that contain
digested blood
14. surgical opening between an organ
and the surface of the body
15. passage of bloody feces
16. expelling matter from the stomach
through the mouth
17. impaired digestion or intestinal
absorption
18. to examine by hand

Exercise 39

Spelling Exercise; see text p. 501.

Exercise 40

1. endoscopic retrograde
cholangiopancreatography
2. endoscopic ultrasound
3. nausea and vomiting
4. irritable bowel syndrome
5. percutaneous endoscopic
gastrostomy
6. upper gastrointestinal
7. uvulopalatopharyngoplasty
8. gastroesophageal reflux disease
9. gastrointestinal
10. *Helicobacter pylori*
11. barium enema
12. esophagogastroduodenoscopy
13. abdominoperineal resection
14. fecal occult blood test

Exercise 41

A. 1. endoscopy
2. nausea
3. dyspepsia
4. hematemesis
5. melena
6. esophagogastroduodenoscopy
7. gastroscope
8. reflux

9. *H. pylori*
10. ulcers
11. gastritis
12. duodenal

B.
1. d
2. b
3. a
4. d

C.
1. a
2. d
3. d

D. Online Exercise

Exercise 42

1. cholelithiasis
2. cholecystectomy

3. anastomoses
4. ulcerative colitis
5. proctoptosis
6. adhesion
7. peptic ulcers
8. upper GI series, esophagogastroduodenoscopy
9. gastrectomy, pyloroplasty, vagotomy
10. dyspepsia
11. gavage
12. abdominoperineal resection and colostomy
13. colonoscopy
14. ileus
15. fecal occult blood test
16. stomata

Exercise 43

Reading Exercise

Exercise 44

1. c
2. *T*
3. *T*
4. *F*, vomiting blood is not a warning sign of colorectal cancer.

Outline

Objectives

Upon completion of this chapter you will be able to:

1   Identify organs and structures of the eye.

2   Define and spell word parts related to the eye.

3   Define, pronounce, and spell disease and disorder terms related to the eye.

4   Define, pronounce, and spell surgical terms related to the eye.

5   Define, pronounce, and spell diagnostic terms related to the eye.

6   Define, pronounce, and spell complementary terms related to the eye.

7   Interpret the meaning of abbreviations related to the eye.

8   Interpret, read, and comprehend medical language in simulated medical statements, documents, and electronic health records.

ANATOMY

Function

The eyes are organs of vision and are located in a bony protective cavity of the skull called the orbit. Only a small portion of the eye is visible from the exterior (Figures 12-1 and 12-2).

Structures of the Eye

TERM	DEFINITION
sclera	outer protective layer of the eye; the portion seen on the anterior portion of the eyeball is referred to as the **white of the eye**
cornea	transparent anterior part of the sclera, which is anterior to the aqueous humor and lies over the iris. It allows the light rays to enter the eye.
choroid	middle layer of the eye, which is interlaced with many blood vessels that supply nutrients to the eye
iris	pigmented muscular structure that regulates the amount of light entering the eye by controlling the size of the pupil
pupil	opening in the center of the iris
lens	lies directly behind the pupil; its function is to focus and bend light
retina	innermost layer of the eye, which contains the vision receptors (Figure 12-3)
aqueous humor	watery liquid found in the anterior cavity of the eye. It provides nourishment to nearby structures and maintains shape in the anterior part of the eye.
vitreous humor	jellylike substance found behind the lens in the posterior cavity of the eye that maintains its shape
meibomian glands	oil glands found in the upper and lower edges of the eyelids that help lubricate the eye
lacrimal glands and ducts	produce and drain tears
optic nerve	carries visual impulses from the retina to the brain
conjunctiva	mucous membrane lining the eyelids and covering the anterior portion of the sclera

🏛 **IRIS**

was the special messenger of the Queen of Heaven according to Greek mythology. In this role she passed from heaven to earth over the rainbow while dressed in rainbow hues. Her name was applied to the **circular eye muscle** because of its varied colors.

A & P Booster

For more anatomy and physiology, go to evolve.elsevier.com.

Select: **Extra Contents**, A & P Booster, Chapter 12.

Refer to p. 10 for your Evolve Access Information.

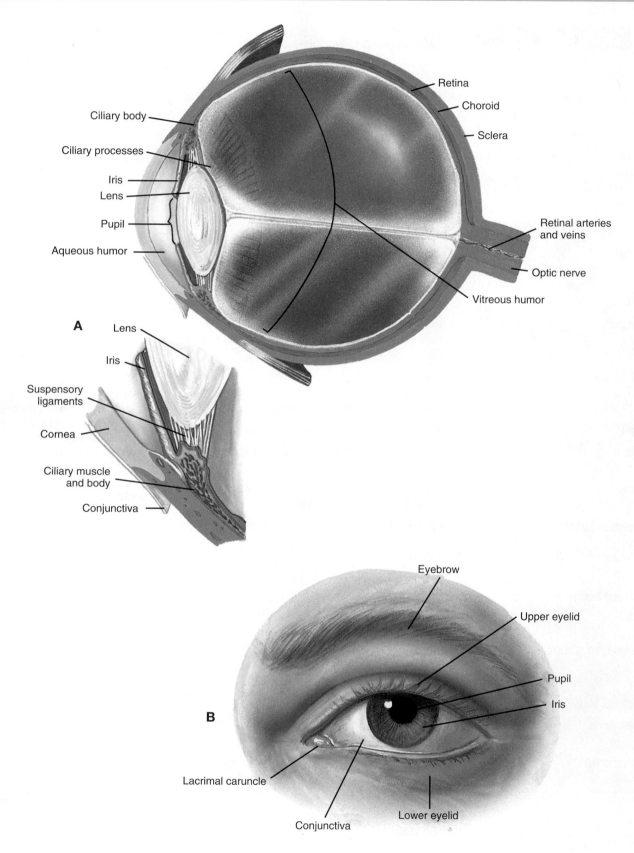

FIGURE 12-1
A, Anatomy of the eye. **B,** Visible surface of the eye.

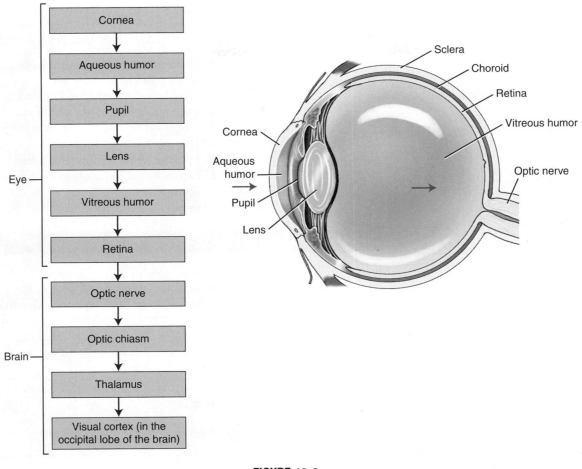

FIGURE 12-2
Pathway of light.

To watch animations, go to evolve.elsevier.com. Select:
Chapter 12, **Animations**, Anatomy of the Eye.

Refer to p. 10 for your Evolve Access Information.

EXERCISE 1

Match the anatomic terms in the first column with the correct definitions in the second column. *To check your answers to the exercises in this chapter, go to Answers, p. 551, at the end of the chapter.*

_____ 1. aqueous humor
_____ 2. choroid
_____ 3. conjunctiva
_____ 4. cornea
_____ 5. iris
_____ 6. lacrimal glands
_____ 7. lens

a. lies directly behind the pupil
b. pigmented muscular structure
c. middle layer of the eye
d. watery liquid found in the anterior cavity of the eye
e. produce tears
f. mucous membrane lining the eyelids
g. jellylike substance behind the lens in the posterior cavity
h. transparent anterior part of the sclera

EXERCISE 2

Match the anatomic terms in the first column with the correct definitions in the second column.

_____ 1. meibomian glands
_____ 2. optic nerve
_____ 3. pupil
_____ 4. retina
_____ 5. sclera
_____ 6. vitreous humor

a. outer protective layer of the eye
b. innermost layer of the eye
c. jellylike substance found behind the lens in the posterior cavity of the eye
d. oil glands in eyelids that help lubricate the eye
e. opening in the center of the iris
f. carries visual impulses from the retina to the brain
g. middle layer of the eye

WORD PARTS

Combining Forms of the Eye

Word parts you need to learn to complete this chapter are listed on the following pages. The exercises at the end of each list will help you learn their definitions and spellings.

> Use the flashcards accompanying this text or electronic flashcards to assist you in memorizing the word parts for this chapter.

> e To use electronic flashcards, go to evolve.elsevier.com.
> Select: Chapter 12, **Flashcards.**
>
> Refer to p. 10 for your Evolve Access Information.

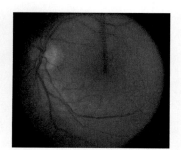

FIGURE 12-3
Ophthalmoscopic view of the retina.

COMBINING FORM	DEFINITION
blephar/o	eyelid
conjunctiv/o	conjunctiva
cor/o, core/o, pupill/o (NOTE: pupil has one l; the combining form has two l's)	pupil
corne/o, kerat/o (NOTE: kerat/o also means hard or horny tissue; see Chapter 4)	cornea
dacry/o, lacrim/o	tear, tear duct
ir/o, irid/o	iris
ocul/o, ophthalm/o	eye
opt/o	vision
phac/o, phak/o	lens
retin/o	retina (Figure 12-3)
scler/o	sclera

> ☀ **SPELLING** *ophthalm*
> Look closely at the spelling of the word root **ophthalm.** Medical terms containing **ophthalm** are often misspelled by omitting the first h; **ph** gives the **f** sound followed by the sound of **thal.** Think pronunciation when spelling terms that contain **ophthalm,** as in ophthalmology (of[ph]-thal-MOL-o-jē).

EXERCISE 3

Write the definitions of the following combining forms.

1. ocul/o_____
2. blephar/o_____
3. corne/o_____
4. lacrim/o_____
5. retin/o_____
6. pupill/o_____
7. scler/o_____
8. irid/o_____
9. conjunctiv/o_____

10. cor/o_____
11. ophthalm/o_____
12. kerat/o_____
13. ir/o_____
14. core/o_____
15. opt/o_____
16. dacry/o_____
17. phac/o, phak/o_____

EXERCISE FIGURE A

Diagrams of the eye. Fill in the blanks with combining forms. *To check your answers, go to p. 551.*

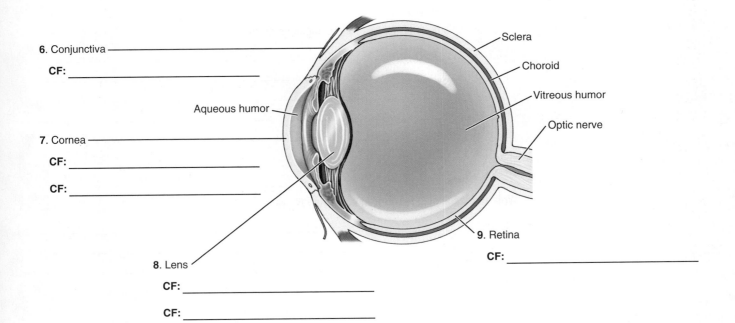

1. Eye

   CF:_____

   CF:_____

2. Eyelid

   CF:_____

3. Pupil

   CF:_____

   CF:_____

   CF:_____

4. Sclera

   CF:_____

5. Iris

   CF:_____

   CF:_____

Lacrimal sac

Sclera

Choroid

Vitreous humor

Aqueous humor

Optic nerve

6. Conjunctiva

   CF:_____

7. Cornea

   CF:_____

   CF:_____

8. Lens

   CF:_____

   CF:_____

9. Retina

   CF:_____

EXERCISE 4

Write the combining form for each of the following terms.

1. eye
   a. _____
   b. _____

2. cornea
   a. _____
   b. _____

3. conjunctiva _____

4. tear, tear duct
   a. _____
   b. _____

5. eyelid _____

6. pupil
   a. _____
   b. _____
   c. _____

7. sclera _____

8. retina _____

9. iris
   a. _____
   b. _____

10. vision _____

11. lens
    a. _____
    b. _____

Combining Forms Commonly Used with the Eye

COMBINING FORM	DEFINITION
cry/o	cold
dipl/o	two, double
is/o	equal
phot/o	light
ton/o	tension, pressure

EXERCISE 5

Write the definitions of the following combining forms.

1. ton/o _____
2. phot/o _____
3. cry/o _____
4. dipl/o _____
5. is/o _____

EXERCISE 6

Write the combining form for each of the following.

1. cold _____
2. tension, pressure _____
3. two, double _____
4. light _____
5. equal _____

Prefixes and Suffixes

PREFIXES	DEFINITION
bi-, bin-	two
SUFFIXES	**DEFINITIONS**
-opia	vision (condition)
-phobia	abnormal fear of or aversion to specific things
-plegia	paralysis

Refer to **Appendix A** and **Appendix B** for a complete listing of word parts.

EXERCISE 7

Write the definition of the following prefixes and suffixes.

1. -opia _____

2. bi- _____

3. -plegia _____

4. -phobia _____

5. bin- _____

EXERCISE 8

Write the prefixes or suffixes for each of the following definitions.

1. paralysis _____

2. two   a. _____

         b. _____

3. abnormal fear of or aversion to specific things _____

4. vision (condition) _____

For review and/or assessment, go to evolve.elsevier.com. Select:
Chapter 12, **Activities**, Word Parts
Chapter 12, **Games**, Name that Word Part

Refer to p. 10 for your Evolve Access Information.

Fill in the blanks to label the diagram.

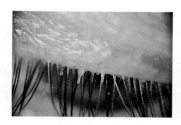

_____ / _____
eyelid / inflammation
with thickened lids and crusts
around the lashes.

Fill in the blanks to label the diagram.

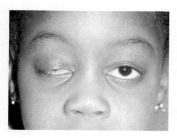

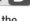

_____ / __ / _____
eyelid / cv / drooping

Fill in the blanks to label the diagram.

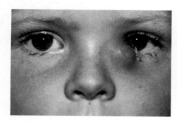

____ / __ / ___ / _____
tear / cv / sac / inflammation

💬 MEDICAL TERMS

The terms you need to learn to complete this chapter are listed on the following pages. The exercises following each list will help you learn the definition and the spelling of each word.

Disease and Disorder Terms
Built from Word Parts

The following terms are built from word parts you have already learned and can be translated literally to find their meanings. Further explanation of terms beyond the definition of their word parts, if needed, is included in parentheses.

TERM	DEFINITION
aphakia (a-FĀ-kē-a)	condition of without a lens (may be congenital, though often is the result of extraction of a cataract without the placement of an intraocular lens)
blepharitis (*blef*-a-RĪ-tis)	inflammation of the eyelid (Exercise Figure B)
blepharoptosis (*blef*-ar-op-TŌ-sis)	drooping of the eyelid (Exercise Figure C) (commonly called **ptosis**)
conjunctivitis (kon-*junk*-ti-VĪ-tis)	inflammation of the conjunctiva (commonly called **pinkeye**)
dacryocystitis (*dak*-rē-ō-sis-TĪ-tis)	inflammation of the tear (lacrimal) sac (Exercise Figure D)
diplopia (di-PLŌ-pē-a)	double vision
endophthalmitis (*en*-dof-thal-MĪ-tis) (*NOTE: the* o *in endo is dropped*)	inflammation within the eye
iridoplegia (*īr*-i-dō-PLĒ-ja)	paralysis of the iris
iritis (*ī*-RĪ-tis)	inflammation of the iris
keratitis (*ker*-a-TĪ-tis)	inflammation of the cornea
keratomalacia (*ker*-a-tō-ma-LĀ-sha)	softening of the cornea (usually a bilateral condition associated with vitamin A deficiency)
leukocoria (*lū*-kō-KŌ-rē-a)	condition of white pupil
oculomycosis (*ok*-ū-lō-mī-KŌ-sis)	abnormal condition of the eye caused by a fungus
ophthalmalgia (*of*-*thal*-MAL-ja)	pain in the eye
ophthalmoplegia (of-thal-mō-PLĒ-ja)	paralysis of the eye (muscle)

TERM	DEFINITION
phacomalacia (făk-ō-ma-LĀ-sha)	softening of the lens
photophobia (fŏ-tō-FŌ-bē-a)	abnormal fear of (sensitivity to) light
retinoblastoma (ret-i-nō-blas-TŌ-ma)	tumor arising from a developing retinal cell (a congenital, malignant tumor)
retinopathy (ret-i-NOP-a-thē)	(any noninflammatory) disease of the retina (such as **diabetic retinopathy**)
sclerokeratitis (sklēr-ō-ker-a-TĪ-tis)	inflammation of the sclera and the cornea
scleromalacia (sklēr-ō-ma-LĀ-sha)	softening of the sclera
xerophthalmia (zēr-of-THAL-mē-a)	condition of dry eye (conjunctiva and cornea)

EXERCISE 9

Practice saying aloud each of the disease and disorder terms built from word parts.

> To hear the terms, go to evolve.elsevier.com. Select: Chapter 12, **Exercises**, Pronunciation.
>
> Refer to p. 10 for your Evolve Access Information.

☐ Place a check mark in the box when you have completed this exercise.

EXERCISE 10

Analyze and define the following terms.

1. sclerokeratitis _____
2. ophthalmalgia _____
3. blepharoptosis _____
4. diplopia _____
5. conjunctivitis _____
6. leukocoria _____
7. iridoplegia _____
8. scleromalacia _____
9. photophobia _____
10. blepharitis _____
11. oculomycosis _____
12. dacryocystitis _____
13. endophthalmitis _____

14. iritis _____

15. retinoblastoma _____

16. keratitis _____

17. ophthalmoplegia _____

18. retinopathy _____

19. xerophthalmia _____

20. keratomalacia _____

21. phacomalacia _____

22. aphakia _____

EXERCISE 11

Build disease and disorder terms for the following definitions by using the word parts you have learned.

1. inflammation of the conjunctiva

_____ / _____
WR   /   S

2. abnormal eye condition caused by a fungus

_____ / __ / _____ / ____
WR   /CV/   WR   /   S

3. pain in the eye

_____ / _____
WR   /   S

4. double vision

_____ / _____
WR   /   S

5. inflammation of the eyelid

_____ / _____
WR   /   S

6. condition of white pupil

_____ / __ / _____ / ____
WR   /CV/   WR   /   S

7. paralysis of the iris

_____ / __ / _____
WR   /CV/   S

8. drooping of the eyelid

_____ / __ / _____
WR   /CV/   S

9. inflammation of the iris

_____ / _____
WR   /   S

10. tumor arising from a developing retinal cell

_____ / __ / _____ / ____
WR   /CV/   WR   /   S

11. softening of the sclera

_____ / __ / _____
WR   /CV/   S

12. inflammation of a tear (lacrimal) sac

_____ / __ / _____ / ____
WR   /CV/   WR   /   S

13. inflammation of the sclera and cornea

_____ / __ / _____ / ____
WR   /CV/   WR   /   S

14. abnormal fear of
    (sensitivity to) light

    _____
    WR   /CV/   S

15. inflammation of the cornea

    _____
    WR   /   S

16. disease of the retina

    _____
    WR   /CV/   S

17. inflammation within the eye

    _____
    P   / WR   /   S

18. paralysis of the eye (muscle)

    _____
    WR   /CV/   S

19. condition of dry eye

    _____
    WR   / WR   /   S

20. softening of the cornea

    _____
    WR   /CV/   S

21. condition of without a lens

    _____
    P   / WR   /   S

22. softening of the lens

    _____
    WR   /CV/   S

EXERCISE 12

Spell each of the disease and disorder terms built from word parts on pp. 524–525 by having someone dictate them to you.

> To hear and spell the terms, go to evolve.elsevier.com. Select: Chapter 12, **Exercises**, Spelling.
>
> Refer to p. 10 for your Evolve Access Information.

☐ Place a check mark in the box if you have completed this exercise online.

1. _____
2. _____
3. _____
4. _____
5. _____
6. _____
7. _____
8. _____
9. _____
10. _____
11. _____
12. _____
13. _____
14. _____
15. _____
16. _____
17. _____
18. _____
19. _____
20. _____
21. _____
22. _____

Disease and Disorder Terms

Not Built from Word Parts

In some of the following terms, you may recognize word parts you have already learned; however, the full meaning of the terms cannot be discerned by the definition of their word parts.

TERM	DEFINITION
amblyopia (*am*-blē-Ō-pē-a)	reduced vision in one eye caused by disuse or misuse associated with strabismus, unequal refractive errors, or otherwise impaired vision. The brain suppresses images from the impaired eye to avoid double vision (also called **lazy eye**).
astigmatism (Ast) (a-STIG-ma-tizm)	blurred vision caused by irregular curvature of the cornea or lens. Light refracts improperly, resulting in diffused, rather than points of light focusing on the retina. (Figure 12-4, *C*)
cataract (KAT-a-rakt)	clouding of the lens of the eye (Figure 12-5)
chalazion (ka-LĂ-zē-on)	obstruction of an oil gland of the eyelid (also called **meibomian cyst**) (Figure 12-6)
detached retina (RET-in-a)	separation of the retina from the choroid in back of the eye (Figure 12-7)
glaucoma (glaw-KŎ-ma)	eye disorder characterized by increase of intraocular pressure (IOP). If left untreated may progress to optic nerve damage and visual impairment or loss.

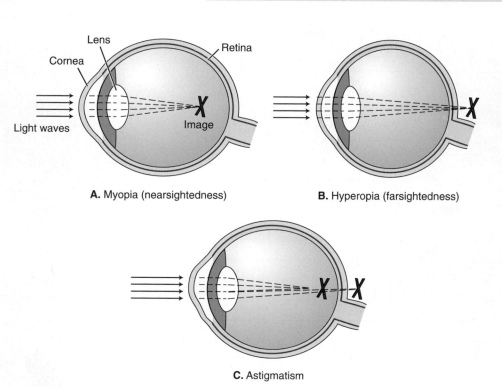

A. Myopia (nearsightedness) **B.** Hyperopia (farsightedness)

C. Astigmatism

FIGURE 12-4

Refraction errors. **A,** Myopia, nearsightedness. **B,** Hyperopia, farsightedness. **C,** Astigmatism.

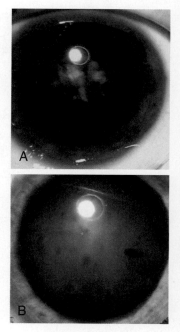

FIGURE 12-5
A, Snowflake cataract.
B, Senile cataract.

TERM	DEFINITION
hyperopia (*hī*-per-Ō-pē-a)	farsightedness (see Figure 12-4, *B*)
macular degeneration (MAC-ū-lar) (dē-*gen*-e-RĀ-shun)	progressive deterioration of the portion of the retina called the **macula lutea**, resulting in loss of central vision (Figure 12-8)
myopia (mī-Ō-pē-a)	nearsightedness (see Figure 12-4, *A*)
nyctalopia (*nik*-ta-LŌ-pē-a)	poor vision at night or in faint light (also called **night blindness**)
nystagmus (nis-TAG-mus)	involuntary, jerking movements of the eyes
pinguecula (ping-GWEH-kū-la)	yellowish mass on the conjunctiva that may be related to exposure to ultraviolet light, dry climates, and dust. A pinguecula that spreads onto the cornea becomes a **pterygium**.
presbyopia (*pres*-bē-Ō-pē-a)	impaired vision as a result of aging

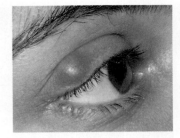

FIGURE 12-6
Chalazion (right upper eyelid).

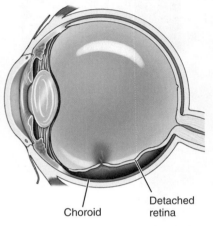

Choroid   Detached retina

FIGURE 12-7
Detached retina. Vitreous fluid has seeped through a tear in the retina, causing the choroid coat and retina to separate.

AGE-RELATED MACULAR DEGENERATION (ARMD)

is the leading cause of legal blindness in persons older than 65 years. Onset occurs between the ages of 50 and 60 (see Figure 12-8).

🍃 CAM TERM

Vitamin therapy is the use of nutrition, through diet and supplements, to promote optimal health and as preventive support, reduce the incidence and progression of disease and symptoms. Current research is yielding suggestive evidence that dietary supplementation may serve to prevent or delay the onset of age-related **macular degeneration**.

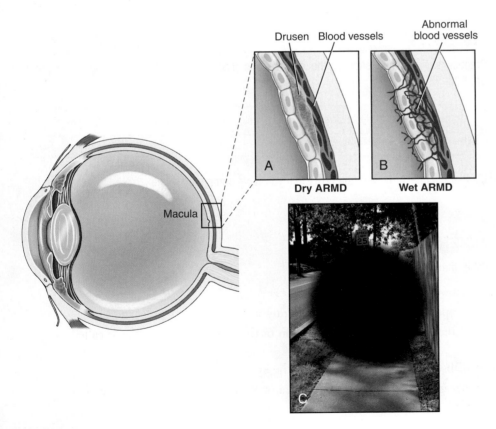

Drusen Blood vessels   Abnormal blood vessels

A **Dry ARMD**   B **Wet ARMD**

Macula

C

FIGURE 12-8
Macular degeneration (AMD or ARMD). **A, Dry macular degeneration,** where blood vessels under the macula become brittle and yellow deposits called drusen form, is the most common form of age-related macular degeneration (ARMD). **B, Wet macular degeneration,** where new abnormal blood vessels form under the macula, is less common though more likely to cause legal blindness. **C, Central vision loss** as may be experienced in ARMD.

Disease and Disorder Terms—cont'd

Not Built from Word Parts

TERM	DEFINITION
pterygium (te-RIJ-ē-um)	thin tissue growing into the cornea from the conjunctiva, usually caused from sun exposure
retinitis pigmentosa (*ret*-i-NĪ-tis) (*pig*-men-TŌ-sa)	hereditary, progressive disease marked by night blindness with atrophy and retinal pigment changes
strabismus (stra-BIZ-mus)	condition in which the eyes look in different directions; caused by dysfunction of the external eye muscles (called **cross-eyed** when one eye turns in)
sty (stī)	infection of an oil gland of the eyelid (Figure 12-9) (also spelled **stye** and also called **hordeolum**)

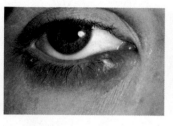

FIGURE 12-9
Sty, stye, or hordeolum.

To watch animations, go to evolve.elsevier.com. Select:
Chapter 12, **Animations**, Retinal Detachment.

Refer to p. 10 for your Evolve Access Information.

EXERCISE 13

Practice saying aloud each of the disease and disorder terms not built from word parts on pp. 528–530.

To hear the terms, go to evolve.elsevier.com. Select: Chapter 12, **Exercises**, Pronunciation.

Refer to p. 10 for your Evolve Access Information.

☐ Place a check mark in the box when you have completed this exercise.

EXERCISE 14

Fill in the blanks with the correct terms.

1. Another name for nearsightedness is _____.
2. Impaired vision as a result of aging is _____.
3. Condition caused by dysfunction of the external eye muscles is called _____.
4. Obstruction of an oil gland of the eyelid is called a(n) _____.
5. Irregular curvature of the cornea or lens causes a condition known as _____.

6. _____ is the name given to involuntary, jerking movements of the eye.

7. Clouding of the lens of the eye is called a(n) _____.

8. _____ is the name given to an infection of an oil gland of the eyelids.

9. Eye disorder characterized by the increase of intraocular pressure is _____.

10. A(n) _____ is a separation of the retina from the choroid in the back of the eye.

11. Another name for farsightedness is _____.

12. _____ is a hereditary, progressive disease causing night blindness with retinal pigment changes and atrophy.

13. Another name for night blindness is _____.

14. Thin tissue growing into the cornea from the conjunctiva is called a(n) _____.

15. _____ is the progressive deterioration of the macula lutea.

16. Another name for lazy eye is _____.

17. _____ may be related to exposure to ultraviolet light, dry climates, and dust and may spread onto the cornea to become a pterygium.

🏛 **CATARACT**
is derived from the Greek **kato,** meaning **down,** and **raktos,** meaning **precipice.** Together, the words were interpreted as **waterfall.** The cataract sufferer sees things as through a watery veil of mist, or waterfall.

🏛 **GLAUCOMA**
is composed of the Greek **glaukos,** meaning **blue-gray** or **sea green,** and **oma,** meaning a morbid condition. The term was given to any condition in which gray or green replaced the black in the pupil.

EXERCISE 15

Match the terms in the first column with the correct definitions in the second column.

_____ 1. astigmatism
_____ 2. cataract
_____ 3. chalazion
_____ 4. detached retina
_____ 5. glaucoma
_____ 6. myopia
_____ 7. nystagmus
_____ 8. hyperopia
_____ 9. presbyopia
_____ 10. strabismus
_____ 11. sty
_____ 12. pterygium
_____ 13. retinitis pigmentosa
_____ 14. nyctalopia
_____ 15. macular degeneration
_____ 16. pinguecula
_____ 17. amblyopia

a. infection of an oil gland of the eyelid
b. deterioration of the macula lutea
c. cross-eyed when one eye turns in
d. involuntary, jerking movements of the eye
e. impaired vision caused by aging
f. irregular curvature of the lens or cornea of the eye
g. clouding of a lens of the eye
h. hereditary, progressive disease marked by night blindness
i. nearsightedness
j. obstruction of an oil gland of the eye
k. usually caused from sun exposure
l. eye disorder characterized by optic nerve damage
m. separation of the retina from the choroid in the back of the eye
n. poor vision at night or in faint light
o. farsightedness
p. double vision
q. yellow mass on the conjunctiva
r. reduced vision in one eye caused by disuse or misuse

EXERCISE 16

Spell each of the disease and disorder terms not built from word parts on pp. 528–530 by having someone dictate them to you.

> To hear and spell the terms, go to evolve.elsevier.com. Select: Chapter 12, **Exercises**, Spelling.
>
> Refer to p. 10 for your Evolve Access Information.
>
> ☐ Place a check mark in the box if you have completed this exercise online.

1. _____
2. _____
3. _____
4. _____
5. _____
6. _____
7. _____
8. _____
9. _____
10. _____
11. _____
12. _____
13. _____
14. _____
15. _____
16. _____
17. _____

Surgical Terms

Built from Word Parts

The following terms are built from word parts you have already learned and can be translated literally to find their meanings. Further explanation of terms beyond the definition of their word parts, if needed, is included in parentheses.

TERM	DEFINITION
blepharoplasty (BLEF-a-rō-*plas*-tē)	surgical repair of the eyelid
cryoretinopexy (*krī*-ō-RE-tin-ō-*pek*-sē)	surgical fixation of the retina by using extreme cold (carbon dioxide)
dacryocystorhinostomy (*dak*-rē-ō-*sis*-tō-rī-NOS-to-mē)	creation of an artificial opening between the tear (lacrimal) sac and the nose (to restore drainage into the nose when the nasolacrimal duct is obstructed or obliterated)
dacryocystotomy (*dak*-rē-ō-sis-TOT-o-mē)	incision of the tear (lacrimal) sac
iridectomy (*ir*-i-DEK-to-mē)	excision (of part) of the iris
iridotomy (*ir*-i-DOT-o-mē)	incision of the iris
keratoplasty (KER-a-tō-*plas*-tē)	surgical repair of the cornea (corneal transplant) (Figure 12-10)
sclerotomy (skle-ROT-o-mē)	incision of the sclera

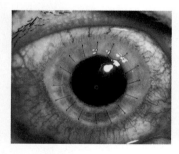

FIGURE 12-10
Appearance of eye after keratoplasty.

EXERCISE 17

Practice saying aloud each of the surgical terms built from word parts.

> To hear the terms, go to evolve.elsevier.com. Select: Chapter 12, **Exercises**, Pronunciation.
>
> Refer to p. 10 for your Evolve Access Information.

☐ Place a check mark in the box when you have completed this exercise.

EXERCISE 18

Analyze and define the following surgical terms.

1. keratoplasty _____
2. sclerotomy _____
3. dacryocystotomy _____
4. cryoretinopexy _____
5. blepharoplasty _____
6. iridectomy _____
7. dacryocystorhinostomy _____
8. iridotomy _____

EXERCISE 19

Build surgical terms for the following definitions by using the word parts you have learned.

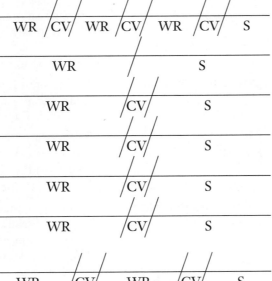

1. creation of an artificial opening between the tear (lacrimal) sac and the nose

   WR /CV/ WR /CV/ WR /CV/ S

2. excision of the iris

   WR / S

3. surgical repair of the cornea

   WR /CV/ S

4. incision of the sclera

   WR /CV/ S

5. incision of the iris

   WR /CV/ S

6. surgical repair of the eyelid

   WR /CV/ S

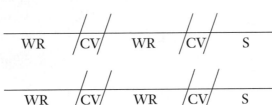

7. surgical fixation of the retina using extreme cold

   WR /CV/ WR /CV/ S

8. incision of the (lacrimal) tear sac

   WR /CV/ WR /CV/ S

EXERCISE 20

Spell each of the surgical terms built from word parts on p. 532 by having someone dictate them to you.

> To hear and spell the terms, go to evolve.elsevier.com. Select: Chapter 12, **Exercises**, Spelling.
>
> (e) Refer to p. 10 for your Evolve Access Information.
>
> ☐ Place a check mark in the box if you have completed this exercise online.

1. _____   5. _____

2. _____   6. _____

3. _____   7. _____

4. _____   8. _____

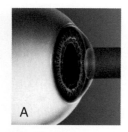

Flap of cornea

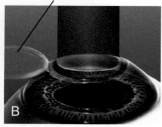

FIGURE 12-11
Excimer laser treatments for near-sightedness. **A, PRK** (photorefractive keratectomy): removes tissue from the surface of the cornea. **B, LASIK** (laser-assisted in situ keratomileusis): reshapes corneal tissue below the surface of the cornea. The Excimer laser was invented in the early 1980s. It is a computer-controlled ultraviolet beam of light that reshapes the cornea. It has replaced **RK** (radial keratotomy), a surgery in which spokelike incisions are made to reshape the cornea.

Surgical Terms

Not Built from Word Parts

In some of the following terms, you may recognize word parts you have already learned; however, the full meaning of the terms cannot be discerned by the definition of their word parts.

TERM	DEFINITION
enucleation (ē-*nū*-klē-Ā-shun)	surgical removal of the eyeball (also, the removal of any organ that comes out clean and whole)
LASIK (laser-assisted in situ keratomileusis) (LĀ-sik) (*ker*-a-tō-mi-LOO-sis)	laser procedure that reshapes the corneal tissue beneath the surface of the cornea to correct astigmatism, hyperopia, and myopia. LASIK is a combination of Excimer laser and lamellar keratoplasty. It differs from PRK in that it reshapes corneal tissue beneath the surface rather than on the surface (Figure 12-11, *B*).
phacoemulsification (PHACO) (*fa*-kō-ē-*mul*-si-fi-KĀ-shun)	method to remove cataracts in which an ultrasonic needle probe breaks up the lens, which is then aspirated
PRK (photorefractive keratectomy) (fŏ-tō-rē-FRAK-tiv) (*ker*-a-TEK-to-mē)	procedure for the treatment of nearsightedness in which an Excimer laser is used to reshape (flatten) the corneal surface by removing a portion of the cornea (Figure 12-11, *A*)
retinal photocoagulation (RET-in-al) (fŏ-tō-kō-*ag*-ū-LĀ-shun)	intense beam of light from a laser condenses retinal tissue to seal leaking blood vessels, to destroy abnormal tissue or lesions, or to bond the retina to the back of the eye. Used to treat retinal tears and detachment, diabetic retinopathy, wet macular degeneration, glaucoma, and intraocular tumors.

TERM	DEFINITION
scleral buckling (SKLER-al) (BUK-ling)	procedure to repair a detached retina. A strip of sclera is resected, or a fold is made in the sclera. An exoplant is used to hold and buckle the sclera (Figure 12-12).
trabeculectomy (tra-*bek*-ū-LEK-to-mē)	surgical creation of an opening that allows aqueous humor to drain out of the eye to underneath the conjunctiva where it is absorbed; used to treat glaucoma by reducing intraocular pressure. (Laser trabeculoplasty may also be used.)
vitrectomy (vi-TREK-to-mē)	surgical removal of all or part of the vitreous humor (used to treat diabetic retinopathy)

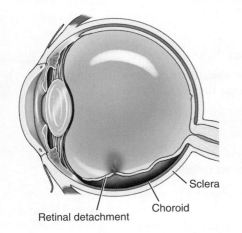 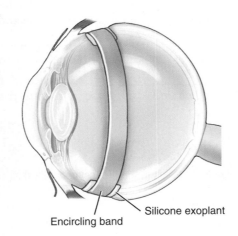

Sclera

Choroid

Retinal detachment

Silicone exoplant

Encircling band

FIGURE 12-12
Scleral buckling. A surgical procedure to repair a detached retina.

To watch animations, go to evolve.elsevier.com. Select:
Chapter 12, **Animations,** LASIK.

Refer to p. 10 for your Evolve Access Information.

EXERCISE 21

Practice saying aloud each of the surgical terms not built from word parts.

To hear the terms, go to evolve.elsevier.com.
Select: Chapter 12, **Exercises**, Pronunciation.

Refer to p. 10 for your Evolve Access Information.

☐ Place a check mark in the box when you have completed this exercise.

EXERCISE 22

Fill in the blank with the correct terms.

1. _____ _____ is the use of a laser beam to condense retinal tissue to seal leaking blood vessels, destroy abnormal tissue, or bond the retina to the back of the eye.

2. Surgical removal of an eyeball is called a(n) _____.

3. _____ is the name given to the procedure that breaks up the lens with ultrasound and then aspirates it.

4. Procedure using the Excimer laser and lamellar keratoplasty to correct hyperopia, myopia, and astigmatism is called _____.

5. _____ is the surgical creation of an opening that allows aqueous humor to drain out of the eye to reduce intraocular pressure.

6. Operation to repair a detached retina in which the sclera is folded or resected and an exoplant is used to buckle and hold the sclera is called

   _____ _____.

7. Surgery to remove vitreous humor from the eye is called _____.

8. _____ is a procedure for the treatment of nearsightedness in which an Excimer laser is used to reshape the corneal surface.

EXERCISE 23

Match the terms in the first column with their correct definitions in the second column.

_____ 1. LASIK

_____ 2. enucleation

_____ 3. trabeculectomy

_____ 4. retinal photocoagulation

_____ 5. phacoemulsification

_____ 6. scleral buckling

_____ 7. vitrectomy

_____ 8. PRK

a. use of a laser beam to repair retinal tears and detachment, as well as other retinopathies

b. surgical creation of an opening to reduce intraocular pressure

c. procedure for the treatment of nearsightedness in which an Excimer laser is used to reshape the corneal surface

d. procedure in which the lens is broken up by ultrasound and aspirated

e. procedure used to correct astigmatism, nearsightedness, and farsightedness by reshaping tissue beneath the corneal surface

f. surgical removal of an eyeball

g. surgical removal of vitreous humor

h. operation in which a cataract is lifted from the eye with an extremely cold probe

i. detached retina surgery in which the sclera is folded and an exoplant is used to buckle and hold the sclera

j. surgical incision of the sclera

EXERCISE 24

Spell each of the surgical terms not built from word parts on pp. 534–535 by having someone dictate them to you.

1. _____   5. _____
2. _____   6. _____
3. _____   7. _____
4. _____   8. _____

Diagnostic Terms

Built from Word Parts

The following terms are built from word parts you have already learned and can be translated literally to find their meanings. Further explanation of terms beyond the definition of their word parts, if needed, is included in parentheses.

TERM	DEFINITION
DIAGNOSTIC IMAGING	
fluorescein angiography (flō-RES-ēn) (*an*-jē-OG-ra-fē)	radiographic imaging of blood vessels (of the eye with fluorescing dye)
OPHTHALMIC EVALUATION	
keratometer (*ker*-a-TOM-e-ter)	instrument used to measure (the curvature of) the cornea (used for fitting contact lenses)
ophthalmoscope (of-THAL-mō-skōp)	instrument used for visual examination (of the interior) of the eye (Exercise Figure E2)
ophthalmoscopy (*of*-thal-MOS-ko-pē)	visual examination of the eye (Exercise Figure E1)
optometry (op-TOM-e-trē)	measurement of vision (visual acuity and the prescribing of corrective lenses)
pupillometer (*pū*-pil-OM-e-ter)	instrument used to measure (the diameter of) the pupil
pupilloscope (pū-PIL-ō-skōp)	instrument used for visual examination of the pupil
retinoscopy (*ret*-i-NOS-ko-pē)	visual examination of the retina
tonometer (tō-NOM-e-ter)	instrument used to measure pressure (within the eye, used to diagnose glaucoma)
tonometry (tō-NOM-e-trē)	measurement of pressure (within the eye)

Fill in the blanks to label the diagram.

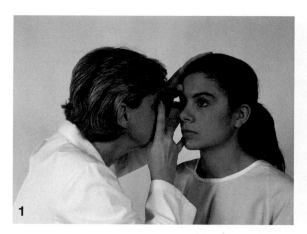

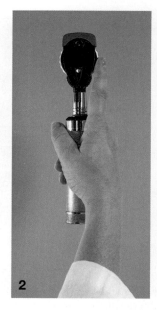

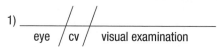

1) _____
   eye / cv / visual examination

2) _____
   eye / cv / instrument used for
                visual examination

EXERCISE **25**

Practice saying aloud each of the diagnostic terms built from word parts on p. 537.

To hear the terms, go to evolve.elsevier.com. Select: Chapter 12, **Exercises**, Pronunciation.
Refer to p. 10 for your Evolve Access Information.

☐ Place a check mark in the box when you have completed this exercise.

EXERCISE **26**

Analyze and define the following diagnostic terms.

1. pupilloscope _____
2. optometry _____
3. ophthalmoscope _____
4. tonometry _____
5. pupillometer _____
6. tonometer _____
7. keratometer _____
8. ophthalmoscopy _____
9. (fluorescein) angiography _____
10. retinoscopy _____

EXERCISE 27

Build diagnostic terms that correspond to the following definitions by using the word parts you have learned.

1. measurement of
   pressure (within the eye)

   _____ /__/ _____
   WR   /CV/   S

2. instrument used to measure
   (the diameter of) the pupil

   _____ /__/ _____
   WR   /CV/   S

3. instrument used to measure
   (the curvature of) the cornea

   _____ /__/ _____
   WR   /CV/   S

4. measurement of vision

   _____ /__/ _____
   WR   /CV/   S

5. instrument used for visual
   examination of the eye

   _____ /__/ _____
   WR   /CV/   S

6. instrument used to measure
   pressure (within the eye)

   _____ /__/ _____
   WR   /CV/   S

7. instrument used for visual
   examination of the pupil

   _____ /__/ _____
   WR   /CV/   S

8. visual examination of the eye

   _____ /__/ _____
   WR   /CV/   S

9. radiographic imaging of
   blood vessels (of the eye with
   fluorescing dye)   fluorescein

   _____ /__/ _____
   WR   /CV/   S

10. visual examination of
    the retina

    _____ /__/ _____
    WR   /CV/   S

EXERCISE 28

Spell each of the diagnostic terms built from word parts on p. 537 by having someone dictate them to you.

> To hear and spell the terms, go to evolve.elsevier.com. Select: Chapter 12, **Exercises**, Spelling.
>
> Refer to p. 10 for your Evolve Access Information.
>
> ☐ Place a check mark in the box if you have completed this exercise online.

1. _____   6. _____
2. _____   7. _____
3. _____   8. _____
4. _____   9. _____
5. _____   10. _____

Complementary Terms

Built from Word Parts

The following terms are built from word parts you have already learned and can be translated literally to find their meanings. Further explanation of terms beyond the definition of their word parts, if needed, is included in parentheses.

TERM	DEFINITION
anisocoria (an-ī-sō-KŌR-ē-a)	condition of absence of equal pupil (size) (unequal size of pupils)
binocular (bin-OK-ū-lar)	pertaining to two or both eyes
corneal (KOR-nē-al)	pertaining to the cornea
intraocular (*in*-tra-OK-ū-lar)	pertaining to within the eye
isocoria (ī-sō-KŌR-ē-a)	condition of equal pupil (size)
lacrimal (LAK-ri-mal)	pertaining to tears
nasolacrimal (*nā*-zō-LAK-ri-mal)	pertaining to the nose and tear ducts
ophthalmic (of-THAL-mik)	pertaining to the eye
ophthalmologist (*of*-thal-MOL-o-jist)	physician who studies and treats diseases of the eye
ophthalmology (Ophth) (*of*-thal-MOL-o-jē)	study of the eye (branch of medicine that deals with treating diseases of the eye)
ophthalmopathy (*of*-thal-MOP-a-thē)	(any) disease of the eye
optic (OP-tik)	pertaining to vision
pseudophakia (*soo*-dō-FĀ-ke-a)	condition of false lens (placement of an intraocular lens during surgery to treat cataracts)
pupillary (PŪ-pi-lar-ē)	pertaining to the pupil
retinal (RET-i-nal)	pertaining to the retina

EXERCISE **29**

Practice saying aloud each of the complementary terms built from word parts.

To hear the terms, go to evolve.elsevier.com. Select: Chapter 12, **Exercises**, Pronunciation.

Refer to p. 10 for your Evolve Access Information.

☐ Place a check mark in the box when you have completed this exercise.

EXERCISE 30

Analyze and define the following complementary terms.

1. ophthalmology _____
2. binocular _____
3. lacrimal _____
4. pupillary _____
5. ophthalmologist _____
6. corneal _____
7. ophthalmic _____
8. nasolacrimal _____

9. optic _____
10. intraocular _____
11. retinal _____
12. ophthalmopathy _____
13. isocoria _____
14. anisocoria _____
15. pseudophakia _____

EXERCISE 31

Build the complementary terms for the following definitions by using the word parts you have learned.

1. study of the eye

    _____ /___/ _____
    WR   CV   S

2. pertaining to two or both eyes

    _____ /___/ _____
    P   WR   S

3. pertaining to the retina

    _____ /___ _____
    WR   S

4. pertaining to within the eye

    _____ /___/ _____
    P   WR   S

5. physician who studies and treats diseases of the eye

    _____ /___/ _____
    WR   CV   S

6. pertaining to tears

    _____ /___ _____
    WR   S

7. pertaining to vision

    _____ /___ _____
    WR   S

8. pertaining to the eye

    _____ /___ _____
    WR   S

9. pertaining to the cornea

    _____ /___ _____
    WR   S

10. pertaining to the nose and tear ducts

    _____ /___/ _____ /___ _____
    WR   CV   WR   S

11. disease of the eye

    _____ /___/ _____
    WR   CV   S

12. pertaining to the pupil

    _____ /___ _____
    WR   S

13. condition of false lens

    _____ /___/ _____ /___ _____
    WR   CV   WR   S

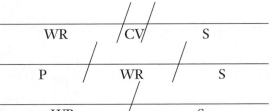
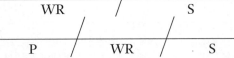
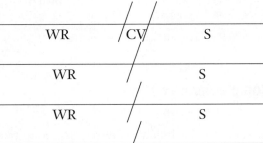
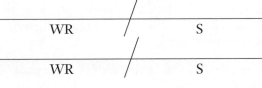
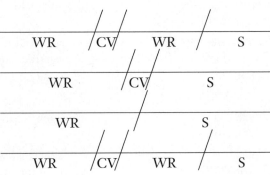

14. condition of equal pupil (size) _____ / ___ / _____ / ___ / ___
                                      WR   /CV/   WR   /   S

15. condition of absence of
    equal pupil (size) ___ / _____ / ___ / _____ / ___ / ___
                       P /   WR   /CV/   WR   /   S

EXERCISE 32

Spell each of the complementary terms built from word parts on p. 540 by having someone dictate them to you.

> To hear and spell the terms, go to evolve.elsevier.com. Select: Chapter 12, **Exercises**, Spelling.
>
> Refer to p. 10 for your Evolve Access Information.
>
> ☐ Place a check mark in the box if you have completed this exercise online.

1. _____   9. _____
2. _____   10. _____
3. _____   11. _____
4. _____   12. _____
5. _____   13. _____
6. _____   14. _____
7. _____   15. _____
8. _____

> For review and/or assessment, go to evolve.elsevier.com. Select:
> Chapter 12, **Activities**, Terms Built from Word Parts
> Chapter 12, **Games**,   Term Storm
>
> Refer to p. 10 for your Evolve Access Information.

Complementary Terms

Not Built from Word Parts

In some of the following terms, you may recognize word parts you have already learned; however, the full meaning of the terms cannot be discerned by the definition of their word parts.

TERM	DEFINITION
emmetropia (Em) (*em*-e-TRŌ-pē-a)	normal refractive condition of the eye
intraocular lens (IOL) (*in*-tra-OK-ū-lar) (lenz)	artificial lens implanted within the eye during cataract surgery
miotic (mī-OT-ik)	agent that constricts the pupil
mydriatic (*mid*-rē-AT-ik)	agent that dilates the pupil
optician (op-TISH-in)	specialist who fills prescriptions for lenses (cannot prescribe lenses)

TERM	DEFINITION
optometrist (op-TOM-e-trist)	health professional who prescribes corrective lenses and/or eye exercises
visual acuity (VA) (VIZH-ū-al) (a-KŪ-i-tē)	sharpness of vision for either distance or near

To watch animations, go to evolve.elsevier.com.
Select: Chapter 12, **Animations**, Visual Acuity.

Refer to p. 10 for your Evolve Access Information.

Refer to **Appendix D** for pharmacology terms related to the eye.

EXERCISE 33

Practice saying aloud each of the complementary terms not built from word parts.

To hear the terms, go to evolve.elsevier.com. Select: Chapter 12, **Exercises**, Pronunciation.

Refer to p. 10 for your Evolve Access Information.

☐ Place a check mark in the box when you have completed this exercise.

EXERCISE 34

Write the definitions for the following complementary terms.

1. optometrist _____
2. mydriatic _____
3. visual acuity _____
4. miotic _____
5. optician _____
6. emmetropia _____
7. intraocular lens _____

EXERCISE 35

Fill in the blanks with the correct terms.

1. Agent that dilates a pupil is a(n) _____.
2. Agent that constricts a pupil is a(n) _____.
3. Health professional who prescribes corrective lenses and/or eye exercises is a(n)

   _____ .
4. Another term for sharpness of vision is _____ _____.
5. Specialist who fills prescriptions for lenses but who cannot prescribe lenses is

   a(n) _____.
6. Normal refractive condition of the eye is called _____.
7. After the removal of the lens by phacoemulsification to treat cataracts, often an
   artificial lens, or _____ _____, is implanted
   within the eye.

EXERCISE 36

Spell each of the complementary terms not built from word parts on pp. 542–543 by having someone dictate them to you.

> To hear and spell the terms, go to evolve.elsevier.com. Select: Chapter 12, **Exercises**, Spelling.
>
> (e) Refer to p. 10 for your Evolve Access Information.
>
> ☐ Place a check mark in the box if you have completed this exercise online.

1. _____   5. _____
2. _____   6. _____
3. _____   7. _____
4. _____

> For review and/or assessment, go to evolve.elsevier.com. Select:
> Chapter 12, **Activities,** Terms Not Built from Word Parts
> Hear It and Type It: Clinical Vignettes
> (e) Chapter 12, **Games,**   Term Explorer
> Termbusters
> Medical Millionaire
>
> Refer to p. 10 for your Evolve access information.

Abbreviations

ABBREVIATION	MEANING
ARMD	age-related macular degeneration
Ast	astigmatism
Em	emmetropia
IOL	intraocular lens
IOP	intraocular pressure
Ophth	ophthalmology
PHACO	phacoemulsification
VA	visual acuity

EXERCISE 37

Write the meaning of the following abbreviations in the spaces provided.

1. VA _____ _____
2. Ast _____
3. IOP _____ _____
4. Em _____
5. Ophth _____
6. ARMD _____ _____ _____
7. PHACO _____
8. IOL _____ _____

> For more practice with abbreviations, go to evolve.elsevier.com. Select:
> Chapter 12, **Flashcards**
> (e) Chapter 12, **Games**, Crossword Puzzle
>
> Refer to p. 10 for your Evolve Access Information.

PRACTICAL APPLICATION

EXERCISE 38 *Interact with Medical Documents and Electronic Health Records*

A. Complete the progress note by writing the medical terms in the blanks. Use the list of definitions with the corresponding numbers.

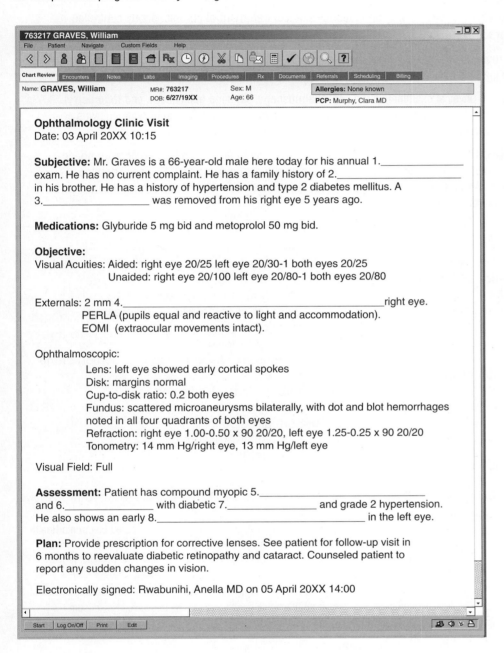

```
763217 GRAVES, William                                                    _ □ X
File    Patient   Navigate    Custom Fields    Help

Chart Review  Encounters   Notes    Labs    Imaging   Procedures   Rx   Documents   Referrals   Scheduling   Billing
Name: GRAVES, William      MR#: 763217      Sex: M       Allergies: None known
                           DOB: 6/27/19XX   Age: 66      PCP: Murphy, Clara MD
```

Ophthalmology Clinic Visit
Date: 03 April 20XX 10:15

Subjective: Mr. Graves is a 66-year-old male here today for his annual 1._____
exam. He has no current complaint. He has a family history of 2._____
in his brother. He has a history of hypertension and type 2 diabetes mellitus. A
3._____ was removed from his right eye 5 years ago.

Medications: Glyburide 5 mg bid and metoprolol 50 mg bid.

Objective:
Visual Acuities: Aided: right eye 20/25 left eye 20/30-1 both eyes 20/25
                 Unaided: right eye 20/100 left eye 20/80-1 both eyes 20/80

Externals: 2 mm 4._____right eye.
           PERLA (pupils equal and reactive to light and accommodation).
           EOMI (extraocular movements intact).

Ophthalmoscopic:

           Lens: left eye showed early cortical spokes
           Disk: margins normal
           Cup-to-disk ratio: 0.2 both eyes
           Fundus: scattered microaneurysms bilaterally, with dot and blot hemorrhages
           noted in all four quadrants of both eyes
           Refraction: right eye 1.00-0.50 x 90 20/20, left eye 1.25-0.25 x 90 20/20
           Tonometry: 14 mm Hg/right eye, 13 mm Hg/left eye

Visual Field: Full

Assessment: Patient has compound myopic 5._____
and 6._____ with diabetic 7._____ and grade 2 hypertension.
He also shows an early 8._____ in the left eye.

Plan: Provide prescription for corrective lenses. See patient for follow-up visit in
6 months to reevaluate diabetic retinopathy and cataract. Counseled patient to
report any sudden changes in vision.

Electronically signed: Rwabunihi, Anella MD on 05 April 20XX 14:00

```
Start    Log On/Off    Print    Edit
```

1. study of the eye
2. eye disorder characterized by the increase of intraocular pressure
3. thin tissue growing into the cornea from the conjunctiva
4. drooping of eyelid
5. irregular curvature of the cornea or lens
6. impaired vision as a result of aging
7. (any noninflammatory) disease of the retina
8. clouding of the lens of the eye

B. Read the following case study and answer the questions that follow.

Case Study

Patient Profile: This 70-year-old woman was admitted for surgical treatment of chronic, poorly controlled **glaucoma** and for **cataract** extraction.

Subjective: The patient reported a progressive loss of **visual acuity** in her right eye; she complained of headaches and problems with glare (particularly at night) and said she perceives halos around lights.

Objective: Vision testing and physical examination (i.e., **ophthalmoscopy,** slit lamp microscopy, and **tonometry**) revealed acuity (unaided) of 10/100 for the right eye and 20/60 for the left eye. Opacification of right lens was evident, as was moderate **corneal** edema.

Therapeutic Management: After a **mydriatic** agent was applied to the right pupil, a combined procedure **phacoemulsification** of the cataract and **trabeculectomy** with releasable sutures (to minimize **IOP**) was performed with the patient under local anesthesia. The patient tolerated the procedure well and returned to her room wearing a 12-hour collagen shield on the treated eye.

---

1. Vision testing and physical examination of the patient revealed opacification of the right lens, confirming the need for:
   a. PRK
   b. phacoemulsification
   c. scleral buckling
   d. enucleation
2. Application of a mydriatic agent would:
   a. reduce tears
   b. produce tears
   c. constrict the pupil
   d. dilate the pupil

3. A trabeculectomy was performed because the patient had a history of:
   a. condition of crossed eyes
   b. disorder characterized by increased intraocular pressure
   c. nearsightedness
   d. progressive deterioration of a portion of the retina
4. The abbreviation IOP stands for:
   a. both eyes
   b. normal vision
   c. intraocular pressure
   d. iris outer pupil

C. Complete the **three medical documents** within the electronic health record (EHR) on Evolve.

> Many healthcare records today are stored and used in an electronic system called **Electronic Health Records (EHR).** Electronic health records contain a collection of health information of an individual patient; the digitally formatted record can be shared through computer networks with patients, physicians, and other health care providers.

> For practice with medical terms using electronic health records, go to evolve.elsevier.com. Select: Chapter 12, **Electronic Health Records.**
>
> Refer to p. 10 for your Evolve Access Information.

EXERCISE 39 *Interpret Medical Terms*

To test your understanding of the terms introduced in this chapter, circle the words that correctly complete the sentences. The italicized words refer to the correct answer.

1. The patient's *pupils* needed to be *dilated*; therefore, the doctor requested that a (**miotic, mydriatic, myopia**) medication be placed in each eye.
2. A person with an *irregular curvature of the cornea or lens* of the eye has (**astigmatism, glaucoma, strabismus**).

3. The doctor diagnosed the patient with the *clouded lens* of the eye as having a(n) (**nystagmus, astigmatism, cataract**).
4. To *measure the pressure within the patient's eye*, the physician used a(n) (**pupillometer, tonometer, keratometer**).
5. A person who is *farsighted* has (**hyperopia, myopia, diplopia**).
6. An *obstruction of an oil gland of the eyelid* is called a (**sty, chalazion, conjunctivitis**).
7. A patient with an *involuntary jerking movement of the eyes* has a condition known as (**astigmatism, strabismus, nystagmus**).
8. The name of the *surgery performed to create an opening to drain aqueous humor* is (**trabeculectomy, iridectomy, phacoemulsification**).
9. The doctor ordered a *radiographic imaging of the blood vessels of the eye* or a(n) (**ophthalmoscopy, fluorescein angiography, optometer**).
10. Vitamin A deficiency is associated with *condition of dry eye* (**oculomycosis, ophthalmoplegia, xerophthalmia**) and also with *night blindness* (**nyctalopia, photophobia, diplopia**) and may progress to *softening of the cornea* (**iridoplegia, keratomalacia, sclerokeratitis**).
11. The surgery schedule indicated the patient being treated for cataracts would undergo right eye *PHACO* (**photorefractive keratectomy, retinal photocoagulation, phacoemulsification**) with *IOL* (**intraocular pressure, intraocular lens**).
12. *Progressive deterioration of the retina, resulting in loss of central vision* (**retinitis pigmentosa, presbyopia, macular degeneration**) may be described as *dry*, where the blood vessels become thin and brittle, or *wet*, where new abnormal vessels develop under the macula lutea.
13. Diabetic *disease of the retina* (**blepharoptosis, retinopathy, ophthalmalgia**), which may involve swelling and leaking of blood vessels or development of new abnormal blood vessels on the surface of the retina, may be surgically treated by *removal of all or part of the vitreous humor* (**trabeculectomy, vitrectomy, iridectomy**) and *intense beam of light from a laser to condense, destroy, or bond tissue* (**retinal photocoagulation, photorefractive keratectomy, phacoemulsification**).

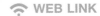 WEB LINK

To learn more about conditions of the eye and vision, visit the **American Optometric Association**'s website at *www.aoa.org*.

EXERCISE 40   *Read Medical Terms in Use*

Practice pronunciation of terms by reading the following medical document. Use the pronunciation key following the medical terms to help you say the word.

To hear these terms, go to evolve.elsevier.com.
Select: Chapter 12, **Exercises**, Read Medical Terms in Use.

Refer to p. 10 for your Evolve Access Information.

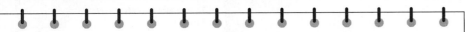

An elderly gentleman visited his **ophthalmologist** (*of*-thal-MOL-o-jist) because of decreased vision. A **tonometry** (tō-NOM-e-trē) examination showed borderline readings. **Visual acuity** (VIZH-ū-al) (a-KŪ-i-tē) measurement indicated a mild degree of **myopia** (mī-Ō-pē–a) and **presbyopia** (*pres*-bē-Ō-pē-a). A diagnosis of **glaucoma** (glaw-KŌ-ma) is suspected in this case and timolol eye drops were prescribed, one drop daily.

A **cataract** (KAT-a-rakt) of the right eye was found. Lens implant surgery, which places an **intraocular lens** (in-tra-OK-ū-lar) (lenz), will be performed when the cataract matures sufficiently. Approximately 5 years ago the patient had a **detached retina** (RET-in-a) of the left eye. A **scleral buckling** (SKLER-al) (BUK-ling) procedure was performed and was successful in halting the progression of retinal detachment.

EXERCISE 41 *Comprehend Medical Terms in Use*

Test your comprehension of terms in the previous medical document by circling the correct answer.

1. T   F   The ophthalmologist used an instrument to measure pressure within the patient's eyes to assist in the diagnosis of increased intraocular pressure.
2. Visual acuity measurement indicated:
   a. farsightedness and impaired vision as a result of aging
   b. nearsightedness and impaired vision as a result of aging
   c. poor night vision and farsightedness
   d. poor night vision and impaired vision because of aging
3. Timolol eye drops were prescribed to address symptoms most likely caused by:
   a. inflammation of the cornea
   b. optic nerve damage caused by increased IOP
   c. separation of the retina from the choroid
   d. clouding of the lens of the eye
4. T   F   A scleral buckling procedure was used to correct clouding of the lens in the right eye.

For a snapshot assessment of your knowledge of medical terms for the eye, go to evolve.elsevier.com.

Select: Chapter 12, **Quick Quizzes.**

Refer to p. 10 for your Evolve Access Information.

CHAPTER REVIEW

Review of Evolve

Keep a record of the online activities you have completed by placing a check mark in the box. You may also record your scores. All activities have been referenced throughout the chapter.

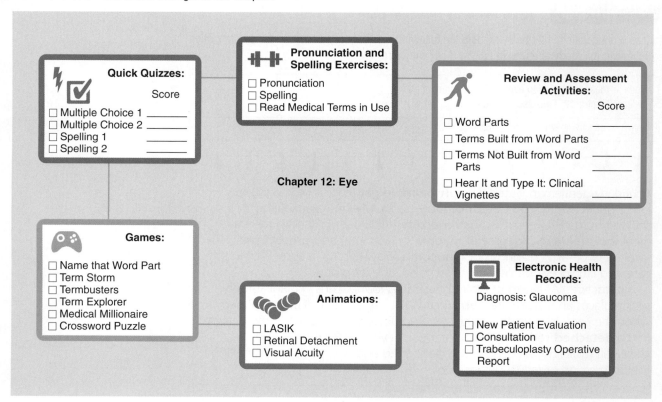

Chapter 12: Eye

Quick Quizzes:
Score
☐ Multiple Choice 1 _____
☐ Multiple Choice 2 _____
☐ Spelling 1 _____
☐ Spelling 2 _____

Pronunciation and Spelling Exercises:
☐ Pronunciation
☐ Spelling
☐ Read Medical Terms in Use

Review and Assessment Activities:
Score
☐ Word Parts _____
☐ Terms Built from Word Parts _____
☐ Terms Not Built from Word Parts _____
☐ Hear It and Type It: Clinical Vignettes _____

Games:
☐ Name that Word Part
☐ Term Storm
☐ Termbusters
☐ Term Explorer
☐ Medical Millionaire
☐ Crossword Puzzle

Animations:
☐ LASIK
☐ Retinal Detachment
☐ Visual Acuity

Electronic Health Records:
Diagnosis: Glaucoma
☐ New Patient Evaluation
☐ Consultation
☐ Trabeculoplasty Operative Report

Review of Word Parts

Can you define and spell the following word parts?

COMBINING FORMS		PREFIXES	SUFFIXES
blephar/o	kerat/o	bi-	-opia
conjunctiv/o	lacrim/o	bin-	-phobia
cor/o	ocul/o		-plegia
core/o	ophthalm/o		
corne/o	opt/o		
cry/o	phac/o		
dacry/o	phak/o		
dipl/o	phot/o		
ir/o	pupill/o		
irid/o	retin/o		
is/o	scler/o		
	ton/o		

Review of Terms

Can you define, pronounce, and spell the following terms *built from word parts?*

DISEASES AND DISORDERS	SURGICAL	DIAGNOSTIC	COMPLEMENTARY
aphakia	blepharoplasty	fluorescein angiography	anisocoria
blepharitis	cryoretinopexy	keratometer	binocular
blepharoptosis	dacryocystorhinostomy	ophthalmoscope	corneal
conjunctivitis	dacryocystotomy	ophthalmoscopy	intraocular
dacryocystitis	iridectomy	optometry	isocoria
diplopia	iridotomy	pupillometer	lacrimal
endophthalmitis	keratoplasty	pupilloscope	nasolacrimal
iridoplegia	sclerotomy	retinoscopy	ophthalmic
iritis		tonometer	ophthalmologist
keratitis		tonometry	ophthalmology (Ophth)
keratomalacia			ophthalmopathy
leukocoria			optic
oculomycosis			pseudophakia
ophthalmalgia			pupillary
ophthalmoplegia			retinal
phacomalacia			
photophobia			
retinoblastoma			
retinopathy			
sclerokeratitis			
scleromalacia			
xerophthalmia			

Can you define, pronounce, and spell the following terms not *built from word parts*?

DISEASES AND DISORDERS		SURGICAL	COMPLEMENTARY
amblyopia	myopia	enucleation	emmetropia (Em)
astigmatism (Ast)	nyctalopia	LASIK (laser-assisted in situ keratomileusis)	intraocular lens (IOL)
cataract	nystagmus	phacoemulsification (PHACO)	miotic
chalazion	pinguecula	PRK (photorefractive keratectomy)	mydriatic
detached retina	presbyopia	retinal photocoagulation	optician
glaucoma	pterygium	scleral buckling	optometrist
hyperopia	retinitis pigmentosa	trabeculectomy	visual acuity (VA)
macular degeneration	strabismus	vitrectomy	
	sty		

ANSWERS

ANSWERS TO CHAPTER 12 EXERCISES
Exercise Figures

Exercise Figure

A. 1. eye: ocul/o, ophthalm/o
2. eyelid: blephar/o
3. pupil: cor/o, core/o, pupill/o
4. sclera: scler/o
5. iris: irid/o, ir/o
6. conjunctiva: conjunctiv/o
7. cornea: corne/o, kerat/o
8. lens: phac/o, phak/o
9. retina: retin/o

Exercise Figure

B. blephar/itis

Exercise Figure

C. blephar/o/ptosis

Exercise Figure

D. dacry/o/cyst/itis

Exercise Figure

E. 1. ophthalm/o/scopy
2. ophthalm/o/scope

Exercise 1
1. d   5. b
2. c   6. e
3. f   7. a
4. h

Exercise 2
1. d   4. b
2. f   5. a
3. e   6. c

Exercise 3
1. eye   10. pupil
2. eyelid   11. eye
3. cornea   12. cornea
4. tear, tear duct   13. iris
5. retina   14. pupil
6. pupil   15. vision
7. sclera   16. tear, tear duct
8. iris   17. lens
9. conjunctiva

Exercise 4
1. a. ocul/o   7. scler/o
   b. ophthalm/o   8. retin/o
2. a. corne/o   9. a. irid/o
   b. kerat/o   b. ir/o
3. conjunctiv/o   10. opt/o
4. a. dacry/o   11. a. phac/o
   b. lacrim/o   b. phak/o
5. blephar/o
6. a. cor/o
   b. core/o
   c. pupill/o

Exercise 5
1. tension, pressure   4. two, double
2. light   5. equal
3. cold

Exercise 6
1. cry/o   4. phot/o
2. ton/o   5. is/o
3. dipl/o

Exercise 7
1. vision (condition)
2. two
3. paralysis
4. abnormal fear of or aversion to specific things
5. two

Exercise 8
1. -plegia   3. -phobia
2. a. bi-   4. -opia
   b. bin-

Exercise 9
Pronunciation Exercise

Exercise 10
Note: The combining form is identified by italic and bold print.
1. WR CV WR S
   scler/o/kerat/itis
      CF
   inflammation of the sclera and the cornea
2. WR   S
   ophthalm/algia
   pain in the eye
3. WR CV S
   blephar/o/ptosis
      CF
   drooping of the eyelid
4. WR S
   dipl/opia
   double vision
5. WR   S
   conjunctiv/itis
   inflammation of the conjunctiva
6. WR CV WR S
   leuk/o/cor/ia
      CF
   condition of white pupil
7. WR CV S
   irid/o/plegia
      CF
   paralysis of the iris

8. WR CV S
   scler/o/malacia
      CF
   softening of the sclera
9. WR CV S
   phot/o/phobia
      CF
   abnormal fear of (sensitivity to) light
10. WR S
   blephar/itis
   inflammation of the eyelid
11. WR CV WR S
   ocul/o/myc/osis
      CF
   abnormal condition of the eye caused by a fungus
12. WR CV WR S
   dacry/o/cyst/itis
      CF
   inflammation of the tear (lacrimal) sac
13. P   WR   S
   end/ophthalm/itis
   inflammation within the eye
14. WR S
   ir/itis
   inflammation of the iris
15. WR CV WR   S
   retin/o/blast/oma
      CF
   tumor arising from a developing retinal cell
16. WR S
   kerat/itis
   inflammation of the cornea
17. WR   CV S
   ophthalm/o/plegia
      CF
   paralysis of the eye (muscles)
18. WR CV S
   retin/o/pathy
      CF
   disease of the retina
19. WR   WR   S
   xer/ophthalm/ia
   condition of dry eye
20. WR CV /malacia
   kerat/o/malacia
      CF
   softening of the cornea
21. WR CV S
   phac/o/malacia
      CF
   softening of the lens

551

22. P WR S
    a/phak/ia
    condition of without a lens

Exercise 11

1. conjunctiv/itis
2. ocul/o/myc/osis
3. ophthalm/algia
4. dipl/opia
5. blephar/itis
6. leuk/o/cor/ia
7. irid/o/plegia
8. blephar/o/ptosis
9. ir/itis
10. retin/o/blast/oma
11. scler/o/malacia
12. dacry/o/cyst/itis
13. scler/o/kerat/itis
14. phot/o/phobia
15. kerat/itis
16. retin/o/pathy
17. end/ophthalm/itis
18. ophthalm/o/plegia
19. xer/ophthalm/ia
20. kerat/o/malacia
21. a/phak/ia
22. phac/o/malacia

Exercise 12
Spelling Exercise; see text p. 527.

Exercise 13
Pronunciation Exercise

Exercise 14

1. myopia
2. presbyopia
3. strabismus
4. chalazion
5. astigmatism
6. nystagmus
7. cataract
8. sty
9. glaucoma
10. detached retina
11. hyperopia
12. retinitis pigmentosa
13. nyctalopia
14. pterygium
15. macular degeneration
16. amblyopia
17. pinguecula

Exercise 15

1. f
2. g
3. j
4. m
5. l
6. i
7. d
8. o
9. e
10. c
11. a
12. k
13. h
14. n
15. b
16. q
17. r

Exercise 16
Spelling Exercise; see text p. 532.

Exercise 17
Pronunciation Exercise

Exercise 18
Note: The combining form is identified by italic and bold print.

1. WR CV S
   ***kerat/o*/plasty**
        CF
   surgical repair of the cornea

2. WR CV S
   ***scler/o*/tomy**
        CF
   incision of the sclera

3. WR CV WR CV S
   ***dacry/o/cyst/o*/tomy**
        CF   CF
   incision of the tear (lacrimal) sac

4. WR CV WR CV S
   ***cry/o/retin/o*/pexy**
       CF   CF
   surgical fixation of the retina by using extreme cold

5. WR CV S
   ***blephar/o*/plasty**
          CF
   surgical repair of the eyelid

6. WR   S
   irid/ectomy
   excision of the iris

7. WR CV WR CV WR CV S
   ***dacry/o/cyst/o/rhin/o*/stomy**
       CF   CF   CF
   creation of an artificial opening between the tear (lacrimal) sac and the nose

8. WR CV S
   ***irid/o*/tomy**
        CF
   incision of the iris

Exercise 19

1. dacry/o/cyst/o/rhin/o/stomy
2. irid/ectomy
3. kerat/o/plasty
4. scler/o/tomy
5. irid/o/tomy
6. blephar/o/plasty
7. cry/o/retin/o/pexy
8. dacry/o/cyst/o/tomy

Exercise 20
Spelling Exercise; see text p. 534.

Exercise 21
Pronunciation Exercise

Exercise 22

1. retinal photocoagulation
2. enucleation
3. phacoemulsification
4. LASIK
5. trabeculectomy
6. scleral buckling
7. vitrectomy
8. PRK

Exercise 23

1. e
2. f
3. b
4. a
5. d
6. i
7. g
8. c

Exercise 24
Spelling Exercise; see text p. 537.

Exercise 25
Pronunciation Exercise

Exercise 26
Note: The combining form is identified by italic and bold print.

1. WR CV S
   ***pupill/o*/scope**
         CF
   instrument used for visual examination of the pupil

2. WR CV S
   ***opt/o*/metry**
        CF
   measurement of vision

3. WR   CV S
   ***ophthalm/o*/scope**
            CF
   instrument used for visual examination of the eye

4. WR CV S
   ***ton/o*/metry**
        CF
   measurement of pressure (within the eye)

5. WR CV S
   ***pupill/o*/meter**
          CF
   instrument used to measure the pupil (diameter)

6. WR CV S
   ***ton/o*/meter**
        CF
   instrument used to measure pressure (within the eye)

7. WR CV S
   ***kerat/o*/meter**
          CF
   instrument used to measure (the curvature of) the cornea

8. WR   CV S
   ***ophthalm/o*/scopy**
            CF
   visual examination of the eye

9.   WR CV S
   (fluorescein) **angi/o**/graphy
            CF
   radiographic imaging of the
   blood vessels (of the eye with
   fluorescing dye)

10. WR CV S
   retin/o/scopy
       CF
   visual examination of the retina

Exercise 27
1. ton/o/metry
2. pupill/o/meter
3. kerat/o/meter
4. opt/o/metry
5. ophthalm/o/scope
6. ton/o/meter
7. pupill/o/scope
8. ophthalm/o/scopy
9. fluorescein angi/o/graphy
10. retin/o/scopy

Exercise 28
Spelling Exercise; see text p. 539.

Exercise 29
Pronunciation Exercise

Exercise 30
Note: The combining form is identified by italic and bold print.
1.   WR   CV S
   ophthalm/o/logy
         CF
   study of the eye
2.   P WR S
   bin/ocul/ar
   pertaining to two or both eyes
3.   WR S
   lacrim/al
   pertaining to tears
4.   WR S
   pupill/ary
   pertaining to the pupil
5.   WR CV S
   ophthalm/o/logist
         CF
   physician who studies and treats
   diseases of the eye
6.   WR S
   corne/al
   pertaining to the cornea
7.   WR   S
   ophthalm/ic
   pertaining to the eye
8. WR CV WR S
   nas/o/lacrim/al
       CF
   pertaining to the nose and tear ducts

9. WR S
   opt/ic
   pertaining to vision
10.   P WR S
   intra/ocul/ar
   pertaining to within the eye
11. WR S
   retin/al
   pertaining to the retina
12.   WR CV S
   ophthalm/o/pathy
        CF
   disease of the eye
13. WRCVWRS
   is/o/cor/ia
     CF
   condition of equal pupil (size)
14. P WRCVWR S
   an/**is/o**/cor/ia
       CF
   condition of absence of equal
   pupil (size)
15.   WR CV WR S
   pseud/o/phak/ia
        CF
   condition of false lens

Exercise 31
1. ophthalm/o/logy
2. bin/ocul/ar
3. retin/al
4. intra/ocul/ar
5. ophthalm/o/logist
6. lacrim/al
7. opt/ic
8. ophthalm/ic
9. corne/al
10. nas/o/lacrim/al
11. ophthalm/o/pathy
12. pupill/ary
13. pseud/o/phak/ia
14. is/o/cor/ia
15. an/is/o/cor/ia

Exercise 32
Spelling Exercise; see text p. 542.

Exercise 33
Pronunciation Exercise

Exercise 34
1. health professional who prescribes corrective lenses and/or eye exercises
2. agent that dilates the pupil
3. sharpness of vision
4. agent that constricts the pupil
5. specialist who fills prescriptions for lenses
6. normal refractive condition of the eye
7. artificial lens implanted within the eye

Exercise 35
1. mydriatic
2. miotic
3. optometrist
4. visual acuity
5. optician
6. emmetropia
7. intraocular lens

Exercise 36
Spelling Exercise; see text p. 544.

Exercise 37
1. visual acuity
2. astigmatism
3. intraocular pressure
4. emmetropia
5. ophthalmology
6. age-related macular degeneration
7. phacoemulsification
8. intraocular lens

Exercise 38
A. 1. ophthalmology
    2. glaucoma
    3. pterygium
    4. blepharoptosis
    5. astigmatism
    6. presbyopia
    7. retinopathy
    8. cataract
B. 1. b
    2. d
    3. b
    4. c
C. Online Exercise

Exercise 39
1. mydriatic
2. astigmatism
3. cataract
4. tonometer
5. hyperopia
6. chalazion
7. nystagmus
8. trabeculectomy
9. fluorescein angiography
10. xerophthalmia, nyctalopia, keratomalacia
11. phacoemulsification, intraocular lens
12. macular degeneration
13. retinopathy, vitrectomy, retinal photocoagulation

Exercise 40
Reading Exercise

Exercise 41
1. *T*
2. b
3. b
4. *F*, scleral buckling was used to correct a detached retina and not a cataract.

Chapter

13   Ear

Objectives

Upon completion of this chapter you will be able to:

1   Identify organs and structures of the ear.

2   Define and spell word parts related to
     the ear.

3   Define, pronounce, and spell disease and
     disorder terms related to the ear.

4   Define, pronounce, and spell surgical terms
     related to the ear.

5   Define, pronounce, and spell diagnostic
     terms related to the ear.

6   Define, pronounce, and spell
     complementary terms related to the ear.

7   Interpret the meaning of abbreviations
     related to the ear.

8   Interpret, read, and comprehend medical
     language in simulated medical statements,
     documents, and electronic health records.

ANATOMY

Function

The two functions of the ear are to hear and to provide the sense of balance. The ear is made up of three parts: the **external ear**, the **middle ear**, and the **inner ear**. The inner ear is also called the **labyrinth** (Figures 13-1 and 13-2). The auricle directs external sound waves to the external auditory canal where they produce vibration in the middle ear structures. The vibration of the stapes results in displacement of the cochlear structure which ultimately produces nerve impulses that are carried to the brain.

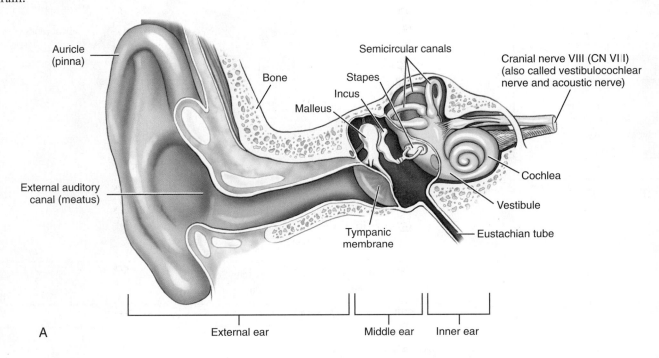

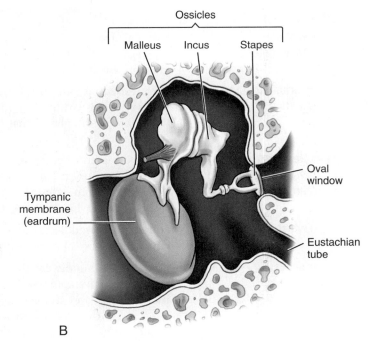

FIGURE 13-1
A, Gross anatomy of the ear. **B,** The middle ear.

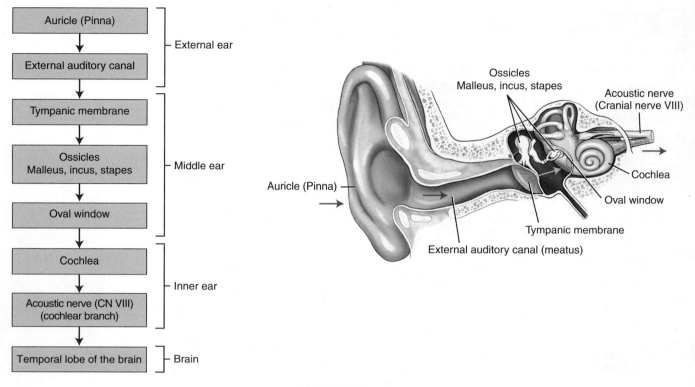

FIGURE 13-2
Perception of sound.

To watch animations, go to evolve.elsevier.com. Select:
Chapter 13, **Animations**, Pathway of Sound.

Refer to p. 10 for your Evolve Access Information.

Structures of the Ear

TERM	DEFINITION
external ear	
auricle (pinna)	external structure located on both sides of the head. The auricle directs sound waves into the external auditory canal.
external auditory canal (meatus)	short tube that ends at the tympanic membrane. The inner part lies within the temporal bone of the skull and contains the glands that secrete earwax (cerumen).
middle ear	
tympanic membrane (eardrum)	semitransparent membrane that separates the external auditory canal and the middle ear cavity. The tympanic membrane transmits sound vibrations to the ossicles (Figure 13-4, *B*, p 562).
eustachian tube	connects the middle ear and the pharynx. It equalizes air pressure on both sides of the eardrum.
ossicles	bones of the middle ear that carry sound vibrations. The ossicles are composed of the **malleus** (hammer), **incus** (anvil), and **stapes** (stirrup). The stapes connects to the **oval window**, which transmits the sound vibrations to the cochlea of the inner ear.
labyrinth (inner ear)	bony spaces within the temporal bone of the skull. It contains the cochlea, semicircular canals, and vestibule.

🏛 **TYMPANIC MEMBRANE**
is derived from the Greek **tympanon,** meaning **drum,** because of its resemblance to a drum or tambourine.

🏛 **STAPES**
is Latin for **stirrup.** The anatomic stapes was so named for its stirrup-like shape.

TERM	DEFINITION
cochlea	snail-shaped and contains the organ of hearing. The cochlea connects to the oval window in the middle ear.
semicircular canals and vestibule	contains receptors and endolymph that help the body maintain its sense of balance (equilibrium)
mastoid bone and cells	located in the skull bone behind the external auditory canal

---

A & P Booster
For more anatomy and physiology, go to evolve.elsevier.com.
Select: **Extra Content**, A & P Booster, Chapter 13.

Refer to p. 10 for your Evolve Access Information.

EXERCISE 1

Match the anatomic terms in the first column with the correct definitions in the second column. *To check your answers to the exercises in this chapter, go to Answers, p. 577, at the end of the chapter.*

_____ 1. auricle

_____ 2. cochlea

_____ 3. eustachian tube

_____ 4. external auditory meatus

_____ 5. labyrinth

_____ 6. mastoid bone

_____ 7. ossicles

_____ 8. semicircular canals and vestibule

_____ 9. tympanic membrane

a. contains receptors and endolymph, which help maintain equilibrium
b. equalizes air pressure on both sides of the eardrum
c. separates the external auditory canal and middle ear cavity
d. malleus, incus, and stapes
e. contains glands that secrete earwax
f. external structure located on each side of the head
g. bony spaces within the temporal bone
h. relays messages to the brain
i. contains the organ of hearing
j. located in the skull behind the external auditory canal

 WORD PARTS

Word parts you need to learn to complete this chapter are as follows. The exercises at the end of each list will help you learn their definitions and spellings.

Use the flashcards accompanying this text or electronic flashcards to assist you in memorizing the word parts for this chapter.

To use electronic flashcards, go to evolve.elsevier.com.
Select: Chapter 13, **Flashcards**.

Refer to p. 10 for your Evolve Access Information.

Combining Forms of the Ear

COMBINING FORM	DEFINITION
audi/o	hearing
aur/i, aur/o, ot/o	ear
cochle/o	cochlea
labyrinth/o	labyrinth (inner ear)

Combining Forms of the Ear—cont'd

COMBINING FORM	DEFINITION
mastoid/o	mastoid bone
myring/o	tympanic membrane (eardrum)
staped/o	stapes (middle ear bone)
tympan/o	tympanic membrane (eardrum), middle ear
vestibul/o	vestibule

Refer to **Appendix A** and **Appendix B** for a complete list of word parts.

EXERCISE FIGURE A

Fill in the blanks with combining forms in this diagram of the ear. *To check your answers, go to p. 577.*

1. Ear

   CF: _____

   CF: _____

   CF: _____

2. Labyrinth (inner ear)

   CF: _____

Auricle

Semicircular canals

Incus

Malleus

Cochlea

Oval window

External auditory
meatus (canal)

Eustachian
tube

3. Stapes

   CF: _____

4. Tympanic membrane (eardrum)

   CF: _____

   CF: _____

5. Mastoid bone

   CF: _____

EXERCISE 2

Write the definitions of the following combining forms.

1. staped/o _____
2. mastoid/o _____
3. audi/o _____
4. aur/i, aur/o, ot/o _____
5. tympan/o _____

6. vestibul/o _____
7. labyrinth/o _____
8. myring/o _____
9. cochle/o _____

EXERCISE 3

Write the combining form for each of the following terms.

1. ear   a. _____

         b. _____

         c. _____

2. mastoid bone _____

3. stapes _____

4. tympanic membrane (eardrum), middle ear _____

5. labyrinth (inner ear) _____

6. hearing _____

7. tympanic membrane (eardrum) _____

8. cochlea _____

9. vestibule _____

For review and/or assessment, go to evolve.elsevier.com. Select:
Chapter 13, **Activities,** Word Parts
Chapter 13, **Games,**   Name that Word Part
_____
Refer to p. 10 for your Evolve Access Information.

🗨 MEDICAL TERMS

The terms you need to learn to complete this chapter are listed on the following pages. The exercises following each list will help you learn the definition and spelling of each word.

Disease and Disorder Terms

Built from Word Parts

The following terms are built from word parts you have already learned and can be translated literally to find their meanings. Further explanation of terms beyond the definition of their word parts, if needed, is included in parentheses.

TERM	DEFINITION
labyrinthitis (*lab*-i-rin-THĪ-tis)	inflammation of the labyrinth (inner ear) (also called **vestibular neuritis**)
mastoiditis (*mas*-toyd-Ī-tis)	inflammation of the mastoid bone
myringitis (*mir*-in-JĪ-tis)	inflammation of the tympanic membrane (eardrum)
otalgia (ō-TAL-ja)	pain in the ear
otomastoiditis (ō-tō-*mas*-toyd-Ī-tis)	inflammation of the ear and the mastoid bone
otomycosis (ō-tō-mī-KŌ-sis)	abnormal condition of fungus in the ear (usually affects the external auditory canal)
otopyorrhea (ō-tō-*pī*-ō-RĒ-a)	discharge of pus from the ear

Disease and Disorder Terms—cont'd

Built from Word Parts

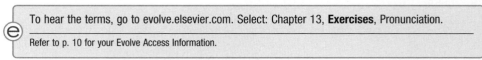

TERM	DEFINITION
otorrhea (ō-tō-RĒ-a)	discharge from the ear (may be serous, bloody, consisting of pus, or containing cerebrospinal fluid)
otosclerosis (ō-tō-skle-RŌ-sis)	hardening of the ear (stapes) (caused by irregular bone development and resulting in hearing loss)

EXERCISE 4

Practice saying aloud each of the disease and disorder terms built from word parts on pp. 559–560.

> 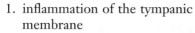 To hear the terms, go to evolve.elsevier.com. Select: Chapter 13, **Exercises**, Pronunciation.
>
> Refer to p. 10 for your Evolve Access Information.

☐ Place a check mark in the box when you have completed this exercise.

EXERCISE 5

Analyze and define the following terms.

1. otomycosis_____
2. otomastoiditis _____
3. otalgia _____
4. labyrinthitis_____
5. myringitis _____
6. otosclerosis _____
7. mastoiditis_____
8. otopyorrhea_____
9. otorrhea_____

EXERCISE 6

Build disease and disorder terms for the following definitions with the word parts you have learned.

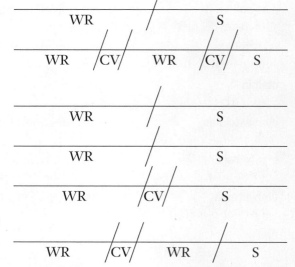

1. inflammation of the tympanic membrane

   _____ / _____
   WR   /   S

2. discharge of pus from the ear

   _____ /CV/ _____ /CV/ ___
   WR   /CV/   WR   /CV/   S

3. inflammation of the mastoid bone

   _____ / _____
   WR   /   S

4. pain in the ear

   _____ / _____
   WR   /   S

5. hardening of the ear (stapes)

   _____ /CV/ _____
   WR   /CV/   S

6. abnormal condition of fungus in the ear

   _____ /CV/ _____ / ___
   WR   /CV/   WR   /   S

7. inflammation of the ear and the mastoid bone

_____ / _____ / _____ / _____
WR / CV / WR / S

8. inflammation of the labyrinth

_____ / _____
WR / S

9. discharge from the ear

_____ / _____ / _____
WR / CV / S

EXERCISE 7

Spell each of the disease and disorder terms built from word parts on pp. 559–560 by having someone dictate them to you.

> To hear and spell the terms, go to evolve.elsevier.com. Select Chapter 13, **Exercises**, Spelling.
>
> Refer to p. 10 for your Evolve Access Information.
>
> ☐ Place a check mark in the box if you have completed this exercise online.

1. _____
2. _____
3. _____
4. _____
5. _____

6. _____
7. _____
8. _____
9. _____

Disease and Disorder Terms

Not Built from Word Parts

In some of the following terms, you may recognize word parts you have already learned; however, the full meaning of the terms cannot be discerned by the definition of their word parts.

TERM	DEFINITION
acoustic neuroma (a-KOOS-tik) (nū-RŌ-ma)	benign tumor within the internal auditory canal growing from the acoustic nerve (cranial nerve VIII, vestibulocochlear nerve); may cause hearing loss and may damage structures of the cerebellum as it grows
ceruminoma (se-_roo_-mi-NŌ-ma)	tumor of a gland that secretes earwax (cerumen)
cholesteatoma (_ko_-le-stē-a-TŌ-ma)	cystlike mass composed of epithelial cells and cholesterol occurring in the middle ear; may be associated with chronic otitis media
Ménière disease (me-NYĀR) (di-ZĒZ)	chronic disease of the inner ear characterized by a sensation of spinning motion (vertigo), ringing in the ear (tinnitus), aural fullness, and fluctuating hearing loss; symptoms are related to a change in volume or composition of fluid within the labyrinth
otitis externa (ō-TĪ-tis) (eks-TER-na)	inflammation of the outer ear (Figure 13-3)
otitis media (OM) (ō-TĪ-tis) (MĒ-dē-a)	inflammation of the middle ear (also called **tympanitis**) (Figure 13-4, _A_)

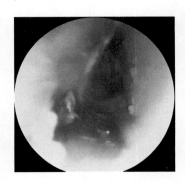

FIGURE 13-3
Otitis externa.

CAM TERM

Music and sound therapy is the use of music or sounds within a therapeutic relationship to address physical, emotional, cognitive, and social needs of individuals. Music and sound therapy studies have shown promising clinical efficacy in the treatment of **tinnitus**.

BENIGN PAROXYSMAL POSITIONAL VERTIGO (BPPV)

is characterized by brief episodes of vertigo associated with a change in the position of the head, such as turning over in bed or sitting up in the morning. In BPPV, normal calcium carbonate crystals called otoconia break loose and shift within the labyrinth, triggering an episode of vertigo.

Disease and Disorder Terms—cont'd

Not Built from Word Parts

TERM	DEFINITION
presbycusis (*prez*-bi-KŪ-sis)	hearing impairment occurring with age
tinnitus (tin-NĪ-tus)	ringing in the ears
vertigo (VER-ti-gō)	sense that either one's own body (subjective vertigo) or the environment (objective vertigo) is revolving; may indicate inner ear disease

 TINNITUS

Note the spelling of **tinnitus**. The ending is **itus** and not **itis**, the ending most familiar to you, meaning *inflammation*.

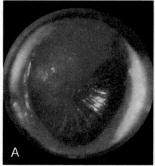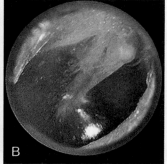

FIGURE 13-4

Otitis media. Signs include bulging, perforated, reddened, or retracted tympanic membrane. **A,** Tympanic membrane demonstrating **acute otitis media (AOM). B,** Normal tympanic membrane.

EXERCISE 8

Practice saying aloud each of the disease and disorder terms not built from word parts on pp. 561–562.

 To hear the terms, go to evolve.elsevier.com. Select: Chapter 13, **Exercises**, Pronunciation.

Refer to p. 10 for your Evolve Access Information.

☐ Place a check mark in the box when you have completed this exercise.

EXERCISE 9

Fill in the blanks with the correct terms.

1. The patient reported that her body seemed to be revolving, or _____, and ringing in the ears, or _____.
2. A chronic ear disease characterized by vertigo, tinnitus, aural fullness, and fluctuating hearing loss is called _____ disease.
3. Inflammation of the middle ear is called _____ _____.
4. _____ is the name given to a tumor of a gland that secretes earwax.
5. _____ _____ means inflammation of the outer ear.

6. A benign tumor arising from the acoustic nerve is called a(n) _____ _____.

7. _____ is hearing impairment occurring with age.

8. _____ may be associated with chronic otitis media.

EXERCISE **10**

Match the terms in the first column with the correct definitions in the second column.

_____ 1. vertigo

_____ 2. ceruminoma

_____ 3. tinnitus

_____ 4. Ménière disease

_____ 5. otitis externa

_____ 6. acoustic neuroma

_____ 7. otitis media

_____ 8. presbycusis

_____ 9. cholesteatoma

a. inflammation of the middle ear
b. tumor of a gland that secretes earwax
c. chronic ear problem characterized by vertigo, tinnitus, and fluctuating hearing loss
d. benign tumor arising from the acoustic nerve
e. sense of revolving of one's own body or the environment
f. hardening of the oval window
g. ringing in the ears
h. inflammation of the outer ear
i. hearing impairment occurring with age
j. mass composed of epithelial cells and cholesterol

EXERCISE **11**

Spell each of the disease and disorder terms not built from word parts on pp. 561–562 by having someone dictate them to you.

> To hear and spell the terms, go to evolve.elsevier.com. Select: Chapter 13, **Exercises**, Spelling.
>
> Ⓔ Refer to p. 10 for your Evolve Access Information.
>
> ☐ Place a check mark in the box if you have completed this exercise online.

1. _____
2. _____
3. _____
4. _____
5. _____

6. _____
7. _____
8. _____
9. _____

> For review and/or assessment, go to evolve.elsevier.com. Select:
> Chapter 13, **Activities**, Terms Not Built from Word Parts
> Ⓔ Chapter 13, **Games**,   Term Explorer
>
> Refer to p. 10 for your Evolve Access Information.

Surgical Terms

Built from Word Parts

The following terms are built from word parts you have already learned and can be translated literally to find their meanings. Further explanation of terms beyond the definition of their word parts, if needed, is included in parentheses.

TERM	DEFINITION
cochlear implant (KŌK-lē-ar) (IM-plant)	pertaining to the cochlea implant (surgically inserted electronic device that converts sound into electrical impulses. The impulses stimulate the auditory nerve to carry the signal to the brain which learns to interpret the signal as sound. The damaged part of the ear is bypassed (Figure 13-5).
labyrinthectomy (*lab*-i-rin-THEK-to-mē)	excision of the labyrinth
mastoidectomy (*mas*-toy-DEK-to-mē)	excision of the mastoid bone
mastoidotomy (*mas*-toy-DOT-o-mē)	incision into the mastoid bone
myringoplasty (mi-RING-gō-*plas*-tē)	surgical repair of the tympanic membrane
myringotomy (*mir*-ing-GOT-o-mē)	incision into the tympanic membrane (performed to release pus or fluid and relieve pressure in the middle ear) (also called **tympanocentesis**) (Exercise Figure B)
stapedectomy (*stā*-pe-DEK-to-mē)	excision of the stapes (performed to restore hearing in cases of otosclerosis; the stapes is replaced by a prosthesis) (Figure 13-6)
tympanoplasty (TIM-pa-nō-*plas*-tē)	surgical repair (of the hearing mechanism) of the middle ear (including the tympanic membrane and the ossicles)

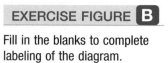

EXERCISE FIGURE B

Fill in the blanks to complete labeling of the diagram.

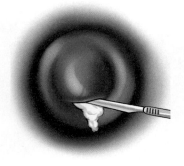

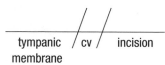

tympanic / cv / incision
membrane

is performed to release pus from the middle ear through the tympanic membrane to treat acute otitis media.

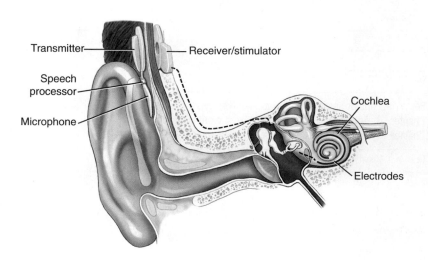

FIGURE 13-5
Cochlear implants are fitted in adults and children who are deaf or severely hard of hearing.

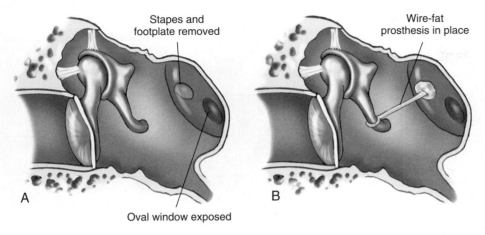

Stapes and
footplate removed

Wire-fat
prosthesis in place

A

B

Oval window exposed

FIGURE 13-6
Stapedectomy. **A,** Stapes is removed. **B,** Prosthesis is in place.

EXERCISE 12

Practice saying aloud each of the surgical terms built from word parts.

> (e) To hear the terms, go to evolve.elsevier.com. Select: Chapter 13, **Exercises**, Pronunciation.
>
> Refer to p. 10 for your Evolve Access Information.

☐ Place a check mark in the box when you have completed this exercise.

EXERCISE 13

Analyze and define the following surgical terms.

1. mastoidectomy _____
2. myringotomy _____
3. labyrinthectomy _____
4. mastoidotomy _____
5. tympanoplasty _____
6. myringoplasty _____
7. stapedectomy _____
8. cochlear implant _____

EXERCISE 14

Build surgical terms for the following definitions by using the word parts you have learned.

1. incision into the mastoid bone _____
   WR   CV   S

2. excision of the labyrinth _____
   WR   S

3. surgical repair (of the hearing
   mechanism) of the middle ear _____
   WR   CV   S

4. excision of the mastoid bone _____
   WR   S

5. incision into the tympanic membrane

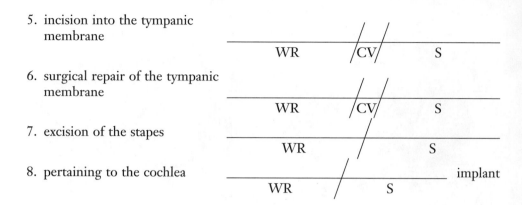

WR   /CV/   S

6. surgical repair of the tympanic membrane

WR   /CV/   S

7. excision of the stapes

WR   /   S

8. pertaining to the cochlea

WR   /   S   implant

EXERCISE 15

Spell each of the surgical terms built from word parts on p. 564 by having someone dictate them to you.

> To hear and spell the terms, go to evolve.elsevier.com. Select: Chapter 13, **Exercises**, Spelling.
>
> Refer to p. 10 for your Evolve Access Information.
>
> ☐ Place a check mark in the box if you have completed this exercise online.

1. _____   5. _____
2. _____   6. _____
3. _____   7. _____
4. _____   8. _____

Diagnostic Terms

Built from Word Parts

The following terms are built from word parts you have already learned and can be translated literally to find their meanings. Further explanation of terms beyond the definition of their word parts, if needed, is included in parentheses.

TERM	DEFINITION
audiogram (AW-dē-ō-*gram*)	(graphic) record of hearing (Figure 13-7, *B*)
audiometer (*aw*-dē-OM-e-ter)	instrument used to measure hearing (Figure 13-7, *A*)
audiometry (*aw*-dē-OM-e-trē)	measurement of hearing
electrocochleography (ē-*lek*-trō-*kok*-lē-OG-ra-fē)	process of recording the electrical activity in the cochlea (in response to sound)
otoscope (Ō-tō-skōp)	instrument used for visual examination of the ear (Exercise Figure C)
otoscopy (ō-TOS-ko-pē)	visual examination of the ear (Exercise Figure C)
tympanometer (*tim*-pa-NOM-e-ter)	instrument used to measure middle ear (function)
tympanometry (*tim*-pa-NOM-e-trē)	measurement (of movement) of the tympanic membrane

PURE-TONE AUDIOGRAM
Frequency (cycles/sec)

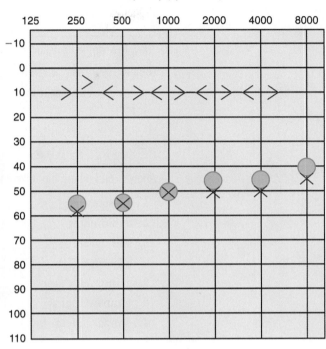

AUDIOGRAM KEY

	Air	Bone
Right	●	<
Left	×	>

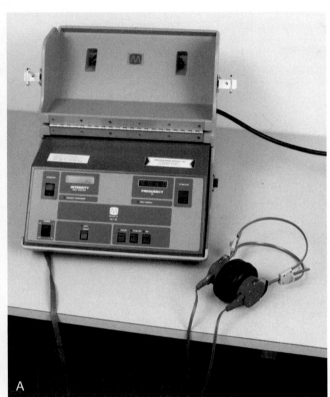

FIGURE 13-7
A, Audiometer. **B,** Audiogram.

EXERCISE FIGURE C

Fill in the blanks to label the diagram.

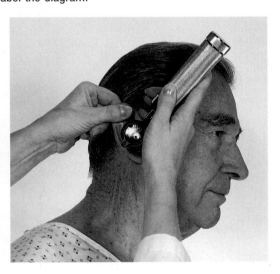

_____ / __ / _____ performed with an _____ / __ / _____
ear / cv / visual examination   ear / cv / instrument used for
                                                    visual examination

EXERCISE 16

Practice saying aloud each of the diagnostic terms built from word parts on p. 566.

> To hear the terms, go to evolve.elsevier.com. Select: Chapter 13, **Exercises**, Pronunciation.
>
> Refer to p. 10 for your Evolve Access Information.
>
> ☐ Place a check mark in the box when you have completed this exercise.

EXERCISE 17

Analyze and define the following diagnostic terms.

1. otoscope _____
2. audiometry _____
3. audiogram _____
4. otoscopy _____
5. audiometer _____
6. tympanometry_____
7. tympanometer_____
8. electrocochleography_____

EXERCISE 18

Build diagnostic terms that correspond to the following definitions by using the word parts you have learned.

1. measurement (of movement)
   of the tympanic membrane   _____ /____/ _____
                                  WR   CV   S

2. instrument used to measure
   hearing   _____ /____/ _____
                                  WR   CV   S

3. visual examination of the ear _____ /____/ _____
                                  WR   CV   S

4. (graphic) record of hearing   _____ /____/ _____
                                  WR   CV   S

5. instrument used for visual
   examination of the ear   _____ /____/ _____
                                  WR   CV   S

6. measurement of hearing   _____ /____/ _____
                                  WR   CV   S

7. instrument used to measure
   middle ear (function)   _____ /____/ _____
                                  WR   CV   S

8. process of recording the
   electrical activity in the cochlea ____ /__/ ____ /__/ __
                                  WR   CV   WR   CV   S

EXERCISE 19

Spell each of the diagnostic terms built from word parts on p. 566 by having someone dictate them to you.

> To hear and spell the terms, go to evolve.elsevier.com. Select: Chapter 13, **Exercises**, Spelling.
>
> Refer to p. 10 for your Evolve Access Information.
>
> ☐ Place a check mark in the box if you have completed this exercise online.

1. _____
2. _____
3. _____
4. _____

5. _____
6. _____
7. _____
8. _____

Complementary Terms

Built from Word Parts

The following terms are built from word parts you have already learned and can be translated literally to find their meanings. Further explanation of terms beyond the definition of their word parts, if needed, is included in parentheses.

TERM	DEFINITION
audiologist (*aw*-dē-OL-o-jist)	one who studies and specializes in hearing
audiology (*aw*-dē-OL-o-jē)	study of hearing
aural (AW-rul)	pertaining to the ear
cochlear (KOK-lē-ar)	pertaining to the cochlea
otologist (ō-TOL-o-jist)	physician who studies and treats diseases of the ear
otology (ō-TOL-o-jē)	study of the ear (a branch of medicine that deals with diseases of the ear)
otorhinolaryngologist (ō-tō-*rī*-nō-*lar*-ing-GOL-o-jist)	physician who studies and treats diseases of the ear, nose, and larynx (throat) (also called **otolaryngologist**)
vestibular (ves-TIB-ū-lar)	pertaining to the vestibule
vestibulocochlear (ves-*tib*-ū-lō-KOK-lē-ar)	pertaining to the vestibule and the cochlea

🔍 Refer to **Appendix D** for pharmacology terms related to the ear.

EXERCISE 20

Practice saying aloud each of the complementary terms built from word parts on p. 569.

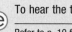 To hear the terms, go to evolve.elsevier.com. Select: Chapter 13, **Exercises**, Pronunciation.

Refer to p. 10 for your Evolve Access Information.

☐ Place a check mark in the box when you have completed this exercise.

EXERCISE 21

Analyze and define the following complementary terms.

1. otology_____
2. audiologist_____
3. otorhinolaryngologist _____
4. audiology_____
5. otologist_____
6. aural_____
7. cochlear_____
8. vestibular_____
9. vestibulocochlear _____

EXERCISE 22

Build the complementary terms for the following definitions by using the word parts you have learned.

1. study of hearing

   _____ / _____ / _____
   WR   CV   S

2. physician who studies and treats diseases of the ear, nose, and larynx (throat)

   _____ / ___ / _____ / ___ / _____ / ___ / ___
   WR   CV   WR   CV   WR   CV   S

3. study of the ear

   _____ / _____ / _____
   WR   CV   S

4. one who studies and specializes in hearing

   _____ / _____ / _____
   WR   CV   S

5. physician who studies and treats diseases of the ear

   _____ / _____ / _____
   WR   CV   S

6. pertaining to the ear

   _____ / _____ / _____
   WR   /   S

7. pertaining to the vestibule and the cochlea

   _____ / ___ / _____ / _____
   WR   CV   WR   /   S

8. pertaining to the vestibule

   _____ / _____ / _____
   WR   /   S

9. pertaining to the cochlea

   _____ / _____ / _____
   WR   /   S

EXERCISE 23

Spell each of the complementary terms built from word parts on p. 569 by having someone dictate them to you.

> To hear and spell the terms, go to evolve.elsevier.com. Select: Chapter 13, **Exercises**, Spelling.
>
> Refer to p. 10 for your Evolve Access Information.
>
> ☐ Place a check mark in the box if you have completed this exercise online.

1. _____   6. _____
2. _____   7. _____
3. _____   8. _____
4. _____   9. _____
5. _____

> For review and/or assessment, go to evolve.elsevier.com. Select:
> Chapter 13, **Activities**, Terms Built from Word Parts
>   Hear It and Type It: Clinical Vignettes
> Chapter 13, **Games,**   Term Storm
>   Termbusters
>   Medical Millionaire
>
> Refer to p. 10 for your Evolve Access Information.

Abbreviations

ABBREVIATION	MEANING
AOM	acute otitis media
EENT	eyes, ears, nose, and throat
ENT	ears, nose, throat
OM	otitis media

EXERCISE 24

Write the meaning of the following abbreviations.

1. ENT _____ _____ _____
2. EENT _____ _____ _____ and _____
3. OM _____ _____
4. AOM _____ _____ _____

> For more practice with abbreviations, go to evolve.elsevier.com. Select:
> Chapter 13, **Flashcards**
> Chapter 13, **Games,** Crossword Puzzle
>
> Refer to p. 10 for your Evolve Access Information.

PRACTICAL APPLICATION

EXERCISE 25   *Interact with Medical Documents and Electronic Health Records*

A. Complete the progress note by writing the medical terms in the blanks. Use the list of definitions with the corresponding numbers.

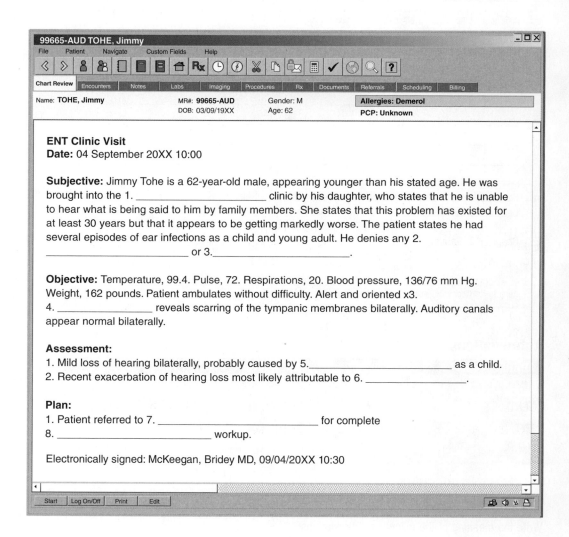

> **99665-AUD TOHE, Jimmy**   _ □ X
> File   Patient   Navigate   Custom Fields   Help
>
> Chart Review | Encounters | Notes | Labs | Imaging | Procedures | Rx | Documents | Referrals | Scheduling | Billing
>
> Name: **TOHE, Jimmy**   MR#: **99665-AUD**   Gender: M   **Allergies: Demerol**
>   DOB: 03/09/19XX   Age: 62   **PCP: Unknown**
>
> **ENT Clinic Visit**
> **Date:** 04 September 20XX 10:00
>
> **Subjective:** Jimmy Tohe is a 62-year-old male, appearing younger than his stated age. He was
> brought into the 1. _____ clinic by his daughter, who states that he is unable
> to hear what is being said to him by family members. She states that this problem has existed for
> at least 30 years but that it appears to be getting markedly worse. The patient states he had
> several episodes of ear infections as a child and young adult. He denies any 2.
> _____ or 3. _____.
>
> **Objective:** Temperature, 99.4. Pulse, 72. Respirations, 20. Blood pressure, 136/76 mm Hg.
> Weight, 162 pounds. Patient ambulates without difficulty. Alert and oriented x3.
> 4. _____ reveals scarring of the tympanic membranes bilaterally. Auditory canals
> appear normal bilaterally.
>
> **Assessment:**
> 1. Mild loss of hearing bilaterally, probably caused by 5. _____ as a child.
> 2. Recent exacerbation of hearing loss most likely attributable to 6. _____.
>
> **Plan:**
> 1. Patient referred to 7. _____ for complete
> 8. _____ workup.
>
> Electronically signed: McKeegan, Bridey MD, 09/04/20XX 10:30
>
> Start | Log On/Off | Print | Edit

1. abbreviation for ears, nose, and throat
2. ringing in the ears
3. sense of one's own body or the environment revolving
4. visual examination of the ear
5. inflammation of the middle ear
6. hearing impairment occurring with age
7. one who studies and specializes in hearing
8. measurement of hearing

B. Read the clinical notes report and answer the questions following it.

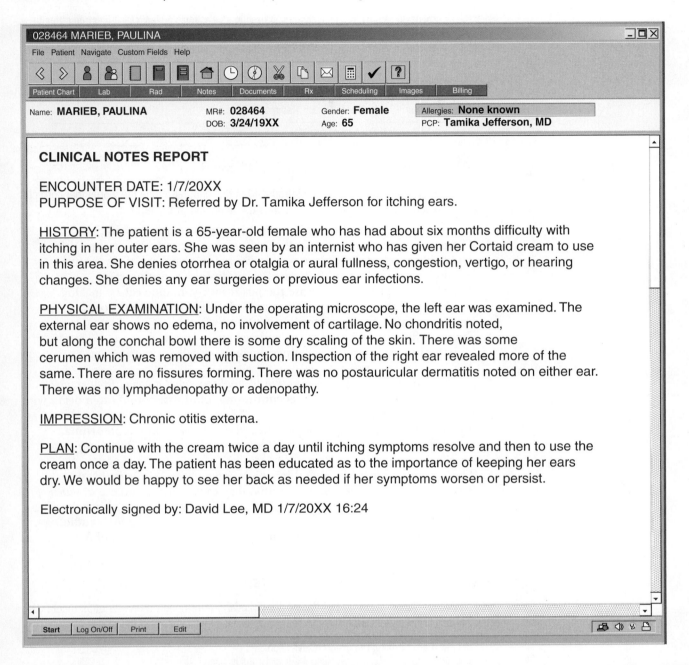

028464 MARIEB, PAULINA

File Patient Navigate Custom Fields Help

| Patient Chart | Lab | Rad | Notes | Documents | Rx | Scheduling | Images | Billing |

Name: **MARIEB, PAULINA** MR#: **028464** Gender: **Female** Allergies: **None known**
DOB: **3/24/19XX** Age: **65** PCP: **Tamika Jefferson, MD**

CLINICAL NOTES REPORT

ENCOUNTER DATE: 1/7/20XX
PURPOSE OF VISIT: Referred by Dr. Tamika Jefferson for itching ears.

HISTORY: The patient is a 65-year-old female who has had about six months difficulty with itching in her outer ears. She was seen by an internist who has given her Cortaid cream to use in this area. She denies otorrhea or otalgia or aural fullness, congestion, vertigo, or hearing changes. She denies any ear surgeries or previous ear infections.

PHYSICAL EXAMINATION: Under the operating microscope, the left ear was examined. The external ear shows no edema, no involvement of cartilage. No chondritis noted, but along the conchal bowl there is some dry scaling of the skin. There was some cerumen which was removed with suction. Inspection of the right ear revealed more of the same. There are no fissures forming. There was no postauricular dermatitis noted on either ear. There was no lymphadenopathy or adenopathy.

IMPRESSION: Chronic otitis externa.

PLAN: Continue with the cream twice a day until itching symptoms resolve and then to use the cream once a day. The patient has been educated as to the importance of keeping her ears dry. We would be happy to see her back as needed if her symptoms worsen or persist.

Electronically signed by: David Lee, MD 1/7/20XX 16:24

Start | Log On/Off | Print | Edit

1. The patient has been experiencing:
   a. itchiness
   b. hearing loss
   c. otalgia
   d. vertigo
2. In the patient's left ear, suction removed:
   a. scaling
   b. cerumen
   c. chondritis
   d. otorrhea

3. The patient's condition has been diagnosed as chronic:
   a. abnormal condition of fungus in the ear
   b. inflammation of the tympanic membrane
   c. hardening of the stapes
   d. inflammation of the outer ear

C. Complete the **three medical documents** within the electronic health record (EHR) on Evolve.

Many healthcare records today are stored and used in an electronic system called **Electronic Health Records (EHR).** Electronic health records contain a collection of health information of an individual patient; the digitally formatted record can be shared through computer networks with patients, physicians, and other health care providers.

For practice with medical terms using electronic health records, go to evolve.elsevier.com.
Select: Chapter 13, **Electronic Health Records.**

Refer to p. 10 for your Evolve Access Information.

EXERCISE 26   *Interpret Medical Terms*

To test your understanding of the terms introduced in this chapter, circle the words that correctly complete the sentences. The italicized phrase is the definition of the term.

1. *Inflammation of the eardrum* is (**labyrinthitis, mastoiditis, myringitis**).
2. The patient reported *ringing in the ears*, or (**tinnitus, vertigo, tympanitis**).
3. The patient seeking a *physician who studies and treats diseases of the ear* for labyrinthitis consulted an (**optometrist, audiologist, otologist**).
4. The physician planned to release the pus from the middle ear by making an *incision in the tympanic membrane*, or performing a (**mastoidotomy, myringotomy, labyrinthectomy**).
5. Tinnitus, fluctuating hearing loss, and vertigo in *chronic disease of the inner ear* (**mastoiditis, Ménière disease, presbycusis**) usually occur in episodes that can last for several days.
6. Manifestations of *benign tumor within the auditory canal growing from cranial nerve VIII* (**acoustic neuroma, ceruminoma, cholesteatoma**) often begin with tinnitus and gradual hearing loss.
7. A *cystlike mass composed of epithelial cells and cholesterol* (**acoustic neuroma, ceruminoma, cholesteatoma**) may destroy adjacent bones, including the ossicles.
8. Thought to be caused by a viral infection, *inflammation of the inner ear* (**labyrinthitis, mastoiditis, myringitis**) may cause sudden intense *sensation of revolving* (**tinnitus, vertigo, presbycusis**), nausea, vomiting, and imbalance.
9. *Process of recording electrical activity in the cochlea in response to sound* (**audiology, electrocochleography, otoscopy**) may be used in the diagnosis of Ménière disease.

EXERCISE 27   *Read Medical Terms in Use*

Practice pronunciation of terms by reading the following information on acute otitis media. Use the pronunciation key following the medical term to assist you in saying the words.

To hear these terms, go to evolve.elsevier.com.
Select: Chapter 13, **Exercises**, Read Medical Terms in Use.

Refer to p. 10 for your Evolve Access Information.

ACUTE OTITIS MEDIA

Acute **otitis media** (ō-TĪ-tis) (MĒ-dē-a) is one of the most common pediatric infections. Most middle ear infections are caused by bacteria, and some by viruses. Symptoms include **otalgia** (ō-TAL-ja), **otorrhea** (ō-tō-RĒ-a), ear pulling, and irritability. The tympanic membrane will be bulging, red in color, with a thickened appearance and reduced translucency. Antibiotics may be ordered if the infection does not resolve on its own. If unresponsive to antibiotic treatment, a **myringotomy** (*mir*-ing-GOT-o-mē) may be performed to identify the causative pathogen, allowing for the appropriate antibiotic treatment to be prescribed.

EXERCISE 28 *Comprehend Medical Terms in Use*

Test your comprehension of terms in the previous passage by answering T for true and F for false.

_____ 1. Inflammation of the outer ear is one of the most common pediatric infections.

_____ 2. Pain and discharge from the ear are symptoms of acute otitis media.

_____ 3. Surgical repair of the tympanic membrane may be performed to identify causative organisms.

For a snapshot assessment of your knowledge of medical terms for the ear, go to evolve.elsevier.com.

Select: Chapter 13, **Quick Quizzes.**

Refer to p. 10 for your Evolve Access Information.

CHAPTER REVIEW

Review of Evolve

Keep a record of the online activities you have completed by placing a check mark in the box. You may also record your scores. All activities have been referenced throughout the chapter.

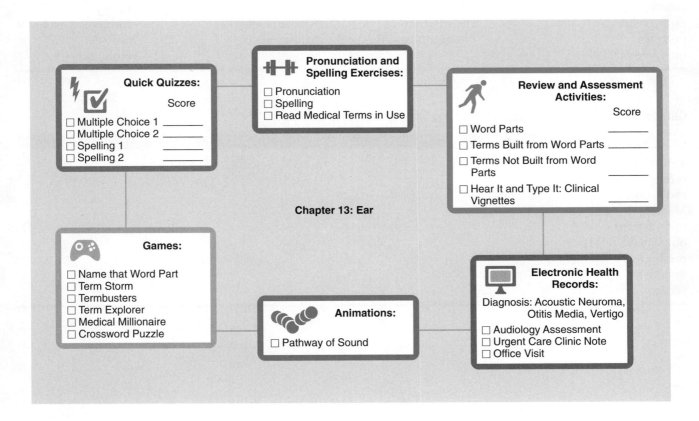

Review of Word Parts

Can you define and spell the following word parts?

COMBINING FORMS

audi/o	myring/o
aur/i	ot/o
aur/o	staped/o
cochle/o	tympan/o
labyrinth/o	vestibul/o
mastoid/o	

Review of Terms

Can you build, analyze, define, pronounce, and spell the following terms *built from word parts*?

DISEASES AND DISORDERS	SURGICAL	DIAGNOSTIC	COMPLEMENTARY
labyrinthitis	cochlear implant	audiogram	audiologist
mastoiditis	labyrinthectomy	audiometer	audiology
myringitis	mastoidectomy	audiometry	aural
otalgia	mastoidotomy	electrocochleography	cochlear
otomastoiditis	myringoplasty	otoscope	otologist
otomycosis	myringotomy	otoscopy	otology
otopyorrhea	stapedectomy	tympanometer	otorhinolaryngologist
otorrhea	tympanoplasty	tympanometry	vestibular
otosclerosis			vestibulocochlear

Can you define, pronounce, and spell the following terms not *built from word parts*?

DISEASES AND DISORDERS

acoustic neuroma
ceruminoma
cholesteatoma
Ménière disease
otitis externa
otitis media (OM)
presbycusis
tinnitus
vertigo

ANSWERS TO CHAPTER 13 EXERCISES
Exercise Figures

Exercise Figure

A. 1. ear: aur/i, aur/o, ot/o
2. labyrinth: labyrinth/o
3. stapes: staped/o
4. tympanic membrane: myring/o, tympan/o
5. mastoid bone: mastoid/o

Exercise Figure

B. myring/o/tomy

Exercise Figure

C. ot/o/scopy, ot/o/scope

Exercise 1

1. f
2. i
3. b
4. e
5. g

6. j
7. d

8. a
9. c

Exercise 2

1. stapes
2. mastoid bone
3. hearing
4. ear
5. tympanic membrane (eardrum), middle ear
6. vestibule
7. labyrinth
8. tympanic membrane (eardrum)
9. cochlea

Exercise 3

1. a. aur/i
   b. aur/o
   c. ot/o
2. mastoid/o
3. staped/o
4. tympan/o
5. labyrinth/o
6. audi/o
7. myring/o
8. cochle/o
9. vestibul/o

Exercise 4

Pronunciation Exercise

Exercise 5

Note: The combining form is identified by italic and bold print.

1. WR CV WR S
   ot/o/myc/osis
     CF
   abnormal condition of fungus in the ear

2. WR CV WR   S
   ot/o/mastoid/itis
     CF
   inflammation of the ear and the mastoid bone

3. WR S
   ot/algia
   pain in the ear

4.   WR   S
   labyrinth/itis
   inflammation of the labyrinth

5.   WR   S
   myring/itis
   inflammation of the tympanic membrane

6. WR CV S
   ot/o/sclerosis
     CF
   hardening of the ear (stapes)

7.   WR   S
   mastoid/itis
   inflammation of the mastoid bone

8. WR CV WR CV S
   ot/o/**py/o**/rrhea
     CF   CF
   discharge of pus from the ear

9. WR CV S
   ot/o/rrhea
     CF
   discharge from the ear

Exercise 6

1. myring/itis
2. ot/o/py/o/rrhea
3. mastoid/itis
4. ot/algia
5. ot/o/sclerosis
6. ot/o/myc/osis
7. ot/o/mastoid/itis
8. labyrinth/itis
9. ot/o/rrhea

Exercise 7

Spelling Exercise; see text p. 561.

Exercise 8

Pronunciation Exercise

Exercise 9

1. vertigo; tinnitus
2. Ménière
3. otitis media
4. ceruminoma
5. otitis externa

6. acoustic neuroma
7. presbycusis
8. cholesteatoma

Exercise 10

1. e
2. b
3. g
4. c
5. h

6. d
7. a
8. i
9. j

Exercise 11

Spelling Exercise; see text p. 563.

Exercise 12

Pronunciation Exercise

Exercise 13

Note: The combining form is identified by italic and bold print.

1.   WR   S
   mastoid/ectomy
   excision of the mastoid bone

2.   WR   CV S
   myring/o/tomy
        CF
   incision into the tympanic membrane

3.   WR   S
   labyrinth/ectomy
   excision of the labyrinth

4.   WR   CV S
   mastoid/o/tomy
        CF
   incision into the mastoid bone

5.   WR   CV   S
   tympan/o/plasty
        CF
   surgical repair of the middle ear

6.   WR   CV   S
   myring/o/plasty
        CF
   surgical repair of the tympanic membrane

7.   WR   S
   staped/ectomy
   excision of the stapes

8.   WR   S
   cochle/ar implant
   pertaining to the cochlea implant

Exercise 14

1. mastoid/o/tomy
2. labyrinth/ectomy

3. tympan/o/plasty
4. mastoid/ectomy
5. myring/o/tomy
6. myring/o/plasty
7. staped/ectomy
8. cochle/ar implant

Exercise 15
Spelling Exercise; see text p. 566.

Exercise 16
Pronunciation Exercise

Exercise 17
Note: The combining form is identified by italic and bold print.
1. WR CV S
   ***ot/o*/**scope
       CF
   instrument used for visual examination of the ear
2. WR CV S
   ***audi/o*/**metry
           CF
   measurement of hearing
3. WR CV S
   ***audi/o*/**gram
          CF
   (graphic) record of hearing
4. WR CV S
   ***ot/o*/**scopy
       CF
   visual examination of the ear
5. WR CV S
   ***audi/o*/**meter
           CF
   instrument used to measure hearing
6. WR CV S
   ***tympan/o*/**metry
              CF
   measurement (of movement) of the tympanic membrane
7. WR CV S
   ***tympan/o*/**meter
              CF
   instrument used to measure middle ear (function)
8. WR CV WR CV S
   ***electr/o*/*cochle/o*/**graphy
           CF   CF
   process of recording the electrical activity in the cochlea

Exercise 18
1. tympan/o/metry
2. audi/o/meter

3. ot/o/scopy
4. audi/o/gram
5. ot/o/scope
6. audi/o/metry
7. tympan/o/meter
8. electr/o/cochle/o/graphy

Exercise 19
Spelling Exercise; see text p. 569.

Exercise 20
Pronunciation Exercise

Exercise 21
Note: The combining form is identified by italic and bold print.
1. WR CV S
   ***ot/o*/**logy
       CF
   study of the ear
2. WR CV S
   ***audi/o*/**logist
           CF
   one who studies and specializes in hearing
3. WR CV WR CV WR CV S
   ***ot/o*/*rhin/o*/*laryng/o*/**logist
       CF   CF   CF
   physician who studies and treats diseases of the ear, nose, and larynx (throat)
4. WR CV S
   ***audi/o*/**logy
           CF
   study of hearing
5. WR CV S
   ***ot/o*/**logist
       CF
   physician who studies and treats diseases of the ear
6. WR S
   aur/al
   pertaining to the ear
7. WR S
   cochle/ar
   pertaining to the cochlea
8. WR S
   vestibul/ar
   pertaining to the vestibule
9. WR CV WR S
   ***vestibul/o*/**cochle/ar
              CF
   pertaining to the vestibule and cochlea

Exercise 22
1. audi/o/logy
2. ot/o/rhin/o/laryng/o/logist
3. ot/o/logy
4. audi/o/logist
5. ot/o/logist
6. aur/al
7. vestibul/o/cochle/ar
8. vestibul/ar
9. cochle/ar

Exercise 23
Spelling Exercise; see text p. 571.

Exercise 24
1. ears, nose, throat
2. eyes, ears, nose, and throat
3. otitis media
4. acute otitis media

Exercise 25
A. 1. ENT
        2. tinnitus
        3. vertigo
        4. otoscopy
        5. otitis media
        6. presbycusis
        7. audiologist
        8. audiometry
B. 1. a
        2. b
        3. d
C. Online Exercise

Exercise 26
1. myringitis
2. tinnitus
3. otologist
4. myringotomy
5. Ménière disease
6. acoustic neuroma
7. cholesteatoma
8. labyrinthitis, vertigo
9. electrocochleography

Exercise 27
Reading Exercise

Exercise 28
1. *F,* inflammation of the middle ear (otitis media) is one of the most common pediatric infection.
2. *T*
3. *F,* myringotomy, incision into the tympanic membrane, would be performed.

Musculoskeletal System

Outline

Objectives

Upon completion of this chapter you will be able to:

1 Identify organs and structures of the
   musculoskeletal system.

2 Identify and define types of body
   movement.

3 Define and spell word parts related to the
   musculoskeletal system.

4 Define, pronounce, and spell disease and
   disorder terms related to the
   musculoskeletal system.

5 Define, pronounce, and spell surgical terms
   related to the musculoskeletal system.

6 Define, pronounce, and spell diagnostic
   terms related to the musculoskeletal
   system.

7 Define, pronounce, and spell
   complementary terms related to the
   musculoskeletal system.

8 Interpret the meaning of abbreviations
   related to the musculoskeletal system.

9 Interpret, read, and comprehend medical
   language in simulated medical statements,
   documents, and electronic health records.

ANATOMY

The musculoskeletal system consists of muscles, bones (Figure 14-1), bone marrow, joints, cartilage, tendons, ligaments, and bursae. The adult human skeleton contains 206 bones (Figure 14-2 and Figure 14-3, *A* and *B*) and more than 600 muscles. Joints are located where two or more bones meet, and contain cartilage and bursae.

Function

The functions of the muscular system are movement, posture, joint stability, and heat production. The functions of the skeletal system are to provide a framework for the body, protect the soft body parts such as the brain, store calcium, and produce blood cells. The organs and structures of the musculoskeletal system work together to protect, support, and move the body.

Bone Structure

PERIOSTEUM

is composed of the prefix **peri-**, meaning **surrounding**, and the word root **oste**, meaning **bone**.

ENDOSTEUM

is composed of the prefix **endo-**, meaning **within**, and the word root **oste**, meaning **bone**.

TERM	DEFINITION
periosteum	outermost layer of the bone, made up of fibrous tissue
compact bone	dense, hard layers of bone tissue that lie underneath the periosteum
cancellous (spongy) bone	contains little spaces like a sponge and is encased in the layers of compact bone
endosteum	membranous lining of the hollow cavity of the bone

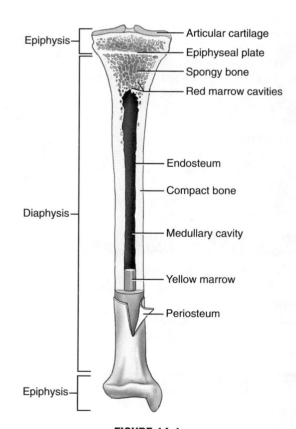

FIGURE 14-1
Bone structure.

TERM	DEFINITION
diaphysis	shaft of the long bones (Figure 14-1)
epiphysis (pl. epiphyses)	end of each long bone (Figure 14-1)
bone marrow	material found in the cavities of bones
red marrow	thick, bloodlike material found in flat bones and the ends of long bones; location of blood cell formation
yellow marrow	soft, fatty material found in the medullary cavity of long bones

Skeletal Bones

TERM	DEFINITION
maxilla	upper jawbone
mandible	lower jawbone
vertebral column	made up of bones called **vertebrae** *(pl.)* or **vertebra** *(sing.)* through which the spinal cord runs. The vertebral column protects the spinal cord, supports the head, and provides points of attachment for ribs and muscles (Figure 14-2).
cervical vertebrae (C1 to C7)	first set of seven bones, forming the neck

🏛 **DIAPHYSIS**

comes from the Greek **diaphusis,** meaning state of growing between.

🏛 **EPIPHYSIS**

has been used in the English language since the 1600s and retains the meaning given to it by a Greco-Roman physician. It means a **portion of bone attached for a time to another bone** by a cartilage, but that later combines with the principal bone. During the period of growth, the epiphysis is separated from the main portion of the bone by cartilage.

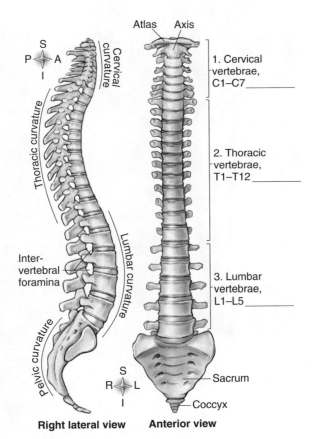

FIGURE 14-2
Vertebral column, right lateral view and anterior view.

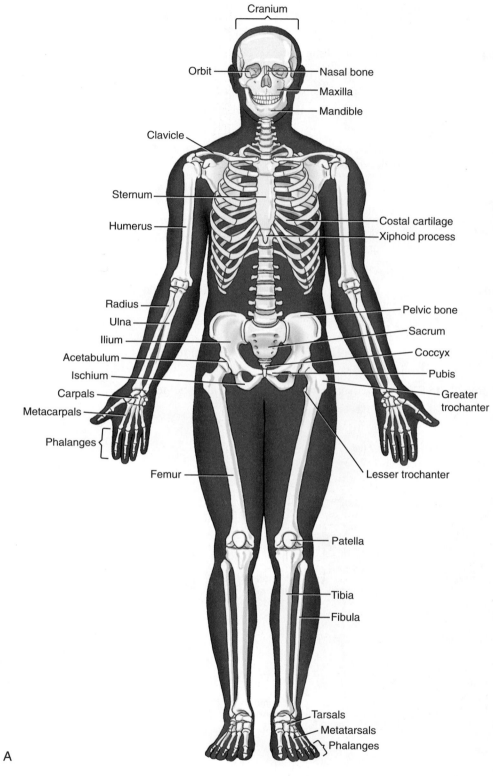

FIGURE 14-3
A, Anterior view of the skeleton.

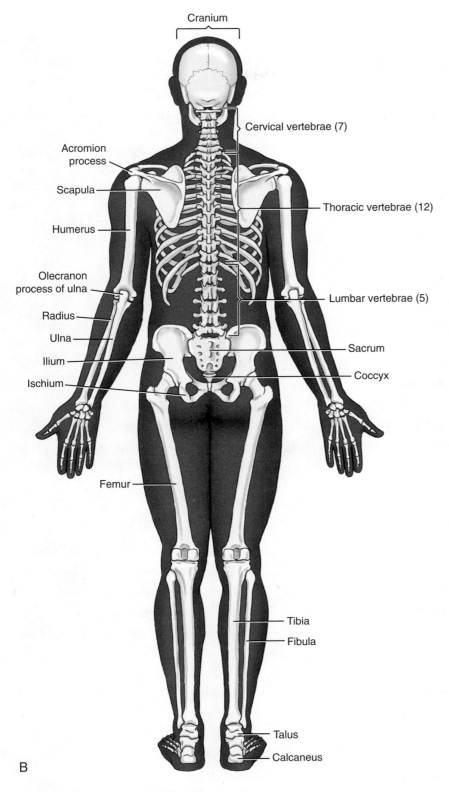

Cranium

Cervical vertebrae (7)

Acromion process

Scapula

Humerus

Thoracic vertebrae (12)

Olecranon process of ulna

Radius

Ulna

Ilium

Ischium

Lumbar vertebrae (5)

Sacrum

Coccyx

Femur

Tibia

Fibula

Talus

Calcaneus

B

FIGURE 14-3, cont'd
B, Posterior view of the skeleton.

Skeletal Bones—cont'd

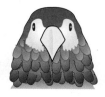

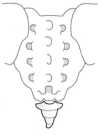

Coccyx is derived from the Greek word *cuckoo* because of its resemblance to a cuckoo's beak.

TERM	DEFINITION
thoracic vertebrae (T1 to T12)	second set of 12 vertebrae. They articulate with the 12 pairs of ribs to form the outward curve of the spine.
lumbar vertebrae (L1 to L5)	third set of five larger vertebrae, which forms the inward curve of the spine
sacrum	next five vertebrae, which fuse together to form a triangular bone positioned between the two hip bones, forming joints called the **sacroiliac joints**
coccyx	four vertebrae fused together to form the tailbone
lamina (pl. laminae)	part of the vertebral arch
clavicle	collarbone
scapula	shoulder blade
acromion process	extension of the scapula, which forms the superior point of the shoulder
sternum	breastbone
xiphoid process	lower portion of the sternum
humerus	upper arm bone
ulna and radius	lower arm bones
olecranon process	projection at the proximal end of the ulna that forms the bony point of the elbow
carpal bones	wrist bones
metacarpal bones	hand bones
phalanges (sing. phalanx)	finger and toe bones
pelvic bone, hip bone	made up of three bones fused together
ischium	lower, posterior portion on which one sits
ilium	upper, wing-shaped part on each side
pubis	anterior portion of the pelvic bone
acetabulum	large socket in the pelvic bone for the head of the femur
femur	upper leg bone
tibia and fibula	lower leg bones
patella (pl. patellae)	kneecap
tarsal bones	ankle bones
calcaneus	heel bone
metatarsal bones	foot bones

EXERCISE 1

Match the definitions in the first column with the correct terms in the second column. *To check your answers to the exercises in this chapter, go to Answers, p. 640, at the end of the chapter.*

_____ 1. shaft of a long bone

_____ 2. hard layer of bone tissue

_____ 3. outermost layer of bone

_____ 4. found in bone cavities

_____ 5. lining of the bone cavity

_____ 6. end of each long bone

_____ 7. contains little spaces

_____ 8. socket in the pelvic bone

_____ 9. heel bone

_____ 10. part of the arch of the vertebra

a. lamina
b. cancellous bone
c. acetabulum
d. diaphysis
e. endometrium
f. calcaneus
g. epiphysis
h. periosteum
i. compact bone
j. endosteum
k. bone marrow

EXERCISE 2

Write the name of the bone to match the definition.

1. shoulder blade _____

2. breastbone_____

3. lower jawbone_____

4. collarbone _____

5. upper arm bone _____

6. lower arm bones   a. _____

                     b. _____

7. ankle bones _____

8. finger, toe bones_____

9. foot bones _____

10. hand bones _____

11. upper leg bone _____

12. lower leg bones   a. _____

                     b. _____

13. kneecap _____

14. neck _____

15. vertebrae of lower back _____

16. anterior portion of the pelvic bone _____

17. five vertebrae fused together_____

18. posterior portion of the pelvic bone _____

19. tailbone _____

20. upper, wing-shaped part of the pelvic bone _____

21. wrist bones _____

Joints

Joints, also called **articulations**, hold our bones together and make movement possible (in most joints) (Figure 14-4).

TERM	DEFINITION
articular cartilage	smooth layer of firm, fibrous tissue covering the contacting surface of joints
meniscus	crescent-shaped cartilage found in the knee
intervertebral disk	cartilaginous pad found between the vertebrae in the spine
pubic symphysis	cartilaginous joint at which two pubic bones come together anteriorly at the midline
synovia	fluid secreted by the synovial membrane and found in joint cavities
bursa (pl. bursae)	fluid-filled sac that allows for easy movement of one part of a joint over another
ligament	flexible, tough band of fibrous connective tissue that attaches one bone to another at a joint
tendon	band of fibrous connective tissue that attaches muscle to bone
aponeurosis	strong sheet of tissue that acts as a tendon to attach muscles to bone

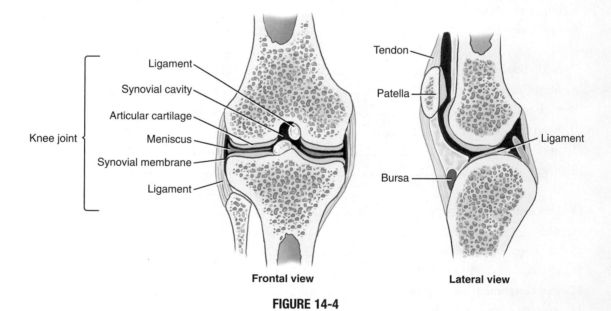

Frontal view   **Lateral view**

FIGURE 14-4
Knee joint.

Muscles

TERM	DEFINITION
skeletal muscles (also known as striated muscles)	attached to bones by tendons and make body movement possible. Skeletal muscles produce action by pulling and by working in pairs. They are also known as **voluntary muscles** because we have control over these muscles (Figure 14-5 and Figure 14-6, *A* and *B*).

TERM	DEFINITION
smooth muscles (also known as unstriated muscles)	located in internal organs such as the walls of blood vessels and the digestive tract. They are also called **involuntary muscles** because they respond to impulses from the autonomic nerves and are not controlled voluntarily (see Figure 14-5, *B*).
cardiac muscle (known as myocardium)	forms most of the wall of the heart. Its involuntary contraction produces the heartbeat (see Figure 14-5, *B*).

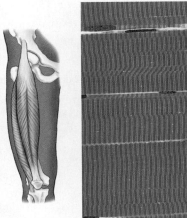
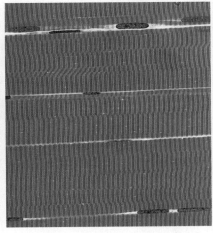
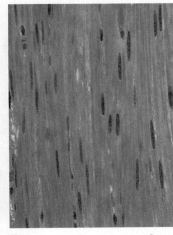
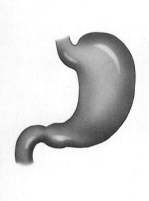

A   Skeletal muscle   B   Smooth muscle

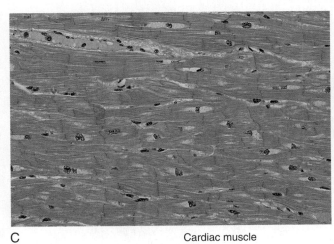
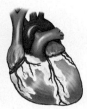

C   Cardiac muscle

FIGURE 14-5
Types of muscle tissue.

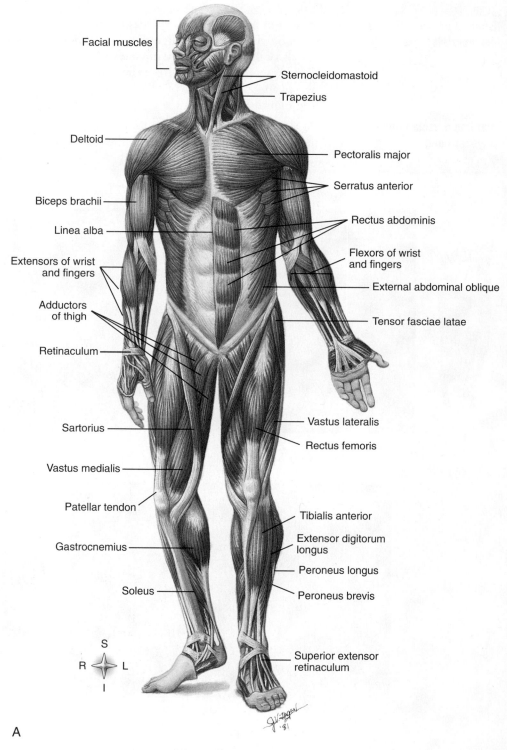

FIGURE 14-6
A, Anterior view of the muscular system.

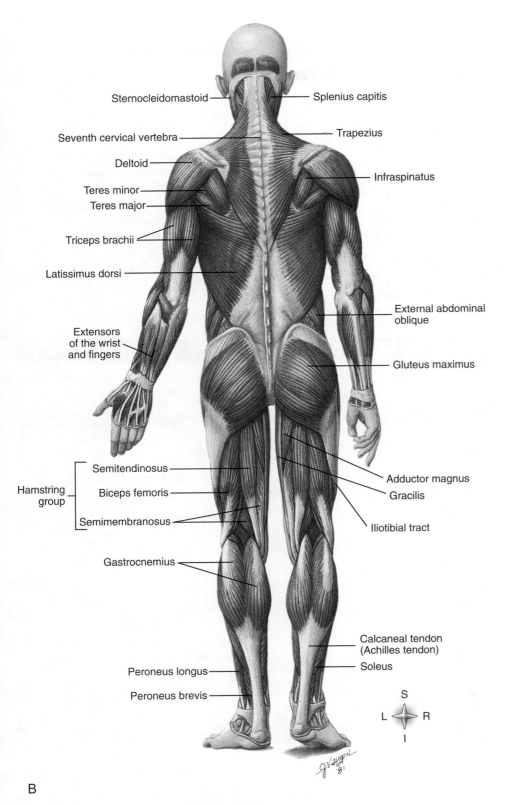

Sternocleidomastoid

Splenius capitis

Seventh cervical vertebra

Trapezius

Deltoid

Infraspinatus

Teres minor

Teres major

Triceps brachii

Latissimus dorsi

External abdominal oblique

Extensors of the wrist and fingers

Gluteus maximus

Adductor magnus

Hamstring group

Semitendinosus

Biceps femoris

Gracilis

Semimembranosus

Iliotibial tract

Gastrocnemius

Calcaneal tendon (Achilles tendon)

Peroneus longus

Soleus

Peroneus brevis

S

L ✦ R

I

B

FIGURE 14-6, cont'd
B, Posterior view of the muscular system.

EXERCISE 3

Match the definitions in the first column with the correct terms in the second column.

_____ 1. attaches muscle to bone
_____ 2. fluid-filled sac
_____ 3. smooth layer of fibrous tissue
_____ 4. voluntary muscles
_____ 5. fluid
_____ 6. located in the internal organs
_____ 7. attaches bone to bone
_____ 8. cartilage found in the knee
_____ 9. pubic bone joint
_____ 10. acts as a tendon
_____ 11. found between each vertebra
_____ 12. produces heartbeat

a. skeletal muscles
b. aponeurosis
c. bursa
d. smooth muscles
e. cartilage
f. intervertebral disk
g. cardiac muscles
h. ligament
i. meniscus
j. periosteum
k. pubic symphysis
l. synovia
m. tendon

🔍 TYPES OF BODY MOVEMENT

Bones and muscles work together to produce various types of body movement. Some are listed below (Figure 14-7).

MIDLINE VS. MIDDLE

The two terms are synonyms, both describing an imaginary line that separates the body, or body part, into equal halves. In medical language, *midline* is the preferred term and is used as a common reference point.

TERM	DEFINITION
abduction (ab-DUK-shun)	moving away from the midline
adduction (ad-DUK-shun)	moving toward the midline
inversion (in-VER-zhun)	turning inward
eversion (ē-VER-zhun)	turning outward
extension (ek-STEN-shun)	movement in which a limb is placed in a straight position, increasing the angle between the bone and the joint
flexion (FLEK-shun)	movement in which a limb is bent, decreasing the angle between the bone and the joint
pronation (prō-NĀ-shun)	movement that turns the palm down
supination (sū-pi-NĀ-shun)	movement that turns the palm up
rotation (rō-TĀ-shun)	turning around its own axis

To watch animations, go to evolve.elsevier.com. Select: Chapter 14, **Animations**, Muscle Range of Motion.

Refer to p. 10 for your Evolve Access Information.

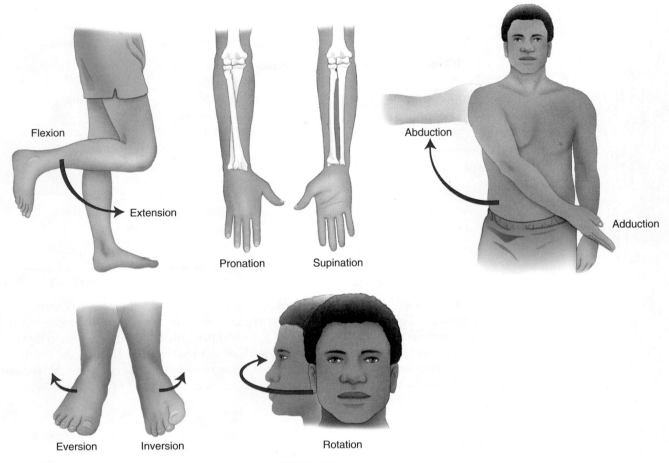

Flexion

Extension

Pronation

Supination

Abduction

Adduction

Eversion   Inversion

Rotation

FIGURE 14-7
Types of body movements.

EXERCISE 4

Write the definitions of the following terms.

1. abduction_____
2. pronation_____
3. supination _____
4. rotation _____
5. extension _____
6. eversion _____
7. adduction_____
8. flexion _____
9. inversion _____

EXERCISE 5

Match the terms in the first column with the correct definitions in the second column.

_____ 1. abduction	a. movement in which the limb is placed in a straight position
_____ 2. adduction	b. movement that turns the palm up
_____ 3. pronation	c. turning outward
_____ 4. rotation	d. moving toward the midline
_____ 5. eversion	e. conveying toward the center
_____ 6. extension	f. turning inward
_____ 7. flexion	g. movement in which the limb is bent
_____ 8. inversion	h. moving away from the midline
_____ 9. supination	i. movement that turns the palm down
	j. turning around its own axis

WORD PARTS

At first glance the number of word parts introduced in this chapter may seem overwhelming, but notice that many of them are names for bones already learned in the anatomic section. The definitions of the word parts include both anatomic terms and commonly used words. For example, both *carpals* and *wrist* are given as the definition of the combining form *carp/o*. Word parts you need to learn to complete this chapter are listed on the following pages. The exercises at the end of each list will help you learn their definitions and spellings.

> Use the flashcards accompanying this text or electronic flashcards to assist you in memorizing the word parts for this chapter.

 To use electronic flashcards, go to evolve.elsevier.com.
Select: Chapter 14, **Flashcards**.

Refer to p. 10 for your Evolve Access Information.

Combining Forms of the Musculoskeletal System

METACARPUS

literally means **beyond the wrist.** It is composed of the prefix **meta-,** meaning **beyond,** and **carpus,** meaning **wrist.**

COMBINING FORM	DEFINITION
carp/o	carpals (wrist)
clavic/o, clavicul/o	clavicle (collarbone)
cost/o	rib
crani/o	cranium (skull)
femor/o	femur (upper leg bone) *(NOTE: The "u" in femur changes to an "o" in the word root femor/.)*
fibul/o	fibula (lower leg bone) (perone/o is also a word root for fibula)
humer/o	humerus (upper arm bone)
ili/o	ilium
ischi/o	ischium
lumb/o	loin, lumbar region of the spine
mandibul/o	mandible (lower jawbone)

COMBINING FORM	DEFINITION
maxill/o	maxilla (upper jawbone)
patell/o	patella (kneecap)
pelv/i, pelv/o *(NOTE: the combining vowels* i *and* o *are used with the word root pelv/)*	pelvis, pelvic bone (also covered in Chapter 9)
phalang/o	phalanges (any bone of the fingers or toes)
pub/o	pubis
rachi/o, spondyl/o, vertebr/o	vertebra, spine, vertebral column
radi/o	radius (lower arm bone)
sacr/o	sacrum
scapul/o	scapula (shoulder blade)
stern/o	sternum (breastbone)
tars/o	tarsals (ankle bones)
tibi/o	tibia (lower leg bone)
uln/o	ulna (lower arm bone)

EXERCISE 6

Write the definitions of the following combining forms.

1. clavic/o _____

2. cost/o _____

3. crani/o _____

4. femor/o _____

5. clavicul/o _____

6. humer/o _____

7. ili/o _____

8. ischi/o _____

9. carp/o _____

10. fibul/o _____

11. mandibul/o _____

12. lumb/o _____

13. pelv/o _____

EXERCISE FIGURE A

Fill in the blanks with combining forms in this diagram of the skeleton, anterior view. *To check your answers, go to p. 640.*

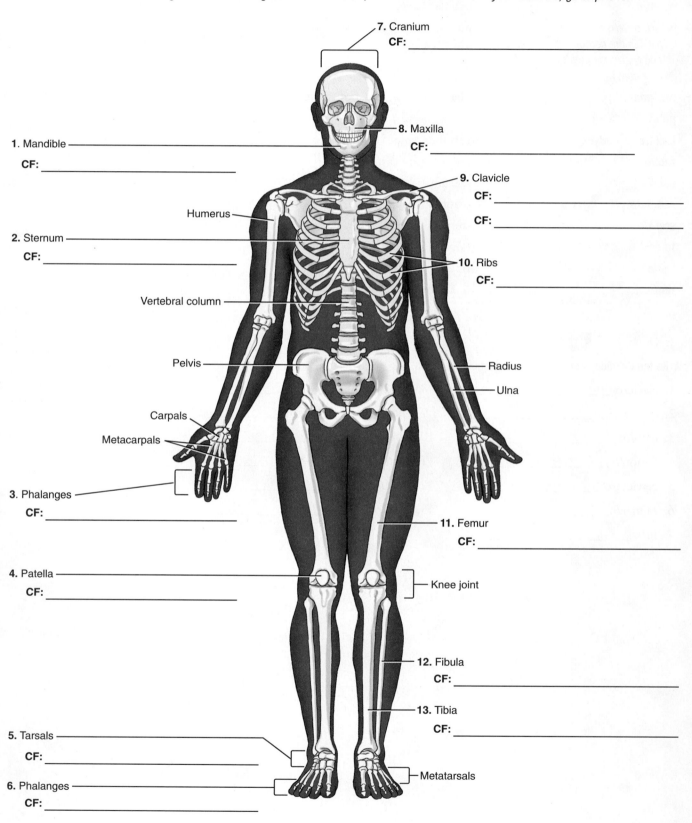

7. Cranium
CF: _____

1. Mandible
   CF: _____

8. Maxilla
   CF: _____

9. Clavicle
   CF: _____
   CF: _____

Humerus

2. Sternum
   CF: _____

10. Ribs
   CF: _____

Vertebral column

Pelvis

Radius

Ulna

Carpals

Metacarpals

3. Phalanges
   CF: _____

11. Femur
   CF: _____

4. Patella
   CF: _____

Knee joint

12. Fibula
   CF: _____

13. Tibia
   CF: _____

5. Tarsals
   CF: _____

Metatarsals

6. Phalanges
   CF: _____

EXERCISE FIGURE B

Fill in the blanks with combining forms in this diagram of the skeleton, posterior view, and the pelvis.

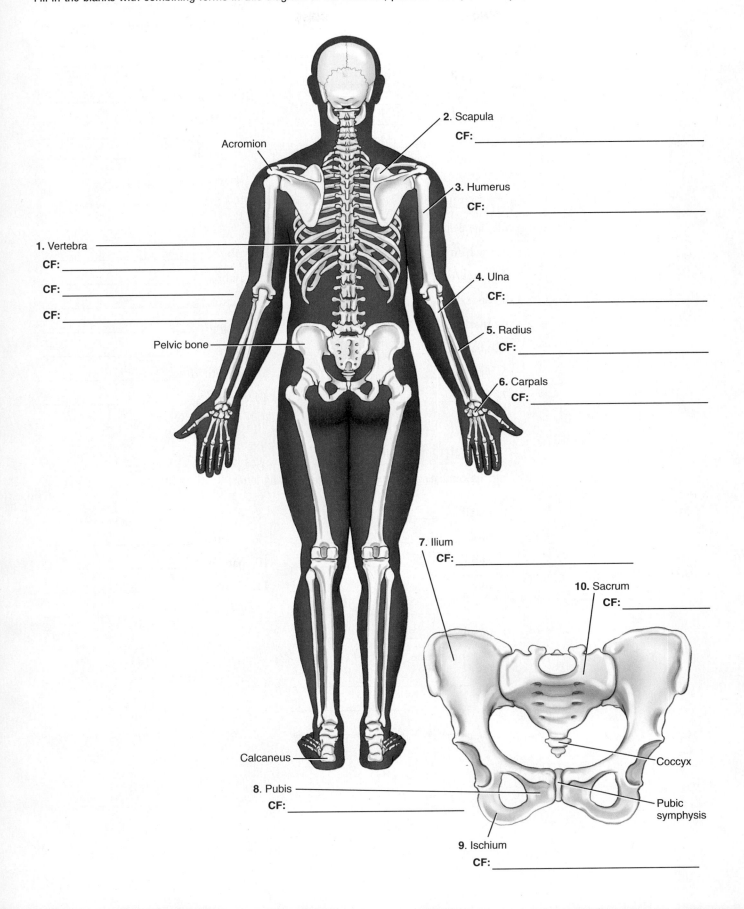

Acromion

2. Scapula

CF: _____

3. Humerus

CF: _____

1. Vertebra

CF: _____

CF: _____

CF: _____

4. Ulna

CF: _____

5. Radius

CF: _____

Pelvic bone

6. Carpals

CF: _____

7. Ilium

CF: _____

10. Sacrum

CF: _____

Coccyx

Pubic symphysis

Calcaneus

8. Pubis

CF: _____

9. Ischium

CF: _____

EXERCISE 7

Write the combining form for each of the following terms.

1. clavicle a. _____
           b. _____
2. rib _____
3. cranium _____
4. femur _____
5. humerus _____
6. carpals _____
7. ischium _____

8. fibula _____
9. ilium _____
10. mandible _____
11. loin, lumbar
    region of the spine _____
12. pelvis, pelvic
    bone a. _____
         b. _____

EXERCISE 8

Write the definitions of the following combining forms.

1. rachi/o _____
2. patell/o _____
3. spondyl/o _____
4. maxill/o _____
5. phalang/o _____
6. uln/o _____
7. radi/o _____

8. tibi/o _____
9. pub/o _____
10. tars/o _____
11. scapul/o _____
12. stern/o _____
13. vertebr/o _____
14. sacr/o _____

EXERCISE 9

Write the combining form for each of the following terms.

1. maxilla _____
2. ulna _____
3. radius _____
4. tibia _____
5. pubis _____
6. tarsals _____
7. vertebra, spine, vertebral column
    a. _____
    b. _____
    c. _____

8. sternum _____
9. scapula _____
10. patella _____
11. phalanges _____
12. sacrum _____

Combining Forms of Joints

COMBINING FORM	DEFINITION
aponeur/o	aponeurosis
arthr/o	joint
burs/o	bursa (cavity)
chondr/o	cartilage
disk/o	intervertebral disk
menisc/o	meniscus (crescent)
synovi/o	synovia, synovial membrane
ten/o, tend/o, tendin/o	tendon

 DISK
is from the Greek diskos, meaning flat plate. A variant spelling, disc, is also used, though chiefly in ophthalmology.

EXERCISE FIGURE C

Fill in the blanks with combining forms on these diagrams of the knee joint.

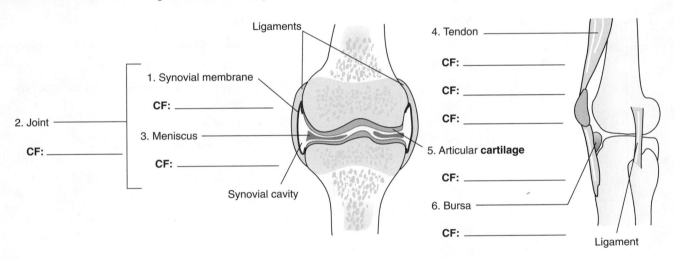

Ligaments

1. Synovial membrane
   CF: _____

2. Joint
   CF: _____

3. Meniscus
   CF: _____

Synovial cavity

4. Tendon
   CF: _____
   CF: _____
   CF: _____

5. Articular **cartilage**
   CF: _____

6. Bursa
   CF: _____

Ligament

EXERCISE 10

Write the definitions of the following combining forms.

1. arthr/o _____

2. aponeur/o _____

3. menisc/o _____

4. tendin/o _____

5. chondr/o _____

6. ten/o _____

7. burs/o _____

8. tend/o _____

9. synovi/o _____

10. disk/o _____

EXERCISE 11

Write the combining form for each of the following terms.

1. meniscus _____

2. aponeurosis _____

3. joint _____

4. cartilage _____

5. tendon   a._____

       b. _____

       c._____

6. bursa _____

7. synovia, synovial membrane _____

8. intervertebral disk _____

Combining Forms Commonly Used with Musculoskeletal System Terms

COMBINING FORM	DEFINITION
ankyl/o	stiff, bent
kinesi/o	movement, motion
kyph/o	hump (increased convexity of the spine)
lamin/o	lamina (thin, flat plate or layer)
lord/o	bent forward (increased concavity of the spine)
my/o, myos/o (NOTE: my/o *was introduced in Chapter 2)*	muscle
myel/o (NOTE: myel/o *also means spinal cord; see Chapter 15)*	bone marrow (also covered in Chapter 10)
oste/o	bone
petr/o (NOTE: lith/o, *also a combining form for* stone, *was introduced in Chapter 6)*	stone
scoli/o	crooked, curved (spine)

EXERCISE 12

Write the definitions of the following combining forms.

1. my/o _____

2. petr/o _____

3. kinesi/o _____

4. oste/o _____

5. lamin/o _____

6. myel/o _____

7. kyph/o _____

8. ankyl/o _____

9. scoli/o _____

10. myos/o _____

11. lord/o _____

EXERCISE 13

Write the combining form for each of the following.

1. muscle   a. _____

          b. _____

2. stone   _____

3. movement, motion   _____

4. bone   _____

5. lamina   _____

6. bone marrow _____

7. hump   _____

8. stiff, bent _____

9. crooked, curved _____

10. bent forward _____

Prefixes

PREFIX	DEFINITION	
inter-	between	
supra-	above	
sym-, syn-	together, joined	

EXERCISE 14

Write the definition of the following prefixes.

1. supra- _____

2. sym-, syn- _____

3. inter- _____

EXERCISE 15

Write the prefix for each of the following definitions.

1. together, joined   a. _____

                      b. _____

2. between _____

3. above _____

Suffixes

SUFFIX	DEFINITION
-asthenia	weakness
-clasia, -clasis, -clast	break
-desis	surgical fixation, fusion
-physis	growth
-schisis	split, fissure

EXERCISE 16

Write the definitions of the following suffixes.

1. -physis _____

2. -clasis _____

3. -desis _____

4. -clast _____

5. -schisis _____

6. -clasia _____

7. -asthenia _____

EXERCISE 17

Write the suffix for each of the following definitions.

1. growth _____

2. weakness _____

3. break   a. _____

         b. _____

         c. _____

4. surgical fixation, fusion _____

5. split, fissure _____

For review and/or assessment, go to evolve.elsevier.com. Select:
Chapter 14, **Activities,** Word Parts
Chapter 14, **Games,**   Name that Word Part

Refer to p. 10 for your Evolve Access Information.

MEDICAL TERMS

Disease and Disorder Terms

Built from Word Parts

The following terms are built from word parts you have already learned and can be translated literally to find their meanings. Further explanation of terms beyond the definition of their word parts, if needed, is included in parentheses.

TERM	DEFINITION
ankylosis (*ang*-ki-LŌ-sis)	abnormal condition of stiffness (often referring to fusion of a joint, such as the result of chronic rheumatoid arthritis)
arthritis (ar-THRĪ-tis)	inflammation of a joint. (The most common forms of arthritis are osteoarthritis and rheumatoid arthritis.) (Figure 14-8)
bursitis (ber-SĪ-tis)	inflammation of a bursa
chondromalacia (*kon*-drō-ma-LĀ-sha)	softening of cartilage
cranioschisis (*krā*-nē-OS-ki-sis)	fissure of the cranium (congenital)
diskitis (dis-KĪ-tis)	inflammation of an intervertebral disk (also spelled **discitis**)
fibromyalgia (*fi*-brō-mī-AL-ja)	pain in the fibrous tissues and muscles (a common condition characterized by widespread pain and stiffness of muscles, fatigue, and disturbed sleep)
kyphosis (kī-FŌ-sis)	abnormal condition of a hump (increased convexity of the thoracic spine as viewed from the side) (also called **hunchback** or **humpback**) (Exercise Figure D2)
lordosis (lōr-DŌ-sis)	abnormal condition of bending forward (increased concavity of the lumbar spine as viewed from the side) (also called **swayback**) (Exercise Figure D1)
maxillitis (*mak*-si-LĪ-tis)	inflammation of the maxilla
meniscitis (*men*-i-SĪ-tis)	inflammation of a meniscus
myasthenia (*mī*-as-THĒ-nē-a)	muscle weakness
myeloma (*mī*-e-LŌ-ma)	tumor of the bone marrow (malignant)
osteitis (*os*-tē-Ĭ-tis)	inflammation of the bone
osteoarthritis (OA) (*os*-tē-ō-ar-THRĪ-tis)	inflammation of the bone and joint (Figure 14-8)
osteochondritis (*os*-tē-ō-kon-DRĪ-tis)	inflammation of the bone and cartilage

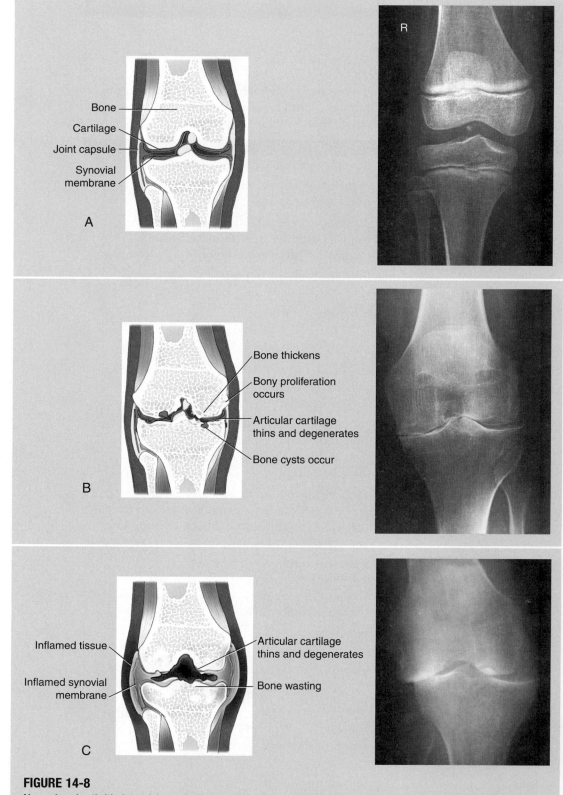

FIGURE 14-8

Normal and arthritic knee joints. **A,** Normal knee joint, illustration and radiograph. **B,** Osteoarthritis of the knee joint, illustration and radiograph. **C,** Rheumatoid arthritis of the knee joint, illustration and radiograph.

Disease and Disorder Terms—cont'd

Built from Word Parts

TERM	DEFINITION
osteofibroma (*os*-tē-ō-fī-BRŌ-ma)	tumor of the bone and fibrous tissue (benign)
osteomalacia (*os*-tē-ō-ma-LĀ-sha)	softening of bone
osteomyelitis (*os*-tē-ō-*mī*-e-LĪ-tis)	inflammation of the bone and bone marrow (caused by bacterial infection)
osteopenia (*os*-tē-ō-PĒ-nē-a)	abnormal reduction of bone mass (caused by inadequate replacement of bone lost to normal bone lysis and can lead to osteoporosis)
osteopetrosis (*os*-tē-ō-pe-TRŌ-sis)	abnormal condition of stonelike bones (marblelike bones caused by defective osteoclast resorption of bone)
osteosarcoma (*os*-tē-ō-sar-KŌ-ma)	malignant tumor of the bone
polymyositis (*pol*-ē-*mī*-ō-SĪ-tis)	inflammation of many muscles
rachischisis (ra-KIS-ki-sis)	fissure of the vertebral column (congenital) (also called **spina bifida**)
rhabdomyolysis (*rab*-dō-*mī*-OL-i-sis)	dissolution of striated muscle (caused by trauma, extreme exertion, or drug toxicity; in severe cases renal failure can result)
sarcopenia (*sar*-kō-PĒ-nē-a)	abnormal reduction of connective tissue (such as loss of skeletal muscle mass in the elderly)
scoliosis (*skō*-lē-Ō-sis)	abnormal condition of (lateral) curved (spine) (Figure 14-9) (Exercise Figure D)
spondylarthritis (*spon*-dil-ar-THRĪ-tis)	inflammation of the vertebral joints (also called **spondyloarthritis**)
spondylosis (*spon*-di-LŌ-sis)	abnormal condition of the vertebrae (a general term used to describe changes to the spine from osteoarthritis or ankylosis)
synoviosarcoma (si-*nō*-vē-ō-sar-KŌ-ma)	malignant tumor of the synovial membrane
tendinitis (*ten*-di-NĪ-tis)	inflammation of a tendon (also spelled **tendonitis**)
tenosynovitis (*ten*-ō-*sin*-ō-VĪ-tis) (NOTE: the i in synovi *is dropped because the suffix begins with an* i)	inflammation of the tendon and synovial membrane

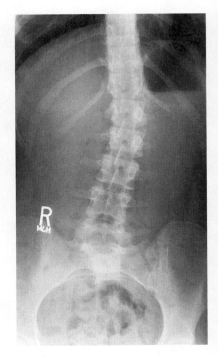

FIGURE 14-9
AP lumbar spine radiograph demonstrating congenital scoliosis.

To watch animations, go to evolve.elsevier.com. Select:
Chapter 14, **Animations**, Osteomyelitis
Scoliosis

Refer to p. 10 for your Evolve Access Information.

EXERCISE 18

Practice saying aloud each of the disease and disorder terms built from word parts on pp. 601 and 603.

 To hear the terms, go to evolve.elsevier.com. Select: Chapter 14, **Exercises**, Pronunciation.

Refer to p. 10 for your Evolve Access Information.

☐ Place a check mark in the box when you have completed this exercise.

EXERCISE FIGURE D

Fill in the blanks to label the diagram.

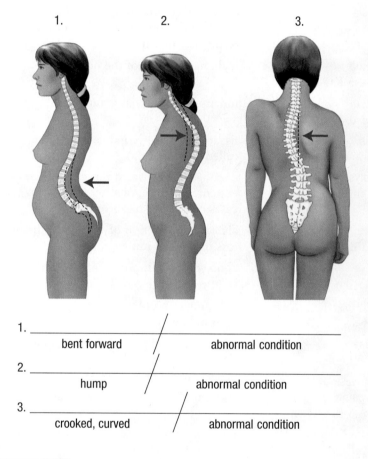

1. _____ / _____
      bent forward   abnormal condition

2. _____ / _____
         hump   abnormal condition

3. _____ / _____
     crooked, curved   abnormal condition

EXERCISE 19

Analyze and define the following disease and disorder terms.

1. osteitis _____

2. osteomyelitis _____

3. osteopetrosis _____

4. osteomalacia _____

5. osteochondritis _____

6. osteofibroma _____

7. arthritis _____

8. rhabdomyolysis _____

9. myeloma _____

10. tendinitis _____

11. osteopenia _____

12. spondylosis _____

13. bursitis _____

14. spondylarthritis_____

15. ankylosis _____

16. kyphosis_____

17. scoliosis _____

18. cranioschisis _____

19. maxillitis _____

20. meniscitis_____

21. rachischisis _____

22. myasthenia _____

23. osteosarcoma_____

24. chondromalacia_____

25. synoviosarcoma_____

26. tenosynovitis _____

27. polymyositis _____

28. diskitis _____

29. lordosis _____

30. osteoarthritis_____

31. fibromyalgia _____

32. sarcopenia _____

EXERCISE 20

Build disease and disorder terms for the following definitions with the word parts you have learned.

1. inflammation of the bone
   and cartilage

   _____ / __ / _____ / _____
   WR   CV   WR   S

2. tumor of the bone and
   fibrous tissue

   _____ / __ / _____ / _____
   WR   CV   WR   S

3. inflammation of a joint

   _____ / _____
   WR   S

4. dissolution of striated muscle

   _____ / __ / _____ / __ / _____
   WR   CV   WR   CV   S

5. tumor of the bone marrow

   _____ / _____
   WR   S

6. inflammation of a tendon

   _____ / _____
   WR   S

7. abnormal condition of the
   vertebrae

   _____ / _____
   WR   S

8. abnormal reduction of
   bone mass

   _____ / _____ / _____
   WR   CV   S

9. inflammation of the bursa

   _____ / _____
   WR   S

10. inflammation of the vertebral
    joints

    _____ / _____ / _____
    WR   WR   S

11. abnormal condition of stiffness

    _____ / _____
    WR   S

12. abnormal condition of a hump
    (increased convexity of thoracic
    spine)

    _____ / _____
    WR   S

13. abnormal condition of (lateral)
    curved (spine)

    _____ / _____
    WR   S

14. fissure of the cranium

    _____ / _____ / _____
    WR   CV   S

15. inflammation of the maxilla

    _____ / _____
    WR   S

16. inflammation of the meniscus

    _____ / _____
    WR   S

17. fissure of the vertebral column

    _____ / _____
    WR   S

18. muscle weakness

    _____ / _____
    WR   S

19. inflammation of the bone

    _____ / _____
    WR   S

20. inflammation of the bone and
    bone marrow

    _____ / _____ / _____ / _____
    WR   CV   WR   S

21. abnormal condition of stonelike
    bones (marblelike bones)

    _____ / _____ / _____ / _____
    WR   CV   WR   S

22. softening of bone

    _____ / _____ / _____
    WR   CV   S

23. inflammation of the tendon
    and synovial membrane

    _____ / _____ / _____ / _____
    WR   CV   WR   S

24. malignant tumor of the
    synovial membrane

    _____ / _____ / _____
    WR   CV   S

25. malignant tumor of the bone

    _____ / _____ / _____
    WR   CV   S

26. softening of cartilage

    _____ / _____ / _____
    WR   CV   S

27. inflammation of an intervertebral disk

_____ / _____ / _____
WR   S

28. inflammation of many muscles

_____ / _____ / _____
P   WR   S

29. abnormal condition of bending forward (increased concavity of lumbar spine)

_____ / _____ / _____
WR   S

30. inflammation of the bone and joint

_____ / CV / _____ / _____
WR   WR   S

31. pain in the fibrous tissues and muscles

_____ / CV / _____ / _____
WR   WR   S

32. abnormal reduction of connective tissue

_____ / CV / _____
WR   S

EXERCISE 21

Spell each of the disease and disorder terms built from word parts on pp. 601 and 603 by having someone dictate them to you.

1. _____   17. _____
2. _____   18. _____
3. _____   19. _____
4. _____   20. _____
5. _____   21. _____
6. _____   22. _____
7. _____   23. _____
8. _____   24. _____
9. _____   25. _____
10. _____   26. _____
11. _____   27. _____
12. _____   28. _____
13. _____   29. _____
14. _____   30. _____
15. _____   31. _____
16. _____   32. _____

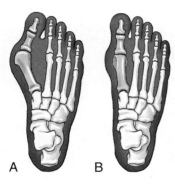

FIGURE 14-10
A, Bunion. **B,** Following
a bunionectomy.

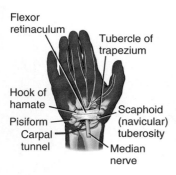

Flexor
retinaculum

Tubercle of
trapezium

Hook of
hamate

Pisiform

Carpal
tunnel

Scaphoid
(navicular)
tuberosity

Median
nerve

FIGURE 14-11
Structures involved with **carpal tunnel syndrome**, which is caused by compression of the median nerve.

Disease and Disorder Terms

Not Built from Word Parts

In some of the following terms, you may recognize word parts you have already learned; however, the full meaning of the terms cannot be discerned by the definition of their word parts.

TERM	DEFINITION
ankylosing spondylitis (*ang*-ki-LŌ-sing) (*spon*-di-LĪ-tis)	form of arthritis that first affects the spine and adjacent structures and that, as it progresses, causes a forward bend of the spine (also called **Strümpell-Marie arthritis** or **disease**, or **rheumatoid spondylitis**)
bunion (BUN-yun)	abnormal prominence of the joint at the base of the great toe, the metatarsal-phalangeal joint. It is a common problem, often hereditary or caused by poorly fitted shoes (also called **hallux valgus**) (Figure 14-10).
carpal tunnel syndrome (CTS) (KAR-pl) (TUN-el) (SIN-drōm)	common nerve entrapment disorder of the wrist caused by compression of the median nerve. Symptoms include pain and paresthesia in portions of the hand and fingers (Figure 14-11).
Colles fracture (KOL-ēz) (FRAK-chur)	type of wrist fracture. The fracture is at the distal end of the radius, the distal fragment being displaced backward. (Figure 14-12 and Figure 14-20, p. 621)
exostosis (*ek*-sos-TŌ-sis)	abnormal benign growth on the surface of a bone (also called **spur**)

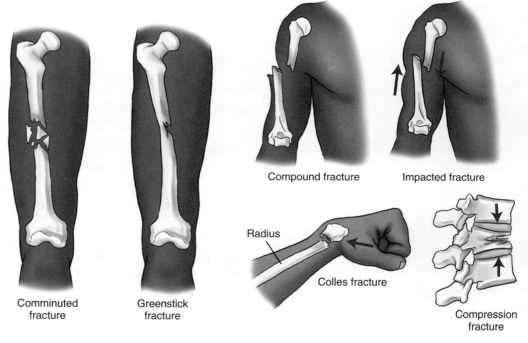

Comminuted
fracture

Greenstick
fracture

Compound fracture

Impacted fracture

Radius

Colles fracture

Compression
fracture

FIGURE 14-12
Types of fractures.

TERM	DEFINITION
fracture (fx) (FRAK-chŭr)	broken bone (see Figure 14-12)
gout (gowt)	disease in which an excessive amount of uric acid in the blood causes sodium urate crystals (**tophi**) to be deposited in the joints, producing arthritis (Figure 14-13, *A*)
herniated disk (HER-nē-*āt*-ed) (disk)	rupture of the intervertebral disk cartilage, which allows the contents to protrude through it, putting pressure on the spinal nerve roots (also called **slipped disk, ruptured disk, herniated intervertebral disk,** or **herniated nucleus pulposus [HNP]**) (Figure 14-14)
Lyme disease (līm) (di-ZĒZ)	an infection caused by a bacterium (*Borrelia burgdorferi*) carried by deer ticks and transmitted to humans by the bite of an infected tick. Symptoms, caused by the body's immune response to the bacteria, vary and may include a rash at the site of the tick bite and flulike symptoms such as fever, headache, joint pain, and fatigue. Lyme disease was first reported in Lyme, Conn., in 1975. The primary treatment is antibiotics. Left untreated, Lyme disease can mimic several musculoskeletal diseases mentioned in this chapter (Figure 14-15).
muscular dystrophy (MD) (MUS-kū-lar) (DIS-tro-fē)	group of hereditary diseases characterized by degeneration of muscle and weakness
myasthenia gravis (MG) (*mī*-as-THĒ-nē-a) (GRA-vis)	chronic disease characterized by muscle weakness and thought to be caused by a defect in the transmission of impulses from nerve to muscle cell. The face, larynx, and throat are frequently affected; no true paralysis of the muscles exists.

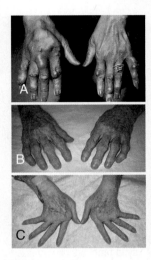

FIGURE 14-13
Types of arthritis, comparison. **A,** Gout. **B,** Osteoarthritis. **C,** Rheumatoid arthritis.

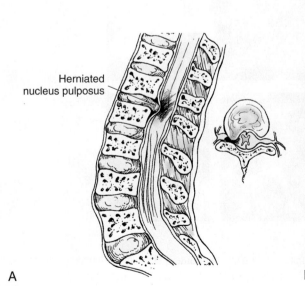

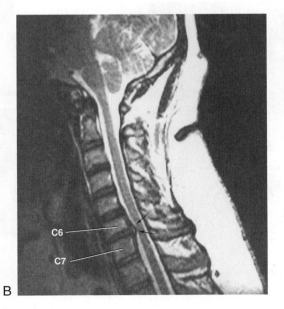

Herniated nucleus pulposus

A

B

FIGURE 14-14
A, Herniated disk. **B,** MRI image of cervical spine, demonstrating herniated disk between C6 and C7.

Disease and Disorder Terms—cont'd

Not Built from Word Parts

REPETITIVE MOTION DISORDERS (RMDs)

are a group of musculoskeletal disorders caused by overuse and repetitive motions performed in the course of normal work or recreational activities. These disorders, which include **tendonitis, bursitis,** and **carpal tunnel syndrome,** are characterized by pain, swelling, numbness, and loss of strength or flexibility and most commonly affect the hands, wrists, elbows, and shoulders. Incorporating rest breaks, stretching, improved posture or ergonomics, antiinflammatory medications, and physical therapy provide the majority of treatment for RMDs. Surgery may be needed as treatment for permanent injuries. These disorders may also be referred to as **repetitive strain syndrome.**

TERM	DEFINITION
osteoporosis (*os*-tē-ō-po-RŌ-sis)	abnormal loss of bone density that may lead to an increase in fractures of the ribs, thoracic and lumbar vertebrae, hips, and wrists after slight trauma (occurs predominantly in postmenopausal women) (Figure 14-16)
plantar fasciitis (PLAN-tar) (fas-ē-Ī-tis)	inflammation of plantar fascia, connective tissue of the sole of the foot, due to repetitive injury; common cause of heel pain
rheumatoid arthritis (RA) (RŪ-ma-toid) (ar-THRĪ-tis)	chronic systemic disease characterized by autoimmune inflammatory changes in the connective tissue throughout the body (see Figure 14-8 and Figure 14-13, *C*)
spinal stenosis (SPĪ-nal) (ste-NŌ-sis)	narrowing of the spinal canal with compression of nerve roots. The condition is either congenital or due to spinal degeneration. Symptoms are pain radiating to the thigh or lower legs and numbness or tingling in the lower extremities (Figure 14-17).
spondylolisthesis (*spon*-di-lō-lis-THĔ-sis)	forward slipping of one vertebra over another (Figure 14-17)

To watch animations, go to evolve.elsevier.com. Select: Chapter 2, **Animations**, Rheumatoid Arthritis.

Refer to p. 10 for your Evolve Access Information.

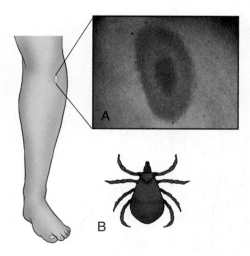

FIGURE 14-15
A, Target lesion of Lyme disease. **B,** Tick that causes Lyme disease.

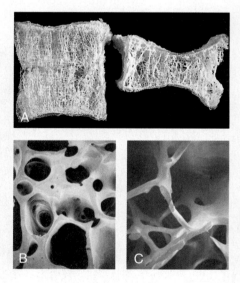

FIGURE 14-16
Osteoporosis. **A,** Comparison of healthy vertebrae (left) with osteoporotic vertebrae (right). The vertebrae with osteoporosis has decreased in size due to compression fractures. **B,** Scanning electron micrograph of normal bone as compared to **C,** bone with osteoporosis.

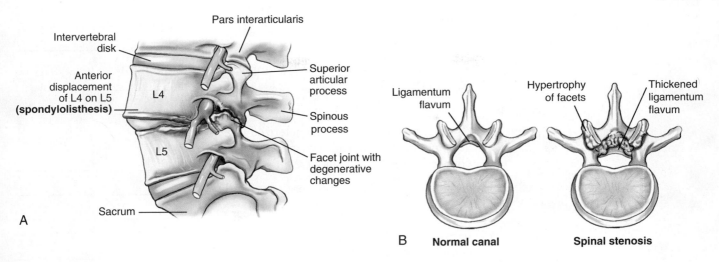

A

B   **Normal canal**   **Spinal stenosis**

FIGURE 14-17
A, Spondylolisthesis showing degenerative changes in the disk and joint. **B,** Normal canal compared with spinal stenosis. Spondylolisthesis may occur with or without spinal stenosis.

EXERCISE 22

Practice saying aloud each of the disease and disorder terms not built from word parts on pp. 608–610.

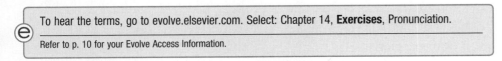

To hear the terms, go to evolve.elsevier.com. Select: Chapter 14, **Exercises**, Pronunciation.

Refer to p. 10 for your Evolve Access Information.

☐ Place a check mark in the box when you have completed this exercise.

EXERCISE 23

Write the term for each of the following definitions.

1. abnormal benign growth on the surface
   of a bone   _____

2. group of hereditary diseases characterized by
   degeneration of muscle and weakness   _____ _____

3. chronic disease characterized by muscle
   weakness and thought to be caused by a
   defect in the transmission of impulses from
   nerve to muscle cell   _____ _____

4. abnormal prominence of the joint at the
   base of the great toe   _____

5. form of arthritis that first affects the spine
   and adjacent structures   _____ _____

6. disease in which an excessive amount of uric
   acid in the blood causes sodium urate crystals
   (tophi) to be deposited in the joints   _____

7. rupture of the intervertebral disk cartilage,
   which allows the contents to protrude through
   it, putting pressure on the spinal nerve roots _____ _____

8. broken bone   _____

9. abnormal loss of bone density   _____

10. a disorder of the wrist caused by compression
   of the median nerve   _____ _____ _____

11. a type of fractured wrist   _____ _____

12. chronic, systemic disease characterized by
   autoimmune inflammatory changes in the
   connective tissue throughout the body   _____ _____

13. forward slipping of one vertebra over another   _____ _____

14. infection transmitted to humans by a deer tick   _____ _____

15. narrowing of the spinal column with
   compression of nerve roots   _____ _____

16. inflammation of plantar fascia due to
   repetitive injury   _____ _____

EXERCISE 24

Write the definitions of the following terms.

1. exostosis_____

2. muscular dystrophy _____

3. myasthenia gravis_____

4. bunion _____

5. ankylosing spondylitis _____

6. osteoporosis _____

7. gout _____

8. herniated disk_____

9. fracture _____

10. carpal tunnel syndrome_____

11. Colles fracture _____

12. rheumatoid arthritis_____

13. Lyme disease_____

14. spondylolisthesis_____

15. spinal stenosis_____

16. plantar fasciitis _____

EXERCISE 25

Spell each of the disease and disorder terms not built from word parts on pp. 608–610 by having someone dictate them to you.

> To hear and spell the terms, go to evolve.elsevier.com. Select: Chapter 14, **Exercises**, Spelling.
>
> Refer to p. 10 for your Evolve Access Information.
>
> ☐ Place a check mark in the box if you have completed this exercise online.

1. _____   9. _____
2. _____   10. _____
3. _____   11. _____
4. _____   12. _____
5. _____   13. _____
6. _____   14. _____
7. _____   15. _____
8. _____   16. _____

Surgical Terms

Built from Word Parts

The following terms are built from word parts you have already learned and can be translated literally to find their meanings. Further explanation of terms beyond the definition of their word parts, if needed, is included in parentheses.

TERM	DEFINITION
aponeurorrhaphy (*ap*-ō-nū-ROR-a-fē)	suturing of an aponeurosis
arthrocentesis (*ar*-thrō-sen-TĒ-sis)	surgical puncture to aspirate fluid from a joint
arthroclasia (*ar*-thrō-KLĀ-zha)	(surgical) breaking of a (stiff) joint
arthrodesis (*ar*-thrō-DĒ-sis)	surgical fixation of a joint (also called **joint fusion**)
arthroplasty (AR-thrō-*plas*-tē)	surgical repair of a joint (Table 14-1)
bursectomy (bur-SEK-to-mē)	excision of a bursa
carpectomy (kar-PEK-to-mē)	excision of a carpal bone
chondrectomy (kon-DREK-to-mē)	excision of a cartilage
chondroplasty (KON-drō-*plas*-tē)	surgical repair of a cartilage
costectomy (kos-TEK-to-mē)	excision of a rib
cranioplasty (KRĀ-nē-ō-*plas*-tē)	surgical repair of the skull

Table 14-1

Types of Arthroplasty

Total hip arthroplasty (THA) is indicated for degenerative joint disease or rheumatoid arthritis. The operation commonly involves replacement of the hip joint with a metallic femoral head and a plastic-coated acetabulum.

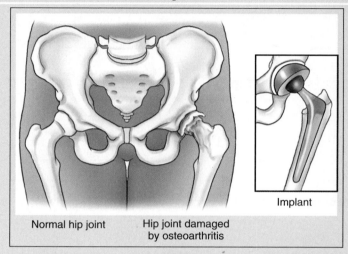

Normal hip joint   Hip joint damaged by osteoarthritis   Implant

Birmingham hip resurfacing is a procedure that provides an option for younger, active patients needing a total hip arthroplasty. The procedure requires the removal of a few millimeters of bone from the femoral head instead of the removal of the entire femoral head required in total hip arthroplasty. A metal cap is then placed on top of the femur, and smooth metal is placed in the acetabulum.

Total knee arthroplasty (TKA) is designed to replace worn surfaces of the knee joint. Various prostheses are used.

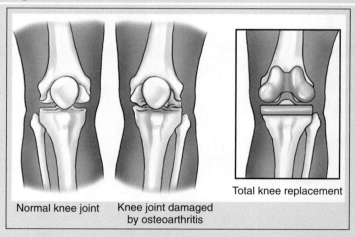

Normal knee joint   Knee joint damaged by osteoarthritis   Total knee replacement

Metatarsal arthroplasty is used to treat deformities associated with rheumatoid arthritis or hallux valgus and to treat painful or unstable joints.

Surgical Terms—cont'd

Built from Word Parts

TERM	DEFINITION
craniotomy (*krā*-nē-OT-o-mē)	incision into the cranium (as for surgery of the brain)
diskectomy (dis-KEK-to-mē)	excision of an intervertebral disk (a portion of the disk is removed to relieve pressure on nerve roots) (also spelled **discectomy**) (Figure 14-18)
laminectomy (*lam*-i-NEK-to-mē)	excision of a lamina (often performed to relieve pressure on the nerve roots in the lower spine caused by a herniated disk and other conditions)
maxillectomy (*mak*-si-LEK-to-mē)	excision of the maxilla
meniscectomy (*men*-i-SEK-to-mē)	excision of the meniscus (performed for a torn cartilage)
myorrhaphy (mī-OR-a-fē)	suturing of a muscle
ostectomy (os-TEK-to-mē) (*NOTE: the* e *is dropped from* oste)	excision of bone
osteoclasis (*os*-tē-OK-la-sis)	(surgical) breaking of a bone (to correct a deformity)
patellectomy (*pat*-e-LEK-to-mē)	excision of the patella
phalangectomy (*fal*-an-JEK-to-mē)	excision of a finger or toe bone
rachiotomy (*rā*-kē-OT-o-mē)	incision into the vertebral column
spondylosyndesis (*spon*-di-lō-sin-DĒ-sis) (*NOTE: the prefix* syn-*appears in the middle of the term*)	fusing together of the vertebrae (also called **spinal fusion**)
synovectomy (*sin*-ō-VEK-to-mē) (*NOTE: the* i *in* synovi *is dropped because the suffix begins with a vowel*)	excision of the synovial membrane (of a joint)
tarsectomy (tar-SEK-to-mē)	excision of (one or more) tarsal bones
tenomyoplasty (*ten*-ō-MĪ-ō-*plas*-tē)	surgical repair of the tendon and muscle
tenorrhaphy (te-NOR-a-fē)	suturing of a tendon
vertebroplasty (VER-te-brō-*plas*-tē)	surgical repair of a vertebra (Table 14-2)

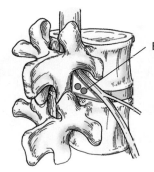

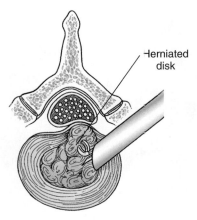

FIGURE 14-18
Microendoscopic diskectomy.

MICROENDOSCOPIC DISKECTOMY (MED)

is a minimally-invasive procedure that uses a fluoroscope and special dilating instrumentation to create a small tunnel to the affected disk area. An endoscopic tool allows the surgeon to visualize and remove the thick, sticky nucleus of the herniated disk. The disk then softens and contracts, relieving severe low back and leg pain. Recovery time is significantly quicker than open diskectomy because of a small incision and less trauma to surrounding tissues.

Table 14-2

Procedures for Treatment of Compression Fractures Caused by Osteoporosis

Percutaneous vertebroplasty (PV) is a minimally invasive operation in which an interventional radiologist places a needle through the skin into the damaged vertebra. A special liquid cement called polymethylmethacrylate is injected into the area through the needle to fill the holes left by osteoporosis. The liquid takes 20 minutes to harden, sealing and stabilizing the fracture and relieving pain.

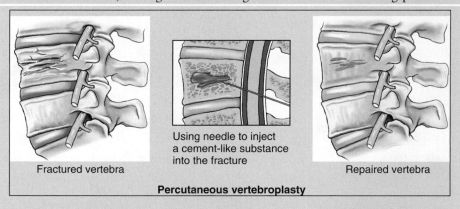

Fractured vertebra

Using needle to inject a cement-like substance into the fracture

Repaired vertebra

Percutaneous vertebroplasty

Kyphoplasty is similar to vertebroplasty except a balloonlike device is used to expand the compressed vertebra before the cement is injected.

To watch animations, go to evolve.elsevier.com. Select: Chapter 14, **Animations,** Repair of Tibial Plateau Fracture.

Refer to p. 10 for your Evolve Access Information.

EXERCISE 26

Practice saying aloud each of the surgical terms built from word parts on pp. 613 and 615.

To hear the terms, go to evolve.elsevier.com. Select: Chapter 14, **Exercises**, Pronunciation.

Refer to p. 10 for your Evolve Access Information.

☐ Place a check mark in the box when you have completed this exercise.

EXERCISE 27

Analyze and define the following surgical terms.

1. osteoclasis _____
2. ostectomy _____
3. arthroclasia _____
4. arthrodesis_____
5. arthroplasty_____
6. chondrectomy_____
7. chondroplasty_____
8. myorrhaphy_____
9. tenomyoplasty_____
10. tenorrhaphy _____

11. costectomy _____

12. patellectomy _____

13. aponeurorrhaphy _____

14. carpectomy _____

15. phalangectomy _____

16. meniscectomy _____

17. spondylosyndesis _____

18. laminectomy _____

19. bursectomy _____

20. craniotomy _____

21. cranioplasty _____

22. maxillectomy _____

23. rachiotomy _____

24. tarsectomy _____

25. synovectomy _____

26. diskectomy _____

27. vertebroplasty _____

28. arthrocentesis _____

EXERCISE 28

Build surgical terms for the following definitions by using the word parts you have learned.

1. (surgical) breaking of a bone (to correct a deformity)

   _____ /CV/ _____
   WR   CV   S

2. excision of bone

   _____ / _____
   WR   S

3. (surgical) breaking of a (stiff) joint

   _____ /CV/ _____
   WR   CV   S

4. surgical fixation of a joint

   _____ /CV/ _____
   WR   CV   S

5. surgical repair of a joint

   _____ /CV/ _____
   WR   CV   S

6. excision of cartilage

   _____ / _____
   WR   S

7. surgical repair of cartilage

   _____ /CV/ _____
   WR   CV   S

8. suturing of a muscle

   _____ /CV/ _____
   WR   CV   S

9. surgical repair of a tendon and muscle

   _____ /CV/ _____ /CV/ _____
   WR   CV   WR   CV   S

10. suturing of a tendon

   _____ /CV/ _____
   WR   CV   S

11. excision of a rib

_____
WR   /   S

12. excision of the patella

_____
WR   /   S

13. suturing of an aponeurosis

_____
WR   /CV/   S

14. excision of a carpal bone

_____
WR   /   S

15. excision of a finger or toe bone

_____
WR   /   S

16. excision of a meniscus

_____
WR   /   S

17. fusing together of the vertebrae

_____
WR   /CV/   P   /   S

18. excision of a lamina

_____
WR   /   S

19. excision of a bursa

_____
WR   /   S

20. incision into the cranium

_____
WR   /CV/   S

21. surgical repair of the skull

_____
WR   /CV/   S

22. excision of the maxilla

_____
WR   /   S

23. incision of the vertebral column

_____
WR   /CV/   S

24. excision of (one or more) tarsal bones

_____
WR   /   S

25. excision of the synovial membrane

_____
WR   /   S

26. excision of an intervertebral disk

_____
WR   /   S

27. surgical repair of a vertebra

_____
WR   /CV/   S

28. surgical puncture to aspirate fluid from a joint

_____
WR   /CV/   S

EXERCISE 29

Spell each of the surgical terms built from word parts on pp. 613 and 615 by having someone dictate them to you.

> ⓔ To hear and spell the terms, go to evolve.elsevier.com. Select: Chapter 14, **Exercises**, Spelling.
>
> Refer to p. 10 for your Evolve Access Information.
>
> ☐ Place a check mark in the box if you have completed this exercise online.

1. _____
2. _____
3. _____
4. _____
5. _____
6. _____
7. _____
8. _____
9. _____
10. _____
11. _____
12. _____
13. _____
14. _____

15. _____
16. _____
17. _____
18. _____
19. _____
20. _____
21. _____
22. _____
23. _____
24. _____
25. _____
26. _____
27. _____
28. _____

Diagnostic Terms

Built from Word Parts

The following terms are built from word parts you have already learned and can be translated literally to find their meanings. Further explanation of terms beyond the definition of their word parts, if needed, is included in parentheses.

TERM	DEFINITION
DIAGNOSTIC IMAGING	
arthrography (ar-THROG-ra-fē)	radiographic imaging of a joint (with contrast media). (Magnetic resonance imaging [MRI] has mostly replaced arthrography as the imaging technique for diarthrodial [movable] joints such as the knee, wrist, hip, and shoulder. Arthrography is still used for specialized functions such as when metal is present in the body.) See Table 14-3 for **diagnostic imaging procedures** for more musculoskeleted system.
ENDOSCOPY	
arthroscopy (ar-THROS-ko-pē)	visual examination of a joint (performed with an endoscope and used for a diarthrodial [movable] joint) (Exercise Figure E)
OTHER	
electromyogram (EMG) (ē-*lek*-trō-MĪ-ō-gram)	record of the (intrinsic) electrical activity in a (skeletal) muscle (Figure 14-19)

EXERCISE FIGURE E

Fill in the blanks to complete labeling of the diagram.

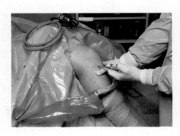

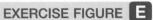

_____ / cv / visual
joint   examination

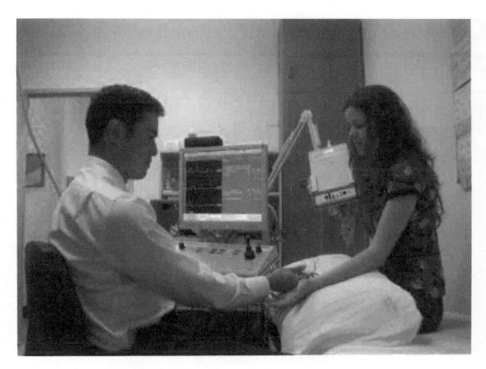

FIGURE 14-19
Patient having an electromyogram (EMG) of the forearm.

EXERCISE 30

Practice saying aloud each of the diagnostic terms built from word parts on p. 619.

> To hear the terms, go to evolve.elsevier.com. Select: Chapter 14, **Exercises**, Pronunciation.
>
> Refer to p. 10 for your Evolve Access Information.
>
> ☐ Place a check mark in the box when you have completed this exercise.

EXERCISE 31

Analyze and define the following diagnostic terms.

1. electromyogram _____
2. arthrography _____
3. arthroscopy _____

EXERCISE 32

Build diagnostic terms for the following definitions using word parts you have learned.

1. radiographic imaging of a joint _____
   WR / CV / S

2. visual examination of a joint _____
   WR / CV / S

3. record of the electrical activity
   of a muscle _____
   WR / CV / WR / CV / S

Table 14-3

Diagnostic Imaging Procedures Used for the Musculoskeletal System

The following diagnostic imaging procedures are commonly used for diagnosing diseases, fractures, strains, and other conditions of the musculoskeletal system.

Radiography (radiographic imaging) of the bones and joints is used to identify fractures or tumors, monitor healing, or identify abnormal structures (Figure 14-20).

Computed tomography (CT) of the bones and joints gives accurate definition of bone structure and demonstrates subtle changes such as linear fractures (Figure 14-21).

Magnetic resonance imaging (MRI) is used to evaluate the soft tissue of the shoulders, hips, elbows, knees, ankles, feet, and spinal cord stenosis, spinal cord defects, and degenerative disk changes (Figure 14-22).

Bone scan (nuclear medicine test) is used to detect the presence of metastatic disease of the bone and to monitor degenerative bone disease (Figure 14-23).

Single-photon emission computed tomography (SPECT) of the bone is an even more sensitive nuclear method for detecting bone abnormalities.

Bone densitometry is a method of determining the density of bone by radiographic techniques used to diagnose osteoporosis. **Dual-energy X-ray absorptiometry (DXA or DEXA)** is commonly used for this test. (Figure 14-24)

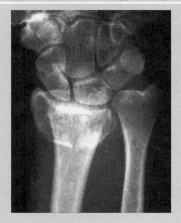

FIGURE 14-20
Radiograph showing a Colles fracture.

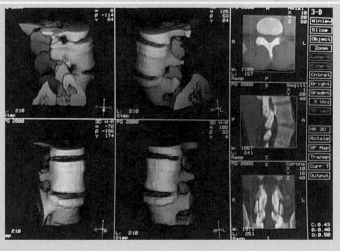

FIGURE 14-21
CT scan showing three-dimensional reconstruction images of the lumbar spine.

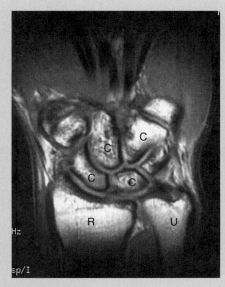

FIGURE 14-22
Coronal MRI of the wrist. Marrow within the carpal bones *(C)*, radius *(R)*, and ulna *(U)*.

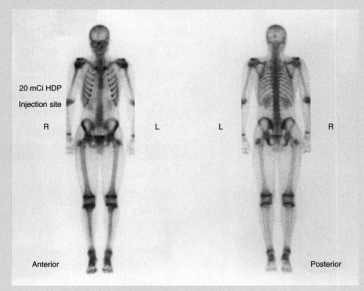

FIGURE 14-23
Whole-body nuclear medicine bone scan.

Table 14-3

Diagnostic Imaging Procedures Used for the Musculoskeletal System—cont'd

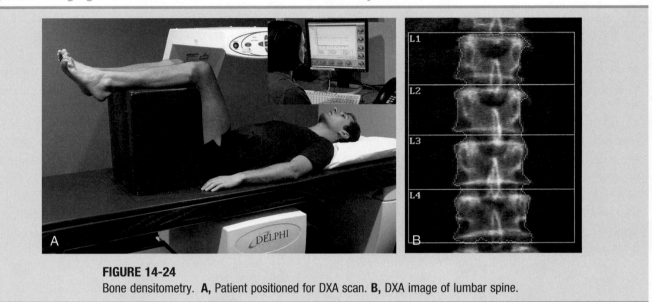

FIGURE 14-24
Bone densitometry. **A,** Patient positioned for DXA scan. **B,** DXA image of lumbar spine.

EXERCISE 33

Spell each of the diagnostic terms built from word parts on p. 619 by having someone dictate them to you.

> To hear and spell the terms, go to evolve.elsevier.com. Select: Chapter 14, **Exercises**, Spelling.
>
> Refer to p. 10 for your Evolve Access Information.
>
> ☐ Place a check mark in the box if you have completed this exercise online.

1. _____   3. _____

2. _____

Complementary Terms

Built from Word Parts

The following terms are built from word parts you have already learned and can be translated literally to find their meanings. Further explanation of terms beyond the definition of their word parts, if needed, is included in parentheses.

TERM	DEFINITION
arthralgia (ar-THRAL-ja)	pain in the joint
atrophy (AT-ro-fē)	without development (process of wasting away)
bradykinesia (*brad*-ē-ki-NĒ-zha)	slow movement
carpal (CAR-pal)	pertaining to the wrist

TERM	DEFINITION
clavicular (kla-VIK-ū-lar)	pertaining to the clavicle
costochondral (KOS-tō-kon-dral)	pertaining to the ribs and cartilage
cranial (KRĂ-nē-al)	pertaining to the cranium
dyskinesia (*dis*-ki-NĒ-zha)	difficult movement
dystrophy (DIS-tro-fē)	abnormal development
femoral (FEM-or-al)	pertaining to the femur
humeral (HŪ-mer-al)	pertaining to the humerus
hyperkinesia (*hī*-per-ki-NĒ-zha)	excessive movement (overactive)
hypertrophy (hī-PER-tro-fē)	excessive development
iliofemoral (*il*-ē-ō-FEM-or-al)	pertaining to the ilium and femur
intercostal (*in*-ter-KOS-tal)	pertaining to between the ribs
intervertebral (*in*-ter-VER-te-bral)	pertaining to between the vertebrae
intracranial (*in*-tra-KRĂ-nē-al)	pertaining to within the cranium
ischiofibular (*is*-kē-ō-FIB-ū-lar)	pertaining to the ischium and fibula
ischiopubic (*is*-kē-ō-PŪ-bik)	pertaining to the ischium and pubis
lumbar (LUM-bar)	pertaining to the loins (the part of the back between the thorax and pelvis)
lumbocostal (*lum*-bō-KOS-tal)	pertaining to the loins and the ribs
lumbosacral (*lum*-bō-SĂ-kral)	pertaining to the lumbar regions (loin) and the sacrum
myalgia (mī-AL-ja)	pain in muscle
osteoblast (OS-tē-ō-*blast*)	developing bone cell
osteocyte (OS-tē-ō-*sīt*)	bone cell
osteonecrosis (*os*-tē-ō-ne-KRŌ-sis)	abnormal condition of bone death (due to lack of blood supply)
pelvic (PEL-vik)	pertaining to the pelvis

Complementary Terms—cont'd

Built from Word Parts

TERM	DEFINITION
pelvisacral (*pel*-vi-SĀ-kral)	pertaining to the pelvis and the sacrum
pubic (PŪ-bik)	pertaining to the pubis
pubofemoral (*pū*-bō-FEM-or-al)	pertaining to the pubis and femur
radial (RĀ-dē-al)	pertaining to the radius
sacral (SĀ-kral)	pertaining to the sacrum
sternoclavicular (*ster*-nō-kla-VIK-ū-lar)	pertaining to the sternum and clavicle
sternoid (STER-noyd)	resembling the sternum
subcostal (sub-KOS-tal)	pertaining to below the rib
submandibular (*sub*-man-DIB-ū-lar)	pertaining to below the mandible
submaxillary (sub-MAK-si-*lar*-ē)	pertaining to below the maxilla
subscapular (sub-SKAP-ū-lar)	pertaining to below the scapula
substernal (sub-STER-nal)	pertaining to under the sternum
suprapatellar (*sū*-pra-pa-TEL-ar)	pertaining to above the patella
suprascapular (*sū*-pra-SKAP-ū-lar)	pertaining to above the scapula
symphysis (SIM-fi-sis)	growing together (as in symphysis pubis)
tibial (TIB-ē-al)	pertaining to the tibia
ulnoradial (ul-nō-RĀ-dē-al)	pertaining to the ulna and radius
vertebrocostal (*ver*-te-brō-KOS-tal)	pertaining to the vertebrae and ribs

EXERCISE 34

Practice saying aloud each of the complementary terms built from word parts on pp. 622–624.

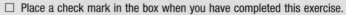

To hear the terms, go to evolve.elsevier.com. Select: Chapter 14, **Exercises**, Pronunciation.

Refer to p. 10 for your Evolve Access Information.

☐ Place a check mark in the box when you have completed this exercise.

EXERCISE 35

Analyze and define the following complementary terms.

1. symphysis _____

2. femoral _____

3. humeral _____

4. intervertebral _____

5. hyperkinesia _____

6. dyskinesia _____

7. bradykinesia _____

8. intracranial _____

9. sternoclavicular _____

10. iliofemoral _____

11. ischiofibular _____

12. submaxillary _____

13. ischiopubic _____

14. submandibular _____

15. pubofemoral _____

16. suprascapular _____

17. subcostal _____

18. vertebrocostal _____

19. subscapular _____

20. osteoblast _____

21. osteocyte _____

22. osteonecrosis _____

23. sternoid _____

24. arthralgia _____

25. carpal _____

26. lumbar _____

27. lumbocostal _____

28. lumbosacral _____

29. sacral _____

30. pubic _____

31. substernal _____

32. suprapatellar _____

33. dystrophy _____

34. atrophy _____

35. hypertrophy _____

36. intercostal _____

37. cranial _____

38. pelvic _____

39. pelvisacral _____

40. clavicular _____

41. tibial _____

42. radial _____

43. ulnoradial _____

44. costochondral _____

45. myalgia _____

EXERCISE 36

Build the complementary terms for the following definitions by using the word parts you have learned.

1. growing together

   _____ / _____
   P   S(WR)

2. pertaining to the femur

   _____ / _____
   WR   S

3. pertaining to the humerus

   _____ / _____
   WR   S

4. pertaining to between the vertebrae

   _____ / _____ / _____
   P   WR   S

5. excessive movement (overactivity)

   _____ / _____ / _____
   P   WR   S

6. difficult movement

   _____ / _____ / _____
   P   WR   S

7. slow movement

   _____ / _____ / _____
   P   WR   S

8. pertaining to within the cranium

   _____ / _____ / _____
   P   WR   S

9. pertaining to the sternum and clavicle

   _____ / _____ / _____ / _____
   WR   CV   WR   S

10. pertaining to the ilium and femur

    _____ / _____ / _____ / _____
    WR   CV   WR   S

11. pertaining to the ischium and fibula

    _____ / _____ / _____ / _____
    WR   CV   WR   S

12. pertaining to below the maxilla

    _____ / _____ / _____
    P   WR   S

13. pertaining to the ischium and pubis

    _____ / _____ / _____ / _____
    WR   CV   WR   S

14. pertaining to below the mandible

    _____ / _____ / _____
    P   WR   S

15. pertaining to the pubis and femur

    _____ / _____ / _____ / _____
    WR   CV   WR   S

16. pertaining to above the scapula ___ P / WR / S

17. pertaining to below the rib ___ P / WR / S

18. pertaining to the vertebrae and ribs ___ WR /CV/ WR / S

19. pertaining to below the scapula ___ P / WR / S

20. developing bone cell ___ WR /CV/ WR

21. bone cell ___ WR /CV/ S

22. abnormal condition of bone death ___ WR /CV/ WR / S

23. resembling the sternum ___ WR / S

24. pain in the joint ___ WR / S

25. pertaining to the wrist ___ WR / S

26. pertaining to the sacrum ___ WR / S

27. pertaining to the loins ___ WR / S

28. pertaining to the pubis ___ WR / S

29. pertaining to the lumbar region (loin) and the sacrum ___ WR /CV/ WR / S

30. pertaining to the loins and ribs ___ WR /CV/ WR / S

31. pertaining to under the sternum ___ P / WR / S

32. pertaining to above the patella ___ P / WR / S

33. abnormal development ___ P / S(WR)

34. without development ___ P / S(WR)

35. excessive development ___ P / S(WR)

36. pertaining to the cranium ___ WR / S

37. pertaining to between the ribs _____
    P / WR / S

38. pertaining to the pelvis _____
    WR / S

39. pertaining to the pelvis and sacrum _____
    WR / CV / WR / S

40. pertaining to the clavicle _____
    WR / S

41. pertaining to the tibia _____
    WR / S

42. pertaining to the radius _____
    WR / S

43. pertaining to the ulna and radius _____
    WR / CV / WR / S

44. pertaining to the ribs and cartilage _____
    WR / CV / WR / S

45. pain in muscle _____
    WR / S

EXERCISE 37

Spell each of the complementary terms built from word parts on pp. 622–624 by having someone dictate them to you.

> To hear and spell the terms, go to evolve.elsevier.com. Select Chapter 14, **Exercises**, Spelling.
>
> (e) Refer to p. 10 for your Evolve Access Information.
>
> ☐ Place a check mark in the box if you have completed this exercise online.

1. _____ 18. _____
2. _____ 19. _____
3. _____ 20. _____
4. _____ 21. _____
5. _____ 22. _____
6. _____ 23. _____
7. _____ 24. _____
8. _____ 25. _____
9. _____ 26. _____
10. _____ 27. _____
11. _____ 28. _____
12. _____ 29. _____
13. _____ 30. _____
14. _____ 31. _____
15. _____ 32. _____
16. _____ 33. _____
17. _____ 34. _____

35. _____   41. _____
36. _____   42. _____
37. _____   43. _____
38. _____   44. _____
39. _____   45. _____
40. _____

> For review and/or assessment, go to evolve.elsevier.com. Select:
> Chapter 14, **Activities**, Terms Built from Word Parts
> Chapter 14, **Games,**   Term Storm
>
> Refer to p. 10 for your Evolve Access Information.

Complementary Terms

Not Built from Word Parts

In some of the following terms, you may recognize word parts you have already learned; however, the full meaning of the terms cannot be discerned by the definition of their word parts.

TERM	DEFINITION
chiropodist, podiatrist (kī-ROP-o-dist) (pō-DĪ-a-trist)	specialist in treating and diagnosing diseases and disorders of the foot, including medical and surgical treatment
chiropractic (kī-rō-PRAK-tik)	system of treatment that consists of manipulation of the vertebral column
chiropractor (KĪ-rō-*prak*-tor)	specialist in chiropractic
crepitus (KREP-i-tus)	crackling sound heard when two bones rub against each other or grating caused by the rubbing together of dry surfaces of a joint. (Crepitus is also used to describe the crackling sound heard with pneumonia or the sound heard from the discharge of gas from the bowel.) (also called **crepitation**)
orthopedics (ortho) (or-thō-PĒ-diks)	branch of medicine dealing with the study and treatment of diseases and abnormalities of the musculoskeletal system
orthopedist (or-thō-PĒ-dist)	physician who specializes in the study and treatment of diseases and abnormalities of the musculoskeletal system
orthotics (or-THOT-iks)	making and fitting of orthopedic appliances, such as arch supports, used to support, align, prevent, or correct deformities
orthotist (or-THOT-ist)	person who specializes in orthotics
osteoclast (OS-tē-ō-*klast*)	type of bone cell involved in absorption and removal of bone minerals. It works in balance with osteoblasts to maintain healthy bone tissue.
osteopath (DO) (OS-tē-ō-path)	physician who specializes in osteopathy

RHEUMATOLOGY & ORTHOPEDICS— WHAT IS THE DIFFERENCE?

While both medical specialties focus on the diagnosis and treatment of disease and disorders of the musculoskeletal system, **rheumatology** focuses on medical management for chronic conditions while **orthopedics** focuses on surgical treatment for acute or chronic conditions. For example, a patient with **rheumatoid arthritis** would see a **rheumatologist** for medications to manage symptoms of the disease and would be referred to an **orthopedist** if joint replacement surgery was warranted.

Complementary Terms—cont'd

Not Built from Word Parts

TERM	DEFINITION
osteopathy (os-tē-OP-a-thē)	system of medicine that uses the usual forms of diagnosis and treatment but places greater emphasis on the relation between body organs and the musculoskeletal system; manipulation may be used in addition to other treatments
prosthesis (pl. prostheses) (pros-THĒ-sis) (pros-THĒ-sēz)	artificial substitute for a missing body part such as a leg, eye, or total hip replacement
rheumatologist (roo-ma-TOL-ō-jist)	physician who specializes in the study and treatment of rheumatic diseases
rheumatology (roo-ma-TOL-ō-jē)	study and treatment of rheumatic diseases and musculoskeletal disorders characterized by inflammation and degeneration of structures

Refer to Appendix D for pharmacology terms related to the musculoskeletal system.

CAM TERM

Tai Chi, often referred to as "meditation in motion," is an ancient Chinese art using slow movements and focused breathing to support mental and physical health. Studies suggest that **improvement in cardiovascular health, muscle strength, and balance** are measurable benefits for the elderly who regularly practice Tai Chi.

EXERCISE 38

Practice saying aloud each of the complementary terms not built from word parts on pp. 629–630.

> To hear the terms, go to evolve.elsevier.com. Select: Chapter 14, **Exercises**, Pronunciation.
>
> Refer to p. 10 for your Evolve Access Information.
>
> ☐ Place a check mark in the box when you have completed this exercise.

EXERCISE 39

Match the definitions in the first column with the correct terms in the second column.

_____ 1. specialist in manipulation of the vertebral column

_____ 2. study and treatment of diseases of the musculoskeletal system

_____ 3. physician who places emphasis on manipulation

_____ 4. foot specialist

_____ 5. substitute for a body part

_____ 6. system of treatment that consists of manipulation of the vertebral column

_____ 7. system of medicine that places greater emphasis on the relation between body organs and the musculoskeletal system

_____ 8. making of orthopedic appliances

_____ 9. skilled in orthotics

_____ 10. crackling or grating sound

_____ 11. physician who specializes in treatment of diseases and abnormalities of the musculoskeletal system

_____ 12. maintains healthy bone tissue with osteoblasts

_____ 13. physician who specializes in the study and treatment of rheumatic diseases

_____ 14. study and treatment of rheumatic diseases

a. chiropodist
b. chiropractic
c. chiropractor
d. osteopath
e. osteopathy
f. orthopedics
g. orthopedist
h. podiatrist
i. orthotics
j. prosthesis
k. orthotist
l. crepitus
m. rheumatologist
n. osteoclast
o. rheumatology

EXERCISE 40

Write the definitions of the following.

1. chiropractor _____
2. chiropractic _____
3. orthopedics _____
4. orthopedist _____
5. chiropodist _____
6. podiatrist _____
7. osteopath _____
8. osteopathy _____
9. orthotics _____
10. prosthesis _____
11. orthotist _____
12. crepitus _____
13. osteoclast _____
14. rheumatologist _____
15. rheumatology _____

EXERCISE 41

Spell each of the complementary terms not built from word parts on pp. 629–630 by having someone dictate them to you.

> To hear and spell the terms, go to evolve.elsevier.com. Select: Chapter 14, **Exercises**, Spelling.
>
> ⓔ Refer to p. 10 for your Evolve Access Information.
>
> ☐ Place a check mark in the box if you have completed this exercise online.

1. _____   9. _____
2. _____   10. _____
3. _____   11. _____
4. _____   12. _____
5. _____   13. _____
6. _____   14. _____
7. _____   15. _____
8. _____

> For review and/or assessment, go to evolve.elsevier.com. Select:
> Chapter 14, **Activities,** Terms Not Built from Word Parts
>   Hear It and Type It: Clinical Vignettes
> ⓔ Chapter 14, **Games,** Term Explorer
>   Termbusters
>   Medical Millionaire
>
> Refer to p. 10 for your Evolve Access Information.

Abbreviations

ABBREVIATION	MEANING
C1-C7	cervical vertebrae
CTS	carpal tunnel syndrome
DO	Doctor of Osteopathy
EMG	electromyogram
fx	fracture
HNP	herniated nucleus pulposus
L1-L5	lumbar vertebrae
MD	muscular dystrophy
MG	myasthenia gravis
OA	osteoarthritis
ortho	orthopedics
RA	rheumatoid arthritis
T1-T12	thoracic vertebrae
THA	total hip arthroplasty

🔍 Refer to **Appendix C** for a complete list of abbreviations.

EXERCISE 42

Write the meaning of the abbreviations in the following sentences.

1. Vertebrae make up the bones of the spinal column. **C1 to C7** _____ _____ are the first set that form the neck. The second set **T1 to T12** _____ _____ articulate with the 12 pairs of ribs that form the outward curve of the spine. **L1 to L5** _____ _____, the third set, are larger and form the inward curve of the spine.

2. Patients with **RA** _____ _____ may experience muscle atrophy and weakness because of inactivity.

3. Water exercise or gentle movement, such as Tai Chi, is recommended for many patients with **OA** _____ , the most common joint disease.

4. **MG** _____ _____ most often affects women and the onset occurs at any age. It is an acquired autoimmune disorder.

5. **EMG** _____ is used to evaluate patients with localized or diffuse muscle weakness, such as polymyositis.

6. **CTS** _____ _____ _____ is a common condition in which, for various reasons, the median nerve in the wrist becomes compressed, causing numbness and pain.

7. Nine types of **MD** _____ _____ have been identified. Because symptoms of the disease are similar to other muscular disorders, diagnosis is often difficult.

8. **HNP** _____ _____ _____ may also be referred to as slipped or ruptured disk or herniated intervertebral disk.

9. **THA** _____ _____ _____ is used to treat severe osteoarthritis of the hip joints.

10. Taking a holistic view of medicine, the **DO** _____ _____ _____ evaluates the patient's musculoskeletal system in relation to overall health.

For more practice with abbreviations, go to evolve. elsevier.com. Select:
Chapter 14, **Flashcard**
Chapter 14, **Games,**
Crossword Puzzle

Refer to p. 10 for your Evolve Access Information.

PRACTICAL APPLICATION

EXERCISE 43 *Interact with Medical Documents and Electronic Health Records*

A. Complete the operative report by writing the medical terms in the blanks. Use the list of definitions with the corresponding numbers.

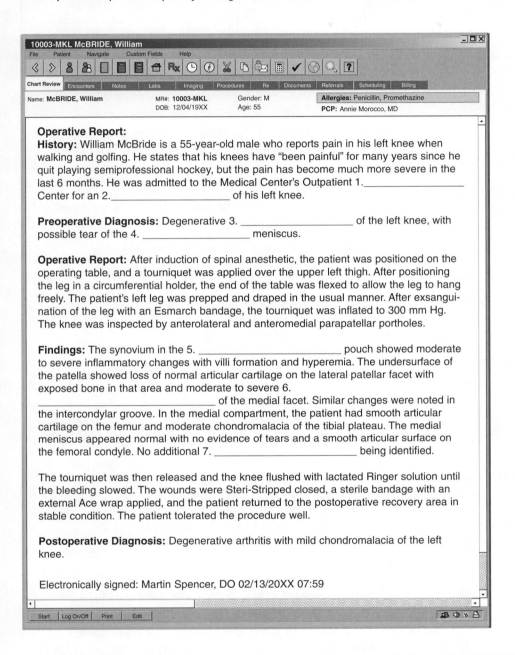

10003-MKL McBRIDE, William

File   Patient   Navigate   Custom Fields   Help

Chart Review | Encounters | Notes | Labs | Imaging | Procedures | Rx | Documents | Referrals | Scheduling | Billing

Name: **McBRIDE, William**   MR#: **10003-MKL**   Gender: M   **Allergies:** Penicillin, Promethazine
                                DOB: 12/04/19XX   Age: 55   **PCP:** Annie Morocco, MD

Operative Report:

History: William McBride is a 55-year-old male who reports pain in his left knee when walking and golfing. He states that his knees have "been painful" for many years since he quit playing semiprofessional hockey, but the pain has become much more severe in the last 6 months. He was admitted to the Medical Center's Outpatient 1._____ Center for an 2._____ of his left knee.

Preoperative Diagnosis: Degenerative 3. _____ of the left knee, with possible tear of the 4. _____ meniscus.

Operative Report: After induction of spinal anesthetic, the patient was positioned on the operating table, and a tourniquet was applied over the upper left thigh. After positioning the leg in a circumferential holder, the end of the table was flexed to allow the leg to hang freely. The patient's left leg was prepped and draped in the usual manner. After exsanguination of the leg with an Esmarch bandage, the tourniquet was inflated to 300 mm Hg. The knee was inspected by anterolateral and anteromedial parapatellar portholes.

Findings: The synovium in the 5. _____ pouch showed moderate to severe inflammatory changes with villi formation and hyperemia. The undersurface of the patella showed loss of normal articular cartilage on the lateral patellar facet with exposed bone in that area and moderate to severe 6. _____ of the medial facet. Similar changes were noted in the intercondylar groove. In the medial compartment, the patient had smooth articular cartilage on the femur and moderate chondromalacia of the tibial plateau. The medial meniscus appeared normal with no evidence of tears and a smooth articular surface on the femoral condyle. No additional 7. _____ being identified.

The tourniquet was then released and the knee flushed with lactated Ringer solution until the bleeding slowed. The wounds were Steri-Stripped closed, a sterile bandage with an external Ace wrap applied, and the patient returned to the postoperative recovery area in stable condition. The patient tolerated the procedure well.

Postoperative Diagnosis: Degenerative arthritis with mild chondromalacia of the left knee.

Electronically signed: Martin Spencer, DO 02/13/20XX 07:59

Start | Log On/Off | Print | Edit

1. branch of medicine dealing with the study and treatment of diseases and abnormalities of the musculoskeletal system
2. visual examination of a joint
3. inflammation of a joint
4. toward the middle or midline
5. pertaining to above the patella
6. softening of the cartilage
7. study of (body changes caused by) disease

B. Read the chart note and answer the questions following it.

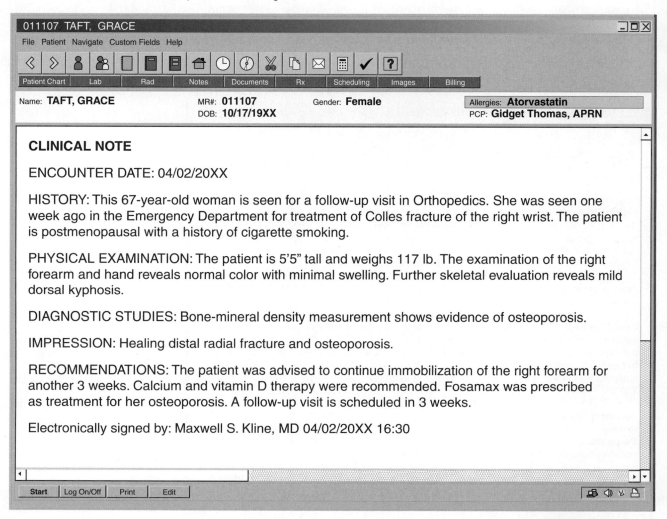

011107 TAFT, GRACE

File Patient Navigate Custom Fields Help

Patient Chart | Lab | Rad | Notes | Documents | Rx | Scheduling | Images | Billing

Name: **TAFT, GRACE**   MR#: **011107**   Gender: **Female**   Allergies: **Atorvastatin**
DOB: **10/17/19XX**   PCP: **Gidget Thomas, APRN**

CLINICAL NOTE

ENCOUNTER DATE: 04/02/20XX

HISTORY: This 67-year-old woman is seen for a follow-up visit in Orthopedics. She was seen one week ago in the Emergency Department for treatment of Colles fracture of the right wrist. The patient is postmenopausal with a history of cigarette smoking.

PHYSICAL EXAMINATION: The patient is 5'5" tall and weighs 117 lb. The examination of the right forearm and hand reveals normal color with minimal swelling. Further skeletal evaluation reveals mild dorsal kyphosis.

DIAGNOSTIC STUDIES: Bone-mineral density measurement shows evidence of osteoporosis.

IMPRESSION: Healing distal radial fracture and osteoporosis.

RECOMMENDATIONS: The patient was advised to continue immobilization of the right forearm for another 3 weeks. Calcium and vitamin D therapy were recommended. Fosamax was prescribed as treatment for her osteoporosis. A follow-up visit is scheduled in 3 weeks.

Electronically signed by: Maxwell S. Kline, MD 04/02/20XX 16:30

Start | Log On/Off | Print | Edit

1. Physical evaluation of the patient revealed:
   a. an abnormal condition of bending forward
   b. an abnormal condition of stiffness
   c. an abnormal hump of the thoracic spine
   d. an abnormal lateral curve of the spine

2. The patient received a diagnosis of:
   a. softening of the cartilage
   b. abnormal reduction of bone mass
   c. stonelike (marblelike) bones
   d. abnormal loss of bone density

C. Complete the **three medical documents** within electronic health record (EHR) on Evolve.

Many healthcare records today are stored and used in an electronic system called **Electronic Health Records (EHR)**. Electronic health records contain a collection of health information of an individual patient documented by various providers at different facilities; the digitally formatted record can be shared through computer networks with patients, physicians, and other health care providers.

For practice with medical terms using electronic health records, go to evolve.elsevier.com. Select: Chapter 14, **Electronic Health Records.**

Refer to p. 10 for your Evolve Access Information.

EXERCISE 44 *Interpret Medical Terms*

To test your understanding of the terms introduced in this chapter, circle the words that correctly complete the sentences. The italicized words refer to the correct answer.

1. The medical term for *hunchback* is (**kyphosis, ankylosis, scoliosis**).
2. The medical term for *excision of cartilage* is (**carpectomy, chondrectomy, costectomy**).
3. *Difficult movement* is (**hyperkinesia, bradykinesia, dyskinesia**).
4. Vitamin D deficiency in adults may cause *osteomalacia*, or (**muscle weakness, marblelike bones, softening of bones**).
5. The *surgical breaking of a bone* to correct a deformity is called (**osteoclasis, arthroclasia, osteoplasty**).
6. The medical term that means *pertaining to below the rib* is (**subscapular, subcostal, substernal**).
7. The medical term for *growing together* is (**diaphysis, epiphysis, symphysis**).
8. A(n) (**orthopedist, podiatrist, chiropractor**) is *competent to treat* a person with a *fractured femur*.
9. (**Osteoporosis, osteopetrosis, osteomyelitis**) is the *abnormal loss of bone density*.
10. A common *disorder of the wrist caused by compression of the median nerve* is called (**lordosis, carpal tunnel syndrome, synoviosarcoma**).
11. Some patients who are taking statin drugs to lower their cholesterol levels may experience a rather rare side effect, *dissolution of striated muscle*, or (**spondylosis, rhabdomyolysis, spondylolisthesis**).
12. During an examination of the patient's left knee, *a crackling sound* (**osteopenia, exostosis, crepitus**) was noted during flexion, extension, and range of motion of the joint.

EXERCISE 45 *Read Medical Terms in Use*

Practice the pronunciation of terms by reading the following statements. Use the pronunciation key following the medical terms to assist you in saying the word.

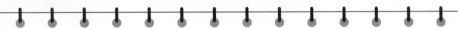

1. The **orthopedist** (or-thō-PĒ-dist) recommended Mr. Shah have an **arthrodesis** (*ar*-thrō-DĒ-sis) to reduce pain caused from an ankle **fracture** (FRAK-chur) he sustained several years ago.
2. Mrs. Diaz severed a tendon by accidentally walking through a glass patio door. A **tenorrhaphy** (te-NOR-a-fē) was performed to repair the tendon.
3. An **electromyogram** (e-*lek*-trō-MĪ-ō-gram) can assist the physician in diagnosing **muscular dystrophy** (MUS-kū-lar) (DIS-trō-fē). **Atrophy** (AT-rō-fē) frequently occurs in patients with this disease.
4. Adjective forms of medical terms are used by health professionals to indicate areas of the body that describe anatomic locations, areas of pain, sites of injections, locations of lesions, and so forth. Below are some examples.
   a. **cranial** (KRĀ-nē-al) laceration
   b. **intercostal** (*in*-ter-KOS-tal) muscles
   c. pain in the **subcostal** (sub-KOS-tal) region
   d. herniation of an **intervertebral** (*in*-ter-VER-te-bral) disk
   e. **intracranial** (*in*-tra-KRĀ-nē-al) pressure
   f. **femoral** (FEM-or-al) artery
   g. strain of the **ischiopubic** (*is*-kē-ō-PŪ-bik) area
   h. degenerative disease of the **sternoclavicular** (*ster*-nō-kla-VIK-ū-lar) joint

To hear these terms, go to evolve.elsevier.com. Select: Chapter 14, **Exercises**, Read Medical Terms in Use.

Refer to p. 10 for your Evolve Access Information.

WEB LINK

For additional information on arthritis, visit the **Arthritis Foundation** at *www.arthritis.org*.

EXERCISE 46 *Comprehend Medical Terms in Use*

Test your comprehension of terms in the previous statements by circling the correct answer.

1. T F A specialist in treating and diagnosing disorders of the foot recommended Mr. Shah for surgical fixation of the ankle joint.
2. A record of electrical activity of muscles is used in the diagnosis of:
   a. an abnormal benign growth on the surface of the body
   b. a group of hereditary diseases involving muscular degeneration and weakness
   c. wrist fracture
   d. form of arthritis that causes a forward bend of the spine
3. Which one of the following corresponds to a statement in number 4?
   a. herniation within the vertebra
   b. degenerative disease of the joint between the scapula and collarbone
   c. laceration of the wrist
   d. pain below the ribs

EXERCISE 47 *Use Plural Endings*

Circle the correct singular or plural term to match the context of the sentence.

1. The (**epiphysis, epiphyses**) are the enlarged ends of the long bone.
2. The distal (**phalanx, phalanges**) of the ring finger was fractured.
3. Osteoporosis was present in four lumbar (**vertebrae, vertebra**).
4. A (**prosthesis, prostheses**) was implanted in the left hip.
5. Many synovial joints contain (**bursa, bursae**).

 For a snapshot assessment of your knowledge of musculoskeletal system terms, go to evolve.elsevier.com.
Select: Chapter 14, **Quick Quizzes.**

Refer to p. 10 for Evolve Access Information.

CHAPTER REVIEW

(e) *Review of Evolve*

Keep a record of the online activities you have completed by placing a check mark in the box. You may also record your scores. All activities have been referenced throughout the chapter.

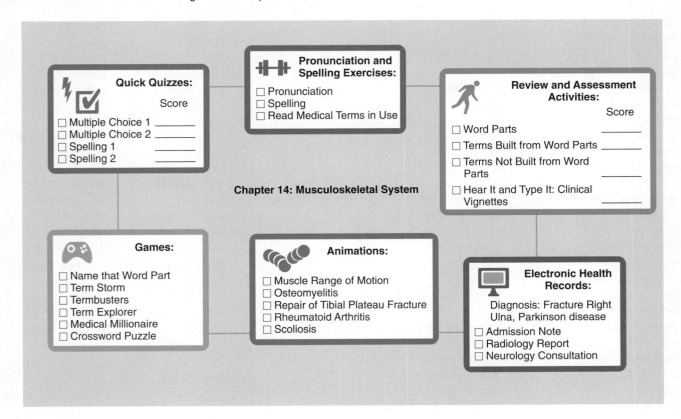

Quick Quizzes:

Score
☐ Multiple Choice 1 _____
☐ Multiple Choice 2 _____
☐ Spelling 1 _____
☐ Spelling 2 _____

Pronunciation and Spelling Exercises:
☐ Pronunciation
☐ Spelling
☐ Read Medical Terms in Use

Review and Assessment Activities:

Score
☐ Word Parts _____
☐ Terms Built from Word Parts _____
☐ Terms Not Built from Word Parts _____
☐ Hear It and Type It: Clinical Vignettes

Chapter 14: Musculoskeletal System

Games:
☐ Name that Word Part
☐ Term Storm
☐ Termbusters
☐ Term Explorer
☐ Medical Millionaire
☐ Crossword Puzzle

Animations:
☐ Muscle Range of Motion
☐ Osteomyelitis
☐ Repair of Tibial Plateau Fracture
☐ Rheumatoid Arthritis
☐ Scoliosis

Electronic Health Records:

Diagnosis: Fracture Right Ulna, Parkinson disease
☐ Admission Note
☐ Radiology Report
☐ Neurology Consultation

Review of Word Parts

Can you define and spell the following word parts?

COMBINING FORMS					PREFIXES	SUFFIXES
ankyl/o	disk/o	lumb/o	petr/o	synovi/o	inter-	-asthenia
aponeur/o	femor/o	mandibul/o	phalang/o	tars/o	supra-	-clasia
arthr/o	fibul/o	maxill/o	pub/o	ten/o	sym-	-clasis
burs/o	humer/o	menisc/o	rachi/o	tend/o	syn-	-clast
carp/o	ili/o	my/o	radi/o	tendin/o		-desis
chondr/o	ischi/o	myel/o	sacr/o	tibi/o		-physis
clavic/o	kinesi/o	myos/o	scapul/o	uln/o		-schisis
clavicul/o	kyph/o	oste/o	scoli/o	vertebr/o		
cost/o	lamin/o	patell/o	spondyl/o			
crani/o	lord/o	pelv/i	stern/o			
		pelv/o				

Review of Terms

Can you define, pronounce, and spell the following terms *built from word parts?*

DISEASES AND DISORDERS	SURGICAL	DIAGNOSTIC	COMPLEMENTARY	
ankylosis	aponeurorrhaphy	arthrography	arthralgia	osteoblast
arthritis	arthrocentesis	arthroscopy	atrophy	osteoclast
bursitis	arthroclasia	electromyogram (EMG)	bradykinesia	osteocyte
chondromalacia	arthrodesis		carpal	osteonecrosis
cranioschisis	arthroplasty		clavicular	pelvic
diskitis	bursectomy		costochondral	pelvisacral
fibromyalgia	carpectomy		cranial	pubic
kyphosis	chondrectomy		dyskinesia	pubofemoral
lordosis	chondroplasty		dystrophy	radial
maxillitis	costectomy		femoral	sacral
meniscitis	cranioplasty		humeral	sternoclavicular
myasthenia	craniotomy		hyperkinesia	sternoid
myeloma	diskectomy		hypertrophy	subcostal
osteitis	laminectomy		iliofemoral	submandibular
osteoarthritis (OA)	maxillectomy		intercostal	submaxillary
osteochondritis	meniscectomy		intervertebral	subscapular
osteofibroma	myorrhaphy		intracranial	substernal
osteomalacia	ostectomy		ischiofibular	suprapatellar
osteomyelitis	osteoclasis		ischiopubic	suprascapular
osteopenia	patellectomy		lumbar	symphysis
osteopetrosis	phalangectomy		lumbocostal	tibial
osteosarcoma	rachiotomy		lumbosacral	ulnoradial
polymyositis	spondylosyndesis		myalgia	vertebrocostal
rachischisis	synovectomy			
rhabdomyolysis	tarsectomy			
sarcopenia	tenomyoplasty			
scoliosis	tenorrhaphy			
spondylarthritis	vertebroplasty			
spondylosis				
synoviosarcoma				
tendinitis				
tenosynovitis				

Can you define, pronounce, and spell the following terms *not built from word parts?*

TYPES OF BODY MOVEMENTS

abduction
adduction
eversion
extension
flexion
inversion
pronation
rotation
supination

DISEASES AND DISORDERS	COMPLEMENTARY
ankylosing spondylitis	chiropodist
bunion	chiropractic
carpal tunnel syndrome (CTS)	chiropractor
Colles fracture	crepitus
exostosis	orthopedics (ortho)
fracture (fx)	orthopedist
gout	orthotics
herniated disk	orthotist
Lyme disease	osteoclast
muscular dystrophy (MD)	osteopath (DO)
myasthenia gravis (MG)	osteopathy
osteoporosis	podiatrist
plantar fasciitis	prosthesis
rheumatoid arthritis (RA)	rheumatologist
spinal stenosis	rheumatology
spondylolisthesis	

ANSWERS

ANSWERS TO CHAPTER 14 EXERCISES

Exercise Figures

Exercise Figure

A.
1. mandible: mandibul/o
2. sternum: stern/o
3. phalanges: phalang/o
4. patella: patell/o
5. tarsals: tars/o
6. phalanges: phalang/o
7. cranium: crani/o
8. maxilla: maxill/o
9. clavicle: clavic/o, clavicul/o
10. ribs: cost/o
11. femur: femor/o
12. fibula: fibul/o
13. tibia: tibi/o

Exercise Figure

B.
1. vertebra: rachi/o, spondyl/o, vertebr/o
2. scapula: scapul/o
3. humerus: humer/o
4. ulna: uln/o
5. radius: radi/o
6. carpals: carp/o
7. ilium: ili/o
8. pubis: pub/o
9. ischium: ischi/o
10. sacrum: sacr/o

Exercise Figure

C.
1. synovial membrane: synovi/o
2. joint: arthr/o
3. meniscus: menisc/o
4. tendon: ten/o, tend/o, tendin/o
5. cartilage: chondr/o
6. bursa: burs/o

Exercise Figure

D.
1. lord/osis
2. kyph/osis
3. scoli/osis

Exercise Figure

E. arthr/o/scopy

Exercise 1
1. d
2. i
3. h
4. k
5. j
6. g
7. b
8. c
9. f
10. a

Exercise 2
1. scapula
2. sternum
3. mandible
4. clavicle
5. humerus
6. a. ulna
   b. radius
7. tarsals
8. phalanges
9. metatarsals
10. metacarpals
11. femur
12. a. fibula
    b. tibia
13. patella
14. cervical vertebrae
15. lumbar
16. pubis
17. sacrum
18. ischium
19. coccyx
20. ilium
21. carpals

Exercise 3
1. m
2. c
3. e
4. a
5. l
6. d
7. h
8. i
9. k
10. b
11. f
12. g

Exercise 4
1. moving away from the midline
2. movement that turns the palm down
3. movement that turns the palm up
4. turning around its own axis
5. movement in which a limb is placed in a straight position
6. turning outward
7. moving toward the midline
8. movement in which a limb is bent
9. turning inward

Exercise 5
1. h
2. d
3. i
4. j
5. c
6. a
7. g
8. f
9. b

Exercise 6
1. clavicle
2. rib
3. cranium (skull)
4. femur
5. clavicle
6. humerus
7. ilium
8. ischium
9. carpals
10. fibula
11. mandible
12. loin, lumbar region of the spine
13. pelvis, pelvic bone

Exercise 7
1. a. clavicul/o
   b. clavic/o
2. cost/o
3. crani/o
4. femor/o
5. humer/o
6. carp/o
7. ischi/o
8. fibul/o
9. ili/o
10. mandibul/o
11. lumb/o
12. a. pelv/i
    b. pelv/o

Exercise 8
1. vertebra
2. patella
3. vertebra
4. maxilla
5. phalanges
6. ulna
7. radius
8. tibia
9. pubis
10. tarsals
11. scapula
12. sternum
13. vertebra
14. sacrum

Exercise 9
1. maxill/o
2. uln/o
3. radi/o
4. tibi/o
5. pub/o
6. tars/o
7. a. rachi/o
   b. spondyl/o
   c. vertebr/o
8. stern/o
9. scapul/o
10. patell/o
11. phalang/o
12. sacr/o

Exercise 10
1. joint
2. aponeurosis
3. meniscus
4. tendon
5. cartilage
6. tendon
7. bursa
8. tendon
9. synovia, synovial membrane
10. intervertebral disk

Exercise 11
1. menisc/o
2. aponeur/o
3. arthr/o
4. chondr/o
5. a. tendin/o
   b. ten/o
   c. tend/o
6. burs/o
7. synovi/o
8. disk/o

Exercise 12
1. muscle
2. stone
3. movement, motion
4. bone
5. lamina
6. bone marrow
7. hump
8. stiff, bent
9. crooked, curved
10. muscle
11. bent forward

Exercise 13
1. a. my/o
   b. myos/o
2. petr/o
3. kinesi/o
4. oste/o
5. lamin/o
6. myel/o
7. kyph/o
8. ankyl/o
9. scoli/o
10. lord/o

Exercise 14
1. above
2. together, joined
3. between

Exercise 15
1. a. syn-
   b. sym-
2. inter-
3. supra-

Exercise 16
1. growth
2. break
3. surgical fixation, fusion
4. break
5. split, fissure
6. break
7. weakness

Exercise 17
1. -physis
2. -asthenia
3. a. -clasis
   b. -clast
   c. -clasia
4. -desis
5. -schisis

Exercise 18
Pronunciation Exercise

Exercise 19
Note: The combining form is identified by italic and bold print.

1. WR S
   oste/itis
   inflammation of the bone

2. WR CV WR S
   oste/o/myel/itis
         CF
   inflammation of the bone and bone marrow

3. WR CV WR S
   oste/o/petr/osis
         CF
   abnormal condition of stonelike bones (marblelike bones)

4. WR CV S
   oste/o/malacia
         CF
   softening of bone

5. WR CV WR   S
   oste/o/chondr/itis
         CF
   inflammation of the bone and cartilage

6. WR CV WR S
   oste/o/fibr/oma
         CF
   tumor of the bone and fibrous tissue

7. WR S
   arthr/itis
   inflammation of a joint

8. WR CV WR CV S
   rhabd/o/my/o/lysis
       CF   CF
   dissolution of striated muscle

9. WR S
   myel/oma
   tumor of the bone marrow

10. WR S
    tendin/itis
    inflammation of a tendon

11. WR CV S
    oste/o/penia
          CF
    abnormal reduction of bone (mass)

12. WR S
    spondyl/osis
    abnormal condition of the vertebrae

13. WR S
    burs/itis
    inflammation of the bursa

14. WR WR S
    spondyl/arthr/itis
    inflammation of the vertebral joints

15. WR S
    ankyl/osis
    abnormal condition of stiffness

16. WR S
    kyph/osis
    abnormal condition of a hump (increased convexity of thoracic spine)

17. WR S
    scoli/osis
    abnormal condition of (lateral) curved (spine)

18. WR CV S
    crani/o/schisis
          CF
    fissure of the cranium

19. WR S
    maxill/itis
    inflammation of the maxilla

20. WR S
    menisc/itis
    inflammation of the meniscus

21. WR S
    rachi/schisis
    fissure of the vertebral column

22. WR S
    my/asthenia
    muscle weakness

23. WR CV S
    oste/o/sarcoma
          CF
    malignant tumor of the bone

24. WR CV S
    chondr/o/malacia
            CF
    softening of cartilage

25. WR CV   S
    synovi/o/sarcoma
            CF
    malignant tumor of the synovial membrane

26. WR CV WR S
    ten/o/synov/itis
         CF
    inflammation of the tendon and synovial membrane

27. P WR S
    poly/myos/itis
    inflammation of many muscles

28. WR S
    disk/itis
    inflammation of an intervertebral disk

29. WR S
    lord/osis
    abnormal condition of bending forward (increased concavity of lumbar spine)

30. WR CV WR S
    oste/o/arthr/itis
          CF
    inflammation of bone and joint

31. WR CV WR S
    fibr/o/my/algia
          CF
    pain in the fibrous tissues and muscles

32. WR CV S
    sarc/o/penia
          CF
    abnormal reduction of connective tissue

Exercise 20
1. oste/o/chondr/itis
2. oste/o/fibr/oma
3. arthr/itis
4. rhabd/o/my/o/lysis
5. myel/oma
6. tendin/itis
7. spondyl/osis
8. oste/o/penia
9. burs/itis
10. spondyl/arthr/itis
11. ankyl/osis
12. kyph/osis
13. scoli/osis
14. crani/o/schisis
15. maxill/itis
16. menisc/itis
17. rachi/schisis

18. my/asthenia
19. oste/itis
20. oste/o/myel/itis
21. oste/o/petr/osis
22. oste/o/malacia
23. ten/o/synov/itis
24. synovi/o/sarcoma
25. oste/o/sarcoma
26. chondr/o/malacia
27. disk/itis
28. poly/myos/itis
29. lord/osis
30. oste/o/arthr/itis
31. fibr/o/my/algia
32. sarc/o/penia

Exercise 21
Spelling Exercise; see text p. 607.

Exercise 22
Pronunciation Exercise

Exercise 23
1. exostosis
2. muscular dystrophy
3. myasthenia gravis
4. bunion
5. ankylosing spondylitis
6. gout
7. herniated disk
8. fracture
9. osteoporosis
10. carpal tunnel syndrome
11. Colles fracture
12. rheumatoid arthritis
13. spondylolisthesis
14. Lyme disease
15. spinal stenosis
16. plantar fasciitis

Exercise 24
1. abnormal benign growth on the surface of a bone
2. group of hereditary diseases characterized by degeneration of muscle and weakness
3. chronic disease characterized by muscle weakness and thought to be caused by a defect in the transmission of impulses from nerve to muscle cell
4. abnormal prominence of the joint at the base of the great toe
5. form of arthritis that first affects the spine and adjacent structures
6. abnormal loss of bone density
7. disease in which an excessive amount of uric acid in the blood causes sodium urate crystals (tophi) to be deposited in the joints

8. rupture of the intervertebral disk cartilage, which allows the contents to protrude through it, putting pressure on the spinal nerve roots
9. broken bone
10. disorder of the wrist caused by compression of the median nerve
11. type of fractured wrist
12. chronic systemic disease characterized by autoimmune inflammatory changes in the connective tissue throughout the body
13. infection transmitted to humans by deer ticks
14. forward slipping of one vertebra over another
15. narrowing of the spinal column with compression of nerve roots
16. inflammation of plantar fascia due to repetitive injury

Exercise 25
Spelling Exercise; see text p. 613.

Exercise 26
Pronunciation Exercise

Exercise 27
Note: The combining form is identified by italic and bold print.

1. WR CV S
   oste/o/clasis
      CF
   (surgical) breaking of a bone
2. WR   S
   ost/ectomy
   excision of bone
3. WR CV S
   arthr/o/clasia
      CF
   (surgical) breaking of a (stiff) joint
4. WR CV S
   arthr/o/desis
      CF
   surgical fixation of a joint
5. WR CV S
   arthr/o/plasty
      CF
   surgical repair of a joint
6. WR   S
   chondr/ectomy
   excision of a cartilage
7. WR CV S
   chondr/o/plasty
      CF
   surgical repair of a cartilage

8. WR CV S
   my/o/rrhaphy
      CF
   suturing of a muscle
9. WR CV WR CV S
   ten/o/my/o/plasty
      CF   CF
   surgical repair of the tendon and muscle
10. WR CV   S
    ten/o/rrhaphy
       CF
    suturing of a tendon
11. WR   S
    cost/ectomy
    excision of a rib
12. WR   S
    patell/ectomy
    excision of the patella
13. WR CV S
    aponeur/o/rrhaphy
       CF
    suturing of an aponeurosis
14. WR   S
    carp/ectomy
    excision of a carpal bone
15. WR   S
    phalang/ectomy
    excision of a finger or toe bone
16. WR   S
    menisc/ectomy
    excision of the meniscus
17. WR   CV P   S
    spondyl/o/syn/desis
       CF
    fusing together of the vertebrae
18. WR   S
    lamin/ectomy
    excision of the lamina
19. WR   S
    burs/ectomy
    excision of a bursa
20. WR CV S
    crani/o/tomy
       CF
    incision into the cranium
21. WR CV S
    crani/o/plasty
       CF
    surgical repair of the skull
22. WR   S
    maxill/ectomy
    excision of the maxilla
23. WR CV S
    rachi/o/tomy
       CF
    incision into the vertebral column

24. WR   S
tars/ectomy
excision of (one or more) tarsal bones

25. WR   S
synov/ectomy
excision of the synovial membrane

26. WR   S
disk/ectomy
excision of an intervertebral disk

27.   WR   CV   S
***vertebr/o*/**plasty
     CF
surgical repair of a vertebra

28. WR CV   S
***arthr/o*/**centesis
     CF
surgical puncture to aspirate fluid from a joint

Exercise 28

1. oste/o/clasis
2. ost/ectomy
3. arthr/o/clasia
4. arthr/o/desis
5. arthr/o/plasty
6. chondr/ectomy
7. chondr/o/plasty
8. my/o/rrhaphy
9. ten/o/my/o/plasty
10. ten/o/rrhaphy
11. cost/ectomy
12. patell/ectomy
13. aponeur/o/rrhaphy
14. carp/ectomy
15. phalang/ectomy
16. menisc/ectomy
17. spondyl/o/syn/desis
18. lamin/ectomy
19. burs/ectomy
20. crani/o/tomy
21. crani/o/plasty
22. maxill/ectomy
23. rachi/o/tomy
24. tars/ectomy
25. synov/ectomy
26. disk/ectomy
27. vertebr/o/plasty
28. arthr/o/centesis

Exercise 29

Spelling Exercise; see text p. 619.

Exercise 30

Pronunciation Exercise

Exercise 31

Note: The combining form is identified by italic and bold print.

1. WR   CV   WR   CV   S
***electr/o*/*my/o*/**gram
     CF   CF
record of the electrical activity in a muscle

2. WR CV   S
***arthr/o*/**graphy
    CF
radiographic imaging of a joint

3. WR CV   S
***arthr/o*/**scopy
    CF
visual examination of a joint

Exercise 32

1. arthr/o/graphy
2. arthr/o/scopy
3. electr/o/my/o/gram

Exercise 33

Spelling Exercise; see text p. 622.

Exercise 34

Pronunciation Exercise

Exercise 35

Note: The combining form is identified by italic and bold print.

1. P   S(WR)
sym/physis
growing together

2. WR   S
femor/al
pertaining to the femur

3. WR   S
humer/al
pertaining to the humerus

4. P   WR   S
inter/vertebr/al
pertaining to between the vertebrae

5. P   WR   S
hyper/kinesi/a
excessive movement (overactivity)

6. P   WR   S
dys/kinesi/a
difficult movement

7. P   WR   S
brady/kinesi/a
slow movement

8. P   WR   S
intra/crani/al
pertaining to within the cranium

9. WR CV WR   S
***stern/o*/**clavicul/ar
       CF
pertaining to the sternum and clavicle

10. WR CV WR   S
***ili/o*/**femor/al
    CF
pertaining to the ilium and femur

11. WR CV WR   S
***ischi/o*/**fibul/ar
     CF
pertaining to the ischium and fibula

12. P   WR   S
sub/maxill/ary
pertaining to below the maxilla

13. WR CV WR S
***ischi/o*/**pub/ic
     CF
pertaining to the ischium and pubis

14. P   WR   S
sub/mandibul/ar
pertaining to below the mandible

15. WR CV   WR   S
***pub/o*/**femor/al
     CF
pertaining to the pubis and femur

16. P   WR   S
supra/scapul/ar
pertaining to above the scapula

17. P   WR   S
sub/cost/al
pertaining to below the rib

18.   WR CV WR   S
***vertebr/o*/**cost/al
       CF
pertaining to the vertebrae and ribs

19. P   WR   S
sub/scapul/ar
pertaining to below the scapula

20. WR CV WR
***oste/o*/**blast
    CF
developing bone (cell)

21. WR CV   S
***oste/o*/**cyte
    CF
bone cell

22. WR CV WR   S
***oste/o*/**necr/osis
    CF
abnormal condition of bone death

23.   WR   S
stern/oid
resembling the sternum

24. WR S
arthr/algia
pain in the joint

25. WR S
carp/al
pertaining to the wrist

26. WR S
lumb/ar
pertaining to the loins

27. WR CV WR S
lumb/o/cost/al
   CF
pertaining to the loins and ribs

28. WR CV WR S
lumb/o/sacr/al
   CF
pertaining to the lumbar region
(loin) and the sacrum

29. WR S
sacr/al
pertaining to the sacrum

30. WR S
pub/ic
pertaining to the pubis

31. P WR S
sub/stern/al
pertaining to under the sternum

32. P WR S
supra/patell/ar
pertaining to above the patella

33. P S(WR)
dys/trophy
abnormal development

34. P S(WR)
a/trophy
without development

35. P S(WR)
hyper/trophy
excessive development

36. P WR S
inter/cost/al
pertaining to between the ribs

37. WR S
crani/al
pertaining to the cranium

38. WR S
pelv/ic
pertaining to the pelvis

39. WR CV WR S
pelv/i/sacr/al
   CF
pertaining to the pelvis and sacrum

40. WR S
clavicul/ar
pertaining to the clavicle

41. WR S
tibi/al
pertaining to the tibia

42. WR S
radi/al
pertaining to the radius

43. WR CV WR S
uln/o/radi/al
pertaining to the ulna and radius

44. WR CV WR S
cost/o/chondr/al
pertaining to ribs and cartilage

45. WR S
my/algia
pain in muscle

Exercise 36

1. sym/physis
2. femor/al
3. humer/al
4. inter/vertebr/al
5. hyper/kinesi/a
6. dys/kinesi/a
7. brady/kinesi/a
8. intra/crani/al
9. stern/o/clavicul/ar
10. ili/o/femor/al
11. ischi/o/fibul/ar
12. sub/maxill/ary
13. ischi/o/pub/ic
14. sub/mandibul/ar
15. pub/o/femor/al
16. supra/scapul/ar
17. sub/cost/al
18. vertebr/o/cost/al
19. sub/scapul/ar
20. oste/o/blast
21. oste/o/cyte
22. oste/o/necr/osis
23. stern/oid
24. arthr/algia
25. carp/al
26. sacr/al
27. lumb/ar
28. pub/ic
29. lumb/o/sacr/al
30. lumb/o/cost/al
31. sub/stern/al
32. supra/patell/ar
33. dys/trophy
34. a/trophy
35. hyper/trophy
36. crani/al
37. inter/cost/al
38. pelv/ic
39. pelv/i/sacr/al
40. clavicul/ar
41. tibi/al
42. radi/al
43. uln/o/radi/al

44. cost/o/chondr/al
45. my/algia

Exercise 37
Spelling Exercise; see text p. 628.

Exercise 38
Pronunciation Exercise

Exercise 39
1. c	8. i
2. f	9. k
3. d	10. l
4. a, h	11. g
5. j	12. n
6. b	13. m
7. e	14. o

Exercise 40

1. specialist in chiropractic
2. system of treatment that consists of manipulation of the vertebral column
3. study and treatment of diseases and abnormalities of the musculoskeletal system
4. physician who specializes in the study and treatment of diseases and abnormalities of the musculoskeletal system
5. specialist in treating and diagnosing diseases and disorders of the foot
6. specialist in treating and diagnosing diseases and disorders of the foot
7. physician who specializes in osteopathy
8. system of medicine in which greater emphasis is on the relation between body organs and the musculoskeletal system
9. making and fitting of orthopedic appliances
10. artificial substitute for a missing body part
11. person who specializes in orthotics
12. crackling sound heard when two bones rub against each other or grating caused by rubbing together of dry surfaces
13. type of bone cell involved in absorption and removal of bone minerals
14. physician who specializes in the study and treatment of rheumatic diseases
15. study and treatment of rheumatic diseases

Exercise 41
Spelling Exercise; see text p. 631.

Exercise 42

1. cervical vertebrae; thoracic vertebrae; lumbar vertebrae
2. rheumatoid arthritis
3. osteoarthritis
4. myasthenia gravis
5. electromyogram
6. carpal tunnel syndrome
7. muscular dystrophy
8. herniated nucleus pulposus
9. total hip arthroplasty
10. Doctor of Osteopathy

Exercise 43

A.
1. orthopedic
2. arthroscopy
3. arthritis
4. medial
5. suprapatellar
6. chondromalacia
7. pathology

B.
1. c
2. d

C. Online Exercise

Exercise 44

1. kyphosis
2. chondrectomy
3. dyskinesia
4. softening of bones
5. osteoclasis
6. subcostal
7. symphysis
8. orthopedist
9. osteoporosis
10. carpal tunnel syndrome
11. rhabdomyolysis
12. crepitus

Exercise 45

Reading Exercise

Exercise 46

1. *F*, an orthopedist and not a podiatrist is treating Mr. Shah.
2. b
3. d

Exercise 47

1. epiphyses
2. phalanx
3. vertebrae
4. prosthesis
5. bursae

Outline

Objectives

Upon completion of this chapter you will be able to:

1   Identify organs and structures of the nervous system.

2   Define and spell word parts related to the nervous system.

3   Define, pronounce, and spell disease and disorder terms related to the nervous system.

4   Define, pronounce, and spell surgical terms related to the nervous system.

5   Define, pronounce, and spell diagnostic terms related to the nervous system.

6   Define, pronounce, and spell complementary terms related to the nervous system.

7   Define, pronounce, and spell behavioral health terms.

8   Interpret the meaning of abbreviations related to the nervous system.

9   Interpret, read, and comprehend medical language in simulated medical statements, documents, and electronic health records.

ANATOMY

The nervous system consists of the brain, spinal cord, and nerves and may be divided into two parts: the **central nervous system** (CNS) and the **peripheral nervous system** (PNS) (Figures 15-1 and 15-2). The central nervous system consists of the brain and spinal cord. The peripheral nervous system is made up of cranial nerves, which carry impulses between the brain and neck and head, and spinal nerves, which carry messages between the spinal cord and abdomen, limbs, and chest.

Function

The nervous system forms a complex communication system allowing for the coordination of body functions and activities. As a whole, the nervous system is designed to detect changes inside and outside the body, to evaluate this sensory information, and to send directions to muscles or glands in response. This system also provides for mental activities such as thought, memory, and emotions.

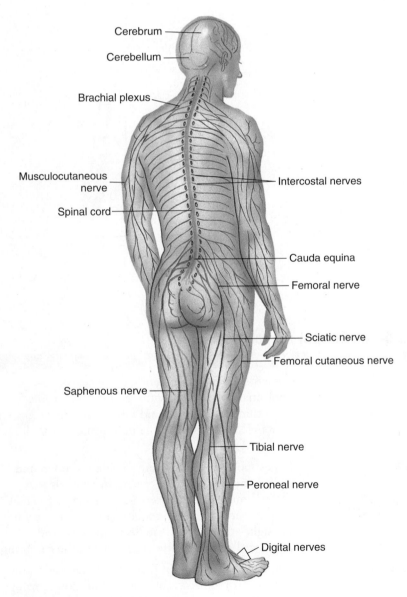

FIGURE 15-1
Simplified view of the nervous system.

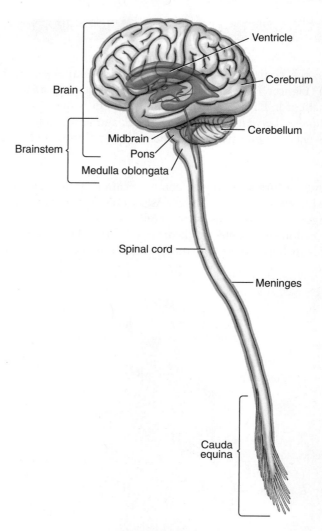

FIGURE 15-2
Brain and spinal cord.

Organs of the Central Nervous System

TERM	DEFINITION
brain	contained within the cranium, the center for coordinating body activities and comprises the cerebrum, cerebellum, and brainstem; the brainstem contains the pons, medulla oblongata, and midbrain (Figure 15-2)
cerebrum	largest portion of the brain, divided into left and right hemispheres. The cerebrum controls the skeletal muscles, interprets general senses (such as temperature, pain, and touch), and contains centers for sight and hearing. Intellect, memory, and emotional reactions also take place in the cerebrum.
ventricles	spaces within the brain that contain **cerebrospinal fluid (CSF)**. The cerebrospinal fluid flows through the subarachnoid space around the brain and spinal cord.

TERM	DEFINITION
cerebellum	located under the posterior portion of the cerebrum; assists in the coordination of skeletal muscles to maintain balance (also called **hindbrain**)
brainstem	stemlike portion of the brain that connects with the spinal cord; contains centers that control respiration and heart rate. Three structures comprise the brainstem: pons, medulla oblongata, and midbrain.
pons	literally means **bridge**. It connects the cerebrum with the cerebellum and brainstem.
medulla oblongata	located between the pons and spinal cord. It contains centers that control respiration, heart rate, and the muscles in the blood vessel walls, which assist in determining blood pressure.
midbrain	most superior portion of the brainstem
cerebrospinal fluid (CSF)	clear, colorless fluid contained in the ventricles that flows through the subarachnoid space around the brain and spinal cord. It cushions the brain and spinal cord from shock, transports nutrients, and clears metabolic waste.
spinal cord	passes through the vertebral canal extending from the medulla oblongata to the level of the second lumbar vertebra. The spinal cord conducts nerve impulses to and from the brain and initiates reflex action to sensory information without input from the brain.
meninges	three layers of membrane that cover the brain and spinal cord (Figure 15-3)
dura mater	tough outer layer of the meninges
arachnoid	delicate middle layer of the meninges. The arachnoid membrane is loosely attached to the pia mater by weblike fibers, which allow for the **subarachnoid space**.
pia mater	thin inner layer of the meninges

🏛 **CEREBELLUM**
was named in the third century BC by Erasistratus, who also named the cerebrum. **Cerebellum** literally means **little brain** and is the diminutive of **cerebrum,** meaning **brain.** Although it was named long ago, its function was not understood until the nineteenth century.

🏛 **MENINGES**
were first named by a Persian physician in the tenth century. When translated into Latin, they became **dura mater,** meaning **hard mother** (because it is a tough membrane), and **pia mater,** meaning **soft mother** (because it is a delicate membrane). **Mater** was used because the Arabians believed that the meninges were the mother of all other body membranes.

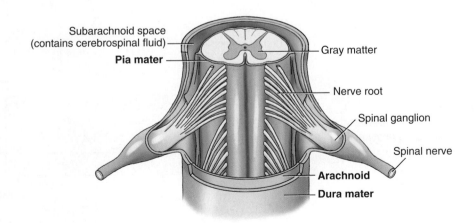

FIGURE 15-3
Layers of meninges.

Organs of the Peripheral Nervous System

TERM	DEFINITION
nerve	cordlike structure made up of fibers that carries impulses from one part of the body to another. There are 12 pairs of cranial nerves and 31 pairs of spinal nerves (see Figures 15-1 and 15-4).
ganglion (pl. ganglia)	group of nerve cell bodies located outside the central nervous system
glia	specialized cells that support and nourish nervous tissue. Some cells assist in the secretion of cerebrospinal fluid and others assist with phagocytosis. They do not conduct impulses. Three types of glia are **astroglia, oligodendroglia,** and **microglia** (also called **neuroglia**).
neuron	nerve cell that conducts nerve impulses to carry out the function of the nervous system. Destroyed neurons cannot be replaced.

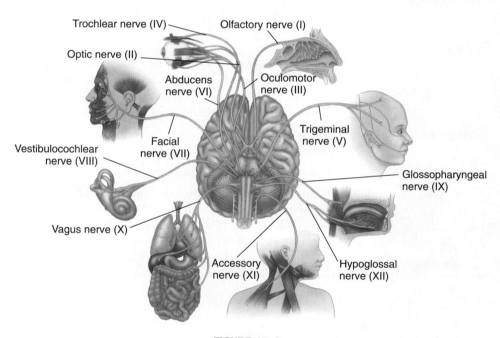

FIGURE 15-4
Cranial nerves.

A & P Booster

For more anatomy and physiology, go to evolve.elsevier.com.
Select: **Extra Content**, A & P Booster, Chapter 15.

Refer to p. 10 for your Evolve Access Information.

EXERCISE 1

Fill in the blanks with the correct terms. *To check your answers to the exercises in this chapter, go to Answers, p. 696, at the end of the chapter.*

The layer of membrane that covers the brain and spinal cord is called the
(1) _____. Three layers that comprise this membrane are
called (2) _____, (3) _____, and
(4) _____. Below the middle layer is a space called the
(5) _____ _____ through which the
(6) _____ flows around the brain and spinal cord.

EXERCISE 2

Match the definitions in the first column with the correct terms in the second column.

_____ 1. coordinates skeletal muscles to maintain
balance

_____ 2. connects the cerebrum with the cerebellum
and brainstem

_____ 3. spaces within the brain

_____ 4. contains the control centers for respiration
and heart rate

_____ 5. carries impulses from one part of the body
to another

_____ 6. conducts impulses to and from the brain and
initiates reflex action to sensory information

_____ 7. group of nerve cell bodies outside the central
nervous system

_____ 8. colorless fluid contained in the ventricles

_____ 9. supports and nourishes nervous tissue

a. nerve
b. ganglion
c. cerebrospinal fluid
d. cerebellum
e. medulla oblongata
f. pons
g. ventricles
h. spinal cord
i. pia mater
j. glia

 WORD PARTS

Word parts you need to learn to complete this chapter are listed on the following
pages. The exercises at the end of each list will help you learn their definitions and
spellings.

 Use the flashcards accompanying this text or electronic flashcards to assist you in memorizing the
word parts for this chapter.

 To use electronic flashcards, go to evolve.elsevier.com.
Select: Chapter 15, **Flashcards**.

Refer to p. 10 for your Evolve Access Information.

Combining Forms of the Nervous System

COMBINING FORM	DEFINITION
cerebell/o	cerebellum
cerebr/o	cerebrum, brain
dur/o	hard, dura mater
encephal/o	brain

Combining Forms of the Nervous System—cont'd

COMBINING FORM	DEFINITION
gangli/o, ganglion/o	ganglion
gli/o	glia, gluey substance
mening/o, meningi/o	meninges
myel/o *(NOTE: myel/o also means bone marrow; see Chapter 14)*	spinal cord
neur/o *(NOTE: neur/o was introduced in Chapter 2)*	nerve
radic/o, radicul/o, rhiz/o	nerve root (proximal end of a peripheral nerve, closest to the spinal cord)

EXERCISE FIGURE **A**

Fill in the blanks with combining forms in this diagram of the brain and spinal cord. *To check your answers, go to p. 696.*

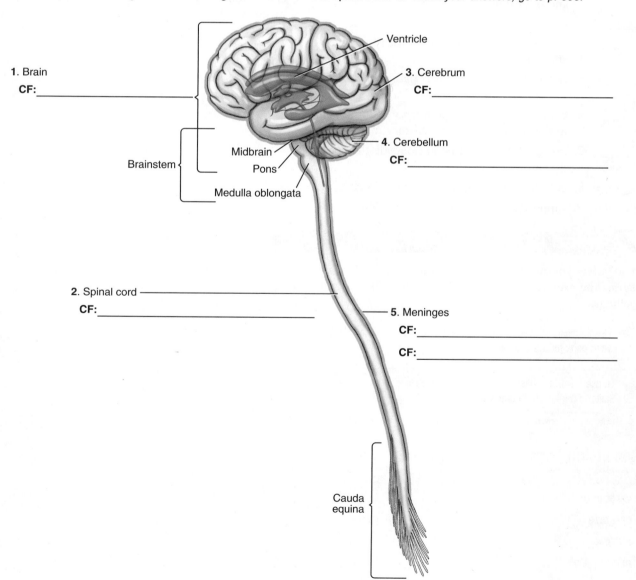

1. Brain
   CF:_____

2. Spinal cord
   CF:_____

Brainstem
Midbrain
Pons
Medulla oblongata

Ventricle

3. Cerebrum
   CF:_____

4. Cerebellum
   CF:_____

5. Meninges
   CF:_____
   CF:_____

Cauda equina

EXERCISE FIGURE B

Fill in the blanks with combining forms in this diagram of the spinal cord and layers of meninges.

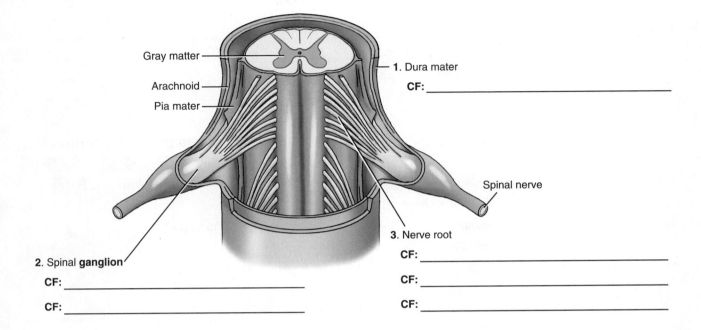

Gray matter

Arachnoid

Pia mater

1. Dura mater

CF: _____

Spinal nerve

3. Nerve root

CF: _____

CF: _____

2. Spinal **ganglion**

CF: _____

CF: _____

CF: _____

EXERCISE 3

Write the definitions of the following combining forms.

1. cerebell/o _____
2. neur/o _____
3. myel/o _____
4. meningi/o, mening/o _____
5. encephal/o _____
6. cerebr/o _____
7. radicul/o _____
8. gangli/o _____
9. radic/o _____
10. dur/o _____
11. ganglion/o _____
12. rhiz/o _____
13. gli/o _____

EXERCISE 4

Write the combining form for each of the following terms.

1. cerebellum _____
2. nerve _____
3. spinal cord _____
4. meninges   a. _____
            b. _____

    5. brain_____

    6. cerebrum, brain _____

    7. nerve root   a._____

                  b._____

                  c._____

    8. hard, dura mater_____

    9. ganglion   a. _____

                  b. _____

  10. glia, gluey substance_____

Combining Forms Commonly Used with Nervous System Terms

COMBINING FORM	DEFINITION
esthesi/o	sensation, sensitivity, feeling
ment/o, psych/o	mind
mon/o	one, single
phas/o	speech
poli/o	gray matter
quadr/i (NOTE: an i is the combining vowel in quadr/i)	four

EXERCISE 5

Write the definitions of the following combining forms.

    1. mon/o _____

    2. psych/o _____

    3. quadr/i_____

    4. ment/o_____

    5. phas/o _____

    6. esthesi/o _____

    7. poli/o_____

EXERCISE 6

Write the combining form for each of the following.

    1. four _____

    2. one, single_____

    3. mind   a. _____

             b. _____

    4. speech _____

    5. gray matter _____

    6. sensation, sensitivity, feeling_____

Suffixes

SUFFIX	DEFINITION
-iatrist	specialist, physician (-*logist* also means specialist)
-iatry	treatment, specialty
-ictal	seizure, attack
-paresis	slight paralysis (-*plegia*, meaning *paralysis*, was covered in Chapter 12)

EXERCISE 7

Write the definitions of the following suffixes.

1. -paresis _____
2. -iatry _____
3. -ictal_____
4. -iatrist _____

EXERCISE 8

Write the suffix for each of the following.

1. slight paralysis _____
2. treatment, specialty _____
3. seizure, attack _____
4. specialist, physician _____

For review and/or assessment, go to evolve.elsevier.com. Select:
Chapter 15, **Activities**, Word Parts
Chapter 15, **Games,** Name that Word Part

Refer to p. 10 for your Evolve Access Information.

💬 MEDICAL TERMS

Disease and Disorder Terms

Built from Word Parts

The following terms are built from word parts you have already learned and can be translated literally to find their meanings. Further explanation of terms beyond the definition of their word parts, if needed, is included in parentheses.

TERM	DEFINITION
cerebellitis (*ser*-e-bel-Ī-tis)	inflammation of the cerebellum
cerebral thrombosis (se-RĒ-bral) (throm-BŌ-sis)	pertaining to the cerebrum, abnormal condition of a clot (blood clot in a blood vessel of the brain). (Onset of symptoms may appear from minutes to days after an obstruction occurs; a cause of **ischemic stroke**) (see Figure 15-12, *A*).

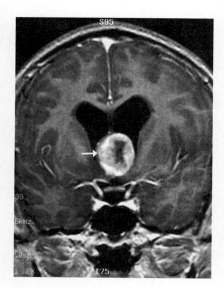

FIGURE 15-5
MRI image of brain demonstrating glioblastoma (arrow).

Disease and Disorder Terms—cont'd

Built from Word Parts

TERM	DEFINITION
duritis (dū-RĪ-tis)	inflammation of the dura mater
encephalitis (en-*sef*-a-LĪ-tis)	inflammation of the brain
encephalomalacia (en-*sef*-a-lō-ma-LĀ-sha)	softening of the brain
encephalomyeloradiculitis (en-*sef*-a-lō-*mī*-e-lō-ra-*dik*-ū-LĪ-tis)	inflammation of the brain, spinal cord, and nerve roots
gangliitis (*gang*-glē-Ī-tis)	inflammation of a ganglion
glioblastoma (*glī*-ō-blas-TŌ-ma)	tumor composed of developing glial tissue (the most malignant and most common primary tumor of the brain) (Figure 15-5)
glioma (glī-Ō-ma)	tumor composed of the glial tissue (glioma is used to describe all primary neoplasms of the brain and spinal cord)
meningioma (me-*nin*-jē-Ō-ma)	tumor of the meninges (benign and slow growing)
meningitis (*men*-in-JĪ-tis)	inflammation of the meninges
meningocele (me-NING-gō-sēl)	protrusion of the meninges (through a defect in the skull or vertebral arch)
meningomyelocele (me-*ning*-gō-MĪ-e-lō-*sēl*)	protrusion of the meninges and spinal cord (through a neural arch defect in the vertebral column) (also called **myelomeningocele**) (see Figure 9-10)
mononeuropathy (*mon*-ō-nū-ROP-a-thē)	disease affecting a single nerve (such as carpal tunnel syndrome)
neuralgia (nū-RAL-ja)	pain in a nerve
neuritis (nū-RĪ-tis)	inflammation of a nerve
neuroarthropathy (*nū*-rō-ar-THROP-a-thē)	disease of nerves and joints

TERM	DEFINITION
neuroma (nū-RŌ-ma)	tumor made up of nerve (cells)
neuropathy (nū-ROP-a-thē)	disease of the nerves (peripheral) (Figure 15-6)
poliomyelitis (pō-lē-ō-*mī*-e-LĪ-tis)	inflammation of the gray matter of the spinal cord. (This infectious disease, commonly referred to as *polio*, is caused by one of three polio viruses.)
polyneuritis (*pol*-ē-nū-RĪ-tis)	inflammation of many nerves
polyneuropathy (*pol*-ē-nū-ROP-a-thē)	disease of many nerves (most often occurs as a side effect of diabetes mellitus, but may also occur as a result of drug therapy, critical illness such as sepsis, or carcinoma; exhibiting symptoms of weakness, distal sensory loss, and burning)
radiculitis (ra-*dik*-ū-LĪ-tis)	inflammation of the nerve roots
radiculopathy (ra-*dik*-ū-LOP-a-thē)	disease of the nerve roots
rhizomeningomyelitis (rī-zō-me-*ning*-gō-*mī*-e-LĪ-tis)	inflammation of the nerve root, meninges, and spinal cord
subdural hematoma (sub-DŪ-ral) (*hē*-ma-TŌ-ma)	pertaining to below the dura mater, tumor of blood (*hematoma*, translated literally, means *blood tumor*; however, a hematoma is a collection of blood resulting from a broken blood vessel) (Figure 15-7)

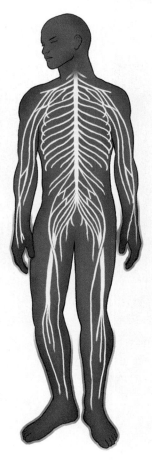

FIGURE 15-6
Peripheral neuropathy.

PERIPHERAL NEUROPATHY

refers to disorders of the peripheral nervous system, including **radiculopathy, neuropathy,** and **mononeuropathy.** The term is often used synonymously with **polyneuropathy.** Signs and symptoms vary and usually begin gradually, starting with tingling and numbness in the toes and spreading to the feet and upwards. Symptoms may be felt only at night, be constant, or be barely noticed by the patient. Other symptoms include numbness, loss of balance, tingling, burning or freezing sensation, and muscle weakness.

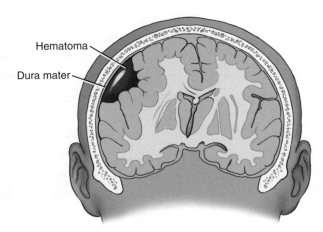

Hematoma
Dura mater

FIGURE 15-7
Subdural hematoma.

> To watch animations, go to evolve.elsevier.com. Select:
> Chapter 15, **Animations**, Cerebral Thrombosis Leading to Stroke
> Meningitis
> Subdural Hematoma
>
> Refer to p. 10 for your Evolve Access Information.

EXERCISE 9

Practice saying aloud each of the disease and disorder terms built from word parts on pp. 655–657.

> To hear the terms, go to evolve.elsevier.com. Select: Chapter 15, **Exercises**, Pronunciation.
>
> Refer to p. 10 for your Evolve Access Information.

☐ Place a check mark in the box when you have completed this exercise.

EXERCISE 10

Analyze and define the following terms.

1. neuritis_____
2. neuroma _____
3. neuralgia _____
4. neuroarthropathy _____
5. meningioma _____
6. encephalomalacia _____
7. encephalitis _____
8. encephalomyeloradiculitis _____
9. meningitis _____
10. meningocele _____
11. meningomyelocele _____
12. radiculitis_____
13. cerebellitis_____
14. gangliitis _____
15. duritis_____
16. polyneuritis_____
17. poliomyelitis_____
18. cerebral thrombosis _____
19. subdural hematoma _____
20. rhizomeningomyelitis _____
21. mononeuropathy _____
22. neuropathy _____
23. radiculopathy _____
24. glioma _____
25. glioblastoma _____
26. polyneuropathy_____

EXERCISE 11

Build disease and disorder terms for the following definitions with the word parts you have learned.

1. inflammation of the nerve   _____ / _____
                                        WR   S

2. tumor made up of nerve (cells) _____ / _____
                                        WR   S

3. pain in a nerve   _____ / _____
                                        WR   S

4. disease of nerves and joints _____ /CV/ _____ /CV/ ____
                                    WR   WR   S

5. disease of the nerve roots   _____ /CV/ _____
                                        WR   S

6. softening of the brain   _____ /CV/ _____
                                        WR   S

7. inflammation of the brain   _____ / _____
                                        WR   S

8. inflammation of the brain,   ____ /CV/ ____ /CV/ ____ / ____
   spinal cord, and nerve roots   WR   WR   WR   S

9. inflammation of the meninges _____ / _____
                                        WR   S

10. protrusion of the meninges   _____ /CV/ _____
    (through a defect in the skull   WR   S
    or vertebral column)

11. protrusion of the meninges   _____ /CV/ _____ /CV/ ____
    and spinal cord (through the   WR   WR   S
    vertebral column)

12. inflammation of the (spinal) _____ / _____
    nerve roots   WR   S

13. inflammation of the cerebellum _____ / _____
                                        WR   S

14. inflammation of the ganglion _____ / _____
                                        WR   S

15. inflammation of the dura mater _____ / _____
                                        WR   S

16. inflammation of many nerves _____ / _____ / _____
                                     P   WR   S

17. inflammation of the gray   _____ /CV/ _____ / ____
    matter of the spinal cord   WR   WR   S

18. pertaining to the cerebrum; _____ / ____   _____ / ____
    abnormal condition of a clot   WR   S   WR   S

19. pertaining to below the dura mater; tumor of blood

___ / ___ / ___   ___ / ___
P / WR / S   WR / S

20. inflammation of the nerve root, meninges, and spinal cord

___ / ___ / ___ / ___ / ___ / ___
WR / CV / WR / CV / WR / S

21. tumor of the meninges

___ / ___
WR / S

22. disease affecting a single nerve

___ / ___ / ___ / ___ / ___
WR / CV / WR / CV / S

23. disease of the nerves

___ / ___ / ___
WR / CV / S

24. tumor composed of glial tissue

___ / ___
WR / S

25. tumor composed of developing glial tissue

___ / ___ / ___ / ___
WR / CV / WR / S

26. disease of many nerves

___ / ___ / ___ / ___
P / WR / CV / S

EXERCISE 12

Spell each of the disease and disorder terms built from word parts on pp. 655–657 by having someone dictate them to you.

> To hear and spell the terms, go to evolve.elsevier.com. Select: Chapter 15, **Exercises**, Spelling.
>
> (e) Refer to p. 10 for your Evolve Access Information.
>
> ☐ Place a check mark in the box if you have completed this exercise online.

1. _____
2. _____
3. _____
4. _____
5. _____
6. _____
7. _____
8. _____
9. _____
10. _____
11. _____
12. _____
13. _____
14. _____
15. _____
16. _____
17. _____
18. _____
19. _____
20. _____
21. _____
22. _____
23. _____
24. _____
25. _____
26. _____

Disease and Disorder Terms

Not Built from Word Parts

In some of the following terms, you may recognize word parts you have already learned; however, the full meaning of the terms cannot be discerned by the definition of their word parts.

TERM	DEFINITION
Alzheimer disease (AD) (AWLTZ-hī-mer) (di-ZĒZ)	disease characterized by early dementia, confusion, loss of recognition of persons or familiar surroundings, restlessness, and impaired memory (Figure 15-8)
amyotrophic lateral sclerosis (ALS) (ā-mī-ō-TRŌ-fik) (LAT-er-al) (skle-RŌ-sis)	progressive muscle atrophy caused by degeneration and scarring of neurons along the lateral columns of the spinal cord that control muscles (also called **Lou Gehrig disease**)
Bell palsy (bel) (PAWL-zē)	paralysis of muscles on one side of the face caused by inflammation or compression of the facial nerve—cranial nerve VII. Signs include a sagging mouth on the affected side and nonclosure of the eyelid; paralysis is usually temporary (Figure 15-9).
cerebral aneurysm (se-RĒ-bral) (AN-ū-rizm)	aneurysm in the cerebrum (See Figure 15-12, *A*)
cerebral embolism (se-RĒ-bral) (EM-bō-lizm)	an embolus (usually a blood clot or a piece of atherosclerotic plaque arising from a distant site) lodges in a cerebral artery, causing sudden blockage of blood supply to the brain tissue. Atrial fibrillation is a common cause of cerebral embolism, which can lead to **ischemic stroke** (See Figure 15-12, *B*).
cerebral palsy (CP) (se-RĒ-bral) (PAWL-zē)	condition characterized by lack of muscle control and partial paralysis, caused by a brain defect or lesion present at birth or shortly after

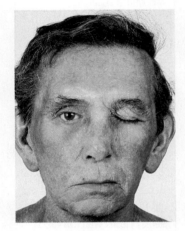

FIGURE 15-9
Bell palsy.

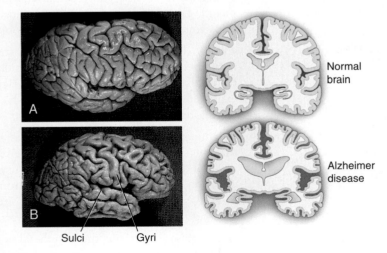

Normal brain

Alzheimer disease

Sulci   Gyri

FIGURE 15-8
Alzheimer disease. **A,** Normal brain—image and cross-section, age matched. **B,** Brain showing changes of Alzheimer disease—image and cross-section. Note brain atrophy, narrowed gyri, and wider sulci compared with normal brain.

Disease and Disorder Terms—cont'd

Not Built from Word Parts

TERM	DEFINITION
dementia (de-MEN-sha)	cognitive impairment characterized by loss of intellectual brain function. Patients have difficulty in various ways, including difficulty in performing complex tasks, reasoning, learning and retaining new information, orientation, word finding, and behavior. Dementia has several causes and is not considered part of normal aging (see Table 15-1).
epilepsy (EP-i-lep-sē)	condition characterized by recurrent seizures; a general term given to a group of neurologic disorders, all characterized by abnormal electrical activity in the brain
hydrocephalus (*hī*-drō-SEF-a-lus)	congenital or acquired disorder caused by obstructed circulation of cerebrospinal fluid, resulting in dilated cerebral ventricles and impaired brain function. For infants, hydrocephalus can cause enlargement of the cranium.
intracerebral hemorrhage (*in*-tra-SER-e-bral) (HEM-o-rij)	bleeding into the brain as a result of a ruptured blood vessel within the brain. Symptoms vary depending on the location of the hemorrhage; acute symptoms include dyspnea, dysphagia, aphasia, diminished level of consciousness, and hemiparesis. The symptoms often develop suddenly. Intracerebral hemorrhage, a cause of **hemorrhagic stroke,** is frequently associated with high blood pressure (see Figure 15-12, *A*).
multiple sclerosis (MS) (MUL-ti-pl) (skle-RŌ-sis)	chronic degenerative disease characterized by sclerotic patches along the brain and spinal cord; signs and symptoms fluctuate over the course of the disease; more common symptoms include fatigue, balance and coordination impairments, numbness, and vision problems
Parkinson disease (PD) (PAR-kin-sun) (di-ZĒZ)	chronic degenerative disease of the central nervous system. Signs and symptoms include resting tremors of the hands and feet, rigidity, expressionless face, and shuffling gait. It usually occurs after the age of 50 years.
sciatica (sī-AT-i-ka)	inflammation of the sciatic nerve, causing pain that travels from the thigh through the leg to the foot and toes; can be caused by injury, infection, arthritis, herniated disk, or from prolonged pressure on the nerve from sitting for long periods (Figure 15-10)
shingles (SHING-gelz)	viral disease that affects the peripheral nerves and causes blisters on the skin that follow the course of the affected nerves (also called **herpes zoster** [Figure 15-11])

🏛 **EPILEPSY**

was written about by Hippocrates, in 400 BC, in a book titled **Sacred Disease.** It was believed at one time that epilepsy was a punishment for offending the gods. The Greek **epilepsia** meant **seizure** and is derived from **epi,** meaning **upon,** and **lambanein,** meaning **to seize.** The term literally means **seized upon** (by the gods).

🏛 **HYDROCEPHALUS**

literally means **water in the head** and is made of the word parts **hydro,** meaning **water,** and **cephal,** meaning **head.** The condition was first described around 30 AD in the book **De Medicina.**

🏛 **PARKINSON DISEASE**

is also called **parkinsonism, paralysis agitans,** and **shaking palsy.** Since James Parkinson, an English professor, described the disease in 1817 in his **Essay on the Shaking Palsy,** it has often been referred to as **Parkinson disease.**

TERM	DEFINITION
stroke (strōk)	occurs when there is an interruption of blood supply to a region of the brain, depriving nerve cells in the affected area of oxygen and nutrients. The cells cannot perform and may be damaged or die within minutes. The parts of the body controlled by the involved cells will experience dysfunction. Speech, movement, memory, and other CNS functions may be affected in varying degrees. **Ischemic stroke** is a result of a blocked blood vessel. **Hemorrhagic stroke** is a result of bleeding. (also called **cerebrovascular accident [CVA]**, or **brain attack** [Figure 15-12])
subarachnoid hemorrhage (SAH) (*sub*-e-RAK-noid) (HEM-o-rij)	bleeding caused by a ruptured blood vessel just outside the brain (usually a ruptured cerebral aneurysm) that rapidly fills the space between the piamater and arachnoid layers of the meninges (subarachnoid space) with blood. The patient may experience an intense, sudden headache accompanied by nausea, vomiting, and neck pain (a cause of **hemorrhagic stroke**) (see Figure 15-12).
transient ischemic attack (TIA) (TRAN-sē-ent) (is-KĒ-mik) (a-TAK)	sudden deficient supply of blood to the brain lasting a short time. The symptoms may be similar to those of stroke, but with TIA the symptoms are temporary and the usual outcome is complete recovery. TIAs are often warning signs for eventual occurrence of a stroke (Figure 15-13).

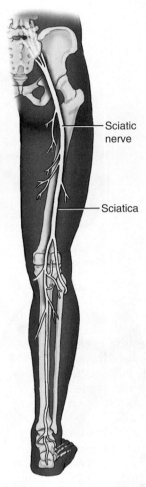

- Sciatic nerve
- Sciatica

FIGURE 15-10
Sciatica. The sciatic nerve, the longest in the body, travels through the hip from the spine to the thigh and continues with branches throughout the lower leg and foot. Sciatica is the inflammation of the nerve along its course.

POSTHERPETIC NEURALGIA

is a complication of **shingles** (herpes zoster) and is caused by damage to the nerve fibers. Severe pain and hyperesthesia persist after the skin lesions disappear and may last months or even years.

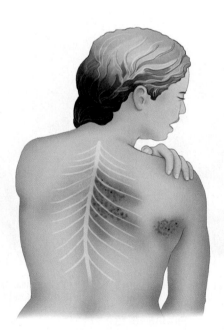

FIGURE 15-11
Shingles. This viral disease, a second outbreak of the chicken pox virus, causes painful blisters on the skin that follow the course of affected nerves.

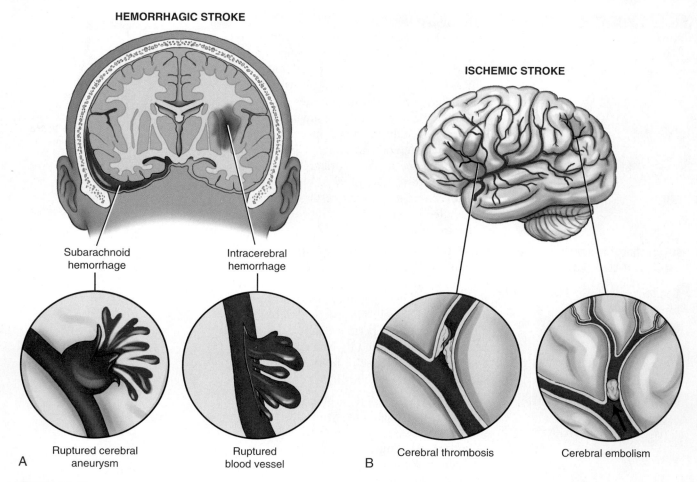

HEMORRHAGIC STROKE

ISCHEMIC STROKE

Subarachnoid hemorrhage

Intracerebral hemorrhage

A

Ruptured cerebral aneurysm

Ruptured blood vessel

B

Cerebral thrombosis

Cerebral embolism

FIGURE 15-12

Causes of stroke. **A,** Hemorrhagic stroke is the result of bleeding caused by a **subarachnoid hemorrhage** or an **intracerebral hemorrhage,** usually a result of a ruptured cerebral aneurysm or ruptured blood vessel. **B,** Ischemic stroke is the result of a blocked blood vessel caused by a **cerebral thrombosis** or **cerebral embolism.**

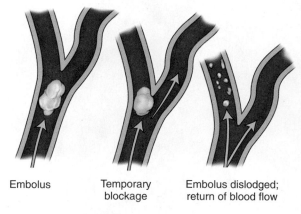

Embolus

Temporary blockage

Embolus dislodged; return of blood flow

FIGURE 15-13

Transient ischemic attack (TIA).

Table 15-1

Types of Dementia

Alzheimer disease	the most common type of dementia, making up 60% to 80% of all cases. The disease, the cause of which is unknown, is a progressive neurodegenerative disorder characterized by diffuse brain atrophy and the presence of senile plaques and neurofibrillary tangles within the brain cortex. Women are affected more than men, and the disease usually occurs after the age of 60. The disease is slowly progressive and usually results in profound dementia in 5 to 10 years.
Vascular or multiple infarct dementia	affects approximately 10% to 20% of patients with dementia. It is secondary to cerebrovascular disease and usually occurs in older patients.
Central nervous system infection dementia	may be caused by herpes simplex encephalitis or may be seen in patients with AIDS
Lewy body dementia	usually a rapidly progressive form of dementia seen with Parkinson syndrome
Parkinson disease	may develop in patients with advanced disease
Wernicke-Korsakoff syndrome	a form of dementia found with chronic alcoholism
Normal pressure hydrocephalus	may cause dementia in elderly individuals and can be treated with a ventricular peritoneal shunt

EXERCISE 13

Practice saying aloud each of the disease and disorder terms not built from word parts on pp. 661–663.

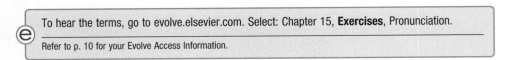

To hear the terms, go to evolve.elsevier.com. Select: Chapter 15, **Exercises**, Pronunciation.

Refer to p. 10 for your Evolve Access Information.

☐ Place a check mark in the box when you have completed this exercise.

EXERCISE 14

Fill in the blanks with correct terms.

1. A stroke occurs when there is a disruption of blood supply to a region of the brain. Four causes of stroke are a) _____ _____, b) _____ _____, c) _____ _____, and d) _____ _____.

2. A ruptured _____ _____ is often the cause of a subarachnoid hemorrhage.

3. _____ _____ is the paralysis of muscles on one side of the face.

4. The term to describe obstructed circulation of cerebrospinal fluid causing dilated ventricles of the brain is _____.

5. Inflammation of the nerve that travels from the thigh to the toes is called _____.

6. A viral disease that affects peripheral nerves is _____.

7. The symptoms of a _____ _____ _____ are similar to a stroke but temporary and the patient usually experiences complete recovery.

8. A degenerative disease of the central nervous system usually occurring after the age of 50 years is called _____ _____.

9. A condition with the main symptom being recurring seizures is _____.

10. _____ _____ _____ is caused by degeneration and scarring of the nerve tissue along the lateral columns of the spinal cord.

11. _____ _____ is characterized by early dementia, confusion, impaired memory, and loss of recognition.

12. _____ _____ is characterized by lack of muscle coordination and partial paralysis and is present at birth or shortly after.

13. A chronic disease characterized by sclerotic patches along the brain and spinal cord is called _____ _____.

14. A type of cognitive impairment that is not considered part of normal aging is called _____.

EXERCISE 15

Match the diseases in the first column with the corresponding phrases in the second column.

_____ 1. cerebral embolism
_____ 2. sciatica
_____ 3. transient ischemic attack
_____ 4. Parkinson disease
_____ 5. cerebral palsy
_____ 6. hydrocephalus
_____ 7. dementia
_____ 8. stroke
_____ 9. Alzheimer disease
_____ 10. intracerebral hemorrhage
_____ 11. epilepsy
_____ 12. multiple sclerosis
_____ 13. shingles
_____ 14. amyotrophic lateral sclerosis
_____ 15. Bell palsy
_____ 16. cerebral aneurysm
_____ 17. subarachnoid hemorrhage

a. causes pain from the thigh to the toes
b. blocking of a cerebral artery by a blood clot or plaque
c. paralysis of muscles on one side of the face
d. sclerotic patches along the brain and spinal cord
e. cognitive impairment characterized by loss of intellectual brain function
f. aneurysm in the cerebrum
g. occurs when there is an interruption of blood supply to the brain
h. blisters on the skin caused by viral disease
i. disease characterized by early dementia
j. resting tremors of the hands and feet and rigidity
k. inflammation of the spinal cord
l. partial paralysis at birth
m. bleeding within the brain tissue
n. deficient supply of blood to the brain lasting a short time
o. also called Lou Gehrig disease
p. obstructed circulation of cerebrospinal fluid
q. recurring seizures
r. bleeding that fills space between the piamater and arachnoid layers of the meninges

EXERCISE 16

Spell each of the disease and disorder terms not built from word parts on pp. 661–663 by having someone dictate them to you.

> To hear and spell the terms, go to evolve.elsevier.com. Select: Chapter 15, **Exercises**, Spelling.
>
> Refer to p. 10 for your Evolve Access Information.
>
> ☐ Place a check mark in the box if you have completed this exercise online.

1. _____
2. _____
3. _____
4. _____
5. _____
6. _____
7. _____
8. _____
9. _____

10. _____
11. _____
12. _____
13. _____
14. _____
15. _____
16. _____
17. _____

EXERCISE FIGURE C

Fill in the blanks to complete labeling of this diagram.

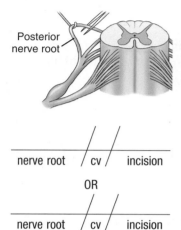

Posterior
nerve root

_____ / / _____
nerve root / cv / incision

OR

_____ / / _____
nerve root / cv / incision

STEREOTACTIC RADIOSURGERY

is used to treat patients with **brain tumors or arteriovenous malformations (AVMs).** A special frame is mounted on the patient's head. Images of the brain are produced by MRI. A high-powered computer uses the images to design a plan for high-intensity radiation that matches the exact size and shape of the tumor. Radiation is then delivered directly to the tumor only, sparing surrounding tissue. This procedure may also be called **Gamma-knife radiosurgery**.

Surgical Terms

Built from Word Parts

The following terms are built from word parts you have already learned and can be translated literally to find their meanings. Further explanation of terms beyond the definition of their word parts, if needed, is included in parentheses.

TERM	DEFINITION
ganglionectomy (*gang*-glē-o-NEK-to-mē)	excision of a ganglion (also called **gangliectomy**)
neurectomy (nū-REK-to-mē)	excision of a nerve
neurolysis (nū-ROL-i-sis)	dissolution of a nerve (for pain management)
neuroplasty (NŪR-ō-*plas*-tē)	surgical repair of a nerve
neurorrhaphy (nū-ROR-a-fē)	suturing of a nerve
neurotomy (nū-ROT-o-mē)	incision into a nerve
radicotomy, rhizotomy (*rad*-i-KOT-o-mē), (rī-ZOT-o-mē)	incision into a nerve root (Exercise Figure C)

EXERCISE 17

Practice saying aloud each of the surgical terms built from word parts.

To hear the terms, go to evolve.elsevier.com. Select: Chapter 15, **Exercises**, Pronunciation.
Refer to p. 10 for your Evolve Access Information.

☐ Place a check mark in the box when you have completed this exercise.

EXERCISE 18

Analyze and define the following surgical terms.

1. radicotomy _____

2. neurectomy _____

3. neurorrhaphy _____

4. ganglionectomy _____

5. neurotomy _____

6. neurolysis _____

7. neuroplasty _____

8. rhizotomy _____

EXERCISE 19

Build surgical terms for the following definitions by using the word parts you have learned.

1. incision into a nerve root   a._____
                        WR   CV   S

                        b._____
                        WR   CV   S

2. excision of a nerve   _____
                        WR   S

3. suturing of a nerve   _____
                        WR   CV   S

4. excision of a ganglion   _____
                        WR   S

5. incision into a nerve   _____
                        WR   CV   S

6. separating or dissolution of a nerve   _____
                        WR   CV   S

7. surgical repair of a nerve   _____
                        WR   CV   S

EXERCISE 20

Spell each of the surgical terms built from word parts by having someone dictate them to you.

> To hear and spell the terms, go to evolve.elsevier.com. Select: Chapter 15, **Exercises**, Spelling.
>
> ℮ Refer to p. 10 for your Evolve Access Information.
>
> ☐ Place a check mark in the box if you have completed this exercise online.

1. _____   5. _____

2. _____   6. _____

3. _____   7. _____

4. _____   8. _____

EXERCISE FIGURE D

EXERCISE FIGURE

Fill in the blanks to complete labeling of the diagram.

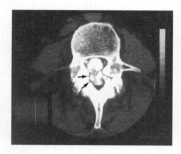

CT _____ / ___ / _____
   spinal   / cv / process of
    cord   recording

Diagnostic Terms

Built from Word Parts

The following terms are built from word parts you have already learned and can be translated literally to find their meanings. Further explanation of terms beyond the definition of their word parts, if needed, is included in parentheses.

TERM	DEFINITION
DIAGNOSTIC IMAGING	
cerebral angiography (se-RĒ-bral) (*an*-jē-OG-ra-fē)	process of recording (scan) of the (blood) vessels of the cerebrum (after an injection of contrast medium) (Figure 15-14)
CT myelography (*mī*-e-LOG-ra-fē)	process of recording (scan) the spinal cord (after an injection of a contrast agent into the subarachnoid space by lumbar puncture. Size, shape, and position of the spinal cord and nerve roots are demonstrated.) (Exercise Figure D)
NEURODIAGNOSTIC PROCEDURES	
electroencephalogram (EEG) (ē-*lek*-trō-en-SEF-a-lō-gram)	record of electrical activity of the brain
electroencephalograph (ē-*lek*-trō-en-SEF-a-lō-graf)	instrument used to record electrical activity of the brain
electroencephalography (ē-*lek*-trō-en-*sef*-a-LOG-ra-fē)	process of recording the electrical activity of the brain

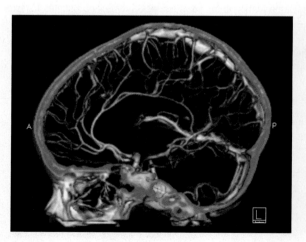

FIGURE 15-14
Cerebral angiogram. CT imaging of cerebral arterial and venous circulation.

EXERCISE 21

Practice saying aloud each of the diagnostic terms built from word parts.

 To hear the terms, go to evolve.elsevier.com. Select: Chapter 15, **Exercises**, Pronunciation.

Refer to p. 10 for your Evolve Access Information.

☐ Place a check mark in the box when you have completed this exercise.

EXERCISE 22

Analyze and define the following diagnostic terms.

1. electroencephalogram _____
2. electroencephalograph _____
3. electroencephalography _____
4. CT myelography _____
5. cerebral angiography _____

EXERCISE 23

Build diagnostic terms that correspond to the following definitions by using the word parts you have learned.

1. record of electrical activity of the brain

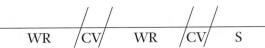
WR / CV / WR / CV / S

2. instrument used to record electrical activity of the brain

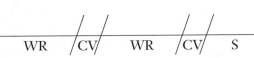
WR / CV / WR / CV / S

3. process of recording the electrical activity of the brain

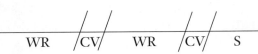
WR / CV / WR / CV / S

4. process of recording (scan) the spinal cord

CT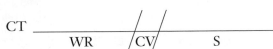
WR / CV / S

5. process of recording (scan) of the (blood) vessels of the cerebrum

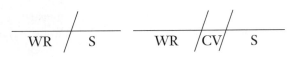
WR / S   WR / CV / S

EXERCISE 24

Spell each of the diagnostic terms built from word parts on p. 670 by having someone dictate them to you.

> To hear and spell the terms, go to evolve.elsevier.com. Select: Chapter 15, **Exercises**, Spelling.
>
> Refer to p. 10 for your Evolve Access Information.
>
> ☐ Place a check mark in the box if you have completed this exercise online.

1. _____   4. _____

2. _____   5. _____

3. _____

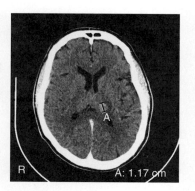

FIGURE 15-15
CT scan of the brain demonstrating a tumor, measured at 1.17 cm.

Diagnostic Terms

Not Built from Word Parts

TERM	DEFINITION
DIAGNOSTIC IMAGING	
computed tomography (CT) of the brain (com-PŪ-td) (tō-MOG-ra-fē)	computerized radiographic process producing a series of sectional images (slices) of brain tissue. Useful in diagnosing brain tumors (Figure 15-15).
magnetic resonance imaging (MRI) of the brain or spine (mag-NET-ik) (REZ-ō-nans) (IM-a-jing)	high-strength computer-controlled magnetic fields producing a series of sectional images (slices) of the soft tissues of the brain or spine. Used to visualize tumors, edema, multiple sclerosis, and herniated disks (Figure 15-16).
positron emission tomography (PET) scan of the brain (POZ-i-tron) (ē-MISH-un) (tō-MOG-ra-fē)	nuclear medicine procedure combining CT and radioactive chemicals producing sectional images of the brain to examine blood flow and metabolic activity. (Figure 15-17).
NEURODIAGNOSTIC PROCEDURES	
evoked potential studies (EP studies) (i-VŌKD) (pō-TEN-shal)	group of diagnostic tests that measure changes and responses in brain waves elicited by visual, auditory, or somatosensory stimuli. Visual evoked response (VER) is a response to visual stimuli. Auditory evoked response (AER) is a response to auditory stimuli.
OTHER	
lumbar puncture (LP) (LUM-bar) (PUNK-chur)	diagnostic procedure performed by insertion of a needle into the subarachnoid space usually between the third and fourth lumbar vertebrae; performed for many reasons, including the removal of cerebrospinal fluid (also called **spinal tap**) (Figure 15-18)

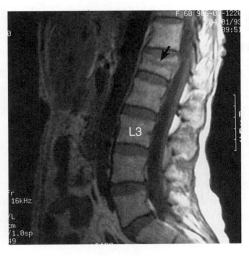

FIGURE 15-16
Sagittal MRI section of the lumbar spine demonstrating a compression fracture of L1 caused by trauma (arrow).

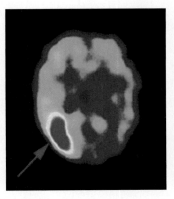

FIGURE 15-17
Positron emission tomography (PET) scan of an infant with seizures. The arrow points to the area of increased brain metabolism, indicating the seizure focus.

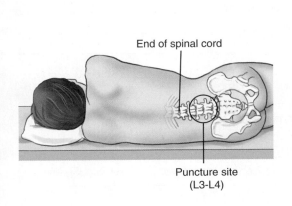

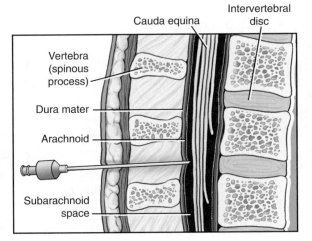

FIGURE 15-18
Lumbar puncture (spinal tap).

EXERCISE 25

Practice saying aloud each of the diagnostic terms not built from word parts.

To hear the terms, go to evolve.elsevier.com. Select: Chapter 15, **Exercises**, Pronunciation.

Refer to p. 10 for your Evolve Access Information.

☐ Place a check mark in the box when you have completed this exercise.

EXERCISE 26

Fill in the blanks with the correct terms.

1. A computer and radiation are used to produce images during

   _____ _____ of the brain.

2. A needle is inserted into the subarachnoid space and cerebrospinal fluid is

   removed during a(n) _____ _____.

3. _____ _____

   _____ produces images to examine blood flow and
   metabolic activity of the brain.

4. Uses a strong magnetic field to produce images of the brain or spine:

   _____ _____

   _____.

5. Measures responses in brain waves from stimuli: _____

   _____ _____.

EXERCISE 27

Write the definitions of the following terms.

1. lumbar puncture_____
2. computed tomography of the brain _____
3. magnetic resonance imaging of the brain or spine _____
4. positron emission tomography of the brain _____
5. evoked potential studies_____

EXERCISE 28

Spell each of the diagnostic terms not built from word parts on p. 672 by having someone dictate
them to you.

> To hear and spell the terms, go to evolve.elsevier.com. Select: Chapter 15, **Exercises**, Spelling.
>
> (e) Refer to p. 10 for your Evolve Access Information.
>
> ☐ Place a check mark in the box if you have completed this exercise online.

1. _____   4. _____
2. _____   5. _____
3. _____

Complementary Terms

Built from Word Parts

The following terms are built from word parts you have already learned and can be translated literally to find their meanings. Further explanation of terms beyond the definition of their word parts, if needed, is included in parentheses.

TERM	DEFINITION
anesthesia (*an*-es-THĒ-zha)	without (loss of) feeling or sensation
aphasia (a-FĀ-zha)	condition of without speaking (loss or impairment of the ability to speak)
cephalalgia (*sef*-el-AL-ja)	pain in the head (headache) (also called **cephalgia**)
cerebral (se-RĔ-bral)	pertaining to the cerebrum
craniocerebral (*krā*-nē-ō-su-RĔ-bral)	pertaining to the cranium and cerebrum
dysphasia (dis-FĀ-zha)	condition of difficulty speaking
encephalosclerosis (en-*sef*-a-lō-skle-RŌ-sis)	hardening of the brain
gliocyte (GLĬ-ō-sīt)	glial cell
hemiparesis (*hem*-ē-pa-RĒ-sis)	slight paralysis of half (right or left side of the body)
hemiplegia (*hem*-ē-PLĒ-ja)	paralysis of half (right or left side of the body); (stroke is the most common cause of hemiplegia) (Exercise Figure E)
hyperesthesia (*hī*-per-es-THĒ-zha)	excessive sensitivity (to stimuli)
interictal (*in*-ter-IK-tal)	(occurring) between seizures or attacks
intracerebral (*in*-tra-SER-e-bral)	pertaining to within the cerebrum
mental (MEN-tel)	pertaining to the mind
monoparesis (*mon*-ō-pa-RĒ-sis)	slight paralysis of one (limb)
monoplegia (*mon*-ō-PLĒ-ja)	paralysis of one (limb)
myelomalacia (*mī*-e-lō-ma-LĀ-sha)	softening of the spinal cord
neuroid (NŪ-royd)	resembling a nerve
neurologist (nū-ROL-o-jist)	physician who studies and treats diseases of the nervous system
neurology (nū-ROL-o-jē)	study of nerves (branch of medicine dealing with diseases of the nervous system)

HEADACHES

Migraine, tension headache, and cluster headaches account for nearly 90% of all headaches. Other types of headaches include posttraumatic headaches, giant cell (temporal) arteritis, sinus headaches, brain tumor, and chronic daily headache.

EXERCISE FIGURE **E**

Fill in the blanks to complete labeling of these diagrams of types of paralysis.

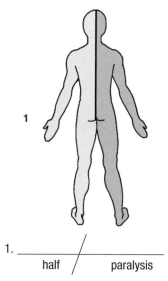

1

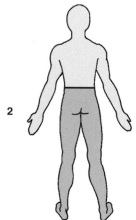

2

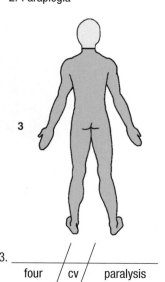

3

1. _____ / _____
   half   paralysis

2. Paraplegia

3. _____ / _____ / _____
   four   cv   paralysis

Complementary Terms—cont'd

Built from Word Parts

TERM	DEFINITION
panplegia (pan-PLĒ-ja)	total paralysis
paresthesia (*par*-es-THĒ-zha) (NOTE: the a is dropped from the prefix para)	abnormal sensation (such as burning, prickling, or tingling sensation, often in the extremities; may be caused by nerve damage or peripheral neuropathy)
postictal (pōst-IK-tal)	(occurring) after a seizure or attack
preictal (prē-IK-tal)	(occurring) before a seizure or attack
quadriplegia (*kwod*-ri-PLĒ-ja)	paralysis of four (limbs) (see Exercise Figure E)
subdural (sub-DŪ-ral)	pertaining to below the dura mater

> To watch animations, go to evolve.elsevier.com. Select:
> Chapter 15, **Animations**, Hemiparesis
>   Quadriplegia
>
> Refer to p. 10 for your Evolve Access Information.

EXERCISE 29

Practice saying aloud each of the complementary terms built from word parts on pp. 675–676.

> To hear the terms, go to evolve.elsevier.com. Select: Chapter 15, **Exercises**, Pronunciation.
> Refer to p. 10 for your Evolve Access Information.

☐ Place a check mark in the box when you have completed this exercise.

EXERCISE 30

Analyze and define the following complementary terms.

1. hemiplegia _____
2. paresthesia _____
3. neurologist _____
4. neurology _____
5. neuroid _____
6. quadriplegia _____
7. cerebral _____
8. monoplegia _____
9. aphasia _____
10. dysphasia _____
11. hemiparesis _____
12. anesthesia _____

13. hyperesthesia_____

14. subdural_____

15. cephalalgia_____

16. craniocerebral_____

17. myelomalacia _____

18. encephalosclerosis _____

19. postictal_____

20. panplegia_____

21. interictal _____

22. monoparesis _____

23. preictal_____

24. intracerebral _____

25. gliocyte _____

26. mental _____

EXERCISE 31

Build the complementary terms for the following definitions by using the word parts you have learned.

1. slight paralysis of half (right or left side of the body)

   _____ / _____
   P   S(WR)

2. without (loss of) feeling or sensation

   _____ / _____ / _____
   P   WR   S

3. excessive sensitivity (to stimuli)

   _____ / _____ / _____
   P   WR   S

4. pertaining to below the dura mater

   _____ / _____ / _____
   P   WR   S

5. pain in the head (headache)

   _____ / _____
   WR   S

6. pertaining to the cranium and cerebrum

   _____ / CV / _____ / _____
   WR   WR   S

7. softening of the spinal cord

   _____ / CV / _____
   WR   S

8. hardening of the brain

   _____ / CV / _____
   WR   S

9. paralysis of half (left or right side) of the body

   _____ / _____
   P   S(WR)

10. physician who studies and treats diseases of the nervous system

    _____ / CV / _____
    WR   S

11. study of nerves (branch of medicine dealing with diseases of the nervous system)

_____ / _____ / _____
WR   CV   S

12. resembling a nerve

_____ / _____
WR   S

13. paralysis of four (limbs)

_____ / _____ / _____
WR   CV   S

14. pertaining to the cerebrum

_____ / _____
WR   S

15. paralysis of one (limb)

_____ / _____ / _____
WR   CV   S

16. condition of without speaking (loss or impairment of the ability to speak)

_____ / _____ / _____
P   WR   S

17. condition of difficulty speaking

_____ / _____ / _____
P   WR   S

18. (occurring) before a seizure or attack

_____ / _____
P   S(WR)

19. slight paralysis of one (limb)

_____ / _____ / _____
WR   CV   S

20. (occurring) after a seizure

_____ / _____
P   S(WR)

21. total paralysis

_____ / _____
P   S(WR)

22. (occurring) between seizures or attacks

_____ / _____
P   S(WR)

23. pertaining to within the cerebrum

_____ / _____ / _____
P   WR   S

24. glial cell

_____ / _____ / _____
WR   CV   S

25. abnormal sensation

_____ / _____ / _____
P   WR   S

26. pertaining to the mind

_____ / _____
WR   S

EXERCISE 32

Spell each of the complementary terms built from word parts on pp. 675–676 by having someone dictate them to you.

> To hear and spell the terms, go to evolve.elsevier.com. Select: Chapter 15, **Exercises**, Spelling.
>
> Refer to p. 10 for your Evolve Access Information.
>
> ☐ Place a check mark in the box if you have completed this exercise online.

1. _____
2. _____
3. _____
4. _____
5. _____
6. _____
7. _____
8. _____
9. _____
10. _____
11. _____
12. _____
13. _____
14. _____
15. _____
16. _____
17. _____
18. _____
19. _____
20. _____
21. _____
22. _____
23. _____
24. _____
25. _____
26. _____

Complementary Terms

Not Built from Word Parts

In some of the following terms you may recognize word parts you have already learned; however, the full meaning of the terms cannot be discerned by the definition of their word parts.

TERM	DEFINITION
afferent (AF-er-ent)	conveying toward a center (for example, afferent nerves carry impulses to the central nervous system)
ataxia (a-TAK-sē-a)	lack of muscle coordination
cognitive (COG-ni-tiv)	pertaining to the mental processes of comprehension, judgment, memory, and reason
coma (KŌ-ma)	state of profound unconsciousness
concussion (kon-KUSH-un)	injury to the brain caused by minor or major head trauma; symptoms include vertigo, headache, and possible loss of consciousness
conscious (KON-shus)	awake, alert, aware of one's surroundings
convulsion (kun-VUL-zhun)	sudden, involuntary contraction of a group of muscles; may be present during a seizure
disorientation (dis-*or*-ē-en-TĀ-shun)	a state of mental confusion as to time, place, or identity

TYPES OF COGNITIVE IMPAIRMENT

Mild cognitive impairment (MCI) is the presence of significant memory difficulty when adjusted for age-related norms. The patient usually has little difficulty performing activities of daily living. This condition may be an early manifestation of Alzheimer disease or other forms of dementia.

Age-associated memory impairment is when memory function tends to decline with aging when compared with young adults. This is not necessarily a forerunner of dementia.

Delirium is potentially reversible acute disturbance of consciousness with impairment of cognition. A number of conditions can cause delirium by interfering with brain metabolism. Drugs, alcohol, systemic infections, head trauma, hypoglycemia, and electrolyte disturbances are common examples.

Pseudodementia is a disorder resembling dementia but is not caused by a brain disease. This can be found in mental illness, such as major depression, and can be reversible with treatment.

Complementary Terms—cont'd

Not Built from Word Parts

TERM	DEFINITION
dysarthria (dis-AR-thrē-a)	the inability to use speech that is distinct and connected because of a loss of muscle control after damage to the peripheral or central nervous system
efferent (EF-er-ent)	conveying away from the center (for example, efferent nerves carry information away from the central nervous system)
gait (gāt)	a manner or style of walking
incoherent (*in*-kō-HĒR-ent)	unable to express one's thoughts or ideas in an orderly, intelligible manner
paraplegia (*par*-a-PLĒ-ja)	paralysis from the waist down caused by damage to the lower level of the spinal cord (see Exercise Figure E)
seizure (SĒ-zher)	sudden, abnormal surge of electrical activity in the brain, resulting in involuntary body movements or behaviors
shunt (shunt)	tube implanted in the body to redirect the flow of a fluid
syncope (SINK-o-pē)	fainting or sudden loss of consciousness caused by lack of blood supply to the cerebrum
unconsciousness (un-KON-shus-nes)	state of being unaware of surroundings and incapable of responding to stimuli as a result of injury, shock, illness, or drugs

> 🏛 **PARAPLEGIA**
>
> is composed of the Greek **para,** meaning **beside,** and **plegia,** meaning **paralysis.** It has been used since Hippocrates' time and at first meant paralysis of any limb or side of the body. Since the nineteenth century, it has been used to mean paralysis from the waist down.

EXERCISE 33

Practice saying aloud each of the complementary terms not built from word parts on pp. 679–680.

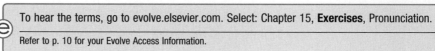

To hear the terms, go to evolve.elsevier.com. Select: Chapter 15, **Exercises**, Pronunciation.

Refer to p. 10 for your Evolve Access Information.

☐ Place a check mark in the box when you have completed this exercise.

EXERCISE 34

Write the term for each of the following definitions.

1. injury to the brain caused by head trauma _____

2. state of being unaware of surroundings and incapable of responding to stimuli as a result of injury, shock, illness, or drugs _____

3. awake, alert, aware of one's surroundings _____

4. sudden, abnormal surge of electrical activity in the brain _____

5. sudden, involuntary contraction
   of a group of muscles   _____

6. tube implanted in the body to redirect
   the flow of a fluid   _____

7. paralysis from the waist down caused
   by damage to the lower level of the
   spinal cord   _____

8. state of profound unconsciousness   _____

9. fainting or sudden loss of consciousness _____

10. lack of muscle coordination   _____

11. manner or style of walking   _____

12. inability to use speech that is distinctive
    and connected   _____

13. unable to express one's thoughts or ideas
    in an orderly, intelligible manner   _____

14. state of mental confusion as to time, place,
    or identity   _____

15. pertaining to the mental processes of
    comprehension, judgment, memory,
    and reason   _____

16. conveying toward the center   _____

17. conveying away from the center   _____

EXERCISE 35

Write the definitions for the following terms.

1. shunt _____

2. paraplegia _____

3. coma _____

4. concussion _____

5. unconsciousness _____

6. conscious _____

7. seizure _____

8. convulsion _____

9. syncope _____

10. ataxia _____

11. dysarthria _____

12. gait _____

13. cognitive _____

14. disorientation _____

15. incoherent _____

16. efferent _____

17. afferent _____

CONCUSSION

is a common type of **traumatic brain injury (TBI),** an umbrella term used to describe mild to severe damage to the brain sustained by a wide range of injuries. Falls, motor vehicle accidents, sports injuries, combat-related injuries or violence may all cause TBI. Bleeding within the brain or skull due to injury, such as **subdural hematoma, intracerebral hemorrhage** and **subarachnoid hemorrhage,** may also be categorized as TBI.

EXERCISE 36

Spell each of the complementary terms not built from word parts on pp. 679–680 by having someone dictate them to you.

> To hear and spell the terms, go to evolve.elsevier.com. Select: Chapter 15, **Exercises**, Spelling.
>
> Refer to p. 10 for your Evolve Access Information.
>
> ☐ Place a check mark in the box if you have completed this exercise online.

1. _____	10. _____
2. _____	11. _____
3. _____	12. _____
4. _____	13. _____
5. _____	14. _____
6. _____	15. _____
7. _____	16. _____
8. _____	17. _____
9. _____	

Behavioral Health

Although the terms below are listed as behavioral health terms, medications, physical changes, substance abuse, and illness may contribute to these conditions.

Built from Word Parts

The following terms are built from word parts you have already learned and can be translated literally to find their meanings. Further explanation of terms beyond the definition of their word parts, if needed, is included in parentheses.

PSYCHIATRIST

is a **physician** who has had **additional training** and experience in prevention, diagnosis, and treatment of mental disorders.

CLINICAL PSYCHOLOGIST

is one who has had **graduate study** in **psychology** and training in clinical psychology and who provides testing and counseling for mental and emotional disorders. A psychologist cannot prescribe medication or medical tests and treatments.

TERM	DEFINITION
psychiatrist (sī-KĪ-a-trist)	physician who studies and treats disorders of the mind
psychiatry (sī-KĪ-a-trē)	specialty of the mind (branch of medicine that deals with the treatment of mental disorders)
psychogenic (sī-kō-JEN-ik)	originating in the mind
psychologist (sī-KOL-o-jist)	specialist of the mind
psychology (sī-KOL-o-jē)	study of the mind (a profession that involves dealing with the mind and mental processes in relation to human behavior)
psychopathy (sī-KOP-a-thē)	(any) disease of the mind
psychosis (pl. psychoses) (sī-KO-sis), (sī-KO-sēz)	abnormal condition of the mind (major mental disorder characterized by extreme derangement, often with delusions and hallucinations)
psychosomatic (sī-kō-sō-MAT-ik)	pertaining to the mind and body (interrelations of)

EXERCISE 37

Practice saying aloud each of the behavioral health terms built from word parts.

> (e) To hear the terms, go to evolve.elsevier.com. Select: Chapter 15, **Exercises**, Pronunciation.
>
> Refer to p. 10 for your Evolve Access Information.

☐ Place a check mark in the box when you have completed this exercise.

EXERCISE 38

Build the behavioral health terms for the following definitions by using the word parts you have learned.

1. specialty of the mind (branch of medicine that deals with the treatment of mental disorders) _____
   WR / S

2. abnormal condition of the mind _____
   WR / S

3. study of the mind (a profession that involves dealing with the mind and mental processes in relation to human behavior) _____
   WR /CV/ S

4. originating in the mind _____
   WR /CV/ S

5. physician who studies and treats disorders of the mind _____
   WR / S

6. specialist of the mind _____
   WR /CV/ S

7. pertaining to the mind and body _____
   WR /CV/ WR / S

8. disease of the mind _____
   WR /CV/ S

EXERCISE 39

Analyze and define the following terms.

1. psychosomatic _____
2. psychopathy _____
3. psychology _____
4. psychiatry _____
5. psychologist _____
6. psychogenic _____
7. psychiatrist _____
8. psychosis _____

EXERCISE 40

Spell each of the behavioral health terms built from word parts on p. 682 by having someone dictate them to you.

> To hear and spell the terms, go to evolve.elsevier.com. Select: Chapter 15, **Exercises**, Spelling.
>
> Refer to p. 10 for your Evolve Access Information.
>
> ☐ Place a check mark in the box if you have completed this exercise online.

1. _____   5. _____

2. _____   6. _____

3. _____   7. _____

4. _____   8. _____

> For review and/or assessment, go to evolve.elsevier.com. Select:
> Chapter 15, **Activities,** Terms Built from Word Parts
> Chapter 15, **Games,**   Term Storm
>
> Refer to p. 10 for your Evolve Access Information.

Behavioral Health

Not Built from Word Parts

In some of the following terms, you may recognize word parts you have already learned; however, the full meaning of the terms cannot be discerned by the definition of their word parts.

TERM	DEFINITION
anorexia nervosa (*an*-ō-REK-sē-a) (ner-VŌ-sa)	eating disorder characterized by a disturbed perception of body image resulting in failure to maintain body weight, intensive fear of gaining weight, pronounced desire for thinness, and, in females, amenorrhea
anxiety disorder (ang-ZĪ-e-tē) (dis-OR-der)	emotional disorder characterized by feelings of apprehension, tension, or uneasiness arising typically from the anticipation of unreal or imagined danger
attention deficit/hyperactivity disorder (ADHD) (a-TEN-shun) (DEF-i-sit) (*hī*-per-ak-TIV-i-tē)	disorder of learning and behavioral problems characterized by marked inattention, distractibility, impulsiveness, and hyperactivity

TERM	DEFINITION
autism (AW-tizm)	spectrum of mental disorders, the features of which include onset during infancy or childhood, preoccupation with subjective mental activity, inability to interact socially, and impaired communication (also referred to as **Autism Spectrum Disorders** [ASD] or **Pervasive Developmental Disorders** [PDD])
bipolar disorder (bī-PŌ-lar) (dis-OR-der)	major psychological disorder typified by a disturbance in mood. The disorder is manifested by manic and depressive episodes that may alternate or elements of both may occur simultaneously.
bulimia nervosa (bū-LĒ-mē-a) (ner-VŌ-sa)	eating disorder characterized by uncontrolled binge eating followed by purging (induced vomiting)
major depression (MĀ-jor) (dē-PRESH-un)	mood disturbance characterized by feelings of sadness, despair, discouragement, hopelessness, lack of joy, altered sleep patterns, and difficulty with decision making and daily function. Depression ranges from normal feelings of sadness (resulting from and proportional to personal loss or tragedy), through dysthymia (chronic depressive neurosis), to major depression (also referred to as **clinical depression, mood disorder**).
obsessive-compulsive disorder (OCD) (ob-SES-iv-kom-PUL-siv) (dis-OR-der)	disorder characterized by intrusive, unwanted thoughts that result in the tendency to perform repetitive acts or rituals (compulsions), usually as a means of releasing tension or anxiety
panic attack (PAN-ik) (a-TAK)	episode of sudden onset of acute anxiety, occurring unpredictably, with feelings of acute apprehension, dyspnea, dizziness, sweating, and/or chest pain, depersonalization, paresthesia and fear of dying, loss of mind or control
phobia (FŌ-bē-a)	marked and persistent fear that is excessive or unreasonable cued by the presence or anticipation of a specific situation or object (such as claustrophobia, the abnormal fear of being in enclosed spaces)
pica (PĪ-ka)	compulsive eating of nonnutritive substances such as clay or ice. This condition is often a result of an iron deficiency. When iron deficiency is the cause of pica the condition will disappear in 1 or 2 weeks when treated with iron therapy.

Behavioral Health—cont'd

Not Built from Word Parts

TERM	DEFINITION
posttraumatic stress disorder (PTSD) (*pōst*-tra-MAT-ik) (stres) (dis-OR-der)	disorder characterized by a chronic, debilitating emotional response to a traumatic event perceived as life threatening or severe emotional stress; may be caused by exposure to repeated physical or emotional trauma, military combat, natural disasters, or serious accidents. Symptoms include anxiety, sleep disturbance, nightmares, difficulty concentrating, and depression.
schizophrenia (*skit*-sō-FRĒ-nē-a)	any one of a large group of psychotic disorders characterized by gross distortions of reality, disturbance of language and communication, withdrawal from social interaction, and the disorganization and fragmentation of thought, perception, and emotional reaction
somatoform disorders (sō-MAT-ō-form)	disorders characterized by physical symptoms for which no known physical cause exists

 CAM TERM

Biofeedback, also referred to as **neurofeedback**, is learned self-control of physiologic responses utilizing electronic devices to provide monitoring information. Current research suggests that biofeedback is a **viable alternative treatment for attention deficit hyperactivity disorder (ADHD)**.

Refer to **Appendix D** for pharmacology terms related to the nervous system and behavioral health.

To learn more behavioral health terms, go to evolve.elsevier.com.
Select: **Extra Content**, Appendices, Appendix H, Behavioral Health Terms.

Refer to p. 10 for your Evolve Access Information.

EXERCISE 41

Practice saying aloud each of the behavioral health terms not built from word parts on pp. 684–686.

To hear the terms, go to evolve.elsevier.com. Select: Chapter 15, **Exercises**, Pronunciation.

Refer to p. 10 for your Evolve Access Information.

☐ Place a check mark in the box when you have completed the exercise.

EXERCISE 42

Match the definitions in the first column with the correct terms in the second column.

_____ 1. manifested by manic and depressive episodes

_____ 2. episode of acute anxiety

_____ 3. characterized by feelings of apprehension and tension

_____ 4. disorder of learning and behavioral problems

_____ 5. mood disturbance characterized by feelings of sadness, despair, and discouragement

_____ 6. marked and persistent fear that is excessive or unreasonable

_____ 7. binge eating followed by purging

_____ 8. physical symptoms for which no known physical cause exists

_____ 9. eating of nonnutritive substances, such as ice

_____ 10. failure to maintain body weight

_____ 11. characterized by gross distortions of reality and disturbance of language and communication

_____ 12. preoccupation with subjective mental activity, inability to interact socially, and impaired communication

_____ 13. chronic, debilitating emotional response to a traumatic event

_____ 14. intrusive unwanted thoughts that result in rituals and/or repetitive acts

a. phobia
b. anxiety disorder
c. attention deficit hyperactivity disorder
d. somatoform disorders
e. schizophrenia
f. anorexia nervosa
g. bulimia nervosa
h. pica
i. bipolar disorder
j. major depression
k. obsessive-compulsive disorder
l. posttraumatic stress disorder
m. panic attack
n. autism

EXERCISE 43

Spell each of the behavioral health terms not built from word parts on pp. 684–686 by having someone dictate them to you.

> To hear and spell the terms, go to evolve.elsevier.com. Select: Chapter 15, **Exercises**, Spelling.
>
> ℮ Refer to p. 10 for your Evolve Access Information.
>
> ☐ Place a check mark in the box if you have completed this exercise online.

1. _____

2. _____

3. _____

4. _____

5. _____

6. _____

7. _____

8. _____

9. _____

10. _____

11. _____

12. _____

13. _____

14. _____

For review and/or assessment, go to evolve.elsevier.com. Select:

Chapter 15, **Activities,** Terms Not Built from Word Parts
Hear It and Type It: Clinical Vignettes

Chapter 15, **Games,** Term Explorer
Termbusters
Medical Millionaire

Refer to p. 10 for your Evolve Access Information.

Abbreviations

ABBREVIATION	MEANING
AD	Alzheimer disease
ADHD	attention deficit hyperactivity disorder
ALS	amyotrophic lateral sclerosis
CNS	central nervous system
CP	cerebral palsy
CSF	cerebrospinal fluid
CVA	cerebrovascular accident
EEG	electroencephalogram
EP studies	evoked potential studies
LP	lumbar puncture
MRI	magnetic resonance imaging
MS	multiple sclerosis
OCD	obsessive-compulsive disorder
PD	Parkinson disease
PET	positron emission tomography
PNS	peripheral nervous system
PTSD	posttraumatic stress disorder
SAH	subarachnoid hemorrhage
TIA	transient ischemic attack

 Refer to **Appendix C** for a complete list of abbreviations.

EXERCISE 44

Write the meaning of the abbreviations in the following sentences.

1. Diagnostic tests used to diagnose patients with diseases of the nervous system include **EEG** _____, **MRI** _____
_____ _____, **PET** _____
_____ _____ **EP studies** _____
_____ _____, and **LP** _____
_____.

2. Diseases that affect the nervous system are **AD** _____
_____, **ALS** _____ _____
_____, **CP** _____ _____,
MS _____ _____, and **PD** _____
_____.

3. Stroke is the disruption of normal blood supply to the brain. It often occurs suddenly. Because of this, Hippocrates used the term *apoplexy*, which literally means *struck down*, to describe the condition. The term *stroke* grew out of the term *apoplexy*. The term *brain attack* is a fairly new term used to signify that a stroke is in progress and an emergency situation exists. **CVA** _____
_____ is also used to describe a stroke. An ischemic stroke, which is caused by a thrombosis or embolus, is frequently preceded by a **TIA**
_____ _____ _____. A ruptured cerebral aneurysm is the most common cause of **SAH** _____
_____, a type of hemorrhagic stroke.

4. The examination of **CSF** _____ _____
may assist in the diagnosis of cerebral hemorrhage, meningitis, encephalitis, and other diseases.

5. Three common psychiatric disorders are **PTSD,** _____
_____ _____, **OCD** _____
_____, and **ADHD** _____
_____ _____
_____.

6. The nervous system may be divided into the **CNS** _____
_____ _____, and the **PNS** _____
_____ _____.

For more practice with abbreviations, go to evolve.elsevier.com. Select:
Chapter 15, **Flashcards**
Chapter 15, **Games,** Crossword Puzzle

Refer to p. 10 for your Evolve Access Information.

PRACTICAL APPLICATION

EXERCISE 45   *Interact with Medical Documents and Electronic Health Records*

A. Complete the progress note by writing the medical terms in the blanks. Use the list of definitions with the corresponding numbers.

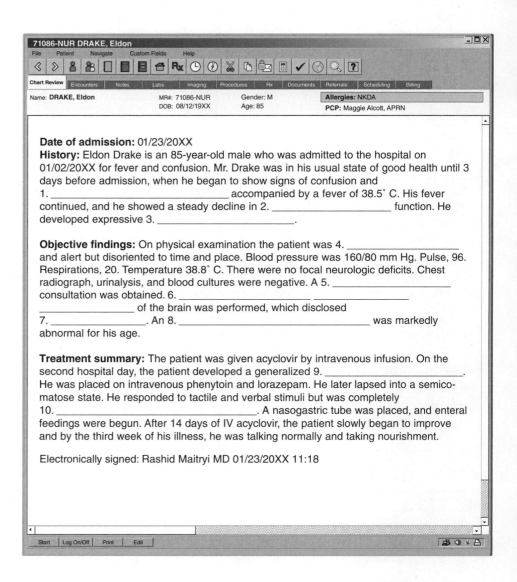

1. a state of mental confusion as to time, place, or identity
2. pertaining to the mental processes of comprehension, judgment, memory, and reason
3. loss of the ability to speak
4. awake, alert, and aware of one's surroundings
5. study of nerves (branch of medicine dealing with diseases of the nervous system)
6. uses high-strength computer-controlled magnetic fields to produce sectional images
7. inflammation of the brain
8. record of electrical impulses of the brain
9. sudden, abnormal surge of electrical activity in the brain
10. unable to express one's thoughts or ideas in an orderly, intelligible manner

B. Read the consultation report and answer the questions following it.

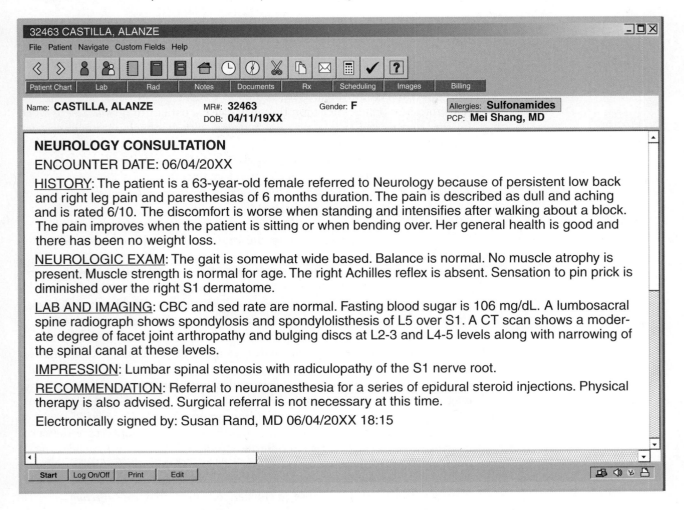

32463 CASTILLA, ALANZE

File Patient Navigate Custom Fields Help

| Patient Chart | Lab | Rad | Notes | Documents | Rx | Scheduling | Images | Billing |

Name: **CASTILLA, ALANZE**   MR#: **32463**   Gender: **F**   Allergies: **Sulfonamides**
DOB: **04/11/19XX**   PCP: **Mei Shang, MD**

NEUROLOGY CONSULTATION

ENCOUNTER DATE: 06/04/20XX

HISTORY: The patient is a 63-year-old female referred to Neurology because of persistent low back and right leg pain and paresthesias of 6 months duration. The pain is described as dull and aching and is rated 6/10. The discomfort is worse when standing and intensifies after walking about a block. The pain improves when the patient is sitting or when bending over. Her general health is good and there has been no weight loss.

NEUROLOGIC EXAM: The gait is somewhat wide based. Balance is normal. No muscle atrophy is present. Muscle strength is normal for age. The right Achilles reflex is absent. Sensation to pin prick is diminished over the right S1 dermatome.

LAB AND IMAGING: CBC and sed rate are normal. Fasting blood sugar is 106 mg/dL. A lumbosacral spine radiograph shows spondylosis and spondylolisthesis of L5 over S1. A CT scan shows a moderate degree of facet joint arthropathy and bulging discs at L2-3 and L4-5 levels along with narrowing of the spinal canal at these levels.

IMPRESSION: Lumbar spinal stenosis with radiculopathy of the S1 nerve root.

RECOMMENDATION: Referral to neuroanesthesia for a series of epidural steroid injections. Physical therapy is also advised. Surgical referral is not necessary at this time.

Electronically signed by: Susan Rand, MD 06/04/20XX 18:15

Start   Log On/Off   Print   Edit

1. Spinal stenosis causes compression of nerve roots demonstrated by which of the following symptoms for the patient?
   a. total paralysis
   b. abnormal sensation of prickling and tingling
   c. paralysis of one limb
   d. slight paralysis

2. The patient's diagnosis is spinal stenosis with:
   a. disease of the nerve roots
   b. disease of peripheral nerves
   c. disease affecting a single nerve
   d. disease of many nerves

C. Complete the **three medical documents** within the electronic health record (EHR) on Evolve.

Many healthcare records today are stored and used in an electronic system called **Electronic Health Records (EHR)**. Electronic health records contain a collection of health information of an individual patient documented by various providers at different facilities; the digitally formatted record can be shared through computer networks with patients, physicians, and other health care providers.

For practice with medical terms using electronic health records, go to evolve.elsevier.com.
Select: Chapter 15, **Electronic Health Records.**

Refer to p. 10 for your Evolve Access Information.

EXERCISE 46   *Interpret Medical Terms*

To test your understanding of the terms introduced in this chapter, circle the words that correctly complete the sentences. The italicized words refer to the correct answer.

1. *Paralysis of all four limbs* is **(paraplegia, monoplegia, hemiplegia, quadriplegia).**
2. The *inability to speak* or **(dysarthria, aphasia, dysphasia, dysphagia)** may be an after-effect of cerebrovascular accident.
3. A symptom of brain concussion that may cause a patient to be *unaware of his or her surroundings and unable to respond to stimuli* is **(subconscious, unconscious, convulsive).**
4. The newborn had *meninges protruding through a defect in his skull,* or a **(meningocele, myelomeningocele, myelomalacia).**
5. *The branch of medicine that deals with the treatment of mental disorders* is **(neurology, psychology, psychiatry).**
6. *Multiple sclerosis* is a disease of the nervous system; it is characterized by **(seizures, sclerotic patches along the brain and spinal cord, muscular tremors).**
7. *The process of recording of electrical activity of the brain,* or **(electroencephalogram, electroencephalograph, electroencephalography),** is used to study brain function and is valuable for diagnosing epilepsy, tumors, and other brain diseases.
8. Cerebral *thrombosis,* or abnormal condition of a(n) **(blood clot, infection, hardened patches),** may cause a stroke.
9. The patient was admitted to the neurology unit of the hospital with a diagnosis of stroke. The physician ordered *a diagnostic procedure to examine blood flow and metabolic activity* or **(computed tomography, positron emission tomography, magnetic resonance imaging).**
10. The patient was diagnosed with **(ganglion, ganglia)** on both wrists.
11. Following a burn injury to the right hand, the patient developed paresthesia of the ring finger related to scarring. Surgery to *separate the nerve from adhesions* **(neurolysis, neuralgia, rhizotomy)** was performed to improve function and provide pain relief.
12. Herpes zoster virus is the cause of chickenpox and *viral disease affecting peripheral nerves* **(sciatica, shingles, polyneuritis).**

EXERCISE 47   *Read Medical Terms in Use*

Practice pronunciation of terms by reading the following document. Use the pronunciation key following the medical term to assist you in saying the word.

To hear these terms, go to evolve.elsevier.com. Select: Chapter 15, **Exercises**, Read Medical Terms in Use.

Refer to p. 10 for your Evolve Access Information.

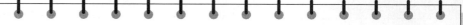

A 78-year-old right-handed male presented to the Emergency Department with a right **hemiparesis** (*hem*-ē-pa-RĒ-sis), expressive **aphasia** (a-FĀ-zha), and no apparent **cognitive** (COG-ni-tiv) decline. He has a history of hypertension and 2 years ago had a **transient ischemic** (is-KĒ-mik) **attack.** A **computed tomography** (tō-MOG-ra-fē) **scan of the brain** was negative for an **intracerebral** (in-tra-SER-e-bral) hemorrhage. A **neurologist** (nū-ROL-o-jist) was consulted. She confirmed the diagnosis of an **ischemic stroke** (strōk) after **magnetic resonance imaging** (mag-NET-ik) (REZ-ō-nans) (IM-a-jing) **of the brain** demonstrated an ischemic area of the left **cerebral** (se-RĒ-bral) cortex caused by a **cerebral embolism** (se-RĒ-bral) (EM-bō-lizm).

EXERCISE 48   *Comprehend Medical Terms in Use*

Test your comprehension of terms in the previous medical document by circling the correct answer.

1. While in the emergency department, the patient had:
   a. inability to swallow and paralysis from the waist down
   b. inability to speak and slight paralysis of the right side of the body
   c. inability to swallow and slight paralysis of the right side of the body
   d. inability to speak and paralysis from the waist down
2. T   F   A diagnosis of stroke was made after an MRI of the brain was performed.
3. The patient had a history of:
   a. sudden deficient supply of blood to the brain
   b. sudden loss of consciousness
   c. slight paralysis of one side
   d. a clot in the cerebrum

> For a snapshot assessment of your knowledge of nervous system and behavioral health terms go to evolve.elsevier.com.
> Select: Chapter 15, **Quick Quizzes**.
>
> Refer to p. 10 for your Evolve Access Information.

CHAPTER REVIEW

Review of Evolve

Keep a record of the online activities you have completed by placing a check mark in the box. You may also record your scores. All activities have been referenced throughout the chapter.

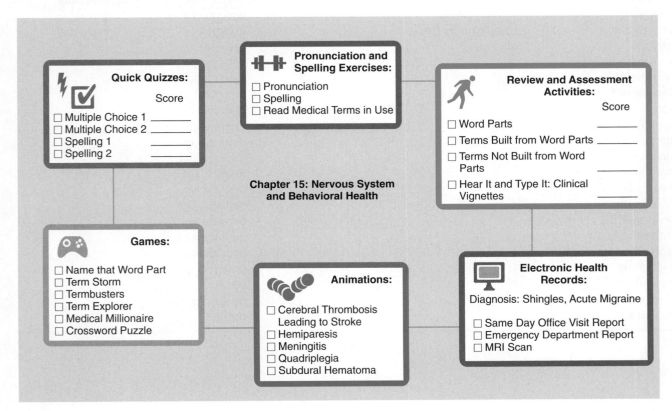

Quick Quizzes:
                                Score
☐ Multiple Choice 1 _____
☐ Multiple Choice 2 _____
☐ Spelling 1 _____
☐ Spelling 2 _____

Pronunciation and Spelling Exercises:
☐ Pronunciation
☐ Spelling
☐ Read Medical Terms in Use

Review and Assessment Activities:
                                Score
☐ Word Parts _____
☐ Terms Built from Word Parts _____
☐ Terms Not Built from Word Parts _____
☐ Hear It and Type It: Clinical Vignettes _____

Games:
☐ Name that Word Part
☐ Term Storm
☐ Termbusters
☐ Term Explorer
☐ Medical Millionaire
☐ Crossword Puzzle

Chapter 15: Nervous System and Behavioral Health

Animations:
☐ Cerebral Thrombosis Leading to Stroke
☐ Hemiparesis
☐ Meningitis
☐ Quadriplegia
☐ Subdural Hematoma

Electronic Health Records:
Diagnosis: Shingles, Acute Migraine

☐ Same Day Office Visit Report
☐ Emergency Department Report
☐ MRI Scan

Review of Word Parts

Can you define and spell the following word parts?

COMBINING FORMS		SUFFIXES
cerebell/o	myel/o	-iatrist
cerebr/o	neur/o	-iatry
dur/o	phas/o	-ictal
encephal/o	poli/o	-paresis
esthesi/o	psych/o	
gangli/o	quadr/i	
ganglion/o	radic/o	
gli/o	radicul/o	
mening/i	rhiz/o	
meningi/o		
ment/o		
mon/o		

Review of Terms

Can you build, analyze, define, pronounce, and spell the following terms *built from word parts?*

DISEASES AND DISORDERS	SURGICAL	DIAGNOSTIC	COMPLEMENTARY	BEHAVIORAL HEALTH
cerebellitis	ganglionectomy	cerebral angiography	anesthesia	psychiatrist
cerebral thrombosis	neurectomy	CT myelography	aphasia	psychiatry
duritis	neurolysis	electroencephalogram	cephalalgia	psychogenic
encephalitis	neuroplasty	(EEG)	cerebral	psychologist
encephalomalacia	neurorrhaphy	electroencephalograph	craniocerebral	psychology
encephalomyeloradiculitis	neurotomy	electroencephalography	dysphasia	psychopathy
gangliitis	radicotomy		encephalosclerosis	psychosis
glioblastoma	rhizotomy		gliocyte	psychosomatic
glioma			hemiparesis	
meningioma			hemiplegia	
meningitis			hyperesthesia	
meningocele			interictal	
meningomyelocele			intracerebral	
mononeuropathy			mental	
neuralgia			monoparesis	
neuritis			monoplegia	
neuroarthropathy			myelomalacia	
neuroma			neuroid	
neuropathy			neurologist	
poliomyelitis			neurology	
polyneuritis			panplegia	
polyneuropathy			paresthesia	
radiculitis			postictal	
radiculopathy			preictal	
rhizomeningomyelitis			quadriplegia	
subdural hematoma			subdural	

Can you define, pronounce, and spell the following terms *not built from word parts?*

DISEASES AND DISORDERS	DIAGNOSTIC	COMPLEMENTARY	BEHAVIORAL HEALTH
Alzheimer disease (AD)	computed tomography (CT) of the brain	afferent	anorexia nervosa
amyotrophic lateral sclerosis (ALS)	evoked potential studies (EP)	ataxia	anxiety disorder
Bell palsy	lumbar puncture (LP)	cognitive	attention deficit/hyperactivity disorder (ADHD)
cerebral aneurysm	magnetic resonance imaging (MRI) of the brain or spine	coma	autism
cerebral embolism	positron emission tomography (PET) of the brain	concussion	bipolar disorder
cerebral palsy (CP)		conscious	bulimia nervosa
dementia		convulsion	major depression
epilepsy		disorientation	obsessive-compulsive disorder (OCD)
hydrocephalus		dysarthria	
intracerebral hemorrhage		efferent	panic attack
multiple sclerosis (MS)		gait	phobia
Parkinson disease (PD)		incoherent	pica
sciatica		paraplegia	posttraumatic stress disorder (PTSD)
shingles		seizure	
stroke		shunt	schizophrenia
subarachnoid hemorrhage (SAH)		syncope	somatoform disorders
transient ischemic attack (TIA)		unconsciousness	

ANSWERS

ANSWERS TO CHAPTER 15 EXERCISES
Exercise Figures

Exercise Figure

A. 1. brain: encephal/o
2. spinal cord: myel/o
3. cerebrum: cerebr/o
4. cerebellum: cerebell/o
5. meninges: meningi/o, mening/o

Exercise Figure

B. 1. dura mater: dur/o
2. ganglion: gangli/o, ganglion/o
3. nerve root: radic/o, radicul/o, rhiz/o

Exercise Figure

C. rhiz/o/tomy or radic/o/tomy

Exercise Figure

D. myel/o/graphy

Exercise Figure

E. 1. hemi/plegia
3. quadr/i/plegia

Exercise 1
1. meninges
2. dura mater
3. arachnoid
4. pia mater
5. subarachnoid space
6. cerebrospinal fluid

Exercise 2
1. d   6. h
2. f   7. b
3. g   8. c
4. e   9. j
5. a

Exercise 3
1. cerebellum
2. nerve
3. spinal cord
4. meninges
5. brain
6. cerebrum, brain
7. nerve root
8. ganglion
9. nerve root
10. hard, dura mater
11. ganglion
12. nerve root
13. glia, gluey substance

Exercise 4
1. cerebell/o
2. neur/o
3. myel/o
4. a. mening/o
   b. meningi/o
5. encephal/o

6. cerebr/o
7. a. radicul/o
   b. radic/o
   c. rhiz/o
8. dur/o
9. a. gangli/o
   b. ganglion/o
10. gli/o

Exercise 5
1. one, single
2. mind
3. four
4. mind
5. speech
6. sensation, sensitivity, feeling
7. gray matter

Exercise 6
1. quadr/i   4. phas/o
2. mon/o   5. poli/o
3. a. psych/o   6. esthesi/o
   b. ment/o

Exercise 7
1. slight paralysis
2. treatment, specialty
3. seizure, attack
4. specialist, physician

Exercise 8
1. -paresis   3. -ictal
2. -iatry   4. -iatrist

Exercise 9
Pronunciation Exercise

Exercise 10
Note: The combining form is identified by italic and bold print.

1. WR   S
   neur/itis
   inflammation of a nerve

2. WR   S
   neur/oma
   tumor made up of nerve (cells)

3. WR   S
   neur/algia
   pain in a nerve

4. WR CV WR CV S
   neur/o/arthr/o/pathy
      CF   CF
   disease of nerves and joints

5. WR   S
   meningi/oma
   tumor of the meninges

6. WR   CV   S
   encephal/o/malacia
      CF
   softening of the brain

7. WR   S
   encephal/itis
   inflammation of the brain

8. WR   CV WR CV   WR   S
   encephal/o/myel/o/radicul/itis
      CF   CF
   inflammation of the brain, spinal cord, and nerve roots

9. WR   S
   mening/itis
   inflammation of the meninges

10. WR   CV   S
    mening/o/cele
       CF
    protrusion of the meninges

11. WR   CV WR CV   S
    mening/o/myel/o/cele
       CF   CF
    protrusion of the meninges and spinal cord

12. WR   S
    radicul/itis
    inflammation of the nerve roots

13. WR   S
    cerebell/itis
    inflammation of the cerebellum

14. WR   S
    gangli/itis
    inflammation of a ganglion

15. WR   S
    dur/itis
    inflammation of the dura mater

16. P   WR   S
    poly/neur/itis
    inflammation of many nerves

17. WR CV WR   S
    poli/o/myel/itis
       CF
    inflammation of the gray matter of the spinal cord

18. WR   S   WR   S
    cerebr/al thromb/osis
    pertaining to the cerebrum, abnormal condition of a clot

19. P   WR S   WR   S
    sub/dur/al hemat/oma
    pertaining to below the dura mater; tumor of blood

20. WR CV   WR CV WR   S
    rhiz/o/mening/o/myel/itis
       CF   CF
    inflammation of the nerve root, meninges, and spinal cord

21. WR CV WR CV S
    ***mon/o/neur/o*/pathy**
       CF   CF
    disease affecting a single nerve
22. WR CV S
    ***neur/o*/pathy**
       CF
    disease of the nerves (peripheral)
23. WR CV S
    ***radicul/o*/pathy**
       CF
    disease of the nerve roots
24. WR S
    gli/oma
    tumor composed of glial tissue
25. WR CV WR S
    ***gli/o*/blast/oma**
       CF
    tumor composed of developing glial tissue
26. P   WR CV S
    poly/***neur/o*/pathy**
          CF
    disease of many nerves

Exercise 11
1. neur/itis
2. neur/oma
3. neur/algia
4. neur/o/arthr/o/pathy
5. radicul/o/pathy
6. encephal/o/malacia
7. encephal/itis
8. encephal/o/myel/o/radicul/itis
9. mening/itis
10. mening/o/cele
11. mening/o/myel/o/cele
12. radicul/itis
13. cerebell/itis
14. gangli/itis
15. dur/itis
16. poly/neur/itis
17. poli/o/myel/itis
18. cerebr/al thromb/osis
19. sub/dur/al hemat/oma
20. rhiz/o/mening/o/myel/itis
21. meningi/oma
22. mon/o/neur/o/pathy
23. neur/o/pathy
24. gli/oma
25. gli/o/blast/oma
26. poly/neur/o/pathy

Exercise 12
Spelling Exercise; see text p. 660.

Exercise 13
Pronunciation Exercise

Exercise 14
1. a. intracerebral hemorrhage
   b. cerebral embolism
   c. subarachnoid hemorrhage
   d. cerebral thrombosis
2. cerebral aneurysm
3. Bell palsy
4. hydrocephalus
5. sciatica
6. shingles
7. transient ischemic attack
8. Parkinson disease
9. epilepsy
10. amyotrophic lateral sclerosis
11. Alzheimer disease
12. cerebral palsy
13. multiple sclerosis
14. dementia

Exercise 15
1. b   10. m
2. a   11. q
3. n   12. d
4. j   13. h
5. l   14. o
6. p   15. c
7. e   16. f
8. g   17. r
9. i

Exercise 16
Spelling Exercise; see text p. 667.

Exercise 17
Pronunciation Exercise

Exercise 18
Note: The combining form is identified by italic and bold print.
1. WR CV S
   ***radic/o*/tomy**
       CF
   incision into a nerve root
2. WR   S
   neur/ectomy
   excision of a nerve
3. WR CV S
   ***neur/o*/rrhaphy**
       CF
   suturing of a nerve
4. WR   S
   ganglion/ectomy
   excision of a ganglion
5. WR CV S
   ***neur/o*/tomy**
       CF
   incision into a nerve
6. WR CV S
   ***neur/o*/lysis**
       CF
   separating or dissolution of a nerve

7. WR CV S
   ***neur/o*/plasty**
       CF
   surgical repair of a nerve
8. WR CV S
   ***rhiz/o*/tomy**
       CF
   incision into a nerve root

Exercise 19
1. a. radic/o/tomy
   b. rhiz/o/tomy
2. neur/ectomy
3. neur/o/rrhaphy
4. ganglion/ectomy
5. neur/o/tomy
6. neur/o/lysis
7. neur/o/plasty

Exercise 20
Spelling Exercise; see text p. 669.

Exercise 21
Pronunciation Exercise

Exercise 22
Note: The combining form is identified by italic and bold print.
1. WR CV WR   CV S
   ***electr/o/encephal/o*/gram**
        CF   CF
   record of the electrical activity of the brain
2. WR CV WR   CV S
   ***electr/o/encephal/o*/graph**
        CF   CF
   instrument used to record the electrical activity of the brain
3. WR CV WR   CV S
   ***electr/o/encephal/o*/graphy**
        CF   CF
   process of recording the electrical activity of the brain
4.   WR CV   S
   CT ***myel/o*/graphy**
         CF
   process of recording (scan) the spinal cord
5. WR   S WR CV S
   cerebr/al ***angi/o*/graphy**
              CF
   process of recording of the (blood) vessels of the cerebrum

Exercise 23
1. electr/o/encephal/o/gram
2. electr/o/encephal/o/graph
3. electr/o/encephal/o/graphy
4. CT myel/o/graphy
5. cerebr/al angi/o/graphy

Exercise 24
Spelling Exercise; see text p. 672.

Exercise 25
Pronunciation Exercise

Exercise 26
1. computed tomography
2. lumbar puncture
3. positron emission tomography
4. magnetic resonance imaging
5. evoked potential studies

Exercise 27
1. diagnostic procedure performed by insertion of a needle into the subarachnoid space
2. computerized radiographic process producing a series of sectional images of brain tissue
3. high-strength computer-controlled magnetic fields producing a series of sectional images of the brain or spine
4. nuclear medicine procedure combining CT and radioactive chemicals producing sectional images of the brain to examine blood flow and metabolic activity
5. group of diagnostic tests that measure changes and responses in brain waves from stimuli

Exercise 28
Spelling Exercise; see text p. 674.

Exercise 29
Pronunciation Exercise

Exercise 30
Note: The combining form is identified by italic and bold print.
1. P S(WR)
   hemi/plegia
   paralysis of half (left or right side of the body)
2. P   WR S
   par/esthesi/a
   abnormal sensation
3. WR CV S
   neur/o/logist
        CF
   physician who studies and treats diseases of the nervous system
4. WR CV S
   neur/o/logy
        CF
   study of nerves (branch of medicine dealing with diseases of the nervous system)

5. WR   S
   neur/oid
   resembling a nerve
6. WR CV S
   quadr/i/plegia
        CF
   paralysis of four (limbs)
7. WR   S
   cerebr/al
   pertaining to the cerebrum
8. WR CV S
   mon/o/plegia
        CF
   paralysis of one (limb)
9. P WR S
   a/phas/ia
   condition of without speaking
10. P WR S
    dys/phas/ia
    condition of difficulty speaking
11. P   S(WR)
    hemi/paresis
    slight paralysis of half (right or left side of the body)
12. P   WR   S
    an/esthesi/a
    without (loss of) feeling or sensation
13. P   WR   S
    hyper/esthesi/a
    excessive sensitivity (to stimuli)
14. P WR S
    sub/dur/al
    pertaining to below the dura mater
15. WR   S
    cephal/algia
    pain in the head (headache)
16. WR CV WR S
    crani/o/cerebr/al
         CF
    pertaining to the cranium and cerebrum
17. WR CV   S
    myel/o/malacia
         CF
    softening of the spinal cord
18. WR   CV   S
    encephal/o/sclerosis
          CF
    hardening of the brain
19. P S(WR)
    post/ictal
    (occurring) after a seizure or attack
20. P S(WR)
    pan/plegia
    total paralysis

21. P S(WR)
    inter/ictal
    (occurring) between seizures or attacks
22. WR CV S
    mon/o/paresis
         CF
    slight paralysis of one (limb)
23. P S(WR)
    pre/ictal
    (occurring) before a seizure or attack
24. P   WR S
    intra/cerebr/al
    pertaining to within the cerebrum
25. WR CV S
    gli/o/cyte
         CF
    glial cell
26. WR   S
    ment/al
    pertaining to the mind

Exercise 31
1. hemi/paresis
2. an/esthesi/a
3. hyper/esthesi/a
4. sub/dur/al
5. cephal/algia
6. crani/o/cerebr/al
7. myel/o/malacia
8. encephal/o/sclerosis
9. hemi/plegia
10. neur/o/logist
11. neur/o/logy
12. neur/oid
13. quadr/i/plegia
14. cerebr/al
15. mon/o/plegia
16. a/phas/ia
17. dys/phas/ia
18. pre/ictal
19. mon/o/paresis
20. post/ictal
21. pan/plegia
22. inter/ictal
23. intra/cerebr/al
24. gli/o/cyte
25. par/esthesi/a
26. ment/al

Exercise 32
Spelling Exercise; see text p. 679.

Exercise 33
Pronunciation Exercise

Exercise 34
1. concussion
2. unconsciousness

3. conscious
4. seizure
5. convulsion
6. shunt
7. paraplegia
8. coma
9. syncope
10. ataxia
11. gait
12. dysarthria
13. incoherent
14. disorientation
15. cognitive
16. afferent
17. efferent

Exercise 35

1. tube implanted in the body to redirect the flow of a fluid
2. paralysis from the waist down caused by damage to the lower level of the spinal cord
3. state of profound unconsciousness
4. injury to the brain caused by head trauma
5. state of being unaware of surroundings and incapable of responding to stimuli as a result of injury, shock, or illness
6. awake, alert, aware of one's surroundings
7. sudden, abnormal surge of electrical activity in the brain
8. sudden involuntary contraction of a group of muscles
9. fainting, or sudden loss of consciousness
10. lack of muscle coordination
11. the inability to use speech that is distinct and connected
12. manner or style of walking
13. pertaining to the mental processes of comprehension, judgment, memory, and reasoning
14. state of mental confusion regarding time, place, and identity
15. unable to express one's thoughts or ideas in an orderly, intelligible manner
16. conveying away from the center
17. conveying toward the center

Exercise 36

Spelling Exercise; see text p. 682.

Exercise 37

Pronunciation Exercise

Exercise 38

1. psych/iatry
2. psych/osis

3. psych/o/logy
4. psych/o/genic
5. psych/iatrist
6. psych/o/logist
7. psych/o/somat/ic
8. psych/o/pathy

Exercise 39

Note: The combining form is identified by italic and bold print.

1. WR CV WR   S
   ***psych/o*/somat/ic**
       CF
   pertaining to the mind and body
2. WR CV   S
   ***psych/o*/pathy**
       CF
   (any) disease of the mind
3. WR CV   S
   ***psych/o*/logy**
       CF
   study of the mind
4. WR   S
   psych/iatry
   specialty of the mind (branch of medicine that deals with the treatment of mental disorders)
5. WR CV   S
   ***psych/o*/logist**
       CF
   specialist of the mind
6. WR CV   S
   ***psych/o*/genic**
       CF
   originating in the mind
7. WR   S
   psych/iatrist
   physician who studies and treats disorders of the mind
8. WR   S
   psych/osis
   abnormal condition of the mind

Exercise 40

Spelling Exercise; see text p. 684.

Exercise 41

Pronunciation Exercise

Exercise 42

1. i	8. d
2. m	9. h
3. b	10. f
4. c	11. e
5. j	12. n
6. a	13. l
7. g	14. k

Exercise 43

Spelling Exercise; see text p. 687.

Exercise 44

1. electroencephalogram, magnetic resonance imaging, positron emission tomography, evoked potential studies, lumbar puncture
2. Alzheimer disease, amyotrophic lateral sclerosis, cerebral palsy, multiple sclerosis, Parkinson disease
3. cerebrovascular accident, transient ischemic attack, subarachnoid hemorrhage
4. cerebrospinal fluid
5. posttraumatic stress disorder, obsessive-compulsive disorder, attention deficit hyperactivity disorder
6. central nervous system, peripheral nervous system

Exercise 45

A.
1. disorientation
2. cognitive
3. aphasia
4. conscious
5. neurology
6. magnetic resonance imaging
7. encephalitis
8. electroencephalogram
9. seizure
10. incoherent

B.
1. b
2. a

C. Online Exercise

Exercise 46

1. quadriplegia
2. aphasia
3. unconscious
4. meningocele
5. psychiatry
6. sclerotic patches along brain and spinal cord
7. electroencephalography
8. blood clot
9. positron emission tomography
10. ganglia
11. neurolysis
12. shingles

Exercise 47

Reading Exercise

Exercise 48

1. b
2. *T*
3. a

Outline

Objectives

Upon completion of this chapter you will be able to:

1   Identify organs and structures of the endocrine system.

2   Define and spell word parts related to the endocrine system.

3   Define, pronounce, and spell disease and disorder terms related to the endocrine system.

4   Define, pronounce, and spell surgical terms related to the endocrine system.

5   Define, pronounce, and spell diagnostic terms related to the endocrine system.

6   Define, pronounce, and spell complementary terms related to the endocrine system.

7   Interpret the meaning of abbreviations related to the endocrine system.

8   Interpret, read, and comprehend medical language in simulated medical statements, documents, and electronic health records.

ANATOMY

The endocrine system is composed of endocrine glands distributed throughout the body. The endocrine glands are: pituitary, thyroid, parathyroid, adrenal, pancreas, gonads (ovaries and testes), and thymus.

Function

The endocrine system regulates body activities through the use of chemical messengers called *hormones*, which when released into the bloodstream influence metabolic activities, growth, and development (Figure 16-1). The nervous system also regulates body activities but does so through electrical impulses and activation of glandular secretions. *Hormones* secreted by the *endocrine glands* that make up the endocrine system go directly into the bloodstream and are transported throughout the body. They are referred to as *ductless glands* because they do not have ducts to carry their secretions. In contrast, the *exocrine* or *duct glands* have ducts that carry their secretions from the producing gland to other parts of the body. An example is the parotid gland, which produces saliva that flows through the parotid duct into the mouth. Only those terms related to the major endocrine glands—pituitary, thyroid, parathyroids, adrenals, and the islets of Langerhans in the pancreas—are presented in this chapter. The thymus and the male and female sex glands were discussed in previous chapters.

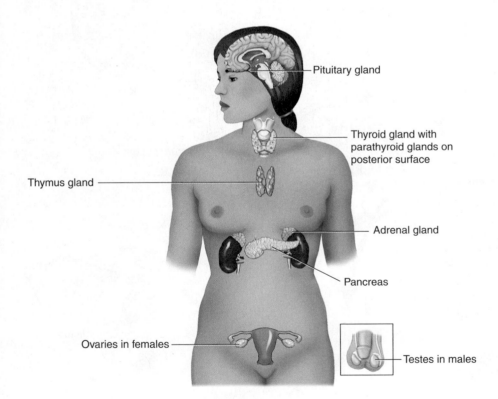

FIGURE 16-1
The endocrine system.

Endocrine Glands

TERM	DEFINITION
pituitary gland or hypophysis cerebri	approximately the size of a pea and located at the base of the brain. The pituitary is divided into two lobes. It is often referred to as the master gland because it produces hormones that stimulate the function of other endocrine glands (Figure 16-2).
anterior lobe or adenohypophysis	produces and secretes the following hormones:
growth hormone (GH)	regulates the growth of the body

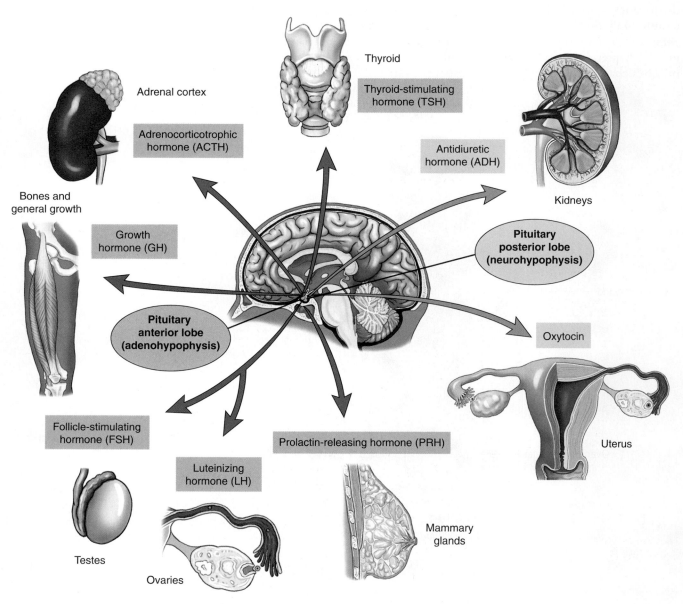

FIGURE 16-2
Pituitary gland, hormones secreted, and target organs.

TERM	DEFINITION
adrenocorticotropic hormone (ACTH)	stimulates the adrenal cortex
thyroid-stimulating hormone (TSH)	stimulates the thyroid gland
gonadotropic hormones	affect the male and female reproductive systems
follicle-stimulating hormone (FSH), luteinizing hormone (LH)	regulate development, growth, and function of the ovaries and testes
prolactin-releasing hormone (PRH), lactogenic hormone	promotes development of glandular tissue during pregnancy and produces milk after birth of an infant
posterior lobe or neurohypophysis	stores and releases antidiuretic hormone and oxytocin
antidiuretic hormone (ADH)	stimulates the kidney to reabsorb water
oxytocin	stimulates uterine contractions during labor and postpartum
hypothalamus	located superior to the pituitary gland in the brain. The hypothalamus secretes "releasing" hormones that function to stimulate or inhibit the release of pituitary gland hormones.
thyroid gland	largest endocrine gland. It is located anteriorly in the neck below the larynx and comprises bilateral lobes connected by an isthmus (see Figure 16-3). The thyroid gland secretes the hormones triiodothyronine (T_3) and thyroxine (T_4), which require iodine for their production. Thyroxine is necessary for body cell metabolism.
parathyroid glands	four small bodies embedded in the posterior aspect of the lobes of the thyroid gland (Figure 16-3). Parathyroid hormone (PTH), the hormone produced by the glands, helps maintain the level of calcium in the blood.
islets of Langerhans	clusters of endocrine tissue found throughout the pancreas, made up of different cell types that secrete various hormones, including insulin and glucagon. Non-endocrine cells found throughout the pancreas produce enzymes that facilitate digestion (Figure 16-4).
adrenal glands or suprarenals	paired glands, one of which is located above each kidney. The outer portion is called the **adrenal cortex,** and the inner portion is called the **adrenal medulla.** The following hormones are secreted by the adrenal glands:

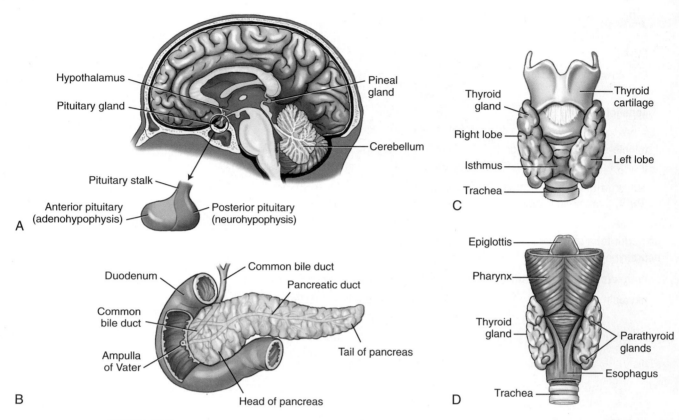

A, Pituitary and pineal glands. B, Pancreas. C, Thyroid gland. D, Parathyroid glands, posterior view.

FIGURE 16-3

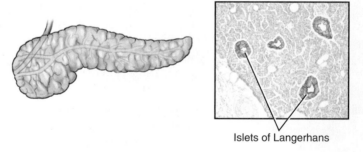

Islets of Langerhans

FIGURE 16-4
Pancreas, with islets of Langerhans.

Endocrine Glands—cont'd

TERM	DEFINITION
cortisol	secreted by the adrenal cortex. It aids the body during stress by increasing glucose levels to provide energy (also called **hydrocortisone**).
aldosterone	secreted by the adrenal cortex. Electrolytes (mineral salts) that are necessary for normal body function are regulated by this hormone.
epinephrine (adrenaline), norepinephrine (noradrenaline)	secreted by the adrenal medulla. These hormones help the body to deal with stress by increasing the blood pressure, heartbeat, and respirations.

A & P Booster
For more anatomy and physiology, go to evolve. elsevier.com.
Select: **Extra Content**, A & P Booster, Chapter 15.

Refer to p. 10 for your Evolve Access Information.

EXERCISE 1

Match the terms in the first column with the correct definitions in the second column. *To check your answers to the exercises in this chapter, go to Answers, p. 732, at the end of the chapter.*

_____ 1. adrenal cortex
_____ 2. adrenal glands
_____ 3. adrenaline
_____ 4. adrenal medulla
_____ 5. adrenocorticotropic hormone
_____ 6. adenohypophysis
_____ 7. aldosterone

a. hormone that stimulates the adrenal cortex
b. tissue that secretes cortisol and aldosterone
c. anterior lobe of pituitary that secretes growth hormone and thyroid-stimulating hormone
d. another name for epinephrine
e. assists in regulating body electrolytes
f. another name for norepinephrine
g. located above each kidney
h. secretes epinephrine and norepinephrine

EXERCISE 2

Match the terms in the first column with the correct phrases in the second column.

_____ 1. antidiuretic hormone
_____ 2. islets of Langerhans
_____ 3. neurohypophysis
_____ 4. parathyroid glands
_____ 5. pituitary gland
_____ 6. thyroid gland

a. portions of the pancreas that secrete insulin
b. glands that maintain the blood calcium level
c. gland located anteriorly in the neck that secretes thyroxine
d. hormone secreted by posterior lobe of the pituitary
e. gland that stores and releases antidiuretic hormone and oxytocin
f. another name for the anterior lobe of the pituitary
g. gland located at the base of the brain

WORD PARTS

Word parts you need to learn to complete this chapter are listed on the following pages. The exercises at the end of each list will help you learn their definitions and spellings.

> Use the flashcards accompanying this text or electronic flashcards to assist you in memorizing the word parts for this chapter.

To use electronic flashcards, go to evolve.elsevier.com.
Select: Chapter 16, **Flashcards**.

Refer to p. 10 for your Evolve Access Information.

Combining Forms of the Endocrine System

COMBINING FORM	DEFINITION
aden/o (NOTE: aden/o was introduced in Chapter 2)	gland
adren/o, adrenal/o	adrenal glands
cortic/o	cortex (the outer layer of a body organ)
endocrin/o	endocrine
parathyroid/o	parathyroid glands
pituitar/o	pituitary gland
thyroid/o, thyr/o	thyroid gland

EXERCISE FIGURE **A**

Fill in the blanks with combining forms in this diagram of the endocrine glands. *To check your answers, go to p. 732.*

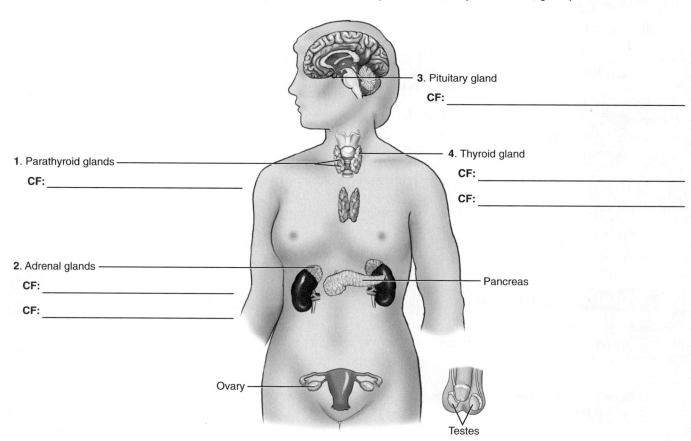

3. Pituitary gland

CF: _____

1. Parathyroid glands —————

CF: _____

4. Thyroid gland

CF: _____

CF: _____

2. Adrenal glands —————

CF: _____

CF: _____

Pancreas

Ovary —

Testes

EXERCISE FIGURE B

Fill in the blank with the combining form in this diagram of adrenal glands (with transverse cross-sectional view).

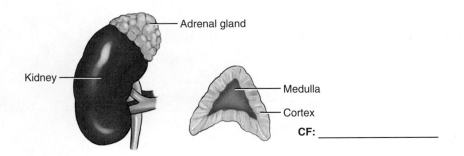

Adrenal gland

Kidney

Medulla

Cortex

CF: _____

EXERCISE 3

Write the definitions of the following combining forms.

1. cortic/o _____
2. adren/o _____
3. parathyroid/o _____
4. thyroid/o _____
5. adrenal/o _____
6. thyr/o _____
7. endocrin/o _____
8. aden/o _____
9. pituitar/o _____

EXERCISE 4

Write the combining form for each of the following terms.

1. adrenal gland   a. _____
                 b. _____
2. thyroid gland   a. _____
                 b. _____
3. endocrine _____
4. cortex _____
5. parathyroid gland _____
6. gland _____
7. pituitary gland _____

Combining Forms Commonly Used with Endocrine System Terms

COMBINING FORM	DEFINITION
acr/o	extremities, height
calc/i (NOTE: the combining vowel is i)	calcium
dips/o	thirst
kal/i (NOTE: the combining vowel is i)	potassium
natr/o	sodium

EXERCISE 5

Write the definitions of the following combining forms.

1. dips/o _____
2. kal/i _____
3. calc/i _____
4. acr/o _____
5. natr/o _____

EXERCISE 6

Write the combining form for each of the following.

1. extremities, height _____
2. calcium _____
3. thirst _____
4. potassium _____
5. sodium _____

Suffix

SUFFIX	DEFINITION
-drome	run, running

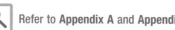 Refer to **Appendix A** and **Appendix B** for a complete list of word parts.

EXERCISE 7

Write the definition of the following word part.

1. -drome _____

EXERCISE 8

Write the suffix for the following.

1. run, running _____

For review and/or assessment, go to evolve.elsevier.com. Select:
Chapter 16, **Activities,** Word Parts
Chapter 16, **Games,**   Name that Word Part

Refer to p. 10 for your Evolve Access Information.

MEDICAL TERMS

The terms you need to learn to complete this chapter are listed below. The exercises following each list will help you learn the definition and spelling of each word.

Disease and Disorder Terms

Built from Word Parts

The following terms are built from word parts you have already learned and can be translated literally to find their meanings. Further explanation of terms beyond the definition of their word parts, if needed, is included in parentheses.

TERM	DEFINITION
acromegaly (ak-rō-MEG-a-lē)	enlargement of the extremities (and bones of the face, hands, and feet caused by excessive production of the growth hormone by the pituitary gland after puberty) (Exercise Figure C)
adenitis (ad-e-NĪ-tis)	inflammation of a gland
adenomegaly (ad-e-nō-MEG-a-lē)	enlargement of a gland
adenosis (ad-e-NŌ-sis)	abnormal condition of a gland
adrenalitis (a-drē-nal-Ī-tis)	inflammation of the adrenal glands
adrenomegaly (a-drē-nō-MEG-a-lē)	enlargement (of one or both) of the adrenal glands
hypercalcemia (hī-per-kal-SĒ-mē-a)	excessive calcium in the blood
hyperglycemia (hī-per-glī-SĒ-mē-a)	excessive sugar in the blood
hyperkalemia (hī-per-ka-LĒ-mē-a)	excessive potassium in the blood
hyperpituitarism (hī-per-pi-TOO-i-ta-rizm)	state of excessive pituitary gland activity (characterized by excessive secretion of pituitary hormones)
hyperthyroidism (hī-per-THĪ-royd-izm)	state of excessive thyroid gland activity (characterized by excessive secretion of thyroid hormones). Signs and symptoms include weight loss, irritability, and heat intolerance.
hypocalcemia (hī-pō-kal-SĒ-mē-a)	deficient calcium in the blood

EXERCISE FIGURE C

Fill in the blanks to complete labeling of this photograph.

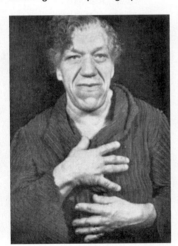

extremities / cv / enlargement

is a metabolic disorder characterized by marked enlargement of the bones of the face, jaw, and extremities.

Disease and Disorder Terms—cont'd

Built from Word Parts

TERM	DEFINITION
hypoglycemia (hī-pō-glī-SĒ-mē-a)	deficient sugar in the blood
hypokalemia (hī-pō-ka-LĒ-mē-a)	deficient potassium in the blood
hyponatremia (hī-pō-na-TRĒ-mē-a)	deficient sodium in the blood
hypopituitarism (hī-pō-pi-TŪ-i-ta-*rizm*)	state of deficient pituitary gland activity (characterized by decreased secretion of one or more of the pituitary hormones, which can affect the function of the target endocrine gland; for example, hypothyroidism can result from decreased secretion of thyroid-stimulating hormone by the pituitary gland)
hypothyroidism (hī-pō-THĪ-royd-izm)	state of deficient thyroid gland activity (characterized by decreased secretion of thyroid hormones. Signs and symptoms include fatigue, weight gain, and cold intolerance.)
panhypopituitarism (pan-hī-pō-pi-TŪ-i-ta-*rizm*) (NOTE: two prefixes contained in this term)	state of total deficient pituitary gland activity (characterized by decreased secretion of all the pituitary hormones; this is a more serious condition than hypopituitarism in that it affects the function of all the other endocrine glands)
parathyroidoma (*par*-a-*thī*-royd-Ō-ma)	tumor of a parathyroid gland
thyroiditis (*thī*-royd-Ī-tis)	inflammation of the thyroid gland

HYPOTHYROIDISM

is the state of deficient thyroid gland activity, resulting in the decreased production of the thyroid hormone called thyroxine. A severe form of hypothyroidism in adults is called **myxedema** and in children is called **congenital hypothyroidism**.

To watch animations, go to evolve.elsevier.com. Select:
Chapter 16, **Animations**, Hyperthyroidism
                                Hypothyroidism

Refer to p. 10 for your Evolve Access Information.

EXERCISE 9

Practice saying aloud each of the disease and disorder terms built from word parts on pp. 709–710.

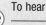 To hear the terms, go to evolve.elsevier.com. Select: Chapter 16, **Exercises**, Pronunciation.

Refer to p. 10 for your Evolve Access Information.

☐ Place a check mark in the box when you have completed this exercise.

EXERCISE 10

Analyze and define the following terms.

1. adrenalitis _____
2. hypocalcemia _____
3. hyperthyroidism _____
4. hyperkalemia _____
5. hyperglycemia _____
6. adrenomegaly _____
7. adenomegaly _____
8. hypothyroidism _____
9. hypokalemia _____
10. adenitis _____
11. parathyroidoma _____
12. acromegaly _____
13. panhypopituitarism _____
14. hypoglycemia _____
15. hypercalcemia _____
16. hyperpituitarism _____
17. hyponatremia _____
18. adenosis _____
19. thyroiditis _____
20. hypopituitarism _____

EXERCISE 11

Build disease and disorder terms for the following definitions with the word parts you have learned.

1. enlargement of (one or both) the adrenal glands

   _____ / CV / _____
   WR   S

2. state of deficient thyroid gland activity

   _____ / _____ / _____
   P   WR   S

3. enlargement of the extremities

   _____ / CV / _____
   WR   S

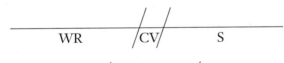

4. deficient sugar in the blood

   _____ / _____ / _____
   P   WR   S

5. excessive potassium in the blood

   _____ / _____ / _____
   P   WR   S

6. deficient calcium in the blood

   _____ / _____ / _____
   P   WR   S

7. state of excessive thyroid gland activity

   _____ / _____ / _____
   P   WR   S

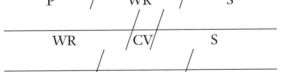

8. state of deficient pituitary
gland activity

_____ / _____ / _____
P   WR   S

9. excessive calcium in the blood

_____ / _____ / _____
P   WR   S

10. state of excessive pituitary
gland activity

_____ / _____ / _____
P   WR   S

11. tumor of a parathyroid gland

_____ / _____
WR   S

12. excessive sugar in the blood

_____ / _____ / _____
P   WR   S

13. abnormal condition of a gland

_____ / _____
WR   S

14. deficient potassium in the
blood

_____ / _____ / _____
P   WR   S

15. inflammation of the adrenal
glands

_____ / _____
WR   S

16. enlargement of a gland

_____ / _____ / _____
WR   CV   S

17. deficient sodium in the blood

_____ / _____ / _____
P   WR   S

18. inflammation of a gland

_____ / _____
WR   S

19. inflammation of the
thyroid gland

_____ / _____
WR   S

20. state of total deficient pituitary
gland activity

_____ / _____ / _____ / _____
P   P   WR   S

EXERCISE 12

Spell each of the disease and disorder terms built from word parts on pp. 709–710 by having someone dictate them to you.

> To hear and spell the terms, go to evolve.elsevier.com. Select: Chapter 16, **Exercises**, Spelling.
>
> (e) Refer to p. 10 for your Evolve Access Information.
>
> ☐ Place a check mark in the box if you have completed this exercise online.

1. _____
2. _____
3. _____
4. _____

5. _____
6. _____
7. _____
8. _____

9. _____   15. _____
10. _____   16. _____
11. _____   17. _____
12. _____   18. _____
13. _____   19. _____
14. _____   20. _____

Disease and Disorder Terms

Not Built from Word Parts

In some of the following terms, you may recognize word parts you have already learned; however, the full meaning of the terms cannot be discerned by the definition of their word parts.

TERM	DEFINITION
acidosis (*as*-i-DŌ-sis)	condition brought about by an abnormal accumulation of acid products of metabolism such as seen in uncontrolled diabetes mellitus
Addison disease (AD-i-sun) (di-ZĒZ)	chronic syndrome resulting from a deficiency in the hormonal secretion of the adrenal cortex. Signs and symptoms may include weakness, darkening of skin, loss of appetite, depression, and other emotional problems.
congenital hypothyroidism (kon-JEN-i-tal) (hī-pō-THĪ-royd-izm)	condition caused by congenital absence or atrophy (wasting away) of the thyroid gland, resulting in hypothyroidism. The disease is characterized by puffy features, mental deficiency, large tongue, and dwarfism (formerly called **cretinism**).
Cushing syndrome (KŪSH-ing) (SIN-drŏm)	group of signs and symptoms attributed to the excessive production of cortisol by the adrenal cortices (*pl.* of cortex). This syndrome may be the result of a pituitary tumor or a primary adrenal cortex hypersecretion. Signs include abnormally pigmented skin, "moon face," pads of fat on the chest and abdomen, "buffalo hump" (fat on the upper back), wasting away of muscle, and hypertension (Figure 16-5).
diabetes insipidus (DI) (*dī*-a-BĒ-tēz) (in-SIP-i-dus)	result of decreased secretion of antidiuretic hormone by the posterior lobe of the pituitary gland. Symptoms include excessive thirst (*polydipsia*), large amounts of urine (*polyuria*), and sodium being excreted from the body.
diabetes mellitus (DM) (*dī*-a-BĒ-tēz) (MEL-li-tus)	chronic disease involving a disorder of carbohydrate metabolism caused by under-activity of the islets of Langerhans and characterized by elevated blood sugar (hyperglycemia). DM can cause chronic renal disease, retinopathy, and neuropathy. In extreme cases the patient may develop ketosis, acidosis, and finally coma.

🏛 **ADDISON DISEASE** was named in **1855** for **Thomas Addison**, an English physician and pathologist. He described the disease as a "morbid state with feeble heart action, anemia, irritability of the stomach, and a peculiar change in the color of the skin."

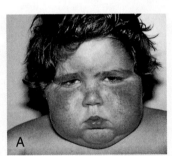

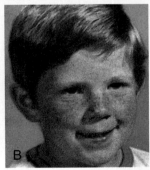

FIGURE 16-5
Cushing syndrome was named for an American neurosurgeon, **Harvey Williams Cushing** (1869–1939), after he described adrenocortical hyperfunction. **A**, At diagnosis. **B**, Four months after treatment.

GIGANTISM AND ACROMEGALY

are both caused by overproduction of growth hormone. **Gigantism** occurs before puberty and before the growing ends of the bones have closed. If untreated, an individual may reach 8 feet tall in adulthood.

Acromegaly occurs after puberty. The bones most affected are those in the hands, feet, and jaw.

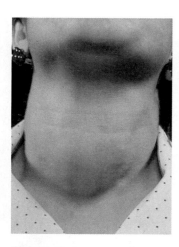

FIGURE 16-6
Goiter. May be caused by Graves disease, thyroiditis, or a thyroid nodule, which is a lump on the thyroid gland. Goiter is a general term for the enlargement of the thyroid gland.

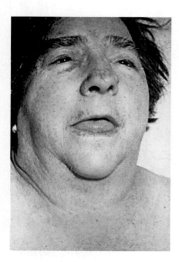

FIGURE 16-7
Myxedema.

Disease and Disorder Terms—cont'd

Not Built from Word Parts

TERM	DEFINITION
gigantism (jī-GAN-tizm)	condition brought about by hypersecretion of growth hormone by the pituitary gland before puberty
goiter (GOY-ter)	enlargement of the thyroid gland (Figure 16-6)
Graves disease (grāvz) (di-ZĒZ)	disorder of the thyroid gland characterized by the presence of hyperthyroidism causing the production of more thyroid hormone than the body needs, goiter, and exophthalmos (abnormal protrusion of the eyeballs)
ketosis (kē-TŌ-sis)	condition resulting from uncontrolled diabetes mellitus, in which the body has an abnormal concentration of ketone bodies resulting from excessive fat metabolism (called **ketoacidosis** if acids accumulate in the blood and tissue as well)
metabolic syndrome (*met*-a-BOL-ik) (SIN-drōm)	group of signs and symptoms including insulin resistance, obesity characterized by excessive fat around the waist and abdomen, hypertension, hyperglycemia, elevated triglycerides, and low levels of the "good" cholesterol HDL. Risks include development of type 2 diabetes, coronary heart disease, or stroke (also called **syndrome X** and **insulin resistance syndrome**).
myxedema (*mik*-se-DĒ-ma)	condition resulting from a deficiency of the thyroid hormone thyroxine; a severe form of hypothyroidism in an adult. Signs include puffiness of the face and hands, coarse and thickened skin, enlarged tongue, slow speech, and anemia (Figure 16-7).
pheochromocytoma (*fĕ*-ō-*krō*-mō-sī-TŌ-ma)	tumor of the adrenal medulla, which is usually non-malignant and characterized by hyper-tension, headaches, palpitations, diaphoresis, chest pain, and abdominal pain. Surgical removal of the tumor is the most common treatment. Though usually curable with early detection, it can be fatal if untreated.
tetany (TET-a-nē)	condition affecting nerves causing muscle spasms as a result of low amounts of calcium in the blood caused by a deficiency of the parathyroid hormone
thyrotoxicosis (*thī*-rō-*tok*-si-KŌ-sis)	condition caused by excessive thyroid hormones

To watch animations, go to evolve.elsevier.com. Select:
Chapter 16, **Animations**, Type 1 Diabetes
                       Type 2 Diabetes
                       Acidosis

Refer to p. 10 for your Evolve Access Information.

EXERCISE 13

Practice saying aloud each of the disease and disorder terms not built from word parts on pp. 713–714.

To hear the terms, go to evolve.elsevier.com. Select: Chapter 16, **Exercises**, Pronunciation.

Refer to p. 10 for your Evolve Access Information.

☐ Place a check mark in the box when you have completed this exercise.

Table 16-1

Diabetes Mellitus

Two major forms of diabetes mellitus are **type 1,** previously called insulin-dependent diabetes mellitus (IDDM) or juvenile-onset diabetes, and **type 2,** previously called noninsulin-dependent diabetes mellitus (NIDDM) or adult-onset diabetes (AODM). Type 2 diabetes mellitus has reached epidemic proportions and is a major cause of cardiovascular disease.

TYPE 1 DIABETES MELLITUS

Cause	the beta cells of the pancreas that produce insulin are destroyed and eventually no insulin is produced
Characteristics	abrupt onset, occurs primarily in childhood or adolescence; patients often are thin
Symptoms	polyuria, polydipsia, weight loss, hyperglycemia, acidosis, and ketosis
Treatment	insulin injections and diet

TYPE 2 DIABETES MELLITUS

Cause	resistance of body cells to the action of insulin, which may eventually lead to a decrease in insulin secretion
Characteristics	slow onset, usually occurs in middle-aged or elderly adults; most patients are obese
Symptoms	fatigue, blurred vision, thirst, and hyperglycemia; may have neural or vascular complications
Treatment	diet, exercise, oral medication, and perhaps insulin

LONG-TERM COMPLICATIONS OF DIABETES MELLITUS

MACROVASCULAR COMPLICATIONS

• coronary artery disease → myocardial infarction

• cerebrovascular disease → stroke

• peripheral artery disease → leg pain when walking (intermittent vascular claudication)

MICROVASCULAR COMPLICATIONS

• diabetic retinopathy → loss of vision

• diabetic nephropathy → chronic renal disease, kidney failure

• neuropathy → loss of feeling in extremities, amputation

🖉 **CAM TERM**

Yoga is the practice of physical postures, conscious breathing, and meditation. The regular practice of yoga has demonstrated efficacy as an adjunct therapy for management of type 2 **diabetes mellitus.**

EXERCISE 14

Match the terms in the first column with the correct definitions in the second column.

_____ 1. acidosis	a. results from a deficiency in the hormonal secretion of the adrenal cortex
_____ 2. Addison disease	b. attributed to the excessive production of cortisol
_____ 3. congenital hypothyroidism	c. chronic disease involving a disorder of carbohydrate metabolism
_____ 4. Cushing syndrome	d. abnormal accumulation of acid products of metabolism
_____ 5. diabetes insipidus	e. enlargement of the thyroid gland
_____ 6. diabetes mellitus	f. results from low blood calcium
_____ 7. gigantism	g. caused by excessive thyroid hormones
_____ 8. goiter	h. result of a decreased amount of antidiuretic hormone
_____ 9. ketosis	i. caused by deficiency of the thyroid hormone thyroxine
_____ 10. myxedema	j. caused by a wasting away of the thyroid gland
_____ 11. tetany	k. abnormal concentration of ketone bodies resulting from excessive fat metabolism
_____ 12. thyrotoxicosis	l. caused by overproduction of the pituitary growth hormone
_____ 13. Graves disease	m. caused by an excessive amount of parahormone
_____ 14. pheochromocytoma	n. characterized by hyperthyroidism, goiter, and exophthalmos
_____ 15. metabolic syndrome	o. tumor of the adrenal medulla
	p. group of signs and symptoms including insulin resistance, excessive fat around the waist and abdomen, hypertension, hyperglycemia, elevated triglycerides, and low HDL

EXERCISE 15

Write the name of the endocrine gland responsible for each of the following conditions.

1. myxedema _____

2. tetany _____

3. ketosis _____

4. gigantism _____

5. goiter _____

6. Addison disease _____

7. diabetes mellitus _____

8. congenital hypothyroidism _____

9. acidosis _____

10. Cushing syndrome _____

11. diabetes insipidus _____

12. Graves disease _____

13. thyrotoxicosis _____

14. pheochromocytoma _____

EXERCISE 16

Spell each of the disease and disorder terms not built from word parts on pp. 713–714 by having someone dictate them to you.

> To hear and spell the terms, go to evolve.elsevier.com. Select: Chapter 16, **Exercises**, Spelling.
>
> Refer to p. 10 for your Evolve Access Information.
>
> ☐ Place a check mark in the box if you have completed this exercise online.

1. _____
2. _____
3. _____
4. _____
5. _____
6. _____
7. _____
8. _____
9. _____
10. _____
11. _____
12. _____
13. _____
14. _____
15. _____

Surgical Terms

Built from Word Parts

The following terms are built from word parts you have already learned and can be translated literally to find their meanings. Further explanation of terms beyond the definition of their word parts, if needed, is included in parentheses.

TERM	DEFINITION
adenectomy (*ad*-en-EK-to-mē)	excision of a gland
adrenalectomy (ad-*rē*-nal-EK-to-mē)	excision of (one or both) adrenal glands
parathyroidectomy (*par*-a-*thī*-royd-EK-to-mē)	excision of (one or more) parathyroid glands
thyroidectomy (*thī*-royd-EK-to-mē)	excision of the thyroid gland
thyroidotomy (*thī*-royd-OT-o-mē)	incision of the thyroid gland
thyroparathyroidectomy (*thī*-rō-*par*-a-*thī*-royd-EK-to-mē)	excision of the thyroid and parathyroid glands

> To watch animations, go to evolve.elsevier.com. Select:
> Chapter 16, **Animations**, Thyroidectomy
>
> Refer to p. 10 for your Evolve Access Information.

EXERCISE 17

Practice saying aloud each of the surgical terms built from word parts on p. 717.

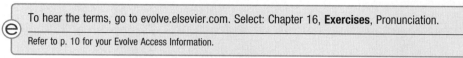

To hear the terms, go to evolve.elsevier.com. Select: Chapter 16, **Exercises**, Pronunciation.

Refer to p. 10 for your Evolve Access Information.

☐ Place a check mark in the box when you have completed this exercise.

EXERCISE 18

Analyze and define the following surgical terms.

1. thyroidotomy _____
2. adrenalectomy_____
3. thyroparathyroidectomy _____
4. thyroidectomy_____
5. parathyroidectomy _____
6. adenectomy_____

EXERCISE 19

Build surgical terms for the following definitions by using the word parts you have learned.

1. excision of the thyroid gland

   _____ / _____
   WR   /   S

2. excision of the thyroid and parathyroid glands

   _____ / CV / _____ / _____
   WR   /CV/   WR   /   S

3. excision of (one or both) adrenal glands

   _____ / _____
   WR   /   S

4. excision of (one or more) parathyroid glands

   _____ / _____
   WR   /   S

5. incision of the thyroid gland

   _____ / CV / _____
   WR   /CV/   S

6. excision of a gland

   _____ / _____
   WR   /   S

EXERCISE 20

Spell each of the surgical terms built from word parts on p. 717 by having someone dictate them to you.

To hear and spell the terms, go to evolve.elsevier.com. Select: Chapter 16, **Exercises**, Spelling.

Refer to p. 10 for your Evolve Access Information.

☐ Place a check mark in the box if you have completed this exercise online.

1. _____   4. _____
2. _____   5. _____
3. _____   6. _____

Diagnostic Terms

Not Built from Word Parts

In some of the following terms, you may recognize word parts you have already learned; however, the full meaning of the terms cannot be discerned by the definition of their word parts.

TERM	DEFINITION
DIAGNOSTIC IMAGING	
radioactive iodine uptake (RAIU) (rā-dē-ō-AK-tiv) (Ī-ō-dīn)	nuclear medicine scan that measures thyroid function. Radioactive iodine is given to the patient orally, after which its uptake into the thyroid gland is measured.
thyroid scan (THĪ-royd)	nuclear medicine test that shows the size, shape, and function of the thyroid gland. The patient is given a radioactive substance to visualize the thyroid gland. An image is recorded as the scanner is passed over the neck area; used to detect tumors and nodules.
thyroid sonography (THĪ-royd) (so-nog-ra-fē)	ultrasound test of the thyroid gland used to indicate whether a thyroid nodule is likely benign or possibly malignant; also used to monitor and evaluate structure.
LABORATORY	
fasting blood sugar (FBS)	blood test to determine the amount of glucose (sugar) in the blood after fasting for 8–10 hours. Elevation may indicate diabetes mellitus.
glycosylated hemoglobin (HbA1C) (glī-KŌ-sa-lāt-ad) (HĒ-mō-glō-bin)	blood test used to diagnose diabetes and monitor its treatment by measuring the amount of glucose (sugar) bound to hemoglobin in the blood. HbA1C provides an indication of blood sugar level over the past three months, covering the 120-day lifespan of the red blood cell (also called **hemoglobin A1C**).
thyroid-stimulating hormone level (TSH) (THĪ-royd)	blood test that measures the amount of thyroid-stimulating hormone in the blood; used to diagnose hypothyroidism and to monitor patients on thyroid replacement therapy.
thyroxine level (T₄) (thī-ROK-sin)	blood test that gives the direct measurement of the amount of thyroxine in the patient's blood. A greater-than-normal amount indicates hyperthyroidism; a less-than-normal amount indicates hypothyroidism.

EXERCISE 21

Practice saying aloud each of the diagnostic terms not built from word parts above.

To hear the terms, go to evolve.elsevier.com. Select: Chapter 16, **Exercises**, Pronunciation.

Refer to p. 10 for your Evolve Access Information.

☐ Place a check mark in the box when you have completed this exercise.

EXERCISE 22

Match the terms in the first column with their correct definitions in the second column.

_____ 1. fasting blood sugar

_____ 2. thyroid scan

_____ 3. thyroxine level

_____ 4. radioactive iodine uptake

_____ 5. thyroid-stimulating hormone level

_____ 6. glycosylated hemoglobin

_____ 7. thyroid sonography

a. nuclear medicine test used to determine the size, shape, and function of the thyroid gland
b. determines the amount of glucose in the blood after fasting for 8–10 hours
c. used to determine hypernatremia
d. uses radioactive iodine to measure thyroid function
e. used to indicate whether a thyroid nodule is likely benign or possibly malignant
f. used to diagnose hypothyroidism and to monitor thyroid replacement therapy
g. measures the amount of thyroxine in the blood
h. provides an indication of blood sugar level over the past three months

EXERCISE 23

Write the name of the procedure that gives information about each of the following.

1. thyroid function _____

2. amount of glucose in the blood at the time of the test _____

3. amount of thyroid-stimulating hormone in the blood_____

4. amount of thyroxine in the blood _____

5. size, shape, and function of the thyroid gland _____

6. amount of hemoglobin coated with sugar_____

7. thyroid nodules, likely benign or possibly malignant _____

EXERCISE 24

Spell each of the diagnostic terms not built from word parts on p. 719 by having someone dictate them to you.

> To hear and spell the terms, go to evolve.elsevier.com. Select: Chapter 16, **Exercises**, Spelling.
>
> (e) Refer to p. 10 for your Evolve Access Information.
>
> ☐ Place a check mark in the box if you have completed this exercise online.

1. _____   5. _____

2. _____   6. _____

3. _____   7. _____

4. _____

Complementary Terms

Built from Word Parts

The following terms are built from word parts you have already learned and can be translated literally to find their meanings. Further explanation of terms beyond the definition of their word parts, if needed, is included in parentheses.

TERM	DEFINITION
adrenocorticohyperplasia (a-*drē*-nō-*kōr*-ti-kō-*hī*-per-PLĀ-zha) (*NOTE:* hyper, *a prefix, appears within this word*)	excessive development of the adrenal cortex
adrenopathy (*ad*-ren-OP-a-thē)	disease of the adrenal gland
cortical (KŌR-ti-kal)	pertaining to the cortex
corticoid (KŌR-ti-koyd)	resembling the cortex
endocrinologist (*en*-dō-kri-NOL-o-jist)	physician who studies and treats diseases of the endocrine (system)
endocrinology (*en*-dō-kri-NOL-o-jē)	study of the endocrine (system) (a branch of medicine dealing with diseases of the endocrine system)
endocrinopathy (*en*-dō-kri-NOP-a-thē)	(any) disease of the endocrine (system)
euglycemia (*ū*-glī-SĒ-mē-a)	normal (level of) sugar in the blood (within normal range)
euthyroid (ū-THĪ-royd)	resembling a normal thyroid gland (normal thyroid function)
glycemia (glī-SĒ-mē-a)	sugar in the blood
polydipsia (*pol*-ē-DIP-sē-a)	abnormal state of much thirst
syndrome (SIN-drōm)	run together (signs and symptoms occurring together that are characteristic of a specific disorder)

EXERCISE 25

Practice saying aloud each of the complementary terms built from word parts above.

To hear the terms, go to evolve.elsevier.com. Select: Chapter 16, **Exercises**, Pronunciation.

Refer to p. 10 for your Evolve Access Information.

☐ Place a check mark in the box when you have completed this exercise.

EXERCISE 26

Analyze and define the following complementary terms.

1. corticoid _____
2. syndrome_____
3. adrenopathy _____
4. endocrinologist_____
5. polydipsia _____
6. euglycemia _____
7. endocrinopathy_____
8. adrenocorticohyperplasia_____
9. euthyroid_____
10. cortical_____
11. endocrinology_____
12. glycemia _____

EXERCISE 27

Build the complementary terms for the following definitions by using the word parts you have learned.

1. (any) disease of the endocrine (system)

   _____ / _____ / _____
       WR   /CV/   S

2. resembling the cortex

   _____ / _____
       WR   /   S

3. run together (signs and symptoms occurring together)

   _____ / _____
       P   /   S(WR)

4. excessive development of the adrenal cortex

   _____ /CV/ _____ /CV/ _____ / _____
     WR /CV/ WR /CV/ P / S

5. study of the endocrine (system)

   _____ / _____ / _____
       WR   /CV/   S

6. abnormal state of much thirst

   _____ / _____ / _____
       P   / WR / S

7. disease of the adrenal gland

   _____ /CV/ _____
       WR   /CV/ S

8. normal (level of) sugar in the blood

   _____ / _____ / _____
       P   / WR / S

9. resembling a normal thyroid gland

   _____ / _____ / _____
       P   / WR / S

10. pertaining to the cortex

   _____ / _____
       WR   / S

11. physician who studies and
    treats diseases of the endocrine
    (system)

         WR   CV   S

12. sugar in the blood

         WR   S

EXERCISE 28

Spell each of the complementary terms built from word parts on p. 721 by having someone dictate them to you.

> To hear and spell the terms, go to evolve.elsevier.com. Select: Chapter 16, **Exercises**, Spelling.
>
> Refer to p. 10 for your Evolve Access Information.
>
> ☐ Place a check mark in the box if you have completed this exercise online.

1. _____
2. _____
3. _____
4. _____
5. _____
6. _____

7. _____
8. _____
9. _____
10. _____
11. _____
12. _____

> For review and/or assessment, go to evolve.elsevier.com. Select:
> Chapter 16, **Activities,** Terms Built from Word Parts
> Chapter 16, **Games,**   Term Storm
>
> Refer to p. 10 for your Evolve Access Information.

Complementary Terms

Not Built from Word Parts

In some of the following terms, you may recognize word parts you have already learned; however, the full meaning of the terms cannot be discerned by the definition of their word parts.

TERM	DEFINITION
exophthalmos (*ek*-sof-THAL-mos)	abnormal protrusion of the eyeball (Figure 16-8)
hormone (HOR-mōn)	chemical substance secreted by an endocrine gland that is carried in the blood to a target tissue
isthmus (IS-mus)	narrow strip of tissue connecting two larger parts in the body, such as the isthmus that connects the two lobes of the thyroid gland (see Figure 16-3, *C*)
metabolism (me-TAB-ō-liz*m*)	sum total of all the chemical processes that take place in a living organism

🏛 **EXOPHTHALMOS**
is derived from the Greek **ex,** meaning **outward,** and **ophthalmos,** meaning **eye.** Protrusion of the eyeball is sometimes a symptom of Graves disease, first described by Dr. Robert Graves, an Irish physician, in 1835.

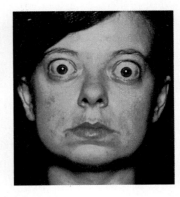

FIGURE 16-8
Abnormal protrusion of eyeballs, exophthalmos, a characteristic of thyroid disease.

EXERCISE 29

Practice saying aloud each of the complementary terms not built from word parts on p. 723.

> (e) To hear the terms, go to evolve.elsevier.com. Select: Chapter 16, **Exercises**, Pronunciation.
>
> Refer to p. 10 for your Evolve Access Information.

☐ Place a check mark in the box when you have completed this exercise.

EXERCISE 30

Fill in the blanks with the correct terms.

1. The sum total of all the chemical processes that take place in a living organism is called its _____.
2. A chemical substance secreted by an endocrine gland is called a(n) _____.
3. A narrow strip of tissue connecting larger parts in the body is called a(n) _____.
4. Abnormal protrusion of the eyeball is called _____.

EXERCISE 31

Write the definitions of the following terms.

1. isthmus _____
2. metabolism _____
3. hormone _____
4. exophthalmos _____

EXERCISE 32

Spell each of the complementary terms not built from word parts on p. 723 by having someone dictate them to you.

> (e) To hear and spell the terms, go to evolve.elsevier.com. Select: Chapter 16, **Exercises**, Spelling.
>
> Refer to p. 10 for your Evolve Access Information.
>
> ☐ Place a check mark in the box if you have completed this exercise online.

1. _____   3. _____
2. _____   4. _____

> 🔍 Refer to **Appendix D** for pharmacology terms related to the endocrine system.

> For review and/or assessment, go to evolve.elsevier.com. Select:
> Chapter 16, **Activities,** Terms Not Built from Word Parts
>   Hear It and Type It: Clinical Vignettes
> (e) Chapter 16, **Games,** Term Explorer
>   Termbusters
>   Medical Millionaire
>
> Refer to p. 10 for your Evolve Access Information.

Abbreviations

ABBREVIATION	MEANING
ACTH	adrenocorticotropic hormone
ADH	antidiuretic hormone
DI	diabetes insipidus
DM	diabetes mellitus
FBS	fasting blood sugar
FSH	follicle-stimulating hormone
GH	growth hormone
HbA1C	glycosylated hemoglobin
LH	luteinizing hormone
PRH	prolactin-releasing hormone
RAIU	radioactive iodine uptake
TSH	thyroid-stimulating hormone
T$_4$	thyroxine level

Refer to **Appendix C** for a complete list of abbreviations.

EXERCISE 33

Write the meaning of the following abbreviations.

1. RAIU _____
2. FBS _____
3. DM _____
4. DI _____
5. T4 _____
6. HbA1C _____
7. TSH _____
8. PRH _____
9. LH _____
10. GH _____
11. FSH _____
12. ADH _____
13. ACTH _____

For more practice with abbreviations, go to evolve.elsevier.com. Select:
Chapter 16, **Flashcards**
Chapter 16, **Games,** Crossword Puzzle

Refer to p. 10 for your Evolve Access Information.

PRACTICAL APPLICATION

EXERCISE 34 *Interact with Medical Documents and Electronic Health Records*

A. Complete the history and physical by writing the medical terms in the blanks. Use the list of definitions with the corresponding numbers.

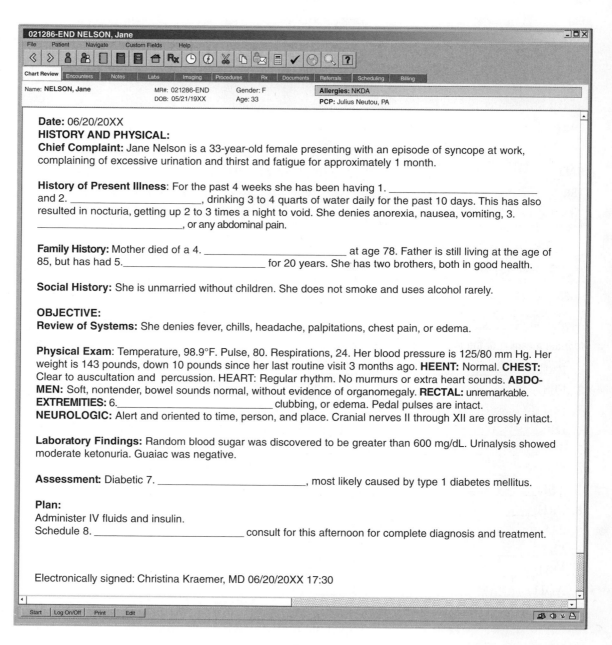

021286-END NELSON, Jane

File   Patient   Navigate   Custom Fields   Help

Chart Review | Encounters | Notes | Labs | Imaging | Procedures | Rx | Documents | Referrals | Scheduling | Billing

Name: **NELSON, Jane**   MR#: 021286-END   Gender: F   **Allergies:** NKDA
                              DOB: 05/21/19XX   Age: 33   **PCP:** Julius Neutou, PA

Date: 06/20/20XX
HISTORY AND PHYSICAL:
Chief Complaint: Jane Nelson is a 33-year-old female presenting with an episode of syncope at work, complaining of excessive urination and thirst and fatigue for approximately 1 month.

History of Present Illness: For the past 4 weeks she has been having 1. _____ and 2. _____, drinking 3 to 4 quarts of water daily for the past 10 days. This has also resulted in nocturia, getting up 2 to 3 times a night to void. She denies anorexia, nausea, vomiting, 3. _____, or any abdominal pain.

Family History: Mother died of a 4. _____ at age 78. Father is still living at the age of 85, but has had 5._____ for 20 years. She has two brothers, both in good health.

Social History: She is unmarried without children. She does not smoke and uses alcohol rarely.

OBJECTIVE:
Review of Systems: She denies fever, chills, headache, palpitations, chest pain, or edema.

Physical Exam: Temperature, 98.9°F. Pulse, 80. Respirations, 24. Her blood pressure is 125/80 mm Hg. Her weight is 143 pounds, down 10 pounds since her last routine visit 3 months ago. **HEENT:** Normal. **CHEST:** Clear to auscultation and percussion. **HEART:** Regular rhythm. No murmurs or extra heart sounds. **ABDOMEN:** Soft, nontender, bowel sounds normal, without evidence of organomegaly. **RECTAL:** unremarkable. **EXTREMITIES:** 6._____ clubbing, or edema. Pedal pulses are intact. **NEUROLOGIC:** Alert and oriented to time, person, and place. Cranial nerves II through XII are grossly intact.

Laboratory Findings: Random blood sugar was discovered to be greater than 600 mg/dL. Urinalysis showed moderate ketonuria. Guaiac was negative.

Assessment: Diabetic 7. _____, most likely caused by type 1 diabetes mellitus.

Plan:
Administer IV fluids and insulin.
Schedule 8. _____ consult for this afternoon for complete diagnosis and treatment.

Electronically signed: Christina Kraemer, MD 06/20/20XX 17:30

Start | Log On/Off | Print | Edit

---

1. excessive urine
2. excessive thirst
3. vomiting of blood
4. interruption of blood supply to a region of the brain
5. chronic disease involving a disorder of carbohydrate metabolism caused by

underactivity of islets of Langerhans and characterized by hyperglycemia
6. abnormal condition of blue (bluish discoloration of skin) caused by inadequate supply of oxygen in the blood
7. abnormal concentration of ketone bodies
8. study of the endocrine system

B. Read the operative report and answer the questions below.

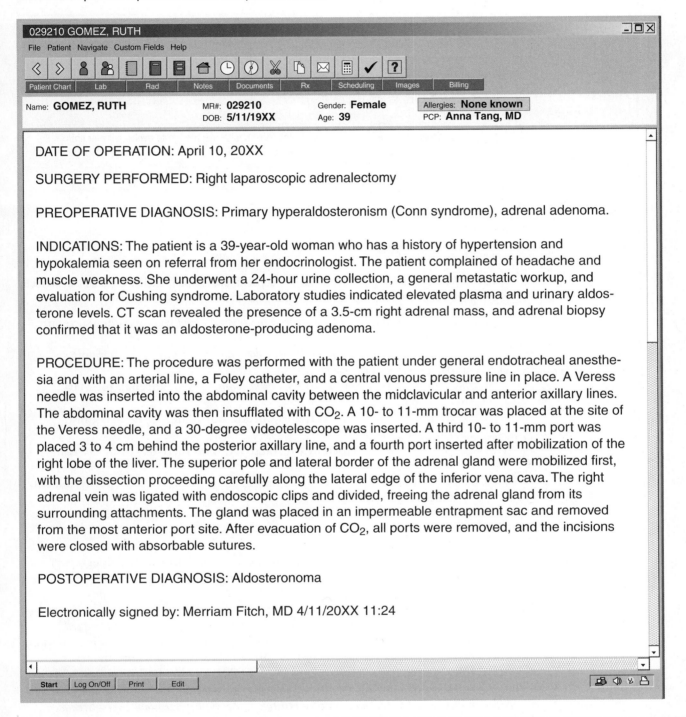

1. Which procedure was performed during surgery:
   a. excision of a parathyroid gland
   b. surgical repair of the thyroid gland
   c. excision of an adrenal gland
   d. surgical repair of the thymus
2. The patient had a history of:
   a. excessive sugar in the blood
   b. deficient potassium in the blood
   c. excessive sodium in the blood
   d. deficient calcium in the blood
3. The patient was evaluated for a:
   a. group of symptoms from the excessive production of cortisol
   b. condition caused by congenital absence of the thyroid gland
   c. syndrome caused by deficient secretion from the adrenal cortex
   d. condition causing muscle spasms resulting from low amounts of calcium

C. Complete the **three medical documents** within the electronic health record (EHR) on Evolve.

> ☀ Many healthcare records today are stored and used in an electronic system called **Electronic Health Records (EHR).** Electronic health records contain a collection of health information of an individual patient documented by various providers at different facilities; the digitally formatted record can be shared through computer networks with patients, physicians, and other health care providers.

> ⓔ For practice with medical terms using electronic health records, go to evolve.elsevier.com. Select: Chapter 16, **Electronic Health Records**
>
> Refer to p. 10 for your Evolve Access Information.

EXERCISE 35 *Interpret Medical Terms*

To test your understanding of the terms introduced in this chapter, circle the words that correctly complete the sentences. The italicized words refer to the correct answer.

1. A patient who has an *enlargement of the thyroid gland* has (**myxedema, tetany, goiter**).
2. A condition that results from *uncontrolled diabetes mellitus* is (**calcipenia, ketosis, tetany**).
3. *Addison disease* is caused by an *underfunctioning* of the (**adrenal, pituitary, thyroid**) gland.
4. *Decreased secretion* of (**ACTH, antidiuretic hormone, TSH**) may cause diabetes insipidus.
5. *Cushing syndrome* is caused by (**overactivity, underactivity**) of the *adrenal cortices.*
6. A *wasting away of the thyroid gland* may result in (**congenital hypothyroidism, myxedema, tetany**).
7. The primary treatment for *tumor of the adrenal medulla* (**pheochromocytoma, adenomegaly, thyrotoxicosis**) is surgical removal of the tumor by laparoscopic *excision of an adrenal gland* (**adenectomy, adrenalectomy, thyroidectomy**).
8. Unlike *the blood test measuring the amount of glucose in the blood at the time of the test* (**fasting blood sugar, glycosylated hemoglobin, radioactive iodine uptake test**), *the test measuring the amount of hemoglobin coated in sugar over the lifespan of the red blood cell* (**fasting blood sugar, glycosylated hemoglobin, radioactive iodine uptake test**) test results are not altered by eating habits the day before the test.
9. Lifestyle changes such as weight loss, regular exercise, healthy eating, and cessation of smoking are central in the treatment and prevention of *a group of health problems including insulin resistance, obesity, hypertension, hyperglycemia, elevated triglycerides and low levels of HDL* (**euglycemia, Addison disease, metabolic syndrome**).

EXERCISE 36 *Read Medical Terms in Use*

Practice pronunciation of the terms by reading the following medical document. Use the pronunciation key following the medical terms to assist you.

> To hear these terms, go to evolve.elsevier.com.
> Select: Chapter 16, **Exercises**, Read Medical Terms in Use.
>
> Refer to p. 10 for your Evolve Access Information.

A 55-year-old female patient presented to her doctor because of a 10-pound weight gain, fatigue, hair loss, dry skin, and cold intolerance. She was referred to an **endocrinologist** (*en*-dō-kri-NOL-o-jist), who established a diagnosis of **hypothyroidism** (*hī*-pō-THĪ-royd-izm) after test results indicated an elevated **thyroid** (THĪ-royd)-**stimulating hormone level** and a low **thyroxine** (thī-ROK-sin) **level.** Thyroid hormone therapy was prescribed. Approximately 20 years ago she was diagnosed with Graves disease characterized by hyperthyroidism, **exophthalmos** (*ek*-sof-THAL-mos), fatigue, irritability, weight loss, and **goiter** (GOY-ter). At this time she had an increased **radioactive iodine** (*ra*-dē-ō-AK-tiv) (Ī-ō-dīn) **uptake** (RAIU). Treatment included a **thyroidectomy** (*thī*-royd-EK-to-mē) with subsequent thyroid hormone therapy. She remained in a **euthyroid** (ū-THĪ-royd) state until she stopped taking the medication 6 months ago. Consequently she became hypothyroid and could easily have developed **myxedema** (*mik*-se-DĒ-ma) if she had not sought treatment.

EXERCISE 37 *Comprehend Medical Terms in Use*

Test your comprehension of terms in the previous medical document by circling the correct answer.

1. On a recent visit to the endocrinologist the patient was diagnosed with:
   a. a state of deficient thyroid gland activity
   b. an enlargement of the thyroid gland
   c. a state of excessive thyroid gland activity
   d. Graves disease
2. After a thyroidectomy the patient remained in a state resembling a:
   a. stressed thyroid gland
   b. normal thyroid gland
   c. hyperactive thyroid gland
   d. hypoactive thyroid gland
3. The patient's earlier diagnosis of Graves disease was characterized by:
   a. thirst, excessive thyroid activity, protruding eyes
   b. protruding eyes, spasms, excessive thyroid activity
   c. excessive thyroid activity, enlargement of the thyroid gland, protruding eyes
   d. enlargement of the extremities, excessive thyroid activities, protruding eyes
4. What type of diagnostic procedure was used to assist in diagnosing hypothyroidism?
   a. computed tomography
   b. nuclear medicine
   c. ultrasound
   d. blood test

> For a snapshot assessment of your knowledge of musculoskeletal system terms go to evolve.elsevier.com.
> Select: Chapter 16, **Quick Quizzes**.
>
> Refer to p. 10 for your Evolve Access Information.

CHAPTER REVIEW

 Review of Evolve

Keep a record of the online activities you have completed by placing a check mark in the box. You may also record your scores. All activities have been referenced throughout the chapter.

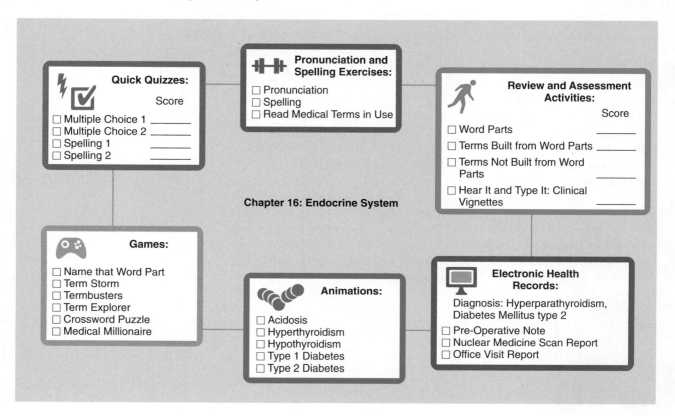

Quick Quizzes:

Score

☐ Multiple Choice 1 _____
☐ Multiple Choice 2 _____
☐ Spelling 1 _____
☐ Spelling 2 _____

Pronunciation and Spelling Exercises:

☐ Pronunciation
☐ Spelling
☐ Read Medical Terms in Use

Review and Assessment Activities:

Score

☐ Word Parts _____
☐ Terms Built from Word Parts _____
☐ Terms Not Built from Word Parts _____
☐ Hear It and Type It: Clinical Vignettes _____

Chapter 16: Endocrine System

Games:

☐ Name that Word Part
☐ Term Storm
☐ Termbusters
☐ Term Explorer
☐ Crossword Puzzle
☐ Medical Millionaire

Animations:

☐ Acidosis
☐ Hyperthyroidism
☐ Hypothyroidism
☐ Type 1 Diabetes
☐ Type 2 Diabetes

Electronic Health Records:

Diagnosis: Hyperparathyroidism, Diabetes Mellitus type 2

☐ Pre-Operative Note
☐ Nuclear Medicine Scan Report
☐ Office Visit Report

Review of Word Parts

Can you define and spell the following word parts?

COMBINING FORMS		SUFFIX
acr/o	endocrin/o	-drome
aden/o	kal/i	
adren/o	natr/o	
adrenal/o	parathyroid/o	
calc/i	pituitar/o	
cortic/o	thyr/o	
dips/o	thyroid/o	

Review of Terms

Can you build, analyze, define, pronounce, and spell the following terms *built from word parts?*

DISEASES AND DISORDERS	SURGICAL	COMPLEMENTARY
acromegaly	adenectomy	adrenocorticohyperplasia
adenitis	adrenalectomy	adrenopathy
adenomegaly	parathyroidectomy	cortical
adenosis	thyroidectomy	corticoid
adrenalitis	thyroidotomy	endocrinologist
adrenomegaly	thyroparathyroidectomy	endocrinology
hypercalcemia		endocrinopathy
hyperglycemia		euglycemia
hyperkalemia		euthyroid
hyperpituitarism		glycemia
hyperthyroidism		polydipsia
hypocalcemia		syndrome
hypoglycemia		
hypokalemia		
hyponatremia		
hypopituitarism		
hypothyroidism		
panhypopituitarism		
parathyroidoma		
thyroiditis		

Can you define, pronounce, and spell the following terms *not built from word parts?*

DISEASES AND DISORDERS	DIAGNOSTIC	COMPLEMENTARY
acidosis	fasting blood sugar (FBS)	exophthalmos
Addison disease	glycosylated hemoglobin (HbA1C)	hormone
congenital hypothyroidism	radioactive iodine uptake (RAIU)	isthmus
Cushing syndrome	thyroid scan	metabolism
diabetes insipidus (DI)	thyroid sonography	
diabetes mellitus (DM)	thyroid-stimulating hormone (TSH) level	
gigantism	thyroxine level (T_4)	
goiter		
Graves disease		
ketosis		
metabolic syndrome		
myxedema		
pheochromocytoma		
tetany		
thyrotoxicosis		

ANSWERS

ANSWERS TO CHAPTER 16 EXERCISES
Exercise Figures

Exercise Figure

A. 1. parathyroid glands: parathyroid/o
2. adrenal glands: adren/o, adrenal/o
3. pituitary gland: pituitar/o
4. thyroid gland: thyroid/o, thyr/o

Exercise Figure

B. cortex: cortic/o

Exercise Figure

C. acr/o/megaly

Exercise 1
1. b
2. g
3. d
4. h
5. a
6. c
7. e

Exercise 2
1. d
2. a
3. e
4. b
5. g
6. c

Exercise 3
1. cortex
2. adrenal glands
3. parathyroid glands
4. thyroid gland
5. adrenal glands
6. thyroid gland
7. endocrine
8. gland
9. pituitary gland

Exercise 4
1. a. adren/o
   b. adrenal/o
2. a. thyroid/o
   b. thyr/o
3. endocrin/o
4. cortic/o
5. parathyroid/o
6. aden/o
7. pituitar/o

Exercise 5
1. thirst
2. potassium
3. calcium
4. extremities, height
5. sodium

Exercise 6
1. acr/o
2. calc/i
3. dips/o
4. kal/i
5. natr/o

Exercise 7
1. run, running

Exercise 8
1. -drome

Exercise 9
Pronunciation Exercise

Exercise 10

Note: The combining form is identified by italic and bold print.

1. WR S
   adrenal/itis
   inflammation of the adrenal glands

2. P WR S
   hypo/calc/emia
   deficient calcium in the blood

3. P WR S
   hyper/thyroid/ism
   state of excessive thyroid gland activity

4. P WR S
   hyper/kal/emia
   excessive potassium in the blood

5. P WR S
   hyper/glyc/emia
   excessive sugar in the blood

6. WR CV S
   adren/o/megaly
      CF
   enlargement of the adrenal glands

7. WR CV S
   aden/o/megaly
      CF
   enlargement of a gland

8. P WR S
   hypo/thyroid/ism
   state of deficient thyroid gland activity

9. P WR S
   hypo/kal/emia
   deficient potassium in the blood

10. WR S
    aden/itis
    inflammation of a gland

11. WR S
    parathyroid/oma
    tumor of a parathyroid gland

12. WR CV S
    acr/o/megaly
       CF
    enlargement of the extremities

13. P P WR S
    pan/hypo/pituitar/ism
    state of total deficient pituitary gland activity

14. P WR S
    hypo/glyc/emia
    deficient sugar in the blood

15. P WR S
    hyper/calc/emia
    excessive calcium in the blood

16. P WR S
    hyper/pituitar/ism
    state of excessive pituitary gland activity

17. P WR S
    hypo/natr/emia
    deficient sodium in the blood

18. WR S
    aden/osis
    abnormal condition of a gland

19. WR S
    thyroid/itis
    inflammation of the thyroid gland

20. P WR S
    hypo/pituitar/ism
    state of deficient pituitary gland activity

Exercise 11
1. adren/o/megaly
2. hypo/thyroid/ism
3. acr/o/megaly
4. hypo/glyc/emia
5. hyper/kal/emia
6. hypo/calc/emia
7. hyper/thyroid/ism
8. hypo/pituitar/ism
9. hyper/calc/emia
10. hyper/pituitar/ism
11. parathyroid/oma
12. hyper/glyc/emia
13. aden/osis
14. hypo/kal/emia
15. adrenal/itis
16. aden/o/megaly
17. hypo/natr/emia
18. aden/itis
19. thyroid/itis
20. pan/hypo/pituitar/ism

Exercise 12
Spelling Exercise; see text pp. 712–713.

Exercise 13
Pronunciation Exercise

Exercise 14
1. d
2. a
3. j
4. b
5. h
6. c
7. l
8. e
9. k
10. i
11. f
12. g
13. n
14. o
15. p

Exercise 15
1. thyroid
2. parathyroid
3. islets of Langerhans (pancreas)
4. pituitary
5. thyroid
6. adrenal
7. islets of Langerhans (pancreas)
8. thyroid
9. islets of Langerhans (pancreas)
10. adrenal
11. pituitary
12. thyroid
13. thyroid
14. adrenal

Exercise 16
Spelling Exercise; see text p. 717.

Exercise 17
Pronunciation Exercise

Exercise 18
Note: The combining form is identified by italic and bold print.

1.   WR CV S
   ***thyroid/o**/tomy*
        CF
   incision of the thyroid gland

2.   WR   S
   adrenal/ectomy
   excision of (one or both) adrenal glands

3.   WR CV   WR   S
   ***thyr/o**/parathyroid/ectomy*
      CF
   excision of the thyroid and parathyroid glands

4.   WR   S
   thyroid/ectomy
   excision of the thyroid gland

5.   WR   S
   parathyroid/ectomy
   excision of (one or more) parathyroid glands

6.   WR   S
   aden/ectomy
   excision of a gland

Exercise 19
1. thyroid/ectomy
2. thyr/o/parathyroid/ectomy
3. adrenal/ectomy
4. parathyroid/ectomy
5. thyroid/o/tomy
6. aden/ectomy

Exercise 20
Spelling Exercise; see text p. 718.

Exercise 21
Pronunciation Exercise

Exercise 22
1. b   5. f
2. a   6. h
3. g   7. e
4. d

Exercise 23
1. radioactive iodine uptake
2. fasting blood sugar
3. thyroid-stimulating hormone level
4. thyroxine level
5. thyroid scan
6. glycosylated hemoglobin
7. thyroid sonography

Exercise 24
Spelling Exercise; see text p. 720.

Exercise 25
Pronunciation Exercise

Exercise 26
Note: The combining form is identified by italic and bold print.

1.   WR   S
   cortic/oid
   resembling the cortex

2.   P   S(WR)
   syn/drome
   run together

3.   WR CV S
   ***adren/o**/pathy*
       CF
   disease of the adrenal glands

4.   WR CV S
   ***endocrin/o**/logist*
         CF
   physician who studies and treats diseases of the endocrine (system)

5.   P WR S
   poly/dips/ia
   abnormal state of much thirst

6.   P WR S
   eu/glyc/emia
   normal (level of) sugar in the blood

7.   WR CV S
   ***endocrin/o**/pathy*
        CF
   (any) disease of the endocrine (system)

8.   WR CV WR CV P   S
   ***adren/o**/**cortic/o**/hyper/plasia*
       CF   CF
   excessive development of the adrenal cortex

9.   P WR   S
   eu/thyr/oid
   resembling normal thyroid gland

10.   WR   S
   cortic/al
   pertaining to the cortex

11.   WR   CV S
   ***endocrin/o**/logy*
         CF
   study of the endocrine (system)

12.   WR   S
   glyc/emia
   sugar in the blood

Exercise 27
1. endocrin/o/pathy
2. cortic/oid
3. syn/drome
4. adren/o/cortic/o/hyper/plasia
5. endocrin/o/logy
6. poly/dips/ia
7. adren/o/pathy
8. eu/glyc/emia
9. eu/thyr/oid
10. cortic/al
11. endocrin/o/logist
12. glyc/emia

Exercise 28
Spelling Exercise; see text p. 723.

Exercise 29
Pronunciation Exercise

Exercise 30
1. metabolism
2. hormone
3. isthmus
4. exophthalmos

Exercise 31
1. narrow strip of tissue connecting two larger parts in the body
2. total of all chemical processes that take place in living organisms
3. chemical substance secreted by an endocrine gland
4. abnormal protrusion of the eyeball

Exercise 32
Spelling Exercise; see text p. 724.

Exercise 33
1. radioactive iodine uptake
2. fasting blood sugar
3. diabetes mellitus
4. diabetes insipidus
5. thyroxine level
6. glycosylated hemoglobin
7. thyroid-stimulating hormone

8. prolactin-releasing hormone
9. luteinizing hormone
10. growth hormone
11. follicle-stimulating hormone
12. antidiuretic hormone
13. adrenocorticotropic hormone

Exercise 34

A. 1. polyuria
2. polydipsia
3. hematemesis
4. stroke
5. diabetes mellitus
6. cyanosis

7. ketosis
8. endocrinology

B. 1. c
2. b
3. a

C. Online Exercise

Exercise 35

1. goiter
2. ketosis
3. adrenal
4. antidiuretic hormone
5. overactivity
6. congenital hypothyroidism

7. pheochromocytoma, adrenalectomy
8. fasting blood sugar, glycosylated hemoglobin
9. metabolic syndrome

Exercise 36
Reading Exercise

Exercise 37

1. a
2. b
3. c
4. d

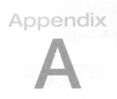
COMBINING FORMS	DEFINITION	CHAPTER
A		
abdomin/o	abdomen, abdominal cavity	11
acr/o	extremities, height	16
aden/o	gland	2, 16
adenoid/o	adenoids	5
adren/o	adrenal glands	16
adrenal/o	adrenal glands	16
albumin/o	albumin	6
alveol/o	alveolus	5
amni/o	amnion, amniotic fluid	9
amnion/o	amnion, amniotic fluid	9
andr/o	male	7
angi/o	vessel (usually refers to blood vessel)	10
ankyl/o	stiff, bent	14
an/o	anus	11
anter/o	front	3
antr/o	antrum	11
aort/o	aorta	10
aponeur/o	aponeurosis	14
appendic/o	appendix	11
append/o	appendix	11
arche/o	first, beginning	8
arteri/o	artery	10
arthr/o	joint	14
atel/o	imperfect, incomplete	5
ather/o	yellowish, fatty plaque	10
atri/o	atrium	10
audi/o	hearing	13
aur/i	ear	13
aur/o	ear	13
aut/o	self	4
azot/o	urea, nitrogen	6
B		
balan/o	glans penis	7
bi/o	life	4

COMBINING FORMS	DEFINITION	CHAPTER
blast/o	developing cell, germ cell	6
blephar/o	eyelid	12
bronch/o	bronchus	5
bronchi/o	bronchus	5
burs/o	bursa (cavity)	14
C		
calc/i	calcium	16
cancer/o	cancer	2
capn/o	carbon dioxide	5
carcin/o	cancer	2
cardi/o	heart	10
carp/o	carpals (wrist)	14
caud/o	tail (downward)	3
cec/o	cecum	11
celi/o	abdomen, abdominal cavity	11
cephal/o	head	3, 9
cerebell/o	cerebellum	15
cerebr/o	cerebrum, brain	15
cervic/o	cervix	8
cheil/o	lip	11
chlor/o	green	2
cholangi/o	bile duct	11
chol/e	gall, bile	11
choledoch/o	common bile duct	11
chondr/o	cartilage	14
chori/o	chorion	9
chrom/o	color	2
clavic/o	clavicle (collarbone)	14
clavicul/o	clavicle (collarbone)	14
cochle/o	cochlea	13
col/o	colon	11
colon/o	colon	11
colp/o	vagina	8
coni/o	dust	4
conjunctiv/o	conjunctiva	12

COMBINING FORMS	DEFINITION	CHAPTER
cor/o	pupil	12
core/o	pupil	12
corne/o	cornea	12
cortic/o	cortex (outer layer of body organ)	16
cost/o	rib	14
crani/o	cranium (skull)	14
cry/o	cold	12
crypt/o	hidden	4
culd/o	cul-de-sac	8
cutane/o	skin	4
cyan/o	blue	2
cyst/o	bladder, sac	6
cyt/o	cell	2
D		
dacry/o	tear, tear duct	12
dermat/o	skin	4
derm/o	skin	4
diaphragmat/o	diaphragm	5
dipl/o	two, double	12
dips/o	thirst	16
disk/o	intervertebral disk	14
dist/o	away (from the point of attachment of a body part)	3
diverticul/o	diverticulum	11
dors/o	back	3
duoden/o	duodenum	11
dur/o	hard, dura mater	15
E		
ech/o	sound	10
electr/o	electricity, electrical activity	10
embry/o	embryo, to be full	9
encephal/o	brain	15
endocrin/o	endocrine	16
enter/o	intestine	11
epididym/o	epididymis	7
epiglott/o	epiglottis	5
episi/o	vulva	8
epitheli/o	epithelium	2

COMBINING FORMS	DEFINITION	CHAPTER
erythr/o	red	2
esophag/o	esophagus	9, 11
esthesi/o	sensation, sensitivity, feeling	15
eti/o	cause (of disease)	2
F		
femor/o	femur (upper leg bone)	14
fet/i	fetus, unborn child	9
fet/o	fetus, unborn child	9
fibr/o	fiber	2
fibul/o	fibula (lower leg bone)	14
G		
gangli/o	ganglion	15
ganglion/o	ganglion	15
gastr/o	stomach	11
gingiv/o	gum	11
gli/o	glia, gluey substance	15
glomerul/o	glomerulus	6
gloss/o	tongue	11
glyc/o	sugar	6
glycos/o	sugar	6
gno/o	knowledge	2
gravid/o	pregnancy	9
gynec/o	woman	8
gyn/o	woman	8
H		
hemat/o	blood	5
hem/o	blood	5
hepat/o	liver	11
herni/o	hernia, or protrusion of an organ through a membrane or cavity wall	11
heter/o	other	4
hidr/o	sweat	4
hist/o	tissue	2
humer/o	humerus (upper arm bone)	14
hydr/o	water	6
hymen/o	hymen	8
hyster/o	uterus	8

COMBINING FORMS	DEFINITION	CHAPTER
I		
iatr/o	physician, medicine (also means treatment)	2
ile/o	ileum	11
ili/o	ilium	14
infer/o	below	3
irid/o	iris	12
ir/o	iris	12
is/o	equal	12
ischi/o	ischium	14
isch/o	deficiency, blockage	10
J		
jejun/o	jejunum	11
K		
kal/i	potassium	16
kary/o	nucleus	2
kerat/o	cornea	12
kerat/o	horny tissue, hard	4
kinesi/o	movement, motion	14
kyph/o	hump (increased convexity of the spine)	14
L		
labyrinth/o	labyrinth (inner ear)	13
lacrim/o	tear, tear duct	12
lact/o	milk	9
lamin/o	lamina (thin, flat plate or layer)	14
lapar/o	abdomen, abdominal cavity	11
laryng/o	larynx	5
later/o	side	3
lei/o	smooth	2
leuk/o	white	2
lingu/o	tongue	11
lip/o	fat	2
lith/o	stone, calculus	6
lob/o	lobe	5
lord/o	bent forward (increased concavity of the spine)	14
lumb/o	loin, lumbar region of the spine	14

COMBINING FORMS	DEFINITION	CHAPTER
lymphaden/o	lymph node	10
lymph/o	lymph, lymph tissue	10
M		
mamm/o	breast	8
mandibul/o	mandible (lower jawbone)	14
mast/o	breast	8
mastoid/o	mastoid bone	13
maxill/o	maxilla (upper jawbone)	14
meat/o	meatus (opening)	6
medi/o	middle	3
melan/o	black	2
meningi/o	meninges	15
mening/o	meninges	15
menisc/o	meniscus (crescent)	14
men/o	menstruation	8
ment/o	mind	15
metr/i	uterus	8
metr/o	uterus	8
mon/o	one, single	15
muc/o	mucus	5
myc/o	fungus	4
myel/o	bone marrow	10, 14
myel/o	spinal cord	15
my/o	muscle	2, 14
myos/o	muscle	14
myring/o	tympanic membrane (eardrum)	13
N		
nas/o	nose	5
nat/o	birth	9
natr/o	sodium	16
necr/o	death (cells, body)	4
nephr/o	kidney	6
neur/o	nerve	2, 15
noct/i	night	6
O		
ocul/o	eye	12
olig/o	scanty, few	6
omphal/o	umbilicus, navel	9
onc/o	tumor, mass	2

COMBINING FORMS	DEFINITION	CHAPTER
onych/o	nail	4
oophor/o	ovary	8
ophthalm/o	eye	12
opt/o	vision	12
orchid/o	testis, testicle	7
orchi/o	testis, testicle	7
orch/o	testis, testicle	7
organ/o	organ	2
or/o	mouth	11
orth/o	straight	5
oste/o	bone	14
ot/o	ear	13
ox/i	oxygen	5
P		
pachy/o	thick	4
palat/o	palate	11
pancreat/o	pancreas	11
parathyroid/o	parathyroid glands	16
par/o	bear, give birth to, labor, childbirth	9
part/o	bear, give birth to, labor, childbirth	9
patell/o	patella (kneecap)	14
path/o	disease	2
pelv/i	pelvis, pelvic bone	9, 14
pelv/o	pelvis, pelvic bone	9, 14
perine/o	perineum	8
peritone/o	peritoneum	11
petr/o	stone	14
phac/o	lens	12
phak/o	lens	12
phalang/o	phalanges (any bone of the fingers or toes)	14
pharyng/o	pharynx	5
phas/o	speech	15
phleb/o	vein	10
phon/o	sound	5
phot/o	light	12
phren/o	diaphragm	5
pituitar/o	pituitary gland	16
plasm/o	plasma	10

COMBINING FORMS	DEFINITION	CHAPTER
pleur/o	pleura	5
pneumat/o	lung, air	5
pneum/o	lung, air	5
pneumon/o	lung, air	5
poli/o	gray matter	15
polyp/o	polyp, small growth	11
poster/o	back, behind	3
prim/i	first	9
proct/o	rectum	11
prostat/o	prostate gland	7
proxim/o	near (the point of attachment of a body part)	3
pseud/o	false	9
psych/o	mind	15
pub/o	pubis	14
puerper/o	childbirth	9
pulmon/o	lung	5
pupill/o	pupil	12
pyel/o	renal pelvis	6
pylor/o	pylorus (pyloric sphincter)	9, 11
py/o	pus	5
Q		
quadr/i	four	15
R		
rachi/o	vertebra, spine, vertebral column	14
radic/o	nerve root	15
radicul/o	nerve root	15
radi/o	radius (lower arm bone)	14
radi/o	x-rays, ionizing radiation	5
rect/o	rectum	11
ren/o	kidney	6
retin/o	retina	12
rhabd/o	rod-shaped, striated	2
rhin/o	nose	5
rhiz/o	nerve root	15
rhytid/o	wrinkles	4
S		
sacr/o	sacrum	14

COMBINING FORMS	DEFINITION	CHAPTER
salping/o	uterine tube (fallopian tube)	8
sarc/o	flesh, connective tissue	2
scapul/o	scapula (shoulder blade)	14
scler/o	sclera	12
scoli/o	crooked, curved (spine)	14
seb/o	sebum (oil)	4
sept/o	septum	5
sial/o	saliva, salivary gland	11
sigmoid/o	sigmoid colon	11
sinus/o	sinus	5
somat/o	body	2
somn/o	sleep	5
son/o	sound	5
sperm/o	spermatozoon, sperm	7
spermat/o	spermatozoon, sperm	7
spir/o	breathe, breathing	5
splen/o	spleen	10
spondyl/o	vertebra, spine, vertebral column	14
staped/o	stapes (middle ear bone)	13
staphyl/o	grapelike clusters	4
steat/o	fat	11
stern/o	sternum (breastbone)	14
stomat/o	mouth	11
strept/o	twisted chains	4
super/o	above	3
synovi/o	synovia, synovial membrane	14
system/o	system	2
T		
tars/o	tarsals (ankle bones)	14
tendin/o	tendon	14
tend/o	tendon	14
ten/o	tendon	14
terat/o	malformations	9
test/o	testis, testicle	7
therm/o	heat	10
thorac/o	thorax, chest, chest cavity	5

COMBINING FORMS	DEFINITION	CHAPTER
thromb/o	clot	10
thym/o	thymus gland	10
thyroid/o	thyroid gland	16
thyr/o	thyroid gland	16
tibi/o	tibia (lower leg bone)	14
tom/o	to cut, section, or slice	5
ton/o	tension, pressure	12
tonsill/o	tonsil	5
trache/o	trachea	5
trich/o	hair	4
tympan/o	tympanic membrane (eardrum), middle ear	13
U		
uln/o	ulna (lower arm bone)	14
ungu/o	nail	4
ureter/o	ureter	6
urethr/o	urethra	6
ur/o	urine, urinary tract	6
urin/o	urine, urinary tract	6
uvul/o	uvula	11
V		
vagin/o	vagina	8
valv/o	valve	10
valvul/o	valve	10
vas/o	vessel, duct	7
ven/o	vein	10
ventricul/o	ventricle	10
ventr/o	belly (front)	3
vertebr/o	vertebra, spine, vertebral column	14
vesic/o	bladder, sac	6
vesicul/o	seminal vesicle	7
vestibul/o	vestibule	13
viscer/o	internal organs	2
vulv/o	vulva	8
X		
xanth/o	yellow	2
xer/o	dry	4

PREFIX	DEFINITION	CHAPTER
a-	absence of, without	5
an-	absence of, without	5
ante-	before	9
bi-	two	3, 12
bin-	two	12
brady-	slow	10
dia-	through, complete	2
dys-	painful, abnormal, difficult, labored	2
endo-	within	5
epi-	on, upon, over	4
eu-	normal, good	5
hemi-	half	11
hyper-	above, excessive	2
hypo-	below, incomplete, deficient, under	2
inter-	between	14
intra-	within	4
meta-	after, beyond, change	2

PREFIX	DEFINITION	CHAPTER
micro-	small	9
multi-	many	9
neo-	new	2
nulli-	none	9
pan-	all, total	10
para-	beside, beyond, around, abnormal	4
per-	through	4
peri-	surrounding (outer)	8
poly-	many, much	5
post-	after	9
pre-	before	9
pro-	before	2
sub-	under, below	4
supra-	above	14
sym-	together, joined	14
syn-	together, joined	14
tachy-	fast, rapid	5
trans-	through, across, beyond	4
uni-	one	3

SUFFIX	DEFINITION	CHAPTER
-a	no meaning	4
-ac	pertaining to	10
-ad	toward	3
-al	pertaining to	2
-algia	pain	5
-amnios	amnion, amniotic fluid	9
-apheresis	removal	10
-ar	pertaining to	5
-ary	pertaining to	5
-asthenia	weakness	14
-atresia	absence of a normal body opening; occlusion; closure	8
-cele	hernia or protrusion	5
-centesis	surgical puncture to aspirate fluid	5
-clasia	break	14
-clasis	break	14
-clast	break	14

SUFFIX	DEFINITION	CHAPTER
-coccus (pl. -cocci)	berry-shaped (form of bacterium)	4
-cyesis	pregnancy	9
-cyte	cell	2
-desis	surgical fixation, fusion	14
-drome	run, running	16
-e	no meaning	9
-eal	pertaining to	5
-ectasis	stretching out, dilation, expansion	5
-ectomy	excision or surgical removal	4
-emia	in the blood	5
-esis	condition	6
-gen	substance or agent that produces or causes	2
-genic	producing, originating, causing	2
-gram	record, radiographic image	5

SUFFIX	DEFINITION	CHAPTER	SUFFIX	DEFINITION	CHAPTER
-graph	instrument used to record; record	5	-physis	growth	14
-graphy	process of recording, radiographic imaging	5	-plasia	condition of formation, development, growth	2
-ia	diseased or abnormal state, condition of	4	-plasm	growth, substance, formation	2
-iasis	condition	6	-plasty	surgical repair	4
-iatrist	specialist, physician	15	-plegia	paralysis	12
-iatry	treatment, specialty	15	-pnea	breathing	5
-ic	pertaining to	2	-poiesis	formation	10
-ictal	seizure, attack	15	-ptosis	drooping, sagging, prolapse	6
-ior	pertaining to	3	-rrhagia	rapid flow of blood	5
-is	no meaning	9	-rrhaphy	suturing, repairing	6
-ism	state of	7	-rrhea	flow, discharge	4
-itis	inflammation	4	-rrhexis	rupture	9
-logist	one who studies and treats (specialist, physician)	2	-salpinx	uterine tube (fallopian tube)	8
-logy	study of	2	-sarcoma	malignant tumor	2
-lysis	loosening, dissolution, separating	6	-schisis	split, fissure	14
			-sclerosis	hardening	10
-malacia	softening	4	-scope	instrument used for visual examination	5
-megaly	enlargement	2			
-meter	instrument used to measure	5	-scopic	pertaining to visual examination	5
-metry	measurement	5	-scopy	visual examination	5
-oid	resembling	2	-sis	state of	2
-oma	tumor, swelling	2	-spasm	sudden, involuntary muscle contraction	5
-opia	vision (condition)	12			
-opsy	view of, viewing	4	-stasis	control, stop, standing	2
-osis	abnormal condition (means increase when used with blood cell word roots)	2	-stenosis	constriction or narrowing	5
			-stomy	creation of an artificial opening	5
-ous	pertaining to	2	-thorax	chest, chest cavity	5
-paresis	slight paralysis	15	-tocia	birth, labor	9
-pathy	disease	2	-tome	instrument used to cut	4
-penia	abnormal reduction (in number)	10	-tomy	cut into, incision	5
			-tripsy	surgical crushing	6
-pepsia	digestion	11	-trophy	nourishment, development	6
-pexy	surgical fixation, suspension	5	-um	no meaning	9
-phagia	eating or swallowing	4	-uria	urine, urination	6
-phobia	abnormal fear of or aversion to specific things	12	-us	no meaning	9

Combining Forms, Prefixes, and Suffixes Alphabetized According to Definition

DEFINITION	COMBINING FORM	CHAPTER
A		
abdomen, abdominal cavity	abdomin/o, lapar/o, celi/o	11
above	super/o	3
adenoids	adenoid/o	5
adrenal glands	adren/o, adrenal/o	16
albumin	albumin/o	6
alveolus	alveol/o	5
amnion, amniotic fluid	amni/o, amnion/o	9
antrum	antr/o	11
anus	an/o	11
aorta	aort/o	10
aponeurosis	aponeur/o	14
appendix	append/o, appendic/o	11
artery	arteri/o	10
atrium	atri/o	10
away (from the point of attachment of a body part)	dist/o	3
B		
back	dors/o	3
back, behind	poster/o	3
bear, give birth to, labor, childbirth	par/o, part/o	9
belly (front)	ventr/o	3
below	infer/o	3
bent forward (increased concavity of the spine)	lord/o	14
bile duct	cholangi/o	11
birth	nat/o	9
black	melan/o	2
bladder, sac	cyst/o, vesic/o	6
blood	hem/o, hemat/o	5
blue	cyan/o	2
body	somat/o	2
bone	oste/o	14
bone marrow	myel/o	10
brain	encephal/o	15

DEFINITION	COMBINING FORM	CHAPTER
breast	mamm/o, mast/o	8
breathe, breathing	spir/o	5
bronchus	bronch/o, bronchi/o	5
bursa (cavity)	burs/o	14
C		
calcium	calc/i	16
cancer	cancer/o, carcin/o	2
carbon dioxide	capn/o	5
carpals (wrist)	carp/o	14
cartilage	chondr/o	14
cause (of disease)	eti/o	2
cecum	cec/o	11
cell	cyt/o	2
cerebellum	cerebell/o	15
cerebrum, brain	cerebr/o	15
cervix	cervic/o	8
childbirth	puerper/o	9
chorion	chori/o	9
clavicle (collarbone)	clavic/o, clavicul/o	14
clot	thromb/o	10
cochlea	cochle/o	13
cold	cry/o	12
colon	col/o, colon/o	11
color	chrom/o	2
common bile duct	choledoch/o	11
conjunctiva	conjunctiv/o	12
cornea	corne/o, kerat/o	12
cortex	cortic/o	16
cranium (skull)	crani/o	14
crooked, curved	scoli/o	14
cul-de-sac	culd/o	8
D		
death (cells, body)	necr/o	4
deficiency, blockage	isch/o	10
developing cell, germ cell	blast/o	6
diaphragm	diaphragmat/o, phren/o	5
disease	path/o	2

DEFINITION	COMBINING FORM	CHAPTER	DEFINITION	COMBINING FORM	CHAPTER
diverticulum	diverticul/o	11	grapelike clusters	staphyl/o	4
dry	xer/o	4	gray matter	poli/o	15
duodenum	duoden/o	11	green	chlor/o	2
dust	coni/o	4	gum	gingiv/o	11
E			**H**		
ear	aur/i, aur/o, ot/o	13	hair	trich/o	4
electricity, electrical activity	electr/o	10	hard, dura mater	dur/o	15
			head	cephal/o	3, 9
embryo, to be full	embry/o	9	hearing	audi/o	13
endocrine	endocrin/o	16	heart	cardi/o	10
epididymis	epididym/o	7	heat	therm/o	10
epiglottis	epiglott/o	5	hernia	herni/o	11
epithelium	epitheli/o	2	hidden	crypt/o	4
equal	is/o	12	horny tissue, hard	kerat/o	4
esophagus	esophag/o	9, 11	humerus (upper arm bone)	humer/o	14
extremities, height	acr/o	16			
eye	ocul/o, ophthalm/o	12	hump (increased convexity of the spine)	kyph/o	14
eyelid	blephar/o	12			
F			hymen	hymen/o	8
false	pseud/o	9	**I**		
fat	lip/o	2	ileum	ile/o	11
fat	steat/o	11	ilium	ili/o	14
femur (upper leg bone)	femor/o	14	imperfect, incomplete	atel/o	5
fetus, unborn child	fet/o, fet/i	9	internal organs	viscer/o	2
fiber	fibr/o	2	intervertebral disk	disk/o	14
fibula (lower leg bone)	fibul/o	14	intestine	enter/o	11
			iris	ir/o, irid/o	12
first	prim/i	9	ischium	ischi/o	14
first, beginning	arche/o	8	**J**		
flesh, connective tissue	sarc/o	2	jejunum	jejun/o	11
			joint	arthr/o	14
four	quadr/i	15	**K**		
front	anter/o	3	kidney	nephr/o, ren/o	6
fungus	myc/o	3	knowledge	gno/o	2
G			**L**		
gall, bile	chol/e	11	labyrinth (inner ear)	labyrinth/o	13
ganglion	gangli/o, ganglion/o	15	lamina (thin, flat plate or layer)	lamin/o	14
gland	aden/o	2, 16			
glans penis	balan/o	7	larynx	laryng/o	5
glia, gluey substance	gli/o	15	lens	phac/o, phak/o	12
glomerulus	glomerul/o	6	life	bi/o	4

DEFINITION	COMBINING FORM	CHAPTER
light	phot/o	12
lip	cheil/o	11
liver	hepat/o	11
lobe	lob/o	5
loin, lumbar region of the spine	lumb/o	14
lung	pulmon/o	5
lung, air	pneum/o, pneumat/o, pneumon/o	5
lymph node	lymphaden/o	10
lymph, lymph tissue	lymph/o	10
M		
male	andr/o	7
malformations	terat/o	9
mandible (lower jawbone)	mandibul/o	14
mastoid bone	mastoid/o	13
maxilla (upper jawbone)	maxill/o	14
meatus (opening)	meat/o	6
meninges	mening/o, meningi/o	15
meniscus (crescent)	menisc/o	14
menstruation	men/o	8
middle	medi/o	3
milk	lact/o	9
mind	ment/o, psych/o	15
mouth	or/o, stomat/o	11
movement, motion	kinesi/o	14
mucus	muc/o	5
muscle	my/o	2, 14
muscle	myos/o	14
N		
nail	onych/o, ungu/o	4
near (the point of attachment of a body part)	proxim/o	3
nerve	neur/o	2, 15
nerve root	radic/o, radicul/o, rhiz/o	15
night	noct/i	6

DEFINITION	COMBINING FORM	CHAPTER
nose	naso, rhin/o	5
nucleus	kary/o	2
O		
one, single	mon/o	15
organ	organ/o	2
other	heter/o	4
ovary	oophor/o	8
oxygen	ox/i	5
P		
palate	palat/o	11
pancreas	pancreat/o	11
parathyroid glands	parathyroid/o	16
patella (kneecap)	patell/o	14
pelvis, pelvic bone	pelv/i, pelv/o	9, 14
perineum	perine/o	8
peritoneum	peritone/o	11
phalanges (any bone of the fingers or toes)	phalang/o	14
pharynx	pharyng/o	5
physician, medicine (also means treatment)	iatr/o	2
plasma	plasm/o	10
pleura	pleur/o	5
polyp, small growth	polyp/o	11
potassium	kal/i	16
pregnancy	gravid/o	9
prostate gland	prostat/o	7
pubis	pub/o	14
pupil	core/o, cor/o, pupill/o	12
pus	py/o	5
pylorus (pyloric sphincter)	pylor/o	9, 11
R		
radius (lower arm bone)	radi/o	14
rectum	proct/o, rect/o	11
red	erythr/o	2
renal pelvis	pyel/o	6
retina	retin/o	12

DEFINITION	COMBINING FORM	CHAPTER	DEFINITION	COMBINING FORM	CHAPTER
rib	cost/o	14	**T**		
rod-shaped, striated	rhabd/o	2	tail (downward)	caud/o	3
S			tarsals (ankle bones)	tars/o	14
sacrum	sacr/o	14	tear, tear duct	dacry/o, lacrim/o	12
saliva, salivary gland	sial/o	11	tendon	ten/o, tend/o, tendin/o	14
scanty, few	olig/o	6	tension, pressure	ton/o	12
scapula (shoulder blade)	scapul/o	14	testis, testicle	orch/o, orchi/o, orchid/o, test/o	7
sclera	scler/o	12	thick	pachy/o	4
sebum (oil)	seb/o	4	thirst	dips/o	16
self	aut/o	4	thorax, chest, chest cavity	thorac/o	5
seminal vesicle	vesicul/o	7	thymus gland	thym/o	10
sensation, sensitivity, feeling	esthesi/o	14	thyroid gland	thyr/o, thyroid/o	16
septum	sept/o	5	tibia (lower leg bone)	tibi/o	14
side	later/o	3	tissue	hist/o	2
sigmoid colon	sigmoid/o	11	to cut, section, or slice	tom/o	5
sinus	sinus/o	5	tongue	gloss/o, lingu/o	11
skin	cutane/o, derm/o, dermat/o	4	tonsil	tonsill/o	5
sleep	somn/o	5	trachea	trache/o	5
smooth	lei/o	2	tumor, mass	onc/o	2
sound	son/o	5	tympanic membrane (eardrum)	myring/o	13
sound	ech/o	10	tympanic membrane (eardrum), middle ear	tympan/o	13
speech	phas/o	15	twisted chains	strept/o	4
spermatozoon, sperm	sperm/o, spermat/o	7	two, double	dipl/o	12
spinal column	rachi/o	14	**U**		
spinal cord	myel/o	15	ulna (lower arm bone)	uln/o	14
spleen	splen/o	10	umbilicus, navel	omphal/o	9
stapes (middle ear bone)	staped/o	13	urea, nitrogen	azot/o	6
stiff, bent	ankyl/o	14	ureter	ureter/o	6
sternum (breast bone)	stern/o	14	urethra	urethr/o	6
stomach	gastr/o	11	urine, urinary tract	ur/o, urin/o	6
stone	petr/o	14	uterine tube (fallopian tube)	salping/o	8
stone, calculus	lith/o	6	uterus	hyster/o, metr/o, metr/i	8
straight	orth/o	5	uvula	uvul/o	11
sugar	glyc/o, glycos/o	6			
sweat	hidr/o	4			
synovia, synovial membrane	synovi/o	14			
system	system/o	2			

DEFINITION	COMBINING FORM	CHAPTER
V		
vagina	colp/o, vagin/o	8
valve	valv/o, valvul/o	10
vein	phleb/o, ven/o	10
ventricle	ventricul/o	10
vertebra, spine, vertebral column	rachi/o, spondyl/o, vertebr/o	14
vessel (usually refers to blood vessel)	angi/o	10
vessel, duct	vas/o	7
vestibule	vestibul/o	13
vision	opt/o	12
vulva	episi/o, vulv/o	8
W		
water	hydr/o	6
white	leuk/o	2
woman	gyn/o, gynec/o	8
wrinkles	rhytid/o	4
X		
x-rays, ionizing radiation	radi/o	5
Y		
yellow	xanth/o	2
yellowish, fatty plaque	ather/o	10

DEFINITION	PREFIX	CHAPTER
absence of, without	a-, an-	5
above	supra-	14
above, excessive	hyper-	2
after	post-	9
after, beyond, change	meta-	2
all, total	pan-	10
before	ante-, pre-	9
before	pro-	2
below, incomplete, deficient, under	hypo-	2
beside, beyond, around, abnormal	para-	4
between	inter-	14
fast, rapid	tachy-	10
half	hemi-	11
many	multi-	9

DEFINITION	COMBINING FORM	CHAPTER
many, much	poly-	5
new	neo-	2
none	nulli-	9
normal, good	eu-	5
on, upon, over	epi-	4
one	uni-	3
painful, abnormal, difficult, labored	dys-	2
slow	brady-	10
small	micro-	9
surrounding (outer)	peri-	8
through	per-	4
through, across, beyond	trans-	4
through, complete	dia-	2
together, joined	syn-, sym-	14
two	bin-	12
two	bi-	3, 12
under, below	sub-	4
within	intra-	4
within	endo-	5

DEFINITION	SUFFIX	CHAPTER
abnormal condition (means increase when used with blood cell word roots)	-osis	2
abnormal fear of or aversion to specific things	-phobia	12
abnormal reduction (in number)	-penia	10
absence of a normal opening; occlusion; closure	-atresia	8
amnion, amniotic fluid	-amnios	9
berry-shaped (form of bacterium)	-coccus (*pl.* -cocci)	4
birth, labor	-tocia	9
break	-clasia, -clasis, -clast	14
breathing	-pnea	5
cell	-cyte	2
chest, chest cavity	-thorax	5
condition	-esis, -iasis	6

DEFINITION	COMBINING FORM	CHAPTER	DEFINITION	COMBINING FORM	CHAPTER
condition of formation, development, growth	-plasia	2	one who studies and treats (specialist, physician)	-logist	2
constriction or narrowing	-stenosis	5	pain	-algia	5
control, stop, standing	-stasis	2	paralysis	-plegia	12
creation of an artificial opening	-stomy	5	pertaining to	-ac	10
cut into, incision	-tomy	5	pertaining to	-ous	2, 6
digestion	-pepsia	11	pertaining to	-ar, -ary, -eal	5
disease	-pathy	2	pertaining to	-al, -ic	2
diseased or abnormal state, condition of	-ia	4	pertaining to	-ior	3
drooping, sagging, prolapse	-ptosis	6	pertaining to visual examination	-scopic	5
eating or swallowing	-phagia	4	pregnancy	-cyesis	9
enlargement	-megaly	2	process of recording, radiographic imaging	-graphy	5
excision or surgical removal	-ectomy	4	producing, originating, causing	-genic	2
flow, discharge	-rrhea	4	rapid flow of blood	-rrhagia	5
formation	-poiesis	10	record, radiographic image	-gram	5
growth	-physis	14	removal	-apheresis	10
growth, substance, formation	-plasm	2	resembling	-oid	2
hardening	-sclerosis	10	run, running	-drome	16
hernia or protrusion	-cele	5	rupture	-rrhexis	9
in the blood	-emia	5	seizure, attack	-ictal	15
inflammation	-itis	4	slight paralysis	-paresis	15
instrument used for visual examination	-scope	5	softening	-malacia	4
instrument used to measure	-meter	5	specialist, physician	-iatrist	15
instrument used to cut	-tome	4	split, fissure	-schisis	14
instrument used to record; record	-graph	5	state of	-ism	7
loosening, dissolution, separating	-lysis	6	state of	-sis	2
malignant tumor	-sarcoma	2	stretching out, dilation, expansion	-ectasis	5
measurement	-metry	5	study of	-logy	2
no meaning	-e	9	substance or agent that produces or causes	-gen	2
nourishment, development	-trophy	6	sudden, involuntary muscle contraction	-spasm	5
			surgical crushing	-tripsy	6
			surgical fixation, fusion	-desis	14

DEFINITION	COMBINING FORM	CHAPTER	DEFINITION	COMBINING FORM	CHAPTER
surgical fixation, suspension	-pexy	5	tumor, swelling	-oma	2
			urine, urination	-uria	6
surgical puncture to aspirate fluid	-centesis	5	uterine tube (fallopian tube)	-salpinx	8
surgical repair	-plasty	4	view of, viewing	-opsy	4
suturing, repairing	-rrhaphy	6	vision (condition)	-opia	12
toward	-ad	3	visual examination	-scopy	5
treatment, specialty	-iatry	15	weakness	-asthenia	14

Topics include:
Common Medical Abbreviations, p. 749
Institute for Safe Medication Practices' (List of Error-Prone Abbreviations, Symbols and Dose Designations, includes The Joint Commission's "do not use" list), p. 756

Abbreviations are written as they appear most commonly in the medical and health care environment. Some may also appear in both capital and small letters and with or without periods.

COMMON MEDICAL ABBREVIATIONS	DEFINITIONS	COMMON MEDICAL ABBREVIATIONS	DEFINITIONS
AB	abortion	AMI	acute myocardial infarction
ABD	abdomen	AML	acute myeloid leukemia
ABE	acute bacterial endocarditis	AMP	ampule
ABGs	arterial blood gases	amt	amount
a.c.	before meals	angio	angiogram, angiography
ACS	acute coronary syndrome	A&O	alert and oriented
ACTH	adrenocorticotropic hormone	ant	anterior
AD	Alzheimer disease	AODM	adult-onset diabetes mellitus
ADH	antidiuretic hormone	AOM	acute otitis media
ADHD	attention deficit hyperactivity disorder	AP	anteroposterior; angina pectoris
ADL	activities of daily living	A&P	auscultation and percussion; anterior and posterior colporrhaphy
ad lib	as desired		
Adm	admission	ARDS	adult respiratory distress syndrome
AFB	acid-fast bacilli	A&P repair	anterior and posterior colporrhaphy
AFib	atrial fibrillation		
AHD	arteriosclerotic heart disease	A&P resection	abdominoperineal resection
AI	aortic insufficiency	ARF	acute renal failure
AICD	automatic implantable cardioverter-defibrillator	ARM	artificial rupture of membranes
AIDS	acquired immunodeficiency syndrome	ARMD	age-related macular degeneration
		ART	assisted reproductive technology
AKA	above-knee amputation	ASA	aspirin (acetylsalicylic acid)
alk phos	alkaline phosphatase	ASCVD	arteriosclerotic cardiovascular disease
ALL	acute lymphoblastic leukemia		
ALS	amyotrophic lateral sclerosis	ASD	atrial septal defect
ALT	alanine aminotransferase	ASHD	arteriosclerotic heart disease
AM	between midnight and noon (or a.m.)	Ast	astigmatism
		as tol	as tolerated
AMA	against medical advice; American Medical Association	AUL	acute undifferentiated leukemia
		AV	atrioventricular, arteriovenous
AMB	ambulate, ambulatory	AVR	aortic valve replacement

COMMON MEDICAL ABBREVIATIONS	DEFINITIONS
ax	axillary
BA	bronchial asthma
BBB	bundle branch block
BC	birth control
BCC	basal cell carcinoma
BE	barium enema
b.i.d.	twice a day
BK	below knee
BKA	below-knee amputation
BM	bowel movement
BOM	bilateral otitis media
BP	blood pressure
BPH	benign prostatic hyperplasia
BR	bedrest
BRP	bathroom privileges
BS	blood sugar; bowel sounds; breath sounds
BSO	bilateral salpingo-oophorectomy
BUN	blood urea nitrogen
Bx or bx	biopsy
c̄	with
C	Celsius
C_1-C_7	cervical vertebrae
Ca	calcium
CA	cancer; carcinoma
CABG	coronary artery bypass graft
CAD	coronary artery disease
CAL	calorie
CA-MRSA	community-associated MRSA infection
CAP	capsule
CAPD	continuous ambulatory peritoneal dialysis
cath	catheterization, catheter
CBC and Diff	complete blood count and differential count
CBR	complete bed rest
CBS	chronic brain syndrome
CC	chief complaint or colony count
CCU	coronary care unit
CDH	congenital dislocation of the hip

COMMON MEDICAL ABBREVIATIONS	DEFINITIONS
CEA	carcinoembryonic antigen
CF	cystic fibrosis
CHB	complete heart block
CHD	coronary heart disease
CHF	congestive heart failure
CHO	carbohydrate
chemo	chemotherapy
chol	cholesterol
CI	coronary insufficiency
circ	circumcision
CIS	carcinoma in situ
Cl	chloride
CKD	chronic kidney disease
CLD	chronic liver disease
CLL	chronic lymphocytic leukemia
cl liq	clear liquid
cm	centimeter
CML	chronic myelogenous leukemia
CNS	central nervous system
c/o	complains of
CO	carbon monoxide
CO_2	carbon dioxide
COB	coordination of benefits
COLD	chronic obstructive lung disease
comp	compound
cond	condition
COPD	chronic obstructive pulmonary disease
CP	cerebral palsy
CPAP	continuous positive airway pressure
CPD	cephalopelvic disproportion
CPK	creatine phosphokinase
CPN	chronic pyelonephritis
CPR	cardiopulmonary resuscitation
CRD	chronic respiratory disease
creat	creatinine
CRF	chronic renal failure
crit	hematocrit (also HCT, Hct)
CRP	C-reactive protein
C&S	culture and sensitivity

COMMON MEDICAL ABBREVIATIONS	DEFINITIONS
C/S, CS, C-section	cesarean section
CSF	cerebrospinal fluid
CT	computed tomography
CTS	carpal tunnel syndrome
Cu	copper
CVA	cerebrovascular accident
CVP	central venous pressure
Cx	cervix
CXR	chest radiograph (x-ray)
DAT	diet as tolerated
D&C	dilation and curettage
DCIS	ductal carcinoma in situ
decub	pressure ulcer
del	delivery
derm	dermatology
DI	diabetes insipidus
DIC	diffuse intravascular coagulation
diff	differential (part of complete blood count)
disch	discharge
DISH	diffuse idiopathic skeletal hyperostosis
DLE	discoid lupus erythematosus
DM	diabetes mellitus
DNA	deoxyribonucleic acid
DND	died natural death
DO	Doctor of Osteopathy
DOA	dead on arrival
DOB	date of birth
DOD	date of death
Dr	dram
DRE	digital rectal examination
DRG	diagnosis-related group
DSA	digital subtraction angiography
DVT	deep vein thrombosis
DW	distilled water
D/W	dextrose in water
Dx	diagnosis
E	enema
EBL	estimated blood loss
ECG	electrocardiogram

COMMON MEDICAL ABBREVIATIONS	DEFINITIONS
ECHO	echocardiogram
ECT	electroconvulsive therapy
ED	erectile dysfunction, emergency department
EDD	expected (estimated) date of delivery
EEG	electroencephalogram
EENT	eyes, ears, nose, and throat
EGD	esophagogastroduodenoscopy
EKG	electrocardiogram
Elix	elixir
Em	emmetropia
EMG	electromyogram
ENG	electronystagmography
ENT	ears, nose, throat
EP	ectopic pregnancy
EP studies	evoked potential studies
ERCP	endoscopic retrograde cholangiopancreatography
ERT	estrogen replacement therapy
ESR	erythrocyte sedimentation rate
ESRD	end-stage renal disease
ESWL	extracorporeal shock wave lithotripsy
etio	etiology
EUS	endoscopic ultrasound
exam	examination
ext	extract; external
F	Fahrenheit
FAS	fetal alcohol syndrome
FBD	fibrocystic breast disease
FBS	fasting blood sugar
FCC	fibrocystic breast condition
Fe	iron
FHT	fetal heart tones
flu	influenza
FOBT	fecal occult blood test
Fr	French (catheter size)
FS	frozen section
FSH	follicle-stimulating hormone
FTT	failure to thrive
FUO	fever of undetermined origin

COMMON MEDICAL ABBREVIATIONS	DEFINITIONS
fx	fracture
g	gram
GC	gonorrhea
GERD	gastroesophageal reflux disease
GH	growth hormone
GI	gastrointestinal
GSW	gunshot wound
gtt	drops
GTT	glucose tolerance test
GU	genitourinary
GYN	gynecology
h	hour
H	hypodermic
HAART	highly active antiretroviral therapy
HA-MRSA	healthcare associated MRSA infection
HB	heart block
HbA1C	glycosylated hemoglobin
HCVD	hypertensive cardiovascular disease
HD	hemodialysis
HHD	hypertensive heart disease
H&H	hemoglobin and hematocrit
HCl	hydrochloric acid
HCO$_3$	bicarbonate
Hct	hematocrit
HD	hemodialysis
HF	heart failure
Hg	mercury
Hgb	hemoglobin
HIV	human immunodeficiency virus
HMD	hyaline membrane disease
HME	Heat/moisture exchanger
HNP	herniated nucleus pulposus
H$_2$O	water
H$_2$O$_2$	hydrogen peroxide (hydrogen dioxide)
HOB	head of bed
H&P	history and physical examination
H. pylori	*Helicobacter pylori*
HPV	human papillomavirus

COMMON MEDICAL ABBREVIATIONS	DEFINITIONS
HRT	hormone replacement therapy
ht	height
HTN	hypertension
Hx	history
hypo	hypodermic
IBS	irritable bowel syndrome
ICD	implantable cardiac defibrillator
ICU	intensive care unit
ID	intradermal
IDDM	insulin-dependent diabetes mellitus
I&D	incision and drainage
IHD	ischemic heart disease
IM	intramuscular
inf	inferior
INR	international normalized ratio
I&O	intake and output
IOL	intraocular lens
IOP	intraocular pressure
IPF	idiopathic pulmonary fibrosis
IPG	impedance plethysmography
IPPB	intermittent positive pressure breathing
IR	interventional radiology
irrig	irrigation
isol	isolation
IUD	intrauterine device
IV	intravenous
IVC	intravenous cholangiogram
IVF	in vitro fertilization
IVP	intravenous pyelogram
IVU	intravenous urogram
K	potassium
KCl	potassium chloride
kg	kilogram
KO	keep open
KUB	kidney, ureter, bladder (radiograph)
KVO	keep vein open
L	liter
L$_1$-L$_5$	lumbar vertebrae
lab	laboratory

COMMON MEDICAL ABBREVIATIONS	DEFINITIONS
LAC	laceration
LAD	left anterior descending (coronary artery)
LAP	laparotomy
lat	lateral
LAVH	laparoscopically-assisted vaginal hysterectomy
L&D	labor and delivery
LDH	lactic dehydrogenase
LE	lupus erythematosus
lg	large
LH	luteinizing hormone
LLL	left lower lobe
LLQ	left lower quadrant
LMP	last menstrual period
LOC	loss of consciousness, level of consciousness
LP	lumbar puncture
LPN	licensed practical nurse
LR	lactated Ringer (IV solution)
lt	left
LTB	laryngotracheobronchitis
LUL	left upper lobe
LUQ	left upper quadrant
mcg	microgram
MCH	mean corpuscular hemoglobin
MCV	mean corpuscular volume
MD	muscular dystrophy
med	medial
mEq	milliequivalent
mets	metastases
mg	milligram
MG	myasthenia gravis
MI	myocardial infarction
mL	milliliter
mm	millimeter
MM	multiple myeloma
MOM	milk of magnesia
MR	mitral regurgitation
MRI	magnetic resonance imaging
MRCP	magnetic resonance cholangiopancreatography

COMMON MEDICAL ABBREVIATIONS	DEFINITIONS
MRSA	methicillin-resistant *Staphylococcus aureus*
MS	multiple sclerosis
multip	multipara
MVP	mitral valve prolapse
Na	sodium
NaCl	sodium chloride (salt)
NAS	no added salt
NB	newborn
neg	negative
neuro	neurology
NG	nasogastric
NICU	neonatal intensive care unit
NIDDM	non-insulin-dependent diabetes mellitus
NIVA	noninvasive vascular assessment
noc	night
noct	night
NPO	nothing by mouth
NPPV	noninvasive positive-pressure ventilator
NS	normal saline
NSAID	nonsteroidal antiinflammatory drug
NSR	normal sinus rhythm
N&V	nausea and vomiting
NVS	neurologic signs
OA	osteoarthritis
O_2	oxygen
OAB	overactive bladder
OB	obstetrics
OCD	obsessive-compulsive disorder
OD	overdose
oint	ointment
OM	otitis media
OOB	out of bed
OP	outpatient
Ophth	ophthalmic or ophthalmology
OR	operating room
Ortho or ortho	orthopedics
OSA	obstructive sleep apnea

COMMON MEDICAL ABBREVIATIONS	DEFINITIONS
OT	occupational therapy
OTC	over-the-counter drugs
oto	otology
oz	ounce
p̄	after
P	phosphorus
P	pulse
PA	physician's assistant or posteroanterior
PAC	premature atrial complex
PAD	peripheral arterial disease
PAT	paroxysmal atrial tachycardia
pc	after meals
PCI	percutaneous coronany intervention
PCU	progressive care unit
PCV	packed cell volume
PD	Parkinson disease
PDA	patent ductus arteriosus
PDR	*Physicians' Desk Reference*
PE	pulmonary embolism
Peds	pediatrics
PEEP	positive end expiratory pressure
PEG	percutaneous endoscopic gastrostomy
per	by
PERRLA	pupils equal, round, reactive to light and accommodation
PET	positron emission tomography
PFM	peak flow meter
PFTs	pulmonary function tests
PHACO	phacoemulsification
PICC	peripherally inserted central catheter
PICU	pediatric intensive care unit
PID	pelvic inflammatory disease
PKU	phenylketonuria
PM	between noon and midnight
PMS	premenstrual syndrome
PNS	peripheral nervous system
po	orally; postoperative; phone order
post-op	postoperatively

COMMON MEDICAL ABBREVIATIONS	DEFINITIONS
PP	postpartum or postprandial (after meals)
PPD	purified protein derivative
pr	per rectum
PRBC	packed red blood cells
pre-op	preoperatively
PRH	prolactin-releasing hormone
primip	primipara
PRN	as needed
PSA	prostate-specific antigen
PSG	polysomnography
pt	patient; pint
PT	physical therapy
PT	prothrombin time
PTCA	percutaneous transluminal coronary angioplasty
PT/INR	prothrombin time/international normalized ratio
PTSD	posttraumatic stress disorder
PTT	partial thromboplastin time
PUL	percutaneous ultrasound lithotripsy
PVC	premature ventricular complex
PVD	peripheral vascular disease
Px	prognosis
q	every
q_h	every (number) hour (e.g., q2h)
qt	quart
R	rectal
RA	rheumatoid arthritis
RAD	reactive airway disease
RAIU	radioactive iodine uptake
RBC	red blood cell
RDS	respiratory distress syndrome
reg	regular
REM	rapid eye movement
resp	respirations
RHD	rheumatic heart disease
RLL	right lower lobe
RLQ	right lower quadrant
RML	right middle lobe

COMMON MEDICAL ABBREVIATIONS	DEFINITIONS
RN	registered nurse
R/O	rule out
ROM	range of motion
ROM	rupture of membranes
RP	radical prostatectomy
RR	recovery room
rt	right; routine
RT	respiratory therapy
RUL	right upper lobe
RUQ	right upper quadrant
Rx	prescription
$\bar{s}$	without
SAB	spontaneous abortion
SAH	subarachnoid hemorrhage
SARS	severe acute respiratory syndrome
SBE	subacute bacterial endocarditis; self-breast examination
SHG	sonohysterography
SG	specific gravity
SI	sacroiliac
SICU	surgical intensive care unit
SIDS	sudden infant death syndrome
SLE	systemic lupus erythematosus
SMAC	Sequential Multiple Analyzer Computer
SMR	submucous resection
SNF	skilled nursing facility
SOB	shortness of breath
SPECT	single-photon emission computed tomography
SqCCA	squamous cell carcinoma
SSE	soapsuds enema
STAPH or staph	staphylococcus
stat	immediately
STD	sexually transmitted disease
STREP or strep	streptococcus
subcut	subcutaneous
subling	sublingual
sup	superior
supp	suppository

COMMON MEDICAL ABBREVIATIONS	DEFINITIONS
surg	surgical
SVD	spontaneous vaginal delivery
SVN	small-volume nebulizer
SWL	shock wave lithotripsy
T_1-T_{12}	thoracic vertebrae
T_4	thyroxine
tab	tablet
TAB	therapeutic abortion
T&A	tonsillectomy and adenoidectomy
TAH	total abdominal hysterectomy
TAH/BSO	total abdominal hysterectomy/bilateral salpingo-oophorectomy
TAT	tetanus antitoxin
TB	tuberculosis
TCDB	turn, cough, deep breathe
TCT	thrombin clotting time
TD	transdermal
TEE	transesophageal echocardiogram
temp	temperature
TENS	transcutaneous electrical nerve stimulation
THA	total hip arthroplasty
THR	total hip replacement
TIA	transient ischemic attack
tid	three times per day
tinct	tincture
TKA	total knee arthroplasty
TPN	total parenteral nutrition
tr	tincture
trach	tracheostomy
TRUS	transrectal ultrasound
TSH	thyroid-stimulating hormone
TSS	toxic shock syndrome
TUIP	transurethral incision of the prostate
TULIP	transurethral laser incision of the prostate
TUMT	transurethral microwave thermotherapy
TURP	transurethral resection of the prostate

COMMON MEDICAL ABBREVIATIONS	DEFINITIONS
TVH	total vaginal hysterectomy
TVS	transvaginal sonography
TWE	tap water enema
Tx	treatment
UA	urinalysis
UAE	uterine artery embolization
UGI	upper gastrointestinal
UGI-SBFT	upper gastrointestinal [series] with small bowel follow through [radiograph]
ung	ointment
UPPP	uvulopalatopharyngoplasty
URI	upper respiratory infection
US	ultrasound
UTI	urinary tract infection
UV	ultraviolet
UVR	ultraviolet radiation
VA	visual acuity
vag	vaginal

COMMON MEDICAL ABBREVIATIONS	DEFINITIONS
VATS	video-assisted thoracic surgery
VBAC	vaginal birth after cesarean section
VCUG	voiding cystourethrogram
VD	venereal disease
VDRL	Venereal Disease Research Laboratory
vent	ventilator
VFib	ventricular fibrillation
VLAP	visual laser ablation of the prostate
VPS	ventilation-perfusion scanning
VS	vital signs
WA	while awake
WBC	white blood cell
W/C	wheelchair
wt	weight
XRT	radiation therapy, x-ray radiotherapy, x-ray therapy

Institute for Safe Medication Practices' List of Error-Prone Abbreviations, Symbols, and Dose Designations

The abbreviations, symbols, and dose designations found in this table have been reported to ISMP through the ISMP Medication Errors Reporting Program (ISMP MERP) as being frequently misinterpreted and involved in harmful medication errors. They should **NEVER** be used when communicating medical information. This includes internal communications, telephone/verbal prescriptions, computer-generated labels, labels for drug storage bins, medication administration records, as well as pharmacy and prescriber computer order entry screens.

The Joint Commission (formerly the Joint Commission on Accreditation of Healthcare Organizations [JCAHO]) has established a National Patient Safety Goal **that specifies that certain abbreviations must appear on an accredited organization's "do not use" list; we have highlighted these items with a double asterisk (**).** However, we hope that you will consider others beyond the minimum requirements. By using and promoting safe practices and by educating one another about hazards, we can better protect our patients.

ABBREVIATIONS	INTENDED MEANING	MISINTERPRETATION	CORRECTION
μg	Microgram	Mistaken as "mg"	Use "mcg"
AD, AS, AU	Right ear, left ear, each ear	Mistaken as OD, OS, OU (right eye, left eye, each eye)	Use "right ear," "left ear," or "each ear"
OD, OS, OU	Right eye, left eye, each eye	Mistaken as AD, AS, AU (right ear, left ear, each ear)	Use "right eye," "left eye," or "each eye"
BT	Bedtime	Mistaken as "BID" (twice daily)	Use "bedtime"
cc	Cubic centimeters	Mistaken as "u" (units)	Use "mL"

ABBREVIATIONS	INTENDED MEANING	MISINTERPRETATION	CORRECTION
D/C	Discharge or discontinue	Premature discontinuation of medications if D/C (intended to mean "discharge") has been misinterpreted as "discontinued" when followed by a list of discharge medications	Use "discharge" and "discontinue"
IJ	Injection	Mistaken as "IV" or "intrajugular"	Use "injection"
IN	Intranasal	Mistaken as "IM" or "IV"	Use "intranasal" or "NAS"
HS hs	Half strength At bedtime, hours of sleep	Mistaken as bedtime Mistaken as half strength	Use "half strength" or "bedtime"
IU**	International unit	Mistaken as IV (intravenous) or 10 (ten)	Use "units"
o.d. or OD	Once daily	Mistaken as "right eye" (OD-oculus dexter), leading to oral liquid medications administered in the eye	Use "daily"
OJ	Orange juice	Mistaken as OD or OS (right or left eye); drugs meant to be diluted in orange juice may be given in the eye	Use "orange juice"
Per os	By mouth, orally	The "os" can be mistaken as "left eye" (OS-oculus sinister)	Use "PO," "by mouth," or "orally"
q.d. or QD**	Every day	Mistaken as q.i.d., especially if the period after the "q" or the tail of the "q" is misunderstood as an "i"	Use "daily"
qhs	Nightly at bedtime	Mistaken as "qhr" or every hour	Use "nightly"
qn	Nightly or at bedtime	Mistaken as "qh" (every hour)	Use "nightly" or "at bedtime"
q.o.d. or QOD**	Every other day	Mistaken as "q.d." (daily) or "q.i.d." (four times daily) if the "o" is poorly written	Use "every other day"
q1d	Daily	Mistaken as q.i.d. (four times daily)	Use "daily"
q6PM, etc.	Every evening at 6 PM	Mistaken as every 6 hours	Use "daily at 6 PM" or "6 PM daily"
SC, SQ, sub q	Subcutaneous	SC mistaken as SL (sublingual); SQ mistaken as "5 every;" the "q" in "sub q" has been mistaken as "every" (e.g., a heparin dose ordered "sub q 2 hours before surgery" misunderstood as every 2 hours before surgery)	Use "subcut" or "subcutaneously"

ABBREVIATIONS	INTENDED MEANING	MISINTERPRETATION	CORRECTION
ss	Sliding scale (insulin) or ½ (apothecary)	Mistaken as "55"	Spell out "sliding scale;" use "one half" or "½"
SSRI **SSI**	Sliding scale regular insulin Sliding scale insulin	Mistaken as selective serotonin reuptake inhibitor Mistaken as Strong Solution of Iodine (Lugol's)	Spell out "sliding scale (insulin)"
i/d	Once daily	Mistaken as "tid"	Use "1 daily"
TIW or tiw	3 times a week	Mistaken as "3 times a day" or "twice in a week"	Use "3 times weekly"
U or u**	Unit	Mistaken as the number 0 or 4, causing a tenfold overdose or greater (e.g., 4U seen as "40" or 4u seen as "44"); mistaken as "cc" so dose given in volume instead of units (e.g., 4u seen as 4cc)	Use "unit"
DOSE DESIGNATIONS AND OTHER INFORMATION	**INTENDED MEANING**	**MISINTERPRETATION**	**CORRECTION**
Trailing zero after decimal point (e.g., 1.0 mg)**	1 mg	Mistaken as 10 mg if the decimal point is not seen	Do not use trailing zeros for doses expressed in whole numbers
"Naked" decimal point (e.g., .5 mg)**	0.5 mg	Mistaken as 5 mg if the decimal point is not seen	Use zero before a decimal point when the dose is less than a whole unit
Drug name and dose run together (especially problematic for drug names that end in "l" such as Inderal 40 mg; Tegretol 300 mg)	Inderal 40 mg Tegretol 300 mg	Mistaken as Inderal 140 mg Mistaken as Tegretol 1300 mg	Place adequate space between the drug name, dose, and unit of measure
Numerical dose and unit of measure run together (e.g., 10 mg, 100 mL)	10 mg 100 mL	The "m" is sometimes mistaken as a zero or two zeros, risking a 10- to 100-fold overdose	Place adequate space between the dose and unit of measure
Abbreviations such as mg. or mL. with a period following the abbreviation	mg mL	The period is unnecessary and could be mistaken as the number 1 if written poorly	Use mg, mL, etc., without a terminal period
Large doses without properly placed commas (e.g., 100000 units; 1000000 units)	100,000 units 1,000,000 units	100000 has been mistaken as 10,000 or 1,000,000; 1000000 has been mistaken as 100,000	Use commas for dosing units at or above 1,000, or use words such as 100 "thousand" or 1 "million" to improve readability

ABBREVIATIONS	INTENDED MEANING	MISINTERPRETATION	CORRECTION
DRUG NAME ABBREVIATIONS	*INTENDED MEANING*	*MISINTERPRETATION*	*CORRECTION*

To avoid confusion, do not abbreviate drug names when communicating medical information. Examples of drug name abbreviations involved in medication errors include:

APAP	acetaminophen	Not recognized as acetaminophen	Use complete drug name
ARA A	vidarabine	Mistaken as cytarabine (ARA C)	Use complete drug name
AZT	zidovudine (Retrovir)	Mistaken as azathioprine or aztreonam	Use complete drug name
CPZ	Compazine (prochlorperazine)	Mistaken as chlorpromazine	Use complete drug name
DPT	Demerol-Phenergan-Thorazine	Mistaken as diphtheria-pertussis-tetanus (vaccine)	Use complete drug name
DTO	Diluted tincture of opium, or deodorized tincture of opium (Paregoric)	Mistaken as tincture of opium	Use complete drug name
HCl	hydrochloric acid or hydrochloride	Mistaken as potassium chloride (the "H" is misinterpreted as "K")	Use complete drug name unless expressed as a salt of a drug
HCT	hydrocortisone	Mistaken as hydrochlorothiazide	Use complete drug name
HCTZ	hydrochlorothiazide	Mistaken as hydrocortisone (seen as HCT250mg)	Use complete drug name
DRUG NAME ABBREVIATIONS	*INTENDED MEANING*	*MISINTERPRETATION*	*CORRECTION*
MgSO₄**	magnesium sulfate	Mistaken as morphine sulfate	Use complete drug name
MS, MSO₄**	morphine sulfate	Mistaken as magnesium sulfate	Use complete drug name
MTX	methotrexate	Mistaken as mitoxantrone	Use complete drug name
PCA	procainamide	Mistaken as patient controlled analgesia	Use complete drug name
PTU	propylthiouracil	Mistaken as mercaptopurine	Use complete drug name
T3	Tylenol with codeine No. 3	Mistaken as liothyronine	Use complete drug name
TAC	triamcinolone	Mistaken as tetracaine, Adrenalin, cocaine	Use complete drug name
TNK	TNKase	Mistaken as "TPA"	Use complete drug name
ZnSO₄	zinc sulfate	Mistaken as morphine sulfate	Use complete drug name
STEMMED DRUG NAMES	*INTENDED MEANING*	*MISINTERPRETATION*	*CORRECTION*
"Nitro" drip	nitroglycerin infusion	Mistaken as sodium nitroprusside infusion	Use complete drug name
"Norflox"	norfloxacin	Mistaken as Norflex	Use complete drug name

ABBREVIATIONS	INTENDED MEANING	MISINTERPRETATION	CORRECTION
"IV Vanc"	intravenous vancomycin	Mistaken as Invanz	Use complete drug name
SYMBOLS	**INTENDED MEANING**	**MISINTERPRETATION**	**CORRECTION**
℥	Dram	Symbol for dram mistaken as "3"	Use metric system
℈ ♏	Minim	Symbol for minim mistaken as "mL"	
x3d	For three days	Mistaken as "3 doses"	Use "for three days"
> and <	Greater than and less than	Mistaken as opposite of intended; mistakenly use incorrect symbol; "< 10" mistaken as "40"	Use "greater than" or "less than"
/ (slash mark)	Separates two doses or indicates "per"	Mistaken as the number 1 (e.g., "25 units/10 units" misread as "25 units and 110" units)	Use "per" rather than a slash mark to separate doses
@	At	Mistaken as "2"	Use "at"
&	And	Mistaken as "2"	Use "and"
+	Plus or and	Mistaken as "4"	Use "and
°	Hour	Mistaken as a zero (e.g., q2° seen as q 20)	Use "hr," "h," or "hour"
Φ or ○	zero, null sign	Mistaken as numerals 4, 6, 8, and 9	Use 0 or zero, or describe intent using whole words

**These abbreviations are included on the Joint Commission's "minimum list" of dangerous abbreviations, acronyms, and symbols that must be included on an organization's "Do Not Use" list, effective Jan. 1, 2004. Visit www.jointcommission.org for more information about this Joint Commission requirement.

Used with permission from the Institute for Safe Medication Practices. Report medication errors or near misses to the ISMP Medication Errors Reporting Program (MERP) at 1-800-FAIL-SAF(E) or online at www.ismp.org.

Pharmacology Terms

Topics include:

GENERAL PHARMACY TERMS	
absorption	the process in which a drug is taken up into the body, organ, tissue, or cell
adverse drug reaction (ADR)	any unintended harmful reaction to a drug administered at a normal dose
ampule (or ampoule)	a small, sterile glass or plastic container that usually holds a single dose of a solution to be administered parenterally
aseptic technique	the method used to minimize the microbial contamination of compounded sterile drugs
bioavailability	the percentage of administered drug available to affect the body and target site(s) after absorption, metabolism, and other factors
capsule (cap)	a small, digestible container (usually made of gelatin) used to hold a dose of medication for oral administration
chemical name	the exact designation of the chemical structure of a drug
chemotherapy (also called *chemo*)	the treatment of cancer with chemical agents
compounding	the act of combining drug ingredients to prepare a customized prescription or drug order for a patient
contraindication	factor that prohibits administration of a drug
controlled substance	a drug that has been identified as having the potential for abuse or addiction; designated as schedule I, II, III, IV, or V under the Controlled Substance Act
cream	a water-based, semisolid preparation that usually contains a drug and is applied topically to external parts of the body
distribution	the uptake pattern of a drug throughout the body to various tissues
dose	the amount of a drug or other substance to be administered at one time
drug	any substance taken by mouth; injected into a muscle, the skin, a blood vessel, or a cavity of the body; or applied topically to treat, cure, prevent, or diagnose a disease or condition
drug-drug interaction (DDI)	a modification of the effect of a drug when administered with another drug; food can also interact with a drug to cause a modification of the drug's effect
elimination	the removal of a substance from the body by any route, including the kidneys, liver, lungs, and sweat glands
elixir	a liquid containing sweeteners, flavorings, water, and/or alcohol in which an oral medication may be dispersed
emulsion	a stable mixture that contains one component suspended within another component that it cannot normally dissolve in or mix with
Food and Drug Administration (FDA)	the U.S. federal agency responsible for the enforcement of federal regulations regarding the manufacturing and distribution of food, drugs, and cosmetics as protection against the sale of impure or dangerous substances

formulary	a listing of drugs and drug information used by health practitioners within an institution to prescribe treatment that is medically appropriate
generic name	the official, established nonproprietary name assigned to a drug
inhaler	a device containing a drug to be breathed in nasally or by mouth
mechanism of action (MOA)	the means by which a drug exerts a desired effect
metabolism	the chemical changes that a drug or other substance undergoes in the body
ointment	an oil-based, semisolid preparation that is applied topically to external parts of the body
over-the-counter (OTC) drug (also called *nonprescription drug*)	a drug that may be purchased without a prescription
pharmaceutical	a drug used for medicinal purposes
pharmacist	a person formally trained to formulate and dispense medications and provide drug information
pharmacodynamics	the study of the actions of a drug on the body
pharmacogenomics	the study of the correlation between genetics and response to a drug
pharmacokinetics	the study of the actions of the body on a drug
pharmacology	the study of the preparation, properties, uses, and actions of drugs
pharmacy	a place for preparing and dispensing drugs
placebo	an inactive substance, prescribed as if it were an effective dose of a needed medication
prescription	an order for medication, therapy, or a therapeutic device given by a properly authorized person for a specified patient
preservative	a substance included in some parenteral and topical medications used to prevent the growth of microorganisms in the product
route of administration	the method in which a drug or agent is given to a patient
side effect	any reaction or result from a medication other than what is the primary intended effect
solution	a homogenous mixture of one or more substances dissolved into another substance
state board of pharmacy	the agency responsible for regulating the practice of pharmacy within the state
suppository	a topical form of drug that is inserted into the rectum, vagina, or penis
suspension	a liquid in which particles of a solid are dispersed, but not dissolved, and in which the dispersal is maintained by stirring or shaking
tablet	a small, solid dose form of a medication
toxicity	the level at which a drug's concentration within the body produces serious adverse effects
trade name (also called *brand name*)	a proprietary name assigned to a drug by its manufacturer that is registered as part of the drug's identity
United States Pharmacopeia (USP)	a compendium, recognized officially by the federal Food and Drug Administration that contains descriptions, uses, strengths, and standards of purity for selected drugs and guidance for related standards of practice

ROUTES OF ADMINISTRATION

enteral	the use of oral ingestion as a mode of drug administration
epidural	injection of a drug into the epidural space of the spine

infusion	the prolonged administration of a fluid substance directly into a vein, artery, or under the skin in which the flow rate is driven by gravity or a mechanical pump
inhalation	a method of drug administration that involves the breathing in of a spray, vapor, or powder via the nose or mouth
injection	the introduction of a substance into the body by using a needle
intramuscular (IM)	the administration of a medication into a muscle
intrathecal	the administration of a drug into the subarachnoid space of the meninges in the spine
intravenous (IV)	the administration of a medication directly into a vein
oral	the administration of a medication by mouth
parenteral	a drug or agent that is administered into the body via a route that bypasses the digestive tract
subcutaneous	the introduction of a medication into the tissue just beneath the skin
sublingual	a form of drug that dissolves under the tongue
topical	a dosage form of a medication that is applied directly to an external area of the body
transdermal	a method of applying a drug to unbroken skin so that it is continuously absorbed through the skin to produce a systemic effect; a transdermal patch is a drug delivery system that controls the rate of absorption through the skin

GENERAL DRUG CATEGORIES

antibacterial	a drug that targets bacteria to kill or halt growth
antibiotic	a drug that targets bacteria, fungi, or protozoa to kill or halt growth
antifungal	a drug that targets fungi to kill or halt growth
antihistamine	a drug that treats allergic and hypersensitivity reactions by blocking histamine-1 receptors
antiinflammatory	a drug that reduces inflammation
antimicrobial	a drug that targets microorganisms to kill or halt growth
antineoplastic agent	a drug used to destroy or slow the rapid replication of cancer cells
antiretroviral	a drug that suppresses the replication of the human immunodeficiency virus (HIV); highly active antiretroviral therapy (HAART) is the combination of three or more of these drugs to treat HIV infection
antiviral	a drug that targets viruses to kill or halt growth
antiadrenergic agent	a drug that blocks adrenergic receptors to reduce sympathetic nervous system activity in the body
bactericidal	the designation for an antimicrobial agent that kills or destroys bacteria
bacteriostatic	the designation for an antimicrobial agent that halts the growth or replication of bacteria but does not kill them
cytotoxic	an agent that causes cell death
dietary supplement	a product that provides nutrients that may be missing from the diet
disinfectant	a chemical agent that can be applied to inanimate objects to destroy microorganisms
herbal supplement	a naturally derived dietary product that is touted to improve well-being and may have some therapeutic effect; rigorous proof of safety and effectiveness is not required because it is not regulated as a drug

immunosuppressant (also called *immunomodulator*)	a drug that reduces the response of the immune system; used in autoimmune diseases and to prepare a patient for an organ transplant
narcotic	a type of drug that has opium-like effects to cause drowsiness, pain relief, and sedation; can be habit-forming and is regulated as a controlled substance
nonsteroidal antiinflammatory drug (NSAID)	a drug that reduces pain, inflammation, and fever
parasympatholytic	an agent that blocks the actions of the parasympathetic nervous system
parasympathomimetic	an agent that enhances the actions of the parasympathetic nervous system
radiopharmaceutical	a drug with a radioactive component; used for diagnosis or treatment
smoking cessation agent	a drug that helps a patient quit smoking; may be a behavioral deterrent or a nicotine substitute
sympatholytic	an agent that blocks the actions of the sympathetic nervous system
sympathomimetic	an agent that enhances the actions of the sympathetic nervous system
vaccine (also called *immunization*)	a preparation of microbial antigen that will confer a degree of immunity to a future infection by that microbial
vitamin	an organic compound essential in small quantities for normal physiologic and metabolic functioning

CHAPTER 2: BODY STRUCTURE, COLOR, AND ONCOLOGY

alkylating agent	a type of antineoplastic agent that binds to cellular DNA to interfere with replication
antimetabolite	a type of antineoplastic agent that interferes with a cell's normal metabolism
antineoplastic agent	a drug used to destroy or slow the replication of cancer cells
chemotherapeutic agent	a drug used to destroy or slow the replication of cancer cells
mitotic inhibitor	a type of antineoplastic agent that interrupts cellular division

CHAPTER 4: INTEGUMENTARY SYSTEM

antibacterial	a drug used to combat an infection caused by bacteria
antifungal	a drug used to combat an infection caused by fungi
antihistamine	a drug used to minimize allergy symptoms by blocking histamine-1 receptors
antipruritic	an agent that reduces itching
antipsoriatic	a drug that treats psoriasis
antiseptic	a chemical agent that can safely be applied to external tissues to halt the growth of microorganisms
astringent	an agent that reduces inflammation and irritation and provides a protective barrier on mucosa and skin by contracting the surface tissue
emollient	an external agent that softens or soothes the skin
keratolytic	an agent that augments the shedding of the top layer of dead skin
pediculicide	an agent that kills lice
retinoid	a derivative of vitamin A that regulates the growth of epithelial cells; often used to treat acne
scabicide	an agent that kills scabies

CHAPTER 5: RESPIRATORY SYSTEM

antitussive	a drug that suppresses coughing
bronchodilator	a drug that expands the airways by relaxing smooth muscle in the lungs
decongestant	a drug that relieves nasal congestion by reducing swelling of mucous membranes

expectorant	a drug that promotes expulsion of mucus from the lungs
leukotriene receptor antagonist (LTRA)	a drug that blocks late-stage regulators of allergic and hypersensitivity reactions to treat allergy-induced asthma
mucolytic	a drug that thins out mucus in the lungs so that it can be expelled more easily

CHAPTER 6: URINARY SYSTEM

aldosterone receptor antagonist (ARA)	a drug that prevents reabsorption of water and sodium; used in chronic heart failure to minimize edema
antispasmodic	a drug that prevents or relieves bladder muscle spasms associated with incontinence
diuretic	a drug that promotes the formation and excretion of urine to reduce the volume of extracellular fluid; used to reduce high blood pressure or edema; commonly referred to as a "water pill"
muscle relaxant	a drug that reduces bladder muscle contractility to relieve spasm-induced pain or uncontrolled urination
urinary alkalinizer	an agent that increases the urine pH to make it more basic to treat acidosis
vasopressin (also called *antidiuretic hormone* or *ADH*)	a drug that increases water retention by the kidneys

CHAPTER 7: MALE REPRODUCTIVE SYSTEM

androgen	a natural or synthetic hormone involved in male reproduction and secondary gender attributes
antiandrogen	a drug that blocks the effects of androgen hormones in the body
phosphodiesterase-5 inhibitor (PDE5 inhibitor)	a drug that blocks the inactivation of cyclic guanosine monophosphate either to increase vasodilation in the penis or to increase cardiac output
spermicide	an agent that kills sperm

CHAPTER 8: FEMALE REPRODUCTIVE SYSTEM

antiestrogen	a drug used to block the action of estrogen hormones in the body
contraceptive	an agent (drug or barrier) used to prevent conception or pregnancy
estrogen	a natural or synthetic hormone involved in female reproduction and secondary gender characteristics
fertility drugs	drugs that enhance a female's ability to conceive a child
hormone replacement therapy (HRT)	a regimen that mimics the body's normal levels of female hormones when they are no longer produced; typically used during menopause
intrauterine device (IUD)	a hormone-containing or metal-based device that is inserted directly in the uterus to prevent pregnancy long-term
oral contraceptive	exogenous hormones taken by mouth to prevent pregnancy
ovulation stimulant	a drug that enhances the release of an egg from the ovary to promote pregnancy
progestin	a synthetic or natural hormone involved in female reproduction and secondary sex characteristics
vaginal ring	a device containing estrogen and progestin hormones that is inserted in the vagina to prevent pregnancy

CHAPTER 9: OBSTETRICS AND NEONATOLOGY

abortifacient	a drug that causes uterine muscles to contract with subsequent abortion of the fetus
oxytocic	a hormone that stimulates the uterine muscles to contract, thereby inducing labor in a pregnant woman

pregnancy category	a level of risk the Food and Drug Administration assigns a drug based on documented problems with the use of that drug during pregnancy; risk categories from safest to most harmful are A, B, C, D, and X
tocolytic	an agent that suppresses labor contractions

CHAPTER 10: CARDIOVASCULAR, IMMUNE, AND LYMPHATIC SYSTEMS AND BLOOD

angiotensin-converting enzyme inhibitor (ACE inhibitor)	a drug that prevents the formation of angiotensin-II, which is a strong vasoconstrictor and major contributor to high blood pressure
angiotensin receptor blocker (ARB) (also called *angiotensin II antagonist*)	a drug that blocks the angiotensin-II molecule from binding to its receptors throughout the body to prevent its effects and to reduce high blood pressure
antianginal	a drug that relieves the chest pain paroxysms caused by lack of oxygen delivery to the heart; typically involves vasodilation
antiarrhythmic	a drug that treats abnormal heart rhythm
anticoagulant	a drug that prevents blood clotting and coagulation
antihypertensive	a drug that lowers blood pressure
antiplatelet agent	a drug that prevents platelet formation or causes platelet destruction
beta-blocker (BB)	a drug that inhibits beta-adrenergic receptors to decrease heart rate and force of contractility; used to treat arrhythmias, hypertension, heart failure, and more
calcium channel blocker (CCB)	a drug that regulates the entry of calcium into muscle cells of the heart and blood vessels; used to treat heart failure, arrhythmias, angina, and hypertension
colony-stimulating factor (CSF)	an agent that promotes the replication of blood cells in the bone marrow
direct thrombin inhibitor (DTI)	a drug that blocks the action of thrombin, thereby reducing blood coagulation
erythropoiesis stimulating agent (ESA)	an agent that stimulates red blood cell production from the bone marrow
hemostatic	a drug that stops bleeding or hemorrhaging
nitrate	a drug that dilates the blood vessels
platelet aggregation inhibitor	a drug that stops platelets from adhering together
renin inhibitor	a drug that blocks renin activity to reduce high blood pressure; renin is the first step in the renin-angiotensin-aldosterone system (RAAS), which is a common contributor to chronic high blood pressure
thrombolytic	a drug that dissolves blood clots
vasodilator	a drug that expands blood vessels to lower blood pressure
vasopressor (also called *vasoconstrictor*)	a drug that contracts blood vessels to raise blood pressure

CHAPTER 11: DIGESTIVE SYSTEM

antacid	a drug that neutralizes acid in the stomach
antidiarrheal	a drug that treats diarrhea by increasing water absorption, decreasing muscle contraction of the intestines, altering electrolyte exchange, or absorbing toxins or microorganisms
antiemetic	a drug that reduces or prevents nausea and vomiting
antihyperlipidemic agent (also called *hypolipidemic agent*)	a drug used to treat high cholesterol by affecting levels of low-density lipoproteins, high-density lipoproteins, total cholesterol, and/or triglycerides, which are collectively called lipids

bile acid sequestrant	a type of antihyperlipidemic agent used to lower high cholesterol levels by increasing the excretion of bile acids
enema	a liquid agent administered rectally to clear the contents of the bowel
fibrate	a type of antihyperlipidemic agent that affects lipid levels by facilitating lipid metabolism
histamine H₂ receptor antagonist (H2RA) (also called *H₂ blocker*)	a drug that reduces production of stomach acid
laxative	a drug that aids the evacuation of the bowel
proton pump inhibitor (PPI)	a drug that blocks acid production in the stomach
statin (also known as *HMG-CoA reductase inhibitor*)	a type of antihyperlipidemic agent that treats dyslipidemia by inhibiting 3-hydroxy-3-methylglutaryl coenzyme A reductase
CHAPTER 12: EYE	
antiglaucoma agent	a drug that treats glaucoma of the eye
miotic	an agent that contracts the pupil
mydriatic	an agent that dilates the pupil
ophthalmic	an agent that is intended to be used in the eye
CHAPTER 13: EAR	
ceruminolytic	an agent that breaks down ear wax
otic	an agent intended to be used in the ear
CHAPTER 14: MUSCULOSKELETAL SYSTEM	
antiarthritic agent	a drug used in the treatment of arthritis
antigout agent	a drug that opposes the buildup of uric acid crystals in the joints to prevent and treat gout attacks
antispasmodic	a drug that prevents or relieves muscle spasms
bisphosphonate	a drug that binds to bone matrix to treat osteoporosis
disease-modifying antirheumatic drug (DMARD)	a drug that slows the progression of rheumatoid arthritis
muscle relaxant	a drug that reduces muscle contractility to relieve tension- or spasm-induced pain
neuromuscular blocking agent (NMBA)	a drug that blocks all nerve stimulation of the skeletal muscles to cause paralysis
CHAPTER 15: NERVOUS SYSTEM AND BEHAVIORAL HEALTH	
adrenergic agonist	a drug that stimulates aspects of the sympathetic nervous system
amphetamine	a drug that stimulates the central nervous system
anticonvulsant (also called *antiepileptic drug*)	a drug that reduces the incidence and severity of seizures and convulsions
analgesic	a drug that relieves pain
anesthetic	a drug that causes numbness or a loss of feeling that can be used locally or systemically; often used systemically to put a patient "to sleep" during extensive procedures
anticholinergic	a drug that blocks the action of acetylcholine and therefore suppresses the parasympathetic nervous system
anticholinesterase	a drug that prevents the breakdown of acetylcholine to yield a cholinergic or parasympathetic effect
antidepressant	a drug used to treat depression

antiparkinsonian agent	a drug that treats Parkinson disease and parkinsonism by affecting levels of dopamine or acetylcholine in the brain
antipsychotic (also called *neuroleptic*)	a drug that treats psychosis disorders by inducing a calming or tranquilizing effect or by adjusting neurotransmitter levels in the brain
antipyretic	a drug that reduces fever
anxiolytic	a drug that relieves anxiety
barbiturate	a drug used to produce relaxation and sleep
benzodiazepine (BZD)	a drug that binds to receptors in the brain to calm and sedate the central nervous system
central nervous system stimulant	a drug that excites the central nervous system; can be used for many brain disorders
cholinergic	an agent that acts like acetylcholine to activate the parasympathetic nervous system
dopaminergic	a drug that acts like dopamine; mostly used to treat Parkinson disease by increasing dopamine-dependent activity in the brain
hypnotic	a drug used to induce sleep; may also be used as a sedative
mood stabilizer	a drug that balances neurotransmitters in the brain to prevent periods of mania or depression
monoamine oxidase inhibitor (MAOI)	a type of antidepressant that prevents the breakdown of many active neurotransmitters in the brain
nonsteroidal antiinflammatory drug (NSAID)	a drug that reduces pain, inflammation, and fever
sedative	a drug that depresses the central nervous system to calm a patient
selective serotonin reuptake inhibitor (SSRI)	a type of antidepressant that maintains a higher level of serotonin in the synapse
tranquilizer	a drug that reduces anxiety or agitation
tricyclic antidepressant (TCA)	a type of antidepressant that maintains a higher level of various neurotransmitters in the synapse

CHAPTER 16: ENDOCRINE SYSTEM

antidiabetic agent	a drug that treats diabetes by controlling blood sugar levels
antithyroid agent	a drug that counters hyperthyroidism by reducing the production of thyroid hormones
corticosteroid	a drug that mimics hormones produced by the adrenal glands and has antiinflammatory and immunosuppressive effects
hypoglycemic agent	a drug that lowers blood sugar levels
thyroid hormone	a replacement hormone to regulate metabolism and endocrine functions

2013 Conn's current therapy, Philadelphia, 2013, Saunders.

American Journal of Nursing, 2008-2013, Lippincott Williams & Wilkins.

Applegate EJ: *The anatomy and physiology learning system*, ed 4, St. Louis, 2010, Saunders.

Ballinger PW, Frank ED: *Merrill's atlas of radiographic positions and radiologic procedures*, ed 12, St. Louis, 2011, Mosby.

Bontrager KL: *Textbook of radiographic positioning and related anatomy*, ed 8, St. Louis, 2013, Mosby.

Chabner D: *The language of medicine*, ed 10, Philadelphia, 2013, Saunders.

Christensen B, Kockrow E: *Foundations of Nursing*, ed 6, St. Louis, 2011, Mosby.

Diehl M: *Medical transcription guide: do's and don'ts*, ed 3, St. Louis, 2005, Saunders.

Diehl M: *Diehl and Fordney's medical transcription, techniques and procedures*, ed 5, 2002, Saunders.

Dorland's illustrated medical dictionary, ed 32, Philadelphia, 2011, Saunders.

Fitzpatrick JE, Aeling JL: *Dermatology secrets in color*, ed 4, Philadelphia, 2010, Mosby.

Frazier M, Drzymkowski JW: *Essentials of human diseases and conditions*, ed 4, Philadelphia, 2009, Elsevier.

Gillingham EA, Seibel, MW: *LaFleur Brooks' health unit coordinating*, ed 7, Philadelphia, 2013, Saunders.

Habif T: *A color guide to diagnosis and therapy, clinical dermatology*, ed 5, Philadelphia, 2010, Mosby.

Haubrich WS: *Medical meanings: a glossary of word origins*, ed 2, Philadelphia, 2004, American College of Physicians.

Health Information, http://www.mayoclinic.com/health -information/,2008-2013, Mayo Foundation for Medical Education and Research.

Herlihy B, Maebius N: *The human body in health and illness*, ed 4, Philadelphia, 2011, Saunders.

Hockenberry MJ, Wilson D: *Wong's nursing care of infants and children*, ed 9, St. Louis, 2011, Mosby.

Huth EJ, Murray TJ: *Medicine in quotations: Views of health and disease through the ages*, Philadelphia, 2006, American College of Physicians.

Ignatavicius DD et al: *Medical-surgical nursing: patient-centered collaborative care*, ed 7, Philadelphia, 2013, Saunders.

Jarvis C: *Physical examination & health assessment*, ed 6, Philadelphia, 2012, Saunders.

LaFleur Brooks M, LaFleur Brooks D: *Basic medical language*, ed 4, St. Louis, 2013, Mosby.

Lewis SM et al: *Medical-surgical nursing*, ed 8, St. Louis, 2011, Mosby.

Littleton LY, Engebretson JC: *Maternal, neonatal, and women's health nursing*, Albany, 2002, Delmar.

Lowdermilk DL et al: *Maternity & women's health care*, ed 10, St. Louis, 2012, Mosby.

Mayo Clinic Health Letter, Rochester, 2008-2013, Mayo Foundation for Medical Education and Research.

Mayo Clinic Women's Health Source, Rochester, 2008-2013, Mayo Foundation for Medical Education and Research.

Medline Plus, http://www.nlm.nih.gov/medlineplus, 2008-2013, National Library of Medicine and the National Institutes of Health.

Mosby's medical, nursing, and allied health dictionary, ed 8, St. Louis, 2009, Mosby.

New England Journal of Medicine, 2008-2013, Massachusetts Medical Society.

Novey D: *Clinicians' complete reference to complementary and alternative medicine*, St. Louis, 2000, Mosby.

Pagana KD, Pagana TJ: *Mosby's manual of diagnostic and laboratory test reference*, ed 4, St. Louis, 2010, Mosby.

Phillips N: *Berry & Kohn's operating room technique*, ed 12, St. Louis, 2013, Mosby.

Rakel D: *Integrative medicine*, ed 3, Philadelphia, 2012, Saunders.

Spencer JW, Jacobs JJ: *Complementary and alternative medicine: an evidence-based approach*, St Louis, 2003, Mosby.

Stedman's abbreviations, acronyms, and symbols, ed 5, Baltimore, 2013, Lippincott Williams & Wilkins.

Thibodeau GA, Patton KT: *Anthony's textbook of anatomy and physiology*, ed 20, St. Louis, 2013, Mosby.

Torpy JM: The metabolic syndrome, *JAMA*, 295 (7), 850, (2006).

UpToDate, http://www.uptodate.com, 2008-2013, Wolters Kluwer Health.

Wein AJ et al: *Campbell-Walsh Urology*, ed 10, Philadelphia, 2012, Elsevier.

Whiteside MM et al: Sensory impairment in older adults: part 2, vision loss, *Consultant*, 106 (11), 52-62, (2006).

ILLUSTRATION CREDITS

Chapter 2

Figure 2-3 from Kamal A, Brockelhurst JC: *Color atlas of geriatric medicine*, ed 2, St. Louis, 1991, Mosby.

Figure 2-4 from LaFleur Brooks M, LaFleur Brooks D: *Basic medical language*, ed 4, St. Louis, 2013, Elsevier.

Figure 2-5 from Damjanov I: *Pathology, A color atlas*, ed 2, St. Louis, 2000, Mosby.

Figure 2-8 from National Cancer Institute (NCI). Courtesy Rhoda Baer (Photographer).

Figure 2-9 from Ballinger PW, Frank ED: *Merrill's atlas of radiographic positions and radiologic procedures*, ed 10, St. Louis, 2003, Mosby.

Exercise Figure A from LaFleur Brooks M, LaFleur Brooks D: *Basic medical language*, ed 4, St. Louis, 2013, Elsevier.

Exercise Figure C from (1) Mace JD: *Radiography pathology*, ed 4, St. Louis, 2004, Elsevier Mosby; (2) Habif TP: *Clinical dermatology*, ed 4, St. Louis, 2004, Elsevier Mosby; (3) Stevens A: *Pathology*, ed 2, London, 2000, Mosby; (4) Damjanov I, Linder J: *Anderson's pathology*, ed 10, St. Louis, 1996, Mosby.

Chapter 3

Table 3-1 figures and Exercise Figure C from Bontrager KL: *Radiographic positioning and related anatomy*, ed 5, St. Louis, 2002, Mosby.

Exercise Figures E, F(2), G from Bontrager KL, Lampignano JP: *Radiographic positioning and related anatomy*, ed 7, St. Louis, 2010, Mosby.

Exercise Figure F(1) from Chapleau W, Pons P: *Emergency medical technician*, ed 1, St. Louis, 2007, Mosby/JEMS.

Chapter 4

Figure 4-2 from Frazier M: *Essentials of human disease and conditions*, ed 3, St. Louis, 2004, Elsevier Mosby.

Dermatology poem courtesy Julia Frank, MD.

Exercise Figure C (1), Figures 4-4 (A), 4-12, 4-13, 4-14 and 4-16 and Unn Fig 4 from Bork K, Brauninger W: *Skin diseases in clinical practice*, ed 2, Philadelphia, 1998, WB Saunders.

Figure 4-4 (B), 4-5 from Callen JP: *Color atlas of dermatology*, ed 2, Philadelphia, 2000, Saunders.

Figure 4-4 (C) from Wilson S, Giddens J: *Health assessment for nursing practice*, ed 4, St. Louis, 2009, Mosby. Courtesy Gary Monheit, MD, University of Alabama at Birmingham School of Medicine.

Figure 4-6 from *Dorland's illustrated medical dictionary*, ed 31, Philadelphia, 2007, Saunders.

Figure 4-7 from Cohen BA: *Pediatric dermatology*, ed 3, St. Louis, 2005, Mosby.

Table 4-1 figures from Frazier M: *Essentials of human disease and conditions*, ed 3, St. Louis, 2004, Elsevier Mosby.

Figure 4-15 and Exercise Figure D (1 and 2) from Shiland B: *Mastering healthcare terminology*, ed 2, St. Louis, 2006, Elsevier Mosby.

Figure 4-4 (D, E), 4-9, 4-11, and Table 4-1 figures from Habif TP: *Clinical dermatology*, ed 4, St. Louis, 2004, Elsevier Mosby.

Chapter 5

Figure 5-3 from Eisenberg RL, Johnson NM: *Comprehensive radiographic pathology*, ed 3, St. Louis, 2003, Mosby.

Figure 5-5 Data from American Cancer Society.

Figure 5-7 from Kumar V et al: *Robbins' basic pathology*, ed 7, Philadelphia, 2003, Saunders.

Figures 5-13 and 5-14 from Ruppel GL: *Manual pulmonary function testing*, ed 7, St. Louis, 1998, Mosby.

Figure 5-15 Courtesy Siemens Medical Systems, Inc., New Jersey.

Figure 5-16 from Ballinger PW, Frank ED: *Merrill's atlas of radiographic positions and radiologic procedures*, ed 10, St. Louis, 2003, Mosby.

Figure 5-17 Courtesy GE Medical Systems, Waukesha, Wis.

Figures 5-18 and 5-19 from Pagana KD, Pagana TJ: *Mosby's manual of diagnostic and laboratory test reference*, ed 7, St. Louis, 2004, Elsevier Mosby.

Exercise Figure H (1, 2) Courtesy Nonin Medical, Inc. Reprinted with permission of Nonin Medical, Inc. © 2013.

Exercise Figure H (3) from Potter PA, Perry AG: *Fundamentals of nursing: concepts, process, and practice*, ed 5, St. Louis, 2001, Mosby.

Figure 5-21 from Cummings N: Perspectives in athletic training, ed 1, St. Louis, 2009, Mosby.

Figure 5-23 from Nelcor Puritan Bennett.

Chapter 6

Figure 6-5 (A), 6-6 from Damjanov I: *Pathology, a color atlas*, ed 2, St. Louis, 2000, Mosby.

Figure 6-8 from Shiland B: *Mastering healthcare terminology*, ed 2, St. Louis, 2006, Elsevier Mosby.

Figure 6-12 from Ballinger PW, Frank ED: *Merrill's atlas of radiographic positions and radiologic procedures*, ed 10, St. Louis, 2003, Mosby.

Figures 6-13, 6-14, 6-18 from Wein A et al: *Campbell-Walsh Urology*, ed 10, 2012, Saunders.

Figure 6-15 from Bontrager KL: *Textbook of radiographic positioning and related anatomy*, ed 6, St. Louis, 2002, Mosby.

Figure 6-19 from James S, Ashwill J: Nursing care of children, ed 3, St. Louis, 2008, Saunders.

Exercise Figure E courtesy Dornier Medical Systems, Kennesaw, Ga.

Chapter 7

Figure 7-10 courtesy EDAP Technomed, Inc., Vaulx-en-Velin, France.

Figure 7-11 (A, B) from Habif TP: *Clinical dermatology*, ed 4, St. Louis, 2004, Elsevier Mosby.

Figure 7-11 (C) from Callen JP: *Color atlas of dermatology*, ed 2, Philadelphia, 2000, Saunders.

Exercise Figure C (1) from Zitelli BJ, David HW: *Atlas of pediatric physical diagnosis*, ed 2, St. Louis, 1992, Mosby.

Exercise Figure B from Bork K, Brauninger W: *Skin diseases in clinical practice*, ed 2, Philadelphia, 1998, WB Saunders.

Chapter 8

Figure 8-10 from Black J, Hawks J: *Medical-surgical nursing*, ed 8, St. Louis, 2009, Elsevier.

Figure 8-14 (A) courtesy Biopsys Medical, Inc, Irvine, Calif.

Figure 8-14 (B, C) from Pagana KD, Pagana TJ: *Mosby's manual of diagnostic and laboratory test reference*, ed 7, St. Louis, 2004, Elsevier Mosby.

Figure 8-16 from Bontrager KL, Lampignano JP: *Radiographic positioning and related anatomy*, ed 6, St. Louis, 2005, Mosby.

Figure 8-20 from Proctor D, Adams A: Kinn's the medical assistant, ed 11, St. Louis, 2011, Saunders.

Chapter 9

Figure 9-2 from Dickason EJ, Schultz MO, Silverman BL: *Maternal-infant nursing care*, ed 3, St. Louis, 1998, Mosby.

Figure 9-6 from from Lowdermilk DL et al: *Maternity and women's health care*, ed 10, St. Louis, 2012, Mosby.

Figure 9-7 from Zitelli BJ, David HW: *Atlas of pediatric physical diagnosis*, ed 4, St. Louis, 2002, Mosby.

Figures 9-9 and 9-14 from Hockenberry M et al: *Wong's nursing care of infants and children*, ed 9, St. Louis, 2011, Elsevier.

Figure 9-10 (B) from Hockenberry M, Wilson D: *Wong's essentials of pediatric nursing*, ed 8, St. Louis, 2009, Elsevier.

Figure 9-12 from Bontrager KL, Lampignano JP: *Radiographic positioning and related anatomy*, ed 6, St. Louis, 2005, Mosby.

Exercise Figure B from Hockenberry M et al: *Wong's nursing care of infants and children*, ed 9, St. Louis, 2011, Elsevier.

Exercise Figure C from Lowdermilk DL, Perry S: *Maternity and women's health care*, ed 9, St. Louis, 2007, Elsevier Mosby.

Chapter 10

Figures 10-1 and 10-5 from LaFleur Brooks M, LaFleur Brooks D: *Basic medical language*, ed 3, St. Louis, 2010, Elsevier.

Figure 10-12 (A) from Thibodeau GA, Patton KT: *Anatomy and physiology*, ed 4, St. Louis, 2001, Mosby.

Figure 10-12 (B) from Bork K, Brauninger W: *Skin diseases in clinical practice*, ed 2, Philadelphia, 1998, WB Saunders.

Figures 10-15 (B), 10-19 (B, C), 10-21, 10-22, 10-23, and 10-25 (B) from Ballinger PW, Frank ED: *Merrill's atlas of radiographic positions and radiologic procedures*, ed 10, St. Louis, 2003, Mosby.

Figure 10-25 (A) courtesy GE Medical Systems, Inc, Waukesha, Wis.

Figure 10-28 from Turgeon M: Linne & Ringsrud's clinical laboratory science, ed 5, St. Louis, 2007, Mosby.

Exercise Figure C from Bolognia JL et al: *Dermatology*, ed 2, St. Louis, 2008, Mosby.

Exercise Figure E from Patton KT, Thibodeau GA: *Anatomy and physiology*, ed 7, St. Louis, 2010, Mosby.

Exercise Figure F from Ignatavicius DM, Workman L: *Medical-surgical nursing*, ed 6, St. Louis, 2010, Saunders.

Chapter 11

Figure 11-11 from Shiland B: *Mastering healthcare terminology*, ed 2, St. Louis, 2006, Elsevier Mosby.

Figure 11-12 (A) from Anderson KN: *Mosby's medical, nursing and allied health dictionary*, St. Louis, 2003, Mosby.

Figure 11-15 from White RA, Klein SR: *Endoscopic surgery*, St. Louis, 1991, Mosby.

Figure 11-18 from Ballinger PW, Frank ED: *Merrill's atlas of radiographic positions and radiologic procedures*, ed 10, St. Louis, 2003, Mosby.

Figure 11-20 from Lewis SM: *Medical-surgical nursing*, ed 7, St. Louis, 2007, Mosby.

Unnumbered Figure 4 from Hagen-Ansert S: *Textbook of diagnostic ultrasonography*, ed 5, St. Louis, 2001, Mosby.

Chapter 12

Figure 12-3 and Exercise Figures B and D from Zitelli BJ, David HW: *Atlas of pediatric physical diagnosis*, ed 4, St. Louis, 2002, Mosby.

Figure 12-5 (A, B) from Seidel H et al: *Mosby's guide to physical examination*, ed 5, St. Louis, 2003, Mosby.

Exercise Figure C from Stein HA, Slatt BJ, Stein RM: *The ophthalmic assistant: fundamentals and clinical practice*, ed 5, St. Louis, 1998, Mosby.

Figure 12-6 from Newell FW: *Ophthalmology*, ed 7, St. Louis, 1992, Mosby.

Figure 12-7 from Apple DJ, Robb MF: *Ocular pathology*, ed 5, St. Louis, 1998, Mosby.

Figure 12-9 from Bedford MA: *Ophthalmological diagnosis*, London, 1986, Wolfe.

Figure 12-10 from Black J, Hawks J: *Medical-surgical nursing*, ed 7, Philadelphia, 2005, Saunders. Courtesy of Ophthalmic Photography at the University of Michigan, WK Kellogg Center, Ann Arbor.

Figure 12-11 courtesy Nidek, Inc., Fremont, Calif.

Exercise Figure E from Jarvis C: Physical examination and health assessment, ed 5, Philadelphia, 2008, Saunders.

Figure 12-13 from Thompson J, Wilson S: *Health assessment for nursing practice*, St. Louis, 1996, Mosby.

Chapter 13

Figure 13-3 from Zitelli BJ, David HW: *Atlas of pediatric physical diagnosis*, ed 4, St. Louis, 2002, Mosby.

Figure 13-4 courtesy Richard A. Buckingham, MD, University of Illinois, Chicago.

Figure 13-7 (A) from Klieger D: *Saunders essentials of medical assisting*, ed 2, St. Louis, 2010, Saunders.

Figure 13-7 (B) from Kliegman R et al: *Nelson textbook of pediatrics*, ed 18, St. Louis, 2008, Saunders.

Exercise Figure C from Jarvis C: *Physical examination and health assessment*, ed 5, Philadelphia, 2008, Saunders.

Chapter 14

Figure 14-5 from Thibodeau GA, Patton KT: *Anatomy and physiology*, ed 5, St. Louis, 2003, Mosby.

Figures 14-8 (A, right) and **14-24** from Bontrager KL, Lampignano JP: *Radiographic positioning and related anatomy*, ed 8, St. Louis, 2014, Mosby.

Figure 14-8 (B, right) from Magee D: *Orthopedic physical assessment*, ed 5, St. Louis, 2008, Saunders.

Figure 14-8 (C, right) from Manaster BJ: *Musculoskeletal imaging*, ed 3, St. Louis, 2007, Mosby.

Figures 14-12 and **14-23** from Mercier LR: *Practical orthopedics*, ed 4, St. Louis, 1995, Mosby.

Figures 14-13 and **14-16** from Patton KT, Thibodeau GA: *Anthony's textbook of anatomy & physiology*, ed 19, St. Louis, 2010, Mosby.

Figure 14-20 from Pagana KD, Pagana TJ: *Mosby's manual of diagnostic and laboratory test reference*, ed 7, St. Louis, 2004, Elsevier Mosby.

Figure 14-21 courtesy Marconi Medical Systems, Cleveland, Ohio.

Figure 14-22 from Ballinger PW, Frank ED: *Merrill's atlas of radiographic positions and radiologic procedures*, ed 10, St. Louis, 2003, Mosby.

Chapter 15

Figure 15-1 and 15-2 from Thibodeau GA, Patton KT: *Anatomy and physiology*, ed 5, St. Louis, 2003, Mosby.

Figure 15-5 from Waldman S: *Atlas of common pain syndromes*, ed 2, Philadelphia, 2008, Saunders.

Figure 15-8 (left images) from Shiland B: *Mastering healthcare terminology*, ed 2, St. Louis, 2006, Elsevier Mosby.

Figure 15-9 from Perkin GD, Hotchberg FH, Miller D: *The atlas of clinical neurology*, St. Louis, 1986, Mosby.

Figure 15-14 from Adam A et al: *Grainger and Allison's diagnostic radiology*, ed 5, London, 2008, Churchill Livingstone.

Figure 15-15 from Bontrager KL, Lampignano JP: *Radiographic positioning and related anatomy*, ed 8, St. Louis, 2014, Mosby.

Figure 15-16 and Exercise Figure D from Ballinger PW, Frank ED: *Merrill's atlas of radiographic positions and radiologic procedures*, ed 10, St. Louis, 2003, Mosby.

Figure 15-17 from Bontrager KL: *Textbook of radiographic positioning and related anatomy*, ed 6, St. Louis, 2002, Mosby.

Chapter 16

Figure 16-5 and Exercise C from Shiland B: *Mastering healthcare terminology*, ed 2, St. Louis, 2006, Elsevier Mosby.

Figure 16-6 courtesy CD Forbes and WF Jackson.

Figure 16-7 from Seidel H et al: *Mosby's guide to physical examination*, ed 5, St. Louis, 2003, Mosby.

Figure 16-8 courtesy Paul W. Ladenson, MD, The Johns Hopkins University and Hospital, Baltimore, Md.

TABLES